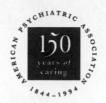

THE AMERICAN JOURNAL OF PSYCHIATRY

The American Journal of Psychiatry, ISSN 0002-953X, is published monthly by the American Psychiatric Association, 1400 K Street, N.W., Washington, DC 20005. Subscriptions (per year): U.S. institutional $85.00, individual $60.00, student $30.00; Canada and foreign institutional $115.00, individual $90.00, student $45.00. Single issues: U.S. $7.00, Canada and foreign $10.00.

Business communications, address changes, and subscription questions from APA members should be directed to the Division of Member Services: (202) 682-6069. Nonmember subscribers should contact the Circulation Department: (202) 682-6158. Authors who wish to contact the *Journal* editorial office should call (202) 682-6020 or fax (202) 682-6016; *Journal* Calendar: (202) 682-6026.

Business Management: Nancy Frey, Director, Periodicals Services; Laura G. Abedi, Advertising Production Manager: (202) 682-6154; Beth Prester, Director, Circulation; Elizabeth Flynn, Promotion Manager; Jackie Coleman Young, Fulfillment Manager.

Advertising Sales: Raymond J. Purkis, Director, 2444 Morris Avenue, Union, NJ 07083; (908) 964-3100.

Pages are produced using Xerox Ventura Publisher, Microsoft Windows version. Printed by The William Byrd Press, Inc., Richmond, VA., on acid-free paper effective with Volume 140, Number 5, May 1983.

Second-class postage paid at Washington, DC, and additional mailing offices. POSTMASTER: Send address changes to *The American Journal of Psychiatry*, Circulation Department, American Psychiatric Association, 1400 K St., N.W., Washington, DC 20005.

Indexed in *Abstracts for Social Workers, Academic Abstracts, Biological Abstracts, Chemical Abstracts, Chicago Psychoanalytic Literature Index, Cumulative Index to Nursing Literature, Excerpta Medica, Hospital Literature Index, Index Medicus, International Nursing Index, Nutrition Abstracts, Psychological Abstracts, Science Citation Index, Social Science Source,* and *Social Sciences Index.* The complete text of the *Journal* is available on the BRS database, BRS Information Technologies, Inc., Latham, NY.

THE AMERICAN JOURNAL OF PSYCHIATRY

Sesquicentennial Anniversary Supplement, 1844–1994

THE

AMERICAN

JOURNAL OF INSANITY,

EDITED BY

THE OFFICERS OF THE NEW YORK STATE
LUNATIC ASYLUM, UTICA.

———————————

VOLUME I.

—————

UTICA:

PRINTED BY BENNETT, BACKUS, & HAWLEY,
1844-5

THE AMERICAN JOURNAL OF PSYCHIATRY
Sesquicentennial Anniversary Supplement

Editor's Introduction

This special supplement of *The American Journal of Psychiatry* celebrates the 150th anniversary of both the American Psychiatric Association and its official journal. *The American Journal of Psychiatry*, at 150 years of age, is the oldest continuously published medical specialty journal in the United States. This commemorative supplemental issue is being distributed to all subscribers as an anniversary gift. We hope that its contents will provide resources for introspection, reappraisal, and growth. As psychiatrists know better than perhaps any other medical specialty, studying the past is the best way to understand the present and to change the future. As we take stock of our profession at its 150th anniversary, we can learn a great deal from the work of our predecessors.

THE HISTORY OF THE AMERICAN JOURNAL OF PSYCHIATRY

When the original founders of the APA decided to join together in 1844 to share ideas about the best way to provide care for the mentally ill in our young country, they needed a way to communicate with one another on a regular basis. *The American Journal of Psychiatry* became that mechanism. One of the founders, Amariah Brigham, assumed responsibility for editing the new journal. Brigham was a self-made and largely self-educated man who apparently aspired from childhood to be a physician, but was nearly deprived of this opportunity through the loss of his father at age 11 and his uncle, a physician who adopted him and began training him, at age 12. He worked at a variety of jobs thereafter and eventually was able to obtain an apprenticeship and then to spend a year attending lectures at the College of Physicians and Surgeons in New York. During that year he also taught himself French! He spent a number of years as a family practitioner, but was eventually called to become superintendent for the Hartford Retreat for the Insane in 1840 and subsequently at the New York State Lunatic Asylum in Utica in 1842. He founded *The American Journal of Insanity* (not given its present name until 1921) while at Utica, publishing it largely at his own expense. The journal soon established itself as the premier scholarly publication in the field of mental illness in the United States.

As will be evident from the selections from Brigham's work that are republished in this supplement, Brigham was an excellent writer, a thoughtful physician, and a compassionate human being. Many of the articles that he wrote in order to help the fledgling journal take flight are models of clinical thinking that would grace any era. They are still fresh and interesting now, 150 years later. After his death in 1849, Brigham was succeeded by T. Romeyn Beck (1849–1854) and subsequently by John P. Gray (1854–1886). Gray was particularly interested in the physical causes of mental illness, took a strong stand against those who argued that mental illnesses were due to sin and more properly treated by the clergy, established the first neuropathology laboratory in the United States at Utica, and published many articles that explored the biology of the brain. His successor, G. Adler Blumer (1886–1894), had a strong interest in rehabilitative therapy, the elimination of the use of restraint, and the creation of a good therapeutic milieu. Blumer was the last of the "Utica editors." In 1894 the journal was sold to the American Medico-Psychological Association (forerunner of our APA) for the sum of $944.50, thereby becoming its official journal. Since its original founding, only 11 individuals have served as editors of *The American Journal of Psychiatry*. The other editors are Richard Dewey (1894–1897, Henry M. Hurd (1897–1904), Edward N. Brush (1904–1931), Clarence B. Farrar (1931–1965), Francis J. Braceland (1965–1978), John C. Nemiah (1978–1993), and myself.

THE CONTENTS OF THE COMMEMORATIVE ISSUE

As the sesquicentennial year approached, the editorial staff of the journal began to address the question of how to honor the long history of the journal and its past editors. After considerable discussion, it was decided that the best way would be to republish some selected examples of its prior contents from the past 150 years. Many of the early articles that were published in the journal, particularly those from its very early years, are available only in a few special libraries and therefore are inaccessible to most subscribers. Reprinting them in a commemorative issue would make them widely available.

But what to choose? A journal that is 150 years old has published thousands of manuscripts in thousands and thousands of pages. While most contributors no doubt viewed their submissions as gems, finding the highest quality diamonds and placing them in the best setting required both thought and effort. Should we sample one article per decade to try to ensure equal representation? Should we stratify by topic? Should we choose a particular topic and trace its history? Should we focus on recent accomplishments and stress the extraordinary progress that has occurred in diagnosis and treatment during the past several decades? Or should we reflect the long sweep of our history, with all its strengths and weaknesses?

Your current editor long ago passed from the healthy state of bibliophilia to the diseased but exhilarating condition of bibliomania. (The diagnostic criteria involve features such as spending large sums on books, buying more than are really necessary, experiencing the aroma of library dust as pleasurable, and endorsing the delusional belief that reading books or scholarly articles is better for the brain than watching television.) She concluded that the best gift to the membership would be to share the inaccessible treasures of the earlier issues by selecting a limited number of especially interesting older articles. This approach would not provide "continuing medical education" about what to do in the here and now, nor would it convey a Panglossian message that we are steadily getting better and better in our progress toward the best of all possible worlds. But it *would* reveal the recurrent themes that have perplexed psychiatrists as they have struggled with defining the structure and purpose of their specialty, both as it relates to other medical disciplines and as it relates to the care of patients. And it would also identify some notable peaks in the broad landscape of a broad medical specialty.

Most of the articles reprinted in this issue are drawn from the first 100 years of *The American Journal of Psychiatry*, since they are least accessible to the average reader. They are reprinted in their original form, including the quirks of language and spelling, as well as the occasional social and cultural biases, that characterize earlier eras. (Lest we feel too smug, we should realize that readers will also find us strange and insensitive 150 years from now, in ways we could not currently predict.) They are divided into four broad categories: Attitudes and Policies, Clinical Description, Research Methods: Mechanisms and Causes, and Developments in Treatment. Each of these four sections is introduced by an overview, written by one of the current members of the journal's Editorial Board.

In general, these categories reflect the contents of *The American Journal of Psychiatry* during its long history. The earliest paper is from the first issue of this journal and was written by Amariah Brigham (1844), while the most recent describe the therapeutic efficacy of lithium (1966) and the reminiscences of John Romano as he contemplated the upcoming sesquicentennial (1990). Some document landmarks in our history, such as the report of methods for measuring cerebral blood flow by Kety (1948), the foundation of the National Institute of Mental Health (1949), and the development of new treatments such as insulin coma (1937) or chlorpromazine (1955). Some reflect the emergence of new nosological conceptualizations, such as catatonia (1877) and schizoaffective disorder (1933). Some describe the desperate cures that were developed to improve patient care in the prepharmacologic era, such as malarial treatment for general paresis and prefrontal leucotomy for psychosis. It is notable that the two Nobel prizes that have been awarded in physiology or medicine for achievements in psychiatric treatment were given to Wagner-Jauregg and Moniz for these two desperate cures, while the achievements of developing antipsychotics, antidepressants, antianxiety agents, and lithium have not been honored, nor have the forward-looking techniques of measuring cerebral blood flow (Kety), nor the introduction of elegant designs for examining gene-environment interactions (Kallman). As we read these works from the past and reflect on the occasional follies of our field, we can take comfort in the fact that we have been far from alone in embracing treatments or ideas that are later recognized as suboptimal.

WHAT CAN WE LEARN FROM OUR HISTORY?

The contents of this issue indicate that many of the struggles we currently confront in psychiatry have been with us throughout most of our history. Many of the themes presented in these articles have been replayed repeatedly.

In one of the earliest articles to appear in the journal, Amariah Brigham discusses the issue of isolation versus mainstreaming of psychiatric patients (and their physicians). Brigham comes down on the side of integration, and Pliny Earle's description of Gheel is an illustration of the benefits and problems of "community treatment" from a mid-nineteenth century perspective. On the other hand, Kirkbride devoted a career to developing ideal designs for hospitals devoted to the exclusive treatment of the mentally ill. Weir Mitchell gives psychiatry a scathing criticism for its isolationism at the time of the 50th anniversary of APA, while Meyerson reflects on our boundaries with neurology and psychology and the special position of psychoanalysis. *Plus ça change, plus c'est la même chose.*

Lest we think that our forefathers represented immutable archetypes of extreme positions, we are also given reminders of their intellectual flexibility. Adolph Meyer wrote repeatedly about the importance of biological approaches to understanding mental illness and even proposed methods for measuring physiognomy (1896). Karl Menninger proposed an infectious disease theory for schizophrenia many years (1925) before the current viral theories became fashionable again.

There are also many indications of the wisdom and prescience of our forefathers and the editors who accepted their articles for publication. (Alas, there were no foremothers in these early years.) Both Brigham and Earle, in a pre-statistical and pre-epidemiological era, argue for the importance of carefully collecting accurate data. Before contemporary health care reform and the emphasis on measuring the "bottom line," they stress the importance of valid measures of outcome and the foolishness of counting patients as "cured" on discharge when they often return again for repeated "cures" on multiple occasions. Davis argues for the value of sound and accurate post-mortem brain data. Boisen and William W. present insights about mental illness based on a patient's personal experience; these reports advocated for the patient's perspective and the value of patient support groups before advocacy became widely organized.

The contents of this issue also serve to remind us that we may be both bigger and better than we sometimes think. Our playing field is large, and we should not forget how large it has historically been. Psychiatrists have traditionally cared for a broad range of patients and illnesses. For example, psychiatrists were the primary physicians to treat general paresis before the development of penicillin. A psychiatrically oriented scientist developed the methods and models that form the foundation for modern techniques for measuring brain metabolism with positron emission tomography or single emission photon computed tomography. (Although not documented here, psychiatrists also developed EEG, the Nissl stain, and Brodmann's maps of brain cytoarchitectonics.)

We also see that major contributions can arise from practicing clinicians and small medical centers, not just from large and powerful research institutions. The best early report of the efficacy of antidepressants in the journal was done by a clinical practitioner at Rochester State Hospital, and the value of curare for modifying ECT was discovered in Nebraska rather than New York or Boston.

Reviewing the contents of *The American Journal of Psychiatry* over the past 150 years in order to select the contents of this issue, while inhaling library dust into the wee hours of the morning, was in fact a source of considerable pleasure. The contents of this issue represent a distillation of that pleasure, chosen to give the gems of wisdom produced by our predecessors back again to our readers. Enjoy.

N.C.A.

I. Attitudes and Policies

INTRODUCTION

I t is 1994, and another turn in the cycle of reform is on the horizon, as it was in 1844, 1894, and 1944. Currently, we await the outcome of the Congressional debate on the President's proposal for health care reform. It is a reform proposal that includes psychiatric services within its scope but also treats these services as somewhat different from other medical services. The opportunity for change is of historic proportion. Psychiatrists look forward to reform with a mix of anticipatory anxiety and hope.

It is entirely fitting to inaugurate this sesquicentennial issue with a section of historic papers that permit a look back at previous reforms. The papers included in this section principally focus on ideas about psychiatric treatment and how to organize mental health services and deliver them to individuals suffering from psychiatric disorders. They reflect the transformation of the first medical specialty organization from the Association of Medical Superintendents of American Institutions for the Insane to the American Medico-Psychological Association to the American Psychiatric Association. These are important papers in the development of the psychiatric profession over the past 150 years. Most of them need little introduction, but some context is offered to identify a thread to guide the reader through a century and a half of reforms and attempts at reform.

The papers in this section on attitudes and policies may be grouped into three subsets, centered on key decades 50 years apart. The initial set of four papers focuses on the first reform movement in American psychiatry, the era of moral treatment and asylum building in the 1840s. This decade also saw the birth of the Association of Medical Superintendents of American Institutions for the Insane (AMSAII). The second set of three papers is from the 1890s, when states began centralizing responsibility for the care of individuals with mental illness. It was the era in which the concepts of mental hygiene were first introduced and in which the AMSAII became the American Medico-Psychological Association. This was also a decade of important advances in general medical science. The third set of five papers spans the 1940s, during which time psychoanalytic and biological psychiatry vied for the attention of a profession moving from hospital-based practice to office-based practice. The ideas discussed in these papers helped to shape the era of community care in which we still practice our profession, represented by an organization renamed the American Psychiatric Association (APA). The section concludes with "Reminiscences: 1938 and Since" by John Romano, a personal look at the last half-century, published in 1990.

THE 1840S AND MORAL TREATMENT

The initial two articles from the 1840s were written by Amariah Brigham, the first editor of *The American Journal of Insanity*, the original name of the journal. These essays focus on "moral treatment," the name for the approach to the care and treatment of mental illness introduced in Europe in the late eighteenth century. Moral treatment was imported to the United States and incorporated into practice in the early nineteenth century. Brigham described the origins of moral treatment and explained its dependence on a combination of what are now called psychosocial and biomedical interventions. He believed that the former were more important than the latter, decrying the excessive use of medicines, physical restraints, and remedies such as bleeding and purging. (In so doing, he gently criticized the revered Dr. Benjamin Rush, widely regarded as the founder of American psychiatry.) Brigham also warned of the dangers of overreliance on manual labor as a remedy, referring to the practice derived from the workhouses and poorhouses of the time. He promoted, instead, "mental activity" and instruction of all kinds in the service of recovery.

In his brief article from 1844, Brigham outlined his strong and well-reasoned opposition to the proposal to build "asylums exclusively for the incurable insane." His arguments reflect the optimism of moral treatment, its egalitarian spirit, and its belief in the power of reason. Brigham raised concerns about the potential for abuse and neglect in such institutions and about the danger of policies motivated primarily by a desire to provide care "at less expense." He also discussed the inaccuracy of determinations of incurability, the dangers of removing hope, the potential for rehabilitation of those "deranged but on one or two subjects," and the problems of monitoring care in a decentralized system of care. The currency of these concerns of 150 years ago is astonishing.

A contrast to the asylum for incurable patients is provided by Pliny Earle's description of the Belgian village of Gheel, a town devoted to the care of individuals who were mentally ill. Held up as a model of the humane treatment of mental disorder, the commune of Gheel in Flanders had for centuries provided care to individuals with mental illness, who were distributed to families throughout the town and its surrounding farms. By the mid-nineteenth century their numbers reached 1,000, among a population of some 10,000 nonpatients. Earle, superintendent of the Northampton (Massachusetts) Asylum, a skeptic and debunker (as reflected in his 1885 article, also reprinted in this issue), provided a generally favorable portrait of Gheel, but not without his trademark concerns.

The final article from the period of moral treatment is the 1845 treatise on the organization of mental hospitals "extracted principally from the reports of Thomas S. Kirkbride, M.D.," physician to the Pennsylvania Hospital for the Insane. The article describes the evolution of that institution from the "insane department" of the Pennsylvania Hospital, the first in the United States, which had been opened in 1752. The separate asylum was opened for patients in 1841 and became a model for the design and organization of mental hospitals throughout the country. These hospitals came to be known as "Kirkbrides" because of their characteristic architectural style, with patient care wards spreading out as wings from a central structure that served as a residence for the superintendent and as a hub for the administration of the hospital.

Originally designed to support moral treatment, hospitals of this efficient design eventually became the model for the ever-enlarging hospitals of the post-moral-treatment era. The warnings of Amariah Brigham and others about the dangers of large institutions, especially for incurable patients, eventually were eclipsed by practical concerns about cost. The first institution for the chronically insane, the Willard (New York) Asylum, opened in 1865 and ushered in an era of asylum growth and pessimism about the curability of mental illness.

THE 1890S AND THE RISE OF MEDICAL SCIENCE AND MENTAL HYGIENE

The quality of care in mental hospitals had deteriorated to a very low level by the occasion of the 50th anniversary of the American Medico-Psychological Association in 1894. Numerous scandals had plagued private as well as public asylums. The association invited a critique by S. Weir Mitchell, a renowned Philadelphia neurologist and novelist, who addressed the assembled profession at its annual meeting "on the dividing year" of its first century. Mitchell's stinging criticism was never published in the journal, probably out of a sense of pique, although the proceedings of the annual meeting contain the speech. The critique is so important as a reflection of turn-of-the century psychiatry that the text of his speech, as it was published in the *Journal of Nervous and Mental Disease*, is included in this section.

Mitchell's analysis of the problems of late nineteenth-century psychiatry are fascinating and have unfortunate relevance today. He provided a brilliant critique of the role of political interference in the management of the mental hospital, but he saved his sharpest comments for the profession itself. He was particularly critical of the lack of scientific progress in the care and treatment of mental illness, due to the separation of the practice of psychiatry from the mainstream of medical practice and research. "Your hospitals are not our hospitals; your ways are not our ways" is the oft-quoted phrase that sums up his critique. He admitted that some advances had been made in recent years, but that progress was the exception rather than the rule and that best practice was not widespread. Mitchell encouraged the profession to leave its isolated hospitals and move into the general hospital and out into the community. Like several other important contemporaries who were "outsiders" to psychiatry (e.g., Clifford Beers and William James), he stimulated the mental hygiene reform movement of the early twentieth century. His call for a scientific basis for psychiatric practice strikes a modern theme, but it is interesting that some of his ideas about technical advances (e.g., the use of faradic stimulation and massage), as well as his obvious class consciousness, appear to the modern reader as smug acceptance of old-fashioned ideas.

Walter Channing of Massachusetts, a reformer who had worked to broaden the definition of the profession and achieved the change in the name of the AMSAII to the Medico-Psychological Association, offered a response to S. Weir Mitchell's address in the journal in 1894. Channing's comments are remarkably nondefensive. He agreed particularly with Mitchell's call for scientific advance, but he reaffirmed the central role of the profession in the management of the hospital. "The medical superintendent . . . deficient in practical ability," he wrote, "though he might write a volume on the cerebral anatomy of a spider, would be of no value whatever." Channing also criticized Mitchell for minimizing the problem faced by running asylums with very limited resources. This is a familiar theme for today's leaders in psychiatry, especially those who are scientists running academic departments with large public service responsibilities.

Adolf Meyer's article "A Short Sketch of the Problems of Psychiatry" was written in 1897, while Meyer was an assistant physician and neuropathologist at the Worcester (Massachusetts) Lunatic Hospital and "docent of psychiatry" at Clark University in Worcester. The essay, the first in this section to use the term "psychiatry," focuses broadly on psychopathology and nosology. It was written comparatively early in Meyer's illustrious career, prior to his moves to the New York State Psychiatric Institute and to the Phipps Clinic at the Johns Hopkins University Medical School and Hospital. Meyer's involvement at Clark University with the psychologist Stanley Hall (who brought Freud to Worcester) reflects both his interest in psychology and his belief in the importance of professional work beyond the walls of the hospital. Although this article emphasizes a "biological conception of man," it also underscores the importance of the "psychological as well as physiological and anatomical methods." Meyer concluded, "A mental disease is a disorder of the person following the laws of general pathology like any other disease." This argument played an important role in the reforms of the mental hygiene movement that Meyer led in the next decade, and it has been a rallying cry in the reforms of our own era.

THE 1940S AND PSYCHIATRIC PLURALISM

Abraham Myerson's two articles provide a transition from the view of psychiatry offered by Meyer to the view presented by William Menninger in his essay in this section. Myerson's own views, as reflected in the two articles, are much closer to those of Meyer. With ideas rooted strongly in a medical and biological understanding of mental illness, Myerson was also a student of psychology who tried to bridge the dualism of body and mind. Writing from the Division of Psychiatric Research at the Boston State Hospital, Myerson, who had also been at the Boston Psychopathic Hospital in its early years, was a scientist and a clinician. He was an empiricist who favored experimental evidence. "Results count," he said in his essay on attitudes toward psychoanalysis, "and where the results are clear-cut, the technique which brings them wins the day." He was troubled by the lack of results from psychoanalysis, so he conducted a survey of neurologists, psychiatrists, and psychologists to learn their opinions about "one of the oldest systems of concepts and of therapeutics in modern medicine." His own results were somewhat confusing, but they were telling and sometimes amusing as he dissected opinions about psychoanalysis.

The same tension between the biological and psychological in the profession is discussed in Myerson's article "Some Trends of Psychiatry," which presented his own review of psychopathology. Again, the emphasis is on science and the "great reality" of "experimental psychiatry." Myerson predicted "that when the history of psychiatry is written for the one hundred fiftieth anniversary of the American Psychiatric Association, the end of the era of therapeutic defeatism will be found to date from the time of the introduction of the shock treatments, and that the advent of these queer and rather barbaric additions to the 'gentle' art of healing will mark the beginning of a real and much better therapeutics."

William Menninger presented a different view in his distinctly post-World War II article "The Role of Psychiatry in the World Today." This essay is as expansive as the title suggests. Menninger's emphasis was on psychiatry as a social science as well as a medical science. His view was broadly social, involving issues of what we now call "family values" (i.e., divorce, single-parent families, working mothers, sexuality, and alcohol and other drug use), as well as the issues of racism, crime, unemployment, and illiteracy. His vision was global, concerned with world war and world peace. And he was optimistic that the profession of psychiatry would have something to offer in the way of greater understanding and help for the ills of the world. Menninger admitted "that we are not now in a position even to deliver much of the available information that we might assemble . . . . We must extend our frontiers of knowledge . . . . We need to develop more medical statesmanship." Menninger was not a passive dreamer; he worked hard to try to improve the position of psychiatry. He described several of these efforts, including the formation of the Group for the Advancement of Psychiatry and the passage of the National Mental Health Act, which ultimately led to the creation of the National Institute of Mental Health.

The psychiatry of the past was a creature of the mental hospital; the psychiatry of the future was to be a community-based practice. The mental hygienists of a half-century before had made some tentative steps into the community; the psychiatrists of the post-World War II era were to become firmly rooted there.

This section concludes with three different but interesting articles. One is a biography of Dr. Benjamin Rush by Clifford B. Farr, written for the APA centennial to honor the first American psychiatrist, who was also a signer of the Declaration of Independence. The other is a post-World War II perspective on "Current Trends in German Psychiatry" by Kurt Schneider of the University of Heidelberg. The perspective of this short report is decidedly biological. John Romano's reminiscences carry us from this era into the present and beyond.

REFORM AND RESEARCH

The one consistent theme in these papers is change; they chronicle the evolution of attitudes and policies. Each of the reforms in psychiatry has been the product of a creative tension between a desire for positive change and the limits of our knowledge about how to effect that change. *The American Journal of Psychiatry* has been a regular vehicle for communicating ideas about reform and for presenting the results of our research. Each of these authors, no matter how optimistic or grand his vision, recognized the need for knowledge. Subsequent sections of this sesquicentennial issue present some of those findings. This section has presented the major themes that shaped that research.

HOWARD H. GOLDMAN, M.D., PH.D.

ASYLUMS EXCLUSIVELY FOR THE INCURABLE INSANE

By Amariah Brigham, M.D.

Superintendent, New York State Lunatic Asylum, Utica, New York

Some benevolent individuals noticing the deplorable situation of the incurable insane, who are confined in poor-houses, and having seen the comfortable condition of deranged persons in well conducted Lunatic Asylums, have proposed that public Asylums should be built on a cheap plan, solely for those supposed to be incurable.

After much consideration we are constrained to oppose such arrangements. Establishments solely for the poor and incurable we believe would soon become objects of but little interest to any one, and in which neglect, abuse and all kinds of misrule would exist, and exist without detection.

We are opposed to them principally on these grounds.

1. No one can determine with much accuracy which patients are, and which are not, incurable. Of those in this Asylum we cannot say of at least one-third to which of these classes they belong. We still indulge hopes of their restoration, but probably shall be disappointed in a majority of them.

But the hope we have and which encourages us in our efforts to cure them would be destroyed by sending them to an incurable establishment. The fact that the chances of recovery would be diminished to even but a few, is enough to make us hesitate before we establish such Asylums.

2. Many that are incurable are monomaniacs. They are deranged but on one or two subjects, and sane on others. Such surely should not be deprived of any comforts that are afforded the curable class, among which the greatest is *hope* of again being restored to society, which would be destroyed if they were sent to an incurable Asylum.

Equally or more strongly does this objection apply to cases of remission, to those numerous cases in which insanity is exhibited for a week and followed by several weeks of sanity. Shall these be told there is no hope for them?

3. Among the incurable insane there would be no certain means of ascertaining the neglect or abuse of them. In all Asylums, the fact that some are well and soon to leave the Asylum is the greatest safeguard against abuse.

4. No possible good could arise from such distinct Asylums, except they might be conducted at less expense. But how, so if they are to have proper officers, physicians, &c., and if they do not, why are they better than poor-houses.

There are no facts in favor of such establishments. As yet we have none in this country. The only one we ever saw, is at Genoa, in Italy. The Hospital of Incurables, when we visited it in 1829, contained two hundred and fifty insane.

They were confined in badly ventilated apartments from which they were never discharged but by death. The quiet, the noisy, and the violent, were all congregated together, and a majority were chained to their beds by their wrists and ancles. No contemplation of human misery ever affected us so much: the howlings, execrations, and clanking of chains, gave to the place the appearance of the infernal regions. Little or no medical treatment was adopted. We hope never to see such institutions in this country. On the contrary, let no Asylum be established but for the curable, and to this the incurable and the rich and the poor should be admitted; let all have the same kind care; and all indulge the same hope, even if delusive to many, of ultimate recovery, but do not drive any to despair, and destroy the little mind they still possess, by consigning them to a house, over the entrance of which, Dante's lines on the gates of hell might well be inscribed,

> "Lasciate ogni speranza
> Voi che intrate qui."

"Leave hope behind, all ye who enter here."

On this subject the Hon. Michael Hoffman thus happily remarked, in the Assembly of the State of New York, during the last session: "To receive," says he, "only incurable insane paupers, would convert the institution into a madhouse—a mad poor-house—a den of filth and misery, and an object of abhorrence and disgust, which nobody would begin to approach. But place those there who have friends of wealth and consequence, and you secure that vigilance, that inducement to look into its entire management, which is necessary to make it a well ordered institution. Make it a poor madhouse and the poor have no feet to travel after them, and the patients would be left to the cold inhuman care of brute officiality, not to be cured but to be cursed. But admit freely the curable and the rich to the institution, and they have kindred who could and would travel after them, relatives who had eyes, aye and voices. They would constitute an active committee of vigilance to look into its affairs, and see they were properly managed."

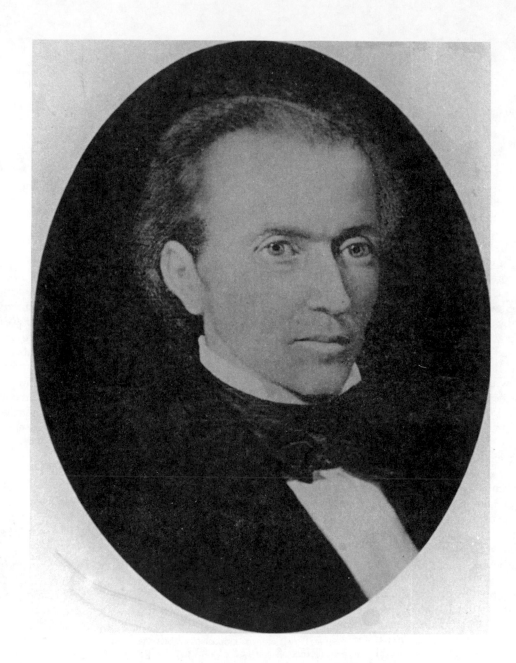

Amariah Brigham, M.D., 1798–1849
Founder and First Editor of *The American Journal of Insanity* (1844–1849)

THE MORAL TREATMENT OF INSANITY

By Amariah Brigham, M.D.

Superintendent, New York State Lunatic Asylum, Utica, New York

The removal of the insane from home and former associations, with respectful and kind treatment under all circumstances, and in most cases manual labor, attendance on religious worship on Sunday, the establishment of regular habits and of self-control, diversion of the mind from morbid trains of thought, are now generally considered as essential in the Moral Treatment of the Insane.

We shall therefore, in this essay, confine ourselves mostly—1st, to a brief historical review of this subject, in order to do at least partial justice to our predecessors, and 2d, notice such new suggestions and new methods of treatment as have come to our knowledge.

Previous to the time of Pinel, the moral treatment of the Insane was fluctuating and unestablished. In some periods and in some countries, a portion of the insane at least, were treated with great kindness, while at the same time, others were neglected and abused. From the most remote periods, insanity was regarded for the most part as a *sacred disease*, as coming direct from heaven, and as a consequence of the possession of a spirit or demon. This was the belief of the Chaldeans and the Jews. Saul was troubled by an evil spirit, and Job by a demon. Hence recourse was had to various moral means of cure. Thus Saul was cured by the music of David. "And it came to pass when the evil spirit from God was upon Saul, that David took a harp and played with his hand; so Saul was refreshed and was well, and the evil spirit departed from him." 1 Sam. xvi. 16.

Similar methods of treatment prevailed in ancient Egypt and Greece; the priests of the former country amused insane persons, and diverted their minds by music, and by pleasant walks in groves and gardens, filled with perfumes and flowers; and Melampus cured the daughters of Pretus, king of Argos, not with Hellebore as some have stated, but by bodily exercise, and by mysterious ceremonies that acted powerfully on the imagination.

But all the insane were not treated in the same manner; while those who were gay, sociable and courageous, were treated with respect and kindness, and even idolized and worshipped as Oracles, many that were timid and melancholy, were considered objects of Heaven's wrath, and driven forth as outcasts, and subjected to the greatest abuse.

The treatment of the insane, has ever varied with the philosophy and intelligence of the age. That they are treated better in modern times, more kindly and judiciously, is not owing to any increase of benevolence, but to an increase of knowledge. Benevolence has ever existed in the heart of man, and compassion for suffering, been manifested from the most remote period. But without knowledge, benevolence may prove to be as injurious as tyranny itself. Hence we find in the ignorant ages, the insane not merely neglected, but abused and persecuted, and in many cases put to death in the most inhuman manner, and not for want of pity and compassion in the human heart, but from ignorance of the nature of insanity. Those thus treated were not considered as diseased, insane or as deserving of pity, but as wicked beings, in league with evil spirits, and meriting punishment.

From the earliest period, some individuals had correct notions on insanity—Celsus who lived at the time of Christ, gave many excellent precepts relating to the moral treatment of the insane, and Caelius Aurelianus, who lived three centuries later, insisted in strong terms on the necessity of acquiring the confidence and esteem of the insane by frankness of manner and by kind treatment.

But the difficulty has ever been to determine who are insane.

Not to go back to times too remote for abundant and correct historical details, we know that from the fourteenth to the eighteenth century, very many thousands of insane persons were put to death, and most of them by order of Courts of Justice. Some were condemned to death or to imprisonment for life as heretics, some were hung for practising witchcraft, and vast numbers were burned as sorcerers, or for being in league with the devil.

These cruelties have for the most part passed away, yet still down even to the present time, there are we believe in most countries, some deranged persons confined with criminals in prisons, and not unfrequently some are put to death for acts committed by them when deprived of their reason.

The burning of Joan of Arc, and the thousands of supposed sorcerers, and which we now look upon with horror, was caused by the ignorance of the times. In fact, ignorance has ever been the worst of all *diseases*, and as relates to insanity much yet remains, and *we* should regard it among our highest duties to endeavor to dispel it, and to diffuse such a knowledge of insanity among all classes, as will prevent the recurrence of the enormities we have mentioned.

Owing to the spread of science, the insane towards the beginning of the last century, ceased to be regarded as witches or sorcerers. Still they continued to be abused and neglected. The most furious were confined in cells and dungeons, and when obstinate or mischievous, were cruelly whipped, and in all respects treated like wild beasts. For many years no other method of treatment was supposed practicable or useful. No one seems to have thought of attempting to cure them.

Undoubtedly there were exceptions, but this was generally the treatment of the insane previous to the time of Pinel, whom we must regard as the founder of the humane, rational, and now generally adopted system of moral treatment.

He had, to be sure, an active assistant, and to some degree a precursor in Pussin; still to Pinel seems fairly due the very great merit which we have mentioned.

He is mostly generally and popularly known in connection with the insane, by his bold act of unchaining above fifty maniacs at one time at the Bicetre Hospital, in 1792. But he had six years previous to this, reduced to practice his mild system of treatment elsewhere.

This system was not the result of an accident or an experiment, but was adopted by Pinel after much reading, observation and reflection. He thoroughly qualified himself for this great work by vast learning,—a knowledge of the languages of other countries, and a thorough acquaintance with all that had been written on the subject of insanity.

Thus prepared, he early matured his system, then tried it in practice on a great scale for several years, and finally published it to the world. His first work on insanity, *Traite Medico-Philosophique*, was published in 1801, and we do not hesitate to say, that we know not of any work on insanity superior to this, especially as improved by Pinel in the last edition;—none more worthy of our daily study. On perusing it, we almost lament to find that very little indeed had been added that may be called improvement in the moral treatment of the insane since his time. This work was early translated, and thus the views of Pinel respecting insanity and the proper treatment of the insane, were soon mad known throughout the civilized world.

Not many years after this, the Retreat, near York in England, was established. It was suggested by Mr. William Tuke, who is generally considered its founder, and was mainly established for insane persons belonging to the Society of Friends, and for the purpose of separating them from the profane and profligate, and placing them under the care of the members of the society, and where they would be kindly treated. Great good resulted from the establishment of this Retreat, although it must be confessed, the original founders did not seem to have had very clear ideas respect[ing] the nature of insanity, or of its proper treatment. Benevolent feelings led them to wish the insane to be kindly treated, and they endeavored to carry their wishes into practice. At first there was no regular medical superintendent, though fortunately in George Jepson, whose name should be ever dear to the insane, and who acted as superintendent, they found a man of an original and vigorous mind, and who having some knowledge of medicine, and having visited other establishments for the insane, was well calculated to introduce and carry out useful reforms. To him we consider the Retreat largely indebted for the success that attended its early administration.

This institution was opened in 1796, four years after Pinel had unchained the Maniacs of the Bicetre. For several years but few patients were admitted, but the success attending their kind treatment, and the notoriety given to the institution, by various publications, made a good impression, and together with the circulation of Pinel's Treatise, translated by Dr. Davis, and published in 1806, had the effect to introduce a milder and better system of moral treatment into many of the institutions for the insane in England. But while we cheerfully admit that great credit is due to the founders of the York Retreat for their humane exertions in behalf of the insane, and freely acknowledge that vast good resulted to other institutions for their exertions, and particularly from the publication and general circulation of Mr. Tuke's description of the Retreat, published in 1813:—historical accuracy will not allow us to say, that they originated what may be called the rational, humane and modern system of moral treatment of the insane.

In this country, the system of Pinel was early introduced, and among those who were most instrumental in establishing it here, we ought to mention Rush, Wyman and Todd.

Dr. Rush was a man of great benevolence as well as great intelligence, and in his published writings on insanity, we find many interesting and valuable facts, and also many useful suggestions respecting the moral treatment of the insane. He inculcates the necessity of mild treatment and kind usage; but still, Dr. Rush can not now be considered as a correct guide for us to follow, either as regards the moral or the medical treatment of the insane.

So great is the authority of his name, and so great the influence which his "*Observations on Diseases of the Mind,*" have exercised on the opinions and practice of medical men in this country, that we deem it not improper to briefly notice some suggestions of his respecting the moral treatment of the insane that we deem erroneous. A prevailing error found in his writings on insanity, is, that the insane are to be disciplined and governed, that those who have the care of them must obtain a dominion over them by fear or by other means that we think improper. Thus he says: "the first object of a physician, when he enters the cell or chamber of the deranged patient, should be, to catch his eye, and look him out of countenance." Again he says, "The conduct of a physician to his patients should be uniformly dignified, if he wishes to acquire their obedience and respect. He should never descend to levity in conversing with them. He should hear with silence their rude or witty answers to his questions, and upon no account ever laugh at them, or with them." After attending to various means for making insane persons obedient, he says, "If these prove ineffectual to establish a government over deranged patients, recourse should be had to certain modes of coercion."

After mentioning a recourse to the strait waistcoat, the tranquilizing chair, (which is an invention of Dr. Rush), the privation of customary pleasant food, and pouring cold water under the coat sleeves, so that it may descend to the arm pits, he adds, "if all these modes of punishment should fail of the intended effect, it will be proper to resort to the fear of death."

I need but mention these remarks of Dr. Rush, to show that he was far behind not only the present age in the moral treatment of the insane, but in arrear of Pinel, whose treatise on insanity had been published several years when Dr. Rush wrote.

Doct. Wyman, the first Physician and Superintendent of the McLean Asylum, though not extensively known by his published writings, was a man of superior qualifications, and admirably qualified for the station he held.

He had much architectural and mechanical ingenuity, and to him we are indebted for some or our best arrangements for the care of the insane. His untiring industry, his constant devotedness to the welfare of those under his charge, his sterling integrity and exactness in everything belonging to the duties of his station, furnished an example that has been in the highest degree salutary.

Having no similar institutions in this country to look to for guidance, he had to depend upon the resources of his own head and heart, and fortunately these were both good, and consequently, most that he devised and suggested, has stood the test of time and experience. Dr. Wyman had, we think, one fault, considering the station he held, and this was excessive modesty or disinclination to make known his improvements and the success that attended his labors. Owing to his extreme sensitiveness on this subject, he is less known, and probably accomplished less good than men of less real merit. That his views of both moral and medical treatment, were what we now deem correct, is evident from the following note to his discourse on "Mental Philosophy as connected with Mental Disease," delivered before the Massachusetts Medical Society. "In mental disorders," he says, "without symptoms of organic disease, a judicious moral management is most successful. It should afford agreeable occupation. It should engage the mind, and exercise the body; as in riding, walking, sewing, embroidery, bowling, gardening, mechanic arts; to which may be added, reading, writing, conversation, &c., the whole to be performed with order and regularity. Even the taking of food, retiring to bed, rising in the morning and at stated times, and conforming to stated rules in almost every thing, is a most salutary discipline. It requires, however, constant attention and vigilance, with the greatest kindness in the attendants upon a lunatic. Moral treatment is indispensable, even in cases arising from organic disease.

In regard to medical treatment, I believe that purging, bleeding, low diet, &c., have been adopted with little discrimination. They are to be resorted to only when there is organic disease, which requires the reducing plan. But these remedies, especially in debilitated subjects, are seldom useful in relieving mental disease. They are usually injurious, and frequently fatal."

Dr. Todd, of Hartford, we also recall with pleasing recollections. He possessed, as Spurzheim said after seeing him, to the writer of this article, "a mountain of benevolence," to which were added a good education, fine personal appearance, most engaging manners, and very superior conversational powers, all of which eminently fitted him for the moral treatment of the insane, in which he particularly excelled. His great merit we conceive, is, his having zealously embraced, and practically introduced into this country, and made extensively known here the moral and medical treatment recommended by Pinel, Tuke and Willis. To use his own words found in his first Report, he made the

"Law of kindness, the all-pervading power of the moral discipline of the Retreat, and required unvaried gentleness and respect to be manifested towards the inmates of the institution, by every member belonging to it."

He early discountenanced depletion, particularly bleeding in insanity, and insisted upon the necessity of generous diet, and recommended a frequent resort to tonics and narcotics in the medical treatment of the insane.

This course of treatment, though it had been recommended by the best writers on insanity in Europe, had not to much extent been resorted to in this country, previous to the time of Dr. Todd, and it was so contrary to that recommended by Dr. Rush, that it required considerable boldness, and much address and management to introduce it, and make it popular in this country, and this, Dr. Todd accomplished.

As already stated, but few improvements in the moral treatment of the insane have been made, since the time of Pinel and Tuke. In their writings, all those methods that we now deem most essential, are clearly pointed out and insisted upon. Still these methods have by the labors of others, become more generally known and established, and in some respects improved.

M. Leuret, the distinguished Physician of the Bicetre Hospital at Paris, in his valuable work, "Du Traitement Moral de la folie," has made many very useful suggestions, and done much good in calling attention to the vast importance of moral treatment in insanity. Most writers previous to Leuret, had considered the moral treatment as auxiliary to the medical, but Leuret considers the latter as of trivial importance compared with the former. He proposes to cure all cases of uncomplicated insanity, solely by moral means. For this purpose, he often excites pain or unpleasant sensations and ideas, in order to prevent and dispel those still more unpleasant.

Unfortunately for the establishment of the many excellent precepts contained in this profound work of M. Leuret, he has created a prejudice against himself and his writings by some of his recommendations, particularly by that of the Douche, which, however valuable it may be in some cases, is, we believe, liable to great abuse. In some of the prisons in this country, where it has been used extensively with refractory criminals, we have been informed on good authority, the use of it has occasionally proved dangerous, and in a few cases, fatal. But apart from this, and this is only one of a great variety of measures which he recommends for exciting the hopes and fears of his patients, dispelling their morbid fancies and teaching them habits of self-control, his work abounds with useful suggestions, and is well worthy of our careful study. He recommends resorting to a great variety of means to direct and engage the attention of patients. He insists on the importance of out door exercise and bodily labor, walking, riding, engaging in active sports, and more particularly on the value of mental labor, such as reading, committing pieces to memory and reciting them, and other school exercises, acting plays, attention to music, &c.

On all these subjects and many others relating to the mental treatment of the insane, more full and useful details will be found in the work of Leuret, than in any other with which we are acquainted.

In the main we coincide with him, that in a majority of

cases of insanity, the moral treatment is of more importance than the medical, and we fear we shall never avail ourselves of the full value of the former, nor cease to do injury to some patients by administering too much medicine, until we heartily embrace this view of the subject.

That some cases of insanity require medical treatment we believe, but we also believe that a large majority of the patients in Lunatic Asylums do not. There is much analogy between many of the patients found in all such institutions, and the passionate, mischievous, and what are called bad boys in a school, and there is about as much propriety in following the example of Mrs. Squeers, and physicing and medicating the latter as the former, in order to cure them or to change their propensities. Rational hopes for the improvement of either, should we believe, be founded on moral management alone.

Bodily labor as a measure for benefiting and curing the insane is generally recommended, and we allude to it now, but to express the hope that better arrangements for this purpose will be made in institutions for the insane, than have hitherto been. Some have an insufficient quantity of land, and are destitute of work shops. We think every such institution should have a good farm attached to it; but still, a farm is not sufficient, as it can afford employment but to comparatively few, and only for part of the year. We think several work shops should be connected with every large establishment for the insane, and be so connected, that the patients of each class can go to them without risk or exposure. One or more rooms in connection with each hall for patients, is needed in order to afford employment to all that would be benefited by it. In such rooms, dressmaking and tailoring, cabinet work, the manufacture of toys, basket-making, shoe-making, painting, printing, bookbinding, and various other employments may be carried on to the advantage of many patients, some of whom can not be employed on the farm or in shops disconnected with the asylum. In the construction of asylums for the insane, we think there should more care be taken to provide convenient rooms for the purposes mentioned.

But however useful bodily labor may be to some, we regard it as less so generally as a curative measure, and less applicable in many cases, than mental occupation or the regular and rational employment of the mind.

In fact, manual labor, we believe, proves more beneficial by producing this result, that is, by engaging the attention and directing the mind to new subjects of thought, than by its direct effect upon the body. Not unfrequently manual labor appears to be injurious, especially in recent cases; it accelerates the circulation, and sometimes reproduces excitement of mind in those that have become quiet and convalescent.

We apprehend many have erroneous views on the subject of manual labor as a remedy for insanity. It is undoubtedly useful of itself in some cases, but it rarely cures. The large majority of patients that recover are restored without it, and most of the work performed by those of this class in lunatic asylums is after convalescence is well established.

It is true, that in many institutions for the insane in this country, and to a greater extent in Europe, a vast amount of manual labor is performed by the patients; but the principal part of this, according to our observation, is done by those that belong to the incurable class; and to these, who constitute the majority in most establishments, manual labor is highly useful, and sometimes necessary for the preservation of the health, and of what mind is still possessed.

But as we have said, the curable class are more benefited by the regular and rational employment of the mind, by pursuits that engage the attention, and tend to the enlargement and the improvement of the mental and moral powers.

For this purpose, asylums should be well supplied with books, maps and apparatus illustrative of different sciences, and also collections in natural history, &c. Schools should be established in every institution for the insane, where patients could engage in reading, writing, drawing, music, arithmetic, geography, history, and also study some of the sciences, as chemistry, mineralogy, conchology, physiology, &c.

To these schools should be attached intelligent instructors, who should spend all their time with the patients, eat at the same table with them, but have no labor or other duty to attend to, than to interest the patients and contribute all they can by their presence and conversation to their contentment and enjoyment. They should join them in their amusements and walks, and be their constant companions.

We are satisfied that an establishment for the insane can be better managed, and with equal economy, by having an arrangement by which some attendants devote their time to the ordinary duties and labors of the halls, while others have nothing to do but to accompany the patients and endeavor to instruct and amuse them. The latter having nothing to do with any coercive measures, the patients do not become prejudiced against, and will readily hearken to their suggestions. Thus they serve as a constant guard, and by their presence and management, prevent outbreaks and disorder and make coercive measures, restraint and seclusion, rarely necessary.

They also by their presence and conversation quiet the timid, console the desponding, and by attention to all, contribute to the contentment and cheerfulness of the patients, and as we believe, essentially aid in curing them. Many cases, we believe, cannot be cured or improved, but by arousing and calling into exercise the dormant faculties of the mind. Hence schools are beneficial, not merely to the curable class of patients, but to the demented and those approaching this condition.

In such, the active state of the disease, which originated the mental disturbance, has passed, and left the brain and faculties of the mind in a torpid state. In these cases, medicine is generally of no use, and they cannot often be much improved, but by exercising the faculties of the mind.

But others are also benefited by devoting a portion of every day to mental improvement. To those who are nearly or quite well, and who remain in an asylum for fear of relapsing at home, or for other reasons, schools afford enjoyment and often means for improvement which are highly valued by the patients themselves.

The melancholy and despairing, and to all those suffering from delusions of mind, and those that are uneasy and nervous, that are constantly restless and disposed to find fault and to annoy the attendants, and quarrel with all about them, because they have nothing else to occupy their minds, are frequently cured by mental occupation and the exercises of a school, by attending to composition, declamation, the writing and acting of dialogues and plays.

Our observations for many years in various lunatic asylums, led us a long time since to regard the want of mental occupation as the greatest want in modern institutions for the insane. Go into any such establishment, and you will find some few, in winter a very few, at work, some playing cards or other games; yet a still larger number will be found sitting about, listless, inactive, doing nothing, saying nothing, taking no interest in anything going on around them; gathered around the stove or place that is heated, looking forward to nothing but the hour for eating and retiring to sleep. For a short time each day, when the physician passes around, they will exhibit a little animation and say a few words, and then relapse into their former condition.

When the weather is pleasant, some of them walk or ride out occasionally for a short time, but this, to many of the class we are describing, after a few times, seems to be a mechanical kind of business and confers but little enjoyment, they notice but little and say but little during the walk or ride, or after it. These patients make no especial trouble in an asylum, and are very apt to be overlooked and neglected, and if not already demented soon become so. They are thought not to require much attention, as they have good bodily health, and are quiet, consequently they generally receive but little notice.

But those belonging to this class require great attention; they need mental exercise; they should attend school and have their minds awakened into activity, for an hour or two every day. Soon, by this course, their memories will improve; they will become interested in singing or in some particular study, and by perseverance a considerable number will be cured, and many, very many, rendered capable of much enjoyment, and be kept from sinking into a state of hopeless dementia.

Various are the methods that may be adopted to awaken into activity the dormant faculties of the mind and to dispel delusions and melancholy trains of thought. A *museum* or collection of minerals, shells, pictures, specimens of ancient and modern art and curiosities of all sorts, should be connected with institutions for the insane. The opportunities are abundant for making interesting and valuable collections of this kind by the aid of the patients that have recovered and their friends.

By means thus indicated Institutions for the care and cure of those affected by mental disorder will be made to resemble those for education, rather than Hospitals for the sick, or prisons for criminals; and when we call to mind that the greater part of those committed to such establishments are not actually sick, and do not require medical treatment, but are suffering from deranged intellect, feelings and passions, it is evident that a judicious course of mental and moral discipline is most essential for their comfort and restoration.

By these remarks we do not however mean to disparage medical treatment as it is in some cases very essential, but we mean to insist upon what we believe to be the fact, that moral treatment including religious instruction and medical advice as to the means of preventing re-attacks, is the most important, and as yet too much neglected;—that institutions in general have not been constructed and arranged in a manner best adapted for carrying into successful operation a complete system of moral treatment.

In conclusion we wish to express the hope that increased attention will be given to this subject, and are confident great good will result. When such a system as we have briefly indicated or rather hinted at, is judiciously introduced into Asylums with convenient rooms and suitable books and apparatus, we apprehend that trivial and objectionable amusements will be abandoned by the inmates themselves for more rational enjoyments—enjoyments which while they serve to dispel the darkness and delusions that affect many, will at the same time have the effect to improve their minds and enable them to leave the institution not only rational, but better qualified by increased intelligence and power of self-control for encountering the troubles and performing the duties of life.

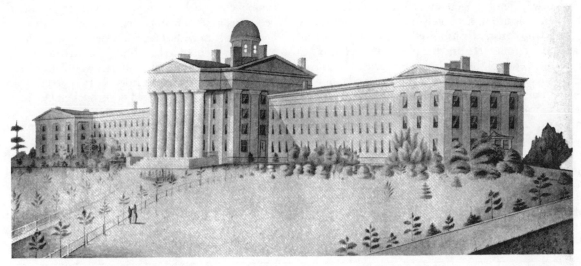

NEW YORK STATE LUNATIC ASYLUM AT UTICA AS IT WAS IN 1844.

—

GHEEL

By Pliny Earle, M.D.

Physician to Bloomingdale Asylum for the Insane, Bloomingdale, New York

No objects of contrast, no extremes or opposites are much more dissimilar than the different sections of country traversed by the Rhine, between Johannesberg and the sea. From the upper extremity of the Rhinegan to "The Castled Crag of Drachenfels," the river is almost uninterruptedly hemmed in by precipitous mountains, while the largest portion of the district farther down, extending through the Netherlands, is an undiversified, monotonous level. The former of these divisions is the region, *par excellence*, of legendary tales. But, although these compositions of mingled fact and fable are mostly concentrated among the mountains, a country best adapted to their romantic spirit, yet even the low lands of Flanders are not wholly destitute of them. The outlines of one of these are as follows.

Sometime in the seventh century there lived, in Ireland, a girl named Dympna, who was no less remarkable for beauty than for piety and chastity. But here loveliness excited the most unholy passions and desires of her father, who, instigated by the devil, determined to gratify them, even though he should accomplish the ruin of his own daughter. Maintaining her virtue, but shocked at the unnatural conduct of her parent, she resolved to fly beyond possible reach of his power. Accordingly, having obtained the companionship of a priest, named Geburnus, she escaped from her native country, and found a place of supposed security in a secluded district of the Netherlands.

The father was greatly angered when he received intelligence of the departure of his lovely daughter. Still incited by the devil, who constantly followed him, whispering evil in his ears, he determined to find her place of refuge, though at the uttermost ends of the earth. He prosecuted enquiries until he discovered the course she had taken, and followed her, the evil one still at his ear. The winds did not dismast his vessel, the waters did not overwhelm it. He landed upon the continent, found his daughter, and immediately caused her to be beheaded. She died and became a Saint. She was buried, and her bones—the bones of Saint Dympna were worshipped.—But, even after her death, the good and benevolent Saint devoted herself to the afflicted of the human race; to the restoration of those whose reason had become alienated.

Geburnus also died, and was buried beside the martyred girl whom, in her flight from an incestuous father, he had

protected. A chapel was erected near the graves, and hither came the insane from all quarters of the land, to intercede with the blessed Saint, and to be healed by her health-restoring power. In process of time, as the fame and influence of the Saint became more and more extended, the people erected a new church, some half-mile distant from the graves of Dympna and Geburnus. It is a massive structure, about two hundred and fifty feet in length, and otherwise correspondingly proportioned.—Nor is it an unimportant testimony to the zeal and devotion of its builders, that the stone of which this large edifice is composed, was drawn more than thirty miles, over a heavy sandy road. They were prodigal of toil until this, the principal church of the commune of Gheel[1] was completed.

At length some Germans came to Gheel, for the purpose of exhuming the remains of Saint Dympna, and removing them to their own country. They excavated the wrong grave and obtained the bones of the priest Geburnus. The Gheelans, excited at the intended outrage, attached the Germans, but were repulsed. The latter, discovering their mistake in regard to the remains, again went to work, and dug to the coffin of Saint Dympna. But, with all the power which could be applied, they could not remove it—could not stir it a hair-breadth. The Gheelans, reinforced, returned, re-attacked the Germans, conquered and drove them from the country.—Thus rid of their enemy, they attempted to remove the coffin of the Saint, but, for a long time, were equally unsuccessful with the Germans. It appeared as if no human power were able to stir the bones of Dympna. When all imaginable devices had failed, and the attempt was about to be relinquished, a deaf and dumb boy, as if by chance, came by. "If you would success," said he, "you must take yonder horse." The people gazed with astonishment. The boy had never spoken before. He never spoke again. These were the only words he ever uttered. The particular horse which he had designated was attached to the coffin, and the remains of the Saint were thus removed, without farther difficulty, to the new church, where they are still preserved in a shrine of silver. The stones of the coffin were deposited in an elegant case, which was placed in the chancel, elevated upon pillars, at a height sufficient for a person to kneel beneath it.

Meanwhile, a knowledge of the miraculously curative power of Saint Dympna circulated more widely, and the

---

[1] Pronounced *Hkale.*

insane from all the surrounding provinces were brought to Gheel for the purpose of obtaining her assistance.—Arrived there, the ceremonies performed, were as follows:—

"The relatives of the patient cause a nine days' offering (*une neuvaine*) to be made in the church of St. Amans.[2] During the nine days the patient is placed in a house attached to the church. He is shut up alone, or with other companions of misfortunes, under the *surveillance* of two old women. A priest comes every day to say mass, and to read prayers. The patients who are tranquil, accompanied by some children of the country, by some devotees, make, during the nine days, the circuit of the church, three times on the outside, and three times within. When the patients are in the chancel, where stands the case enclosing the stones of the Saint's coffin, they kneel and pass under this case three times, that is, at each circuit which they make of the interior. If the patient be furious, a person of the country and some children are paid for making the processions for him.

"While the patient makes the three circuits, his relatives are in the interior, praying to the Saint to effect a restoration. Mass is said on the ninth day, the patient is exorcised, and sometimes a second offering (*neuvaine*) is commenced."[3]

Such is the legend of Gheel. It commences, perhaps, in fable, but terminates in the authentic history of recent years. The place has been, for centuries, known as a resort for persons suffering under mental disorders, and the ceremonies for securing the favor of Saint Dympna, are accurately described.

The principal information in regard to this unique Commune, which has hitherto been received upon this side of the Atlantic, is contained in the description by Esquirol, who visited it in 1821, and published an account of it in 1822, which was afterwards embodied in his large work upon mental diseases. No American has described it, and probably, previous to 1849, no one had visited it. Being in Belgium, in the summer of that year, I determined to obtain a knowledge of it by personal observation.

A diligence runs daily between Antwerp and Gheel, the distance being about twenty-five miles. Upon a beautiful afternoon in July, I took a seat in this conveyance. For several miles we passed through a fertile and highly cultivated district, teeming with a luxuriant vegetation; the road bordered upon both sides with almost uninterrupted rows of trees. Soon after leaving the old town of Sierre, the soil became light and sandy, and vegetation less abundant. Trees no longer bordered the road, but small pines were scattered over the country, and, at length, we traversed an almost sterile plain. As the horses slowly dragged the burdened wheels through the sand, the idea was suggested that this desolation of nature comported well with the mental desolation which I was about to witness; that the change in the face of the earth, during this short journey, was typical of the alteration in a vigorous mind when, by disease, it is transformed into a dreary intellectual waste. As we approached Gheel, however, the landscape again assumed a more cheerful aspect, and rich fields, laden with grass and grain, stretched far and wide around us. Nature resumed her smiles, and the strong mind which had been made a desert

was again restored to reason. We entered the town or city, and stopped at the *Hotel de la Campine*.

The Commune of Gheel is about twelve miles square, and contains a population of ten thousand persons, exclusive of the insane. The city of Gheel has but about three thousand, the remainder being distributed upon farms, and in eighteen small villages, or hamlets, in different sections of the commune. The country is level, the soil in some parts good, and highly cultivated and productive; in others, light and sandy. Agriculture, the care of the insane, and the manufacture of lace, are the principal occupations and sources of revenue of the inhabitants.

The city of Gheel, like most other small towns upon the continent, is as completely built as if it were a portion of one of the larger capitals. The houses are constructed of stone or brick, and but few of them are more than two stories in height. The principal church, the public offices, and the houses for the entertainment of travelers, are upon the limits of a large, open square, near the centre of the city. The accommodations of the *Hotel de la Campine* are quite as comfortable as could be expected in a place so secluded, and of so little trade. Within the square is a public well, with a large pump, the creaking of whose heavy iron handle, as it is moved by the village maids,—*city* maids they must be called, since they are under the government of a Burgomaster—coming, one after another, from various directions, to procure water for domestic use, is almost the only sound which, of a summer afternoon, disturbs the silence of the place.

The house in which patients were formerly kept, while performing the *neuvaine*, is so connected with the church as apparently to form a part of it. Upon either side of its immense fire-place an iron ring is fixed to the wall, and a chair attached. These were used for the confinement of the excited and violent. At the opposite extremity of the church is the case containing the stones of the coffin of Saint Dympna. The floor beneath it, although of stone, is very perceptibly worn away by the persons who have knelt there, in their intercessions to the Saint. In near proximity to the case, there is a small side-chapel. Suspended upon its walls there still exists a well-preserved series of ancient oaken tablets, representing, by figures carved in *alto relievo*, nine scenes in the history of the Saint. The subjects of these may be understood by the following translation of the Latin inscriptions upon the several tablets:—

1. Here Dympna[4] is born of Christ.
2. She is given to an angel to be guarded.
3. She refuses incest with her father.
4. Being virtuous, she leaves her ancient country.
5. Being found, she is given up to her father.
6. She is slain, a victim to chastity.
7. They collect the remains of the angel.
8. They worship the bones of the martyr.
9. She ministers unto many sick people.

The carving is pretty well executed. Wherever the wicked father of the Saint is introduced, the image of the

---

2 This was called the Church of St. Dympna, by the gentleman who conducted me through it.—P. E.
3 Des Maladies Mentales, Par E. Esquirol. Vol. 2d, p. 713–14.
4 Esquirol invariably writes this "Nymphna," but I only heard it spoken, at Gheel, as Dympna. Upon the tablet it is Dimpna.

"unwearied adversary," with an infernal grin, is at his ear. In the last tablet the Saint is represented curing the insane, from the top of the head of one of whom a "devil" is making his egress.

The number of insane of the Commune of Gheel, in the latter part of the last century, was about four hundred. In 1803 it had increased to six hundred. In 1812 there were but five hundred, and, in 1821, four hundred. In 1849, according to Mons. Vygen, the *Commissaire de Police*, there were about one thousand, making the whole population of the Commune eleven thousand, of which the proportion of the insane to the sane, was, of course, as *one to ten*.

There are but three hundred patients in the city of Gheel. The remainder are distributed among the farmers, and in sixteen of the eighteen hamlets. The number of patients in the houses where they are taken is variable, but no person is permitted to have more than five. M. Vygen thinks that, in the city, there are not more than one hundred families which do not receive them.

The accommodations are of various grades. At some houses which I visited, the apartments were very agreeable and commodious, but in none were they furnished in a style nearly so elegant, as that of many of the private institutions for the insane in Belgium, France, England and America. But, at Gheel, much the greater proportion of the patients are supported at the expense of the public, and but about fifty cents a week is paid for the board and care of each of these.

No very great extent of luxury, either in furniture or food, can be supplied at the rate of seven cents a day.—Consequently many of these are placed in garrets, lofts, outhouses and other out-of-the-way nooks and corners where their accommodations can hardly be accurately described by that expressive word—"comfortable."— They appear, however, to be decently clothed and sufficiently well fed, and of all that I saw, in the numerous houses which I visited in Gheel and the surrounding country, I have no recollection of hearing a word of complaint in these respects. On the contrary, one woman, at a large farm-house a mile or two out of the town, was sorely troubled because there was too much food, too much clothing, in short, too much of everything in the world.

A considerable number, though not a large proportion of the patients are permitted to go at large, unaccompanied. A stranger in Gheel, without a knowledge of the fact that he is surrounded by a large number of insane, might, perhaps, pass a day or two before he would suspect it, as those who are abroad are mostly such as betray no very prominent eccentricities of conduct.—Several with whom I conversed in the streets said they were brought to the place because they were thought to be insane. One of them declared himself to be the Emperor of Austria, and another, a woman, claimed to be the daughter of the same sovereign. Within the town, I saw but one patient in the streets upon whom there was any restraining apparatus. His waist was encircled with an iron belt to which his hands were secured by wristlets. In the suburbs and around the farm-houses, however, there were several who were fettered with iron, the chain between the ancles being about eight inches in length. In some cases the rings around the ancles had abraded the skin and occasioned bad ulcers.

The climate of Gheel is said to be favorable to longevity. Mons. Vygen said that many of the patients were over eighty years of age, that a considerable number have died at nearly one hundred, and one, about the year 1845, at one hundred and four. The Asiatic cholera has never visited the place, although it has ravaged some of the surrounding communes.

On the second evening after my arrival in Gheel I attended a meeting of the *Societe d'Harmonie*, a musical association founded by one of the patients resident in the place. He remained a member for several years, and before his decease, saw it a flourishing society, composed of many members, playing upon nearly all kinds of musical instruments and furnished with a spacious hall for the accommodation of themselves and their audiences.

All the insane in the Commune are under the general supervision of a Board of Commissioners consisting of the Burgomaster, four physicians, two surgeons, and three citizens. Until recently the sick were all attended by the physicians of Gheel. The city of Brussels, however, having no less than three hundred and sixty patients here, has sent a physician, Dr. J. Parigot, formerly Professor in the University of Brussels, to have the special oversight of them. To him, as to M. Vygen, I am much indebted, not for verbal information alone, but for their company in visiting the houses in which patients are entertained.

The question whether the welfare of the insane is as much promoted in this Commune as it would be in Asylums or Hospitals has recently been much discussed in Belgium, particularly by medical men and the public authorities of the cities which now send their patients to Gheel. The Gheelans, citizens, medical men and public officers, espouse the opposite side of the question. They maintain that the patients under their care enjoy greater liberty and suffer less coercive restraints, that they breathe a purer air and take more exercise, are more constantly under supervision, and by being so widely distributed, a few in each family, are less subject to disturbance and annoyance from other patients than is possible in large institutions.

I saw nothing, farther than what is herein mentioned, tending to excite a doubt that the patients are kindly treated by their immediate protectors. The Physicians, the *Commissaire de Police* and the other officers whose duties involve a supervision of the insane, have an arduous task, but it is apparently faithfully performed. Notwithstanding all this I believe the *system* is liable to greater abuses than can possibly occur in well ordered institutions, and that the interests of the patients now at Gheel would be advanced if they could be placed in public Asylums, such as have recently been established in America, England, and several of the continental countries.

The work of Mons. Appert, a Frenchman, who recently traveled in Belgium, contains a notice of Gheel from which the following paragraph is translated.

"The greater part of the insane work in the fields with the persons who board them; they sometimes, also, take care of very young children, and, what is very remarkable, there is no instance of any injury (*exces*) committed by them upon these little creatures."[5]

M. Appert, according to the dates in his journal, remained but part of a day in Gheel, and, consequently, had not an opportunity of collecting all the information upon the subject of the insane which the place affords.—I was told, by two or three persons, at different times, that, about two years previous to my visit, one of the patients became strongly attached to a child in the family with which he boarded. Another patient was subsequently received, and, as *he* also became interested in the child, the jealousy of the former was aroused to such an extent that he murdered the little object of his affection.

The modern annals of Gheel furnish another tragedy, no less melancholy in its termination. About four years before my visit, one of the insane men was in the practice of collecting herbs, making infusions of them in beer, and selling this liquid, as medicine, at a high price. He had acquired a somewhat extensive reputation among the people of the vicinity, for his skill as a Physician, and was consequently consulted by many who were suffering from disease. The Burgomaster of Gheel, at that time, was a chemist and druggist, and, as his business was thus interfered with, he be-

came perhaps imprudent in his opposition to the proceedings of the patient. The insane man frequented the beer-shops, where, as in similar places in other countries, political subjects were frequently discussed. He heard much said against the Burgomaster, and hence probably at length believed that officer to be a very general object of dislike. He obtained an old bayonet, sharpened it, met the Burgomaster upon a somewhat secluded cross-path, by which he was accustomed to pass between his house and store, and killed him by repeated stabs.

These occurrences are not related as arguments against the system at Gheel. Incidents equally unfortunate, equally melancholy and fatal have occurred, more than once, in Asylums. Assertions, however, so erroneous as that of M. Appert, although made, undoubtedly, under a conviction of their truth, ought not to be permitted to give a false impression to the public mind. It should be known that at Gheel, as at every other place where there is a large congregation of the insane, there is liability to serious accidents, and that these have not always been avoided.

---

5 Voyage en Belgique. Par B. Appert, 1849.

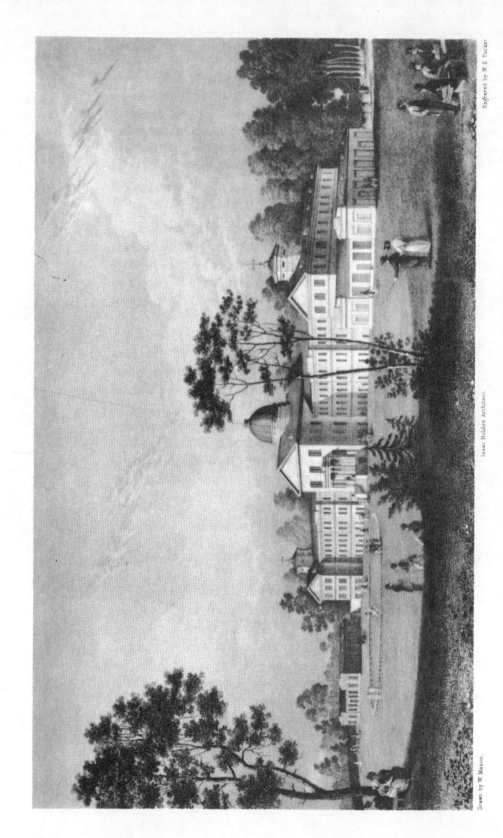

Drawn by W. Mason.

Isaac Holden Architect.

Engraved by W E Tucker

PENNSYLVANIA HOSPITAL FOR THE INSANE.

A Sketch of the History, Buildings, and Organization of the Pennsylvania Hospital for the Insane, Extracted Principally from the Reports of Thomas S. Kirkbride, M.D., Physician to the Institution

HISTORY.—In the year 1751, a number of the benevolent citizens of Philadelphia were incorporated by an act of the Provincial Assembly as "The Contributors to the Pennsylvania Hospital." Their charter was general in its character, and provided for "the relief of the sick and the reception and cure of lunatics."

The distressed condition of the insane of the province, the entire want of accommodations for their reception, and the absence of all judicious treatment were pre-eminently set forth in all the public appeals, and in all the official documents relative to this new undertaking.

From the first opening of the institution, on the 11th of February, 1752, an insane department has always constituted a prominent part of this noble charity, and has claimed a large share of the attention and benevolent labors of its distinguished medical officers and managers.

For a long period of years, it was far in advance of all other receptacles of the insane in the United States; and having the advantage of physicians like Bond, Shippen, Rush, Wistar, Physick and others, of equal celebrity, its wards for this description of patients were constantly filled, and its advantages eagerly sought by patients from the most distant sections of the Union.

From private contributions and legacies this institution has always mainly relied, for its support and for the means of extending its usefulness. Principally from these sources, and from a judicious care of its funds, by its early boards of managers, have arisen the noble buildings, which occupy the square between Spruce and Pine and 8th and 9th sts., in the city of Philadelphia, now used only for medical, surgical and obstetric patients; and those more recently erected, two miles from Philadelphia, devoted entirely to the Insane, and which will be described in detail in the following pages.

The insane were received and treated in the Hospital in the city of Philadelphia till the spring of 1841, and up to that period four thousand three hundred and sixty-six had received the benefits of its care. Of this number, one thousand four hundred and ninety-three were restored to their families perfectly cured; nine hundred and thirteen were discharged improved; nine hundred and ninety-five were removed by their friends without material improvement; two hundred and fifty-six eloped, principally before the square in the city was permanently enclosed; six hundred and ten died; and one hundred and ten were transferred to the new "Pennsylvania Hospital for the Insane."

Although all practicable means had been employed for the comfort and restoration of the insane patients, it became evident long since, that great disadvantages were necessarily attendant upon a city location—in connection with a sick hospital, and without a distinct medical organization. These circumstances had for several years induced the Board of Managers to look forward to a removal of this class of patients from the old building, as soon as sufficient funds could be procured for the construction and endowment of a new Hospital.

For this purpose, the resources of the Hospital were husbanded with great care, and the wise foresight of its early managers, in securing the then vacant lots immediately around the old Institution, ultimately enabled their successors to effect this long cherished object in the most liberal manner.

Several of the lots just adverted to, were purchased at different periods for the sum of eight thousand nine hundred and twenty-seven dollars and twenty-seven cents, and were directed to be sold by the contributors, at special meetings in the years 1832 and 1835. The proceeds of these sales were specially appropriated to the purchase of grounds and the erection of a Hospital for the Insane, and the amount of purchase money and interest received therefrom amounted to about three hundred and twenty-five thousand dollars—with which sum the various improvements, now known as 'THE PENNSYLVANIA HOSPITAL FOR THE INSANE,' have been completed.

The corner stone of the new building was laid on the 22d of June, 1836. It is located on a fine farm of 111 acres, about two miles west of the city of Philadelphia, between the Westchester and Haverford roads, on the latter of which is the gate of entrance. The building was nearly completed by the fall of 1840, when Dr. Thos. S. Kirkbride, who continues to direct its operations, received the appointment of Physician to the Institution. Under his superintendence, its organization and arrangements were completed, and the building opened for the reception of patients on the 1st day of the year 1841.

BUILDINGS.—The centre buildings and main wings of the new Hospital present an eastern front of four hundred and thirty-six feet, and consist of a basement and two principal stories. The basement throughout is surrounded by an area seven feet wide at the bottom, and six feet below the surrounding ground, to which handsomely sodded sloping banks gradually ascend. The area is paved with brick, and at its outer edge is surrounded by permanent gutters, connecting with large culverts.

The centre building is ninety-six feet deep—sixty-three feet wide, east of its junction with the wings—and sixty-seven on its western side. The former, which is the principal front, is built of cut stone and ornamented with a handsome doric portico; the western has also a portico of smaller dimensions, and like the rest of the Hospital is of stone, stuccoed to resemble the eastern front.

Spacious arched halls cross this building at right angles in each of the stories; those passing north and south are twelve feet wide and continuous with the corridors of the wings; the others are fourteen feet wide and contain the stairways, which in the principal stories are six feet wide, and like *all* the stairways leading from the upper story, are, with the exception of the stepping board and hand-rail, constructed entirely of iron and firmly secured to the wall.

In the basement is the kitchen, thirty-six by twenty-two feet, in which are fixtures of approved construction for steaming, baking, &c.,—store-rooms, a family dining room, a similar one for the domestics, and a room for furnaces and the storage of fuel. The kitchen and passage ways are laid with flag-stone embedded in mortar, and under the centre building is a commodious cellar.

In the principal story is the managers' room, (which is also the steward's office,) a family parlour, each twenty-four by nineteen feet, and two large rooms thirty-six by twenty feet, used as reception rooms for visitors, and for collecting the patients on the Sabbath, or on other occasions.

Communicating with the corridors of the wings and with the hall of the centre, are rooms, in which patients can have a private interview with their friends, without exposure, either to other patients or to visitors to the house.

In the second story are the Physician's office,—in which are kept the medicine and the library,—chambers for the officers resident in the Hospital, and two parlors, similar in size to the large rooms on the first floor, handsomely furnished and intended for the better class of convalescent patients.

The centre building is surmounted by a dome of good proportions, in which are placed the iron tanks, from which water is conveyed to every part of the building. The summit of the dome is eighty-five feet above the level of the basement, and from it, the panoramic view is one of great beauty; embracing a large extent of country—several flourishing villages—distant views of the Delaware and Schuylkill rivers, with their shipping—the Girard College, and the city of Philadelphia, with many of its more prominent objects.

The main Hospital is covered throughout with zinc or copper, and all its cornices, window sills, &c., are of cut stone, similar to that used for the front of the centre building. The basement *story* of the centre, and *all* the stories of the wings are thirteen feet six inches high; the two principal stories in the centre are eighteen feet nine inches.

Passing north and south from the centre building are the *main wings*; the north is occupied by the male, and the south by the female patients and they do not differ materially in their structure or arrangements. On the west side of the basement is a passage-way ten feet wide, and laid in cement; opposite to this in each wing, is a dining room forty-two by twenty-four feet—another twenty-four feet square, lodging rooms for the domestics of the establishment, and rooms for

the bath-boilers, for warm-air furnaces, and for the storage of fuel. There is also in the basement a bake house, ironing room, &c.

The principal story consists of a corridor twelve feet wide, with the patients' chambers on each side of it; these rooms are thirty in number, eight by ten feet, and are eleven feet high to the springing line, and twelve and a half feet to the crown of the arch. In each chamber is a glazed window, five feet by three and a half, and over each door is an unglazed iron sash, sixteen by thirty-two inches; by means of which a free circulation of light and air is at all times permitted. At the end of the corridor adjoining the centre building is a private stairway, and at the other is a parlor twenty-nine by twenty-five feet, having by its side one of the main stairways leading to the upper story. The doors at this end of the hall lead to one of the private yards.

There are also, store rooms for the patients' clothing, and a room containing the funnel by which soiled clothes, bedding, &c., are conveyed from both stories to the basement.

Running to the west and at right angles to those just described, are the *return wings*, having a corridor *ten* feet wide, on one side of which are eight chambers, similar to those already mentioned; opposite to these are three rooms each seventeen by thirteen and a half feet, intended for patients who wish superior accommodations, or who have private attendants,—a wash room, water closet, and a bath room, in which is every convenience for the douche, hot, cold, and shower baths. The patients occupying these different divisions, are separated by large folding doors, which can be thrown open at pleasure.

The upper story is similar in its arrangements and fixtures to that just described, except that the main wing is divided, and that the patients occupying one section of it, are intended to have access to the large parlor in the centre building, and pass to the basement by the private stairway.

The basement and passages of the centre building and every part of the wings, except the parlors and some of the lodging rooms below, are arched throughout.

Cast iron window sash, having glass six by fifteen inches, is used in all the patients' chambers, and by its peculiar arrangement, this hospital presents neither bars nor the extra sash which is almost universally met with. The upper and lower sash work in an iron frame, in which they are so exactly balanced, that no difficulty is experienced in moving them. They rise and fall simultaneously to the extent of six inches, when a *stop* prevents their further progress.— Space is thus given for ventilation without the risk of an escape.

Large glass, and wooden sash are used in all the parlors; in those in the wing, a slight wire screen, similar to that frequently seen in private dwellings, is placed on the outside of the lower sash; in those in the centre, ornamental cast iron screens are employed—both being intended to prevent accidents from sudden impulse, and neither offering anything unsightly either on the inside or outside of the building.

Most of the corridors have a handsome carpet, six feet wide, in their whole extent—improving their appearance, and contributing materially to the quiet of the house, by diminishing the sound made by their being used as a promenade during the day—and enabling those who are passing at night, to do so, without disturbing the patients who have retired. The parlors are generally carpeted and neatly furnished; every chamber where the state of the patient will permit it, has a bedstead, straw and hair matrass, table, chair, looking glass, and strip of carpet; and when desired by the friends of patients, still more furniture may be introduced.

Of the bedsteads now in the house, about fifty are of cast iron, neatly made and painted, and so constructed that they can be firmly secured to the floor, and that vermin cannot possibly be harbored in them; the remainder are of wood, and differ in no respect from what are commonly found in boarding houses.

Thirty-one feet, north and south of the main hospital, and nearly on a line with the eastern front of its centre, are placed the *detached buildings*, or *lodges*—one for each sex—which were authorised to be built by the contributors in 1841. They are also of stone, one story high, and built on three sides of a hollow square; the fourth being finished with piers and an open iron railing, giving free access to the air, and a handsome view of the deer park or surrounding scenery. These buildings are ninety-five feet on the west, and seventy-three on the other two sides—have their cellars arched, and a slate roof. Each building contains rooms for the accommodation of eighteen or twenty patients and their attendants,—a complete apparatus for bathing, water closet, &c.

These rooms are arranged specially for the accommodation of noisy and violent patients; they are placed on the outer side of the building, looking into a passage way eight feet wide, and finely lighted by numerous windows opening on the court yard, which is surrounded by a brick pavement, ten feet wide, enclosing a grass plot in its centre.

At the back of each room, near the ceiling, which is eleven feet high, is a glazed window three feet two inches, by eight inches, controlled by a cord which passes over pulleys into the hall. On the inner side of each room, in addition to the door, is a cast iron sash, twenty by thirty-seven inches, which may be glazed, or in front of which may be slid a close, wire, or glazed shutter, according to circumstances.

In each of these buildings, three distinct classes of patients can be accommodated; and from their position and structure, the most noisy will offer no annoyance to the inmates of the main hospital, while their accommodations will be scarcely less comfortable.

These lodges have proved an admirable part of the hospital, they are so near the main building as in no way to diminish the facility of supervision, and yet being entirely disconnected with it, they answer the objects of their erection much better, than any apartments in the main structure could possibly do. Every years experience has gone to confirm, the great value of this species of detached building, with attendants always in them, for certain classes of patients, and to prove that the objections occasionally made, do not exist in practice.

All these buildings have been constructed of the best materials, and in the most substantial and durable manner, and as will have been observed from the description are almost perfectly fire proof.

The *Workshop*, is a handsome frame building twenty by forty feet, two stories high, and situated near the gateway. The lower story is intended for carpenter work, turning, basket making,&c.—the upper room is plastered, and may be used for mattrass making, and other pursuits requiring space or for some of the amusements of the patients.

The buildings which were on the farm at the time of its purchase, (in addition to the residence of the Physician within the enclosure) consist of a comfortable house for the farmer, an adjoining one for the gardener, a spring-house, an ice-house, coach house, barn, &c., outside of the wall, and near the public entrance.

HEATING APPARATUS.—The hospital buildings are warmed by thirty-four air furnaces, burning anthracite coal, and supplied with air to be heated, through openings on the outside of the building. Of these furnaces, twenty-six are placed in the basement story of the main hospital, and four in the cellar of each detached building. By these means, during the severest weather, a regular and pleasant temperature has been given to all the parlors, halls, and chambers, occupied by the patients and their attendants, in every part of the establishment.

By large openings, with valves which regulate the supply, the heated air is freely admitted into all the parlors and corridors; and between the latter and the chambers, there is a free communication by means of the unglazed transom sash over each door, and if desired, during the day, by the doors themselves.

In addition to this, there is provision for giving a further supply of heat to each chamber; on the first floor, from the stone covering the warm air flue, which is about twenty inches wide, and passes along the inner side of each room; and in the second story, by the admission of the heated air through a valve, opening into the room, and out of reach of the patients.

In the Lodges, the warm air is admitted into the passages in a similar manner, and into every room by valves, out of reach of the patients and controlled from the hall.

VENTILATION.—Near the top of each chamber in the main building, is an opening six inches in diameter, from which a flue passes to the attic, and communicates with the external air, by means of numerous openings in the roof. The arrangement of the chamber windows gives for each when open, a free space, twelve by thirty-four inches, and the current of air is carried across the building, through the doorways and the open sash above them. The corridors have either large doors or windows at their terminations, and by opening these, the whole of the wing is thoroughly ventilated in a very short period.

In the detached buildings, each room has one or more openings in the ceiling, six inches square, which communicate with the attic, and thence with the external atmosphere; they are opened and closed by means of a cord which passes over pulleys into the passage.

At each end of each division, (four in all) of this passage way, is an opening similar in design and arrangement. All the ventilators and hot air valves are so constructed, that their position is known at a glance, without entering the patients' rooms.

Fourteen windows, three feet six inches, by four feet nine inches, opening on the courtyard, with the ventilation windows outside, and the door, and iron sash within, give a free ventilation across the building. In addition to the ordinary tight door, there is an open iron one neatly made and painted, at each outer termination of the passage way, by means of which a free current of air is allowed to pass whenever desirable—and the patients restricted to the halls during the summer, are thus given a fine view of the surrounding scenery.

SUPPLY OF WATER.—Near the southeast angle of the hospital property, and more than seven hundred feet from the centre building, is a one story stone structure, sixty-one by twenty-five feet, in which is the pump, driven by horse power, by means of which water is forced into the iron reservoirs in the dome of the centre building. Two horses are able to raise nearly fifteen hundred gallons per hour, through eight hundred and forty-five feet of pipe, to an elevation of one hundred and six feet.

This water is derived from a number of springs which arise on the premises, and empty into a pond one hundred and ninty-five by forty-five feet, and of an average depth of about four feet. From this pond, the water is conveyed by an iron pipe into the large cistern with which the pump communicates. In addition to this source of supply, a small stream passing through the grounds, can at any time be turned into the cistern should circumstances render it necessary. The reservoirs in the dome contain about six thousand gallons, and two small tanks in the return wings, contain about five hundred gallons each, and from them the water is conveyed to every section of the buildings for bathing and other purposes. The average daily consumption is near three thousand gallons.

In the building just described, are all the fixtures for washing and drying clothes, by means of which an abundance of unpleasant effluvium is kept out of the Hospital. Soiled articles are thrown down the *funnels* in the different wards, and are regularly taken from the receiving rooms in the basement to the wash-house, from which they are returned when ready for the ironing-room. The location of this building, and of the ample drying grounds attached to it, is such, that they can scarce be seen from the Hospital.

DRAINAGE.—The Hospital stands upon a high part of the farm, and has a descent from it in every direction. Commencing at the western side of the centre building, is the main culvert, which empties outside of the wall into a small stream of water, forty-five feet below the elevation on which the building stands, and more than three hundred and fifty feet from it. Into this *main*, empty the *branch* culverts, which lead from the western terminations of the return wings, each being about one hundred and seventy-six feet long.

The culverts which drain the yards, the roofs, and all the washings of the *detached buildings*, commence under the bath-rooms, join the *branch* culverts near the commencement, and are each about two hundred and seventy feet long.

All the openings into these various culverts are secured by the most approved apparatus for preventing the escape of effluvium, and the culverts themselves are sufficiently large to allow a man to pass through their whole extent.

PLEASURE GROUND AND FARM.—Of the one hundred and eleven acres in the farm, about forty-one around the Hospital are specially appropriated as a vegetable garden and the pleasure ground of the patients, and are surrounded by a substantial stone-wall. This wall is five thousand four hundred and eighty three feet long, and is ten and a half feet high.

Owing to the favorable character of the ground, the wall has been so placed that it can be seen but in a very small part of its extent, from any one position; and the enclosure is so large, that its presence exerts no unpleasant influence upon those within. Although it is probably sufficient to prevent the escape of a large proportion of the patients, that is a matter of small moment, in comparison with the quiet and privacy which it at all times affords, and the facility with which the patients are enabled to engage in labor, to take exercise, or to enjoy the active scenes which are passing around them, without fear of annoyance from the gaze of idle curiosity or the remarks of unfeeling strangers. Our location gives us the many advantages afforded by a thickly settled district, and proximity to a large city, and the wall obviates most of its disadvantages. Immense utility has been found to result from having such *large pleasure grounds, enclosed, and by a wall so admirably located, and not the slightest objection of any kind.*

Immediately in front of the Hospital, is a lawn forming a segment of a circle, in which is a circular rail-road and extensive flower borders. To the east of this, and passing into the woods, is the *deer-park*, surrounded by a high pallisade, and forming an effectual and not unsightly division of the ground appropriated to the different sexes; from various points of which, and from the whole eastern front of the building, it is seen to much advantage.

The pleasure ground is beautifully undulating, interspersed with clumps and groves of fine forest trees, and from every division of it, as well as from every room in the main Hospital, is a handsome view; either of the surrounding country and villages, the rivers in the distance, or the public roads in its immediate vicinity.

The groves are fitted up with seats, and ornamental summer houses, and are the favorite resort of the patients, during the warm weather. That on the west, from the position of the wall, does not appear to be inclosed, and offers full view of two public roads, of the farm and meadow, a mill race, a fine stream of running water, and two large manufactories. The grove on the east is not less pleasant, and the views from it are equally animated. This last surrounds the pond, in which is found a variety of fish.

On the north and south side of the building are private yards, one hundred and seventeen feet wide, and extending two hundred feet from the return wings which form one of their sides. These yards are enclosed by a tight board fence seven and a half feet high, and are surrounded with a brick pavement, which affords a fine promenade at all seasons.

The fences around these yards, like the wall itself, have been constructed, not so much to confine the patients, as for the sake of privacy, and to protect them from the gaze of visitors.

The remaining seventy acres, outside the wall, are cultivated by the farmer, and, with the grass obtained within it, furnish pasture and hay for the large dairy, which supplies both Hospitals with cream and milk during the whole year. From this source are also obtained some grain, and all the potatoes and other vegetables that are required in large quantities. Ample opportunities for agricultural labor are thus afforded for all patients, for whom it may be deemed beneficial.

ORGANIZATION.—The government of the Pennsylvania Hospital is vested in a Board of twelve Managers, who give their services gratuitously, and who are elected annually by the Contributors.

To this Board is entrusted the general management of the Institution and its funds—the regulation of its domestic economy—the admission and discharge of patients, and the election of Physicians and other officers. In addition to their duties in the city, the attending Managers pay one official visit, weekly, to the Hospital for the Insane, to inspect the accounts, to examine the house and grounds, and to see that the patients receive the proper care and attention.

The Officers of the Hospital for the Insane, are:

1. A *Physician*, who resides upon the premises, to whom is confided the general superintendence of the establishment—the sole direction of the medical, moral and dietetic treatment of the patients, and the selection or approval of all persons employed in their care.

2. An *Assistant Physician*, living in the Hospital, who prepares and dispenses all medicine prescribed for the patients—devotes himself to their care—sees that all directions respecting them are faithfully carried out, and that the attendants, and others employed in the wards, fail not in the performance of their duties.

3. A *Steward*, who takes care that the buildings and grounds are kept in good order—makes all the purchases for the house—receives all monies due the Institution for board, &c.—makes engagements with those employed—pays them for their services, and settles all accounts against the Hospital.

4. A *Matron*, who has the general charge of the domestic economy of the house—the cooking and distribution of the food, and of the female domestics, and attends specially to the comfort of the female patients.

In the wings, the following persons are employed:

1. *Supervisors*, one for each sex, whose duty it is to pass their time among the patients in the different wards and pleasure grounds—to endeavor to interest, employ and amuse them in every way in their power, and to see that all the rules for the attendants in their intercourse with the patients, are rigorously observed. Before retiring at night, the Supervisors furnish the Physician with a written report of whatever has come under their observation during the day.

2. *Attendants*, who have the immediate care of the patients—sleep in the same divisions of the house—attend them in the dining rooms—accompany them in their walks, rides, or amusements—assist them when engaged in manual labor, and take the entire charge of the halls, chambers, and clothing of the patients, as may be directed by the Physician.

The buildings of this Hospital admit of six distinct wards in each wing, making as many complete classes of patients for each sex. To each ward is assigned two attendants—so

that at all times there is one attendant in the presence of the patients, and one who may be walking or riding with them under his care, or performing other duties that may necessarily take him out of his appropriate division. The only exception to this rule is in the two wards of each lodge, where three attendants are found sufficient to keep up the supervision and perform all other duties—two being generally out of doors with a majority of the patients, and the other having the care of those who remain in the wards.

The number of attendants employed, is generally one for every 7 or 8 patients, exclusive of special attendants, the number of whom varies at different times from 2 or 3 to more than double those numbers.

3. A *Watchman*, who attends to the safety of the building on account of fire—visits every part occupied by the *male* patients, frequently during the night—attends to the administration of medicine when required—starts the kitchen fires and rings the bell in the morning—sees that all rules are faithfully observed, and before retiring to rest, makes a written report to the Physician, of his observations during the night. At 6 A.M. his duties as Watchman cease for the day.

4. A *Watch-woman*, who is governed by the same rules as the watchman, and whose duties are similar, except that her time is spent entirely in the wards occupied by the *female* patients.

In addition to those just mentioned, whose duties bring them directly in contact with the patients, there are employed in the Hospital and resident there—a gate-keeper—a coachman—a jobber—a baker—a fireman—one cook—one assistant cook—three attendants in dining rooms—two chambermaids, and four washerwomen. The farmer and gardener reside outside of the enclosure.

TREATMENT.—The *medical* treatment of patients in this institution, is varied of course, according to the peculiar symptoms, presented by each case, and a detail of which would be out of place in a notice like the present. Baths, for which ample provision is made in the different wards, are used very extensively, and all the means of moral treatment in its varied ramifications, are constantly resorted to, for the benefit of the patients. Out door labor in the garden—on the grounds, or farm—mechanical employments of different kinds—riding in the circular railway—ten pins—carriage riding, or long walks to the many objects of interest in and about the city of Philadelphia;—the use of musical instruments—attendance at parties, lectures and concerts—all the usual variety of games—a library of near 1000 volumes, and a great variety of periodicals, are some of the many means which come under this category.

During fine weather at all seasons of the year, the arrangements of this establishment enable a very large part of all the patients to take active exercise, and to spend a large portion of the entire day in the open air.

Those patients who are well enough, attend divine worship in some of the churches in the vicinity, and nearly all attend the reading of the Bible, on the evening of every Sabbath.

RESTRAINT.—Restraining apparatus has very rarely been used in this establishment, and the seclusion of patients to their chambers, is resorted to as little as possible. Several months have frequently elapsed without any form of apparatus being employed, and very often out of from 150 to 170 patients, many days elapse without a single one being confined to their room, even for a single hour.

No restraint is ever employed without the express direction of the physician—no apparatus is ever kept in the wards, and the only form ever used, are the invaluable apparatus for retaining certain classes of patients on their beds at night—the leather mittens and wristbands or some still simpler substitute for the latter. Although cases requiring even these means of restraint are not numerous, still the experience of this institution thus far has been, that they may occasionally be employed with advantage to a patient. Special pains are taken to avoid *long continued seclusion*, the bad effects of which among the insane, are believed often to be still greater than what arise from mechanical means of restraint.

ADMISSION OF PATIENTS.—All classes of insane persons, without regard to the duration of the disease or of its curability, are admitted into this institution, upon securing the payment of a reasonable rate of board, by the obligation of some responsible resident of the city or county of Philadelphia. Cases of *Mania a Potu* are never received into this hospital—but that in the city, exclusively.

In addition to those patients who pay for their board, a limited number from the State of Pennsylvania is received on the free list, and supported by the Institution without charge of any kind. The number thus admitted is regulated by the income of the Corporation, and of this class there is generally from one hundred and twenty to one hundred and fifty under care, in the two Hospitals, of whom about one fourth are insane.

In order to extend as widely as possible the benefits of this charity, it has been deemed advisable to restrict the admission of insane persons on this list, to recent cases and but for a limited period; so that if no indications of recovery are seen after a reasonable trial, they may be discharged to make room for other applicants. If improving when their term is ended, they are generally continued till their restoration is complete.

No person about the Hospital, except the officers, knows who are free patients, and there is no distinction made in their accommodations, but what the character of their disease, or their previous pursuits have rendered necessary.

THE PENNSYLVANIA HOSPITAL FOR THE INSANE, as has been before observed, was opened for the admission of patients on the 1st day of January, 1841, and 93 patients, in a short period, were removed from the Hospital in the city to the new location. A few followed after the completion of the lodges. Of them, nearly all were incurable, and had been residents of the old Institution for various periods from 3 to 40 years. Exclusive of these, the following table shows the number of patients admitted, and the average number and the highest number under care each year since the opening of the Hospital.

	1841	1842	1843	1844
1st Admissions	83	111	140	153
2d. Average number	104	114	132	151
3d. Highest number	116	127	145	163
4th. Total number	176	238	258	285

The number of admissions for the present year, up to this date, (August 1st,) has been 102, and the highest number in the house at one time has been 171. The wing devoted to males has been crowded for two months past, owing mainly however to the unusual preponderance of male patients, during the present summer, as the whole building when completely filled is capable of accommodating 180 patients with their attendants.

AUGUST 1st, 1845.

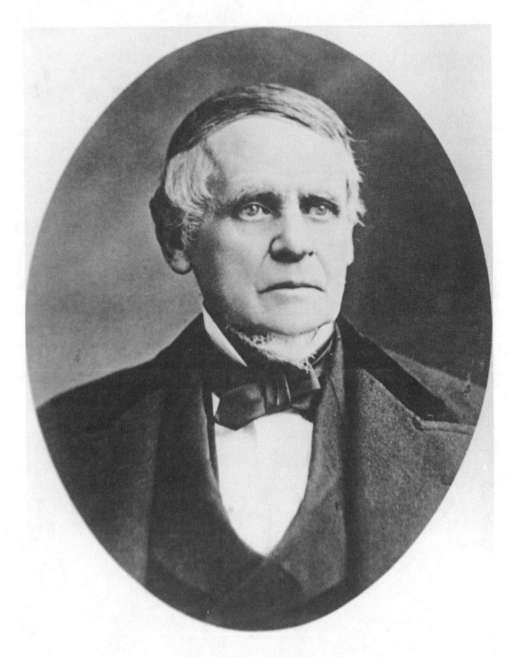

Thomas S. Kirkbride, M.D., 1809–1883
Founding Father, First Secretary, and Officer of the Assoication for 26 Years

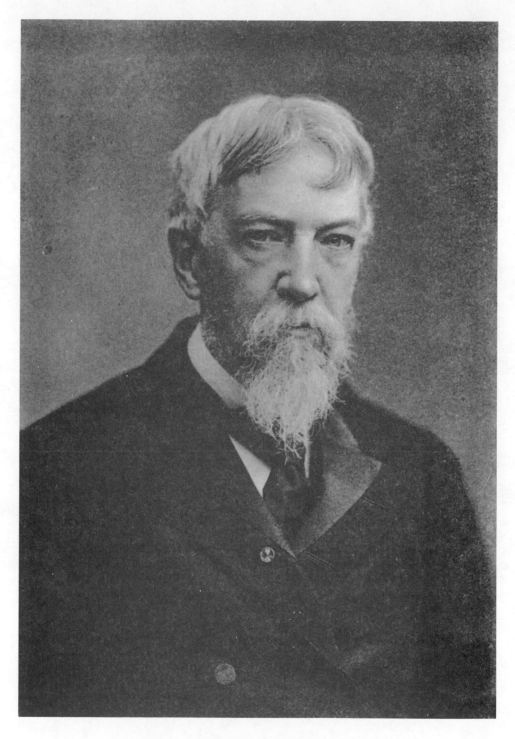

Silas Weir Mitchell, M.D., LL.D., 1829–1914

Founder and First President of the American Neurological Association (1875)

Reprinted from The Journal of Nervous and Mental Disease for July 1894

Address Before the Fiftieth Annual Meeting of the American Medico-Psychological Association, Held in Philadelphia, May 16th, 1894

By S. Weir Mitchell, M.D., LL.D.

Philadelphia, Pennsylvania

I am here to-day under circumstances so unusual, that I may be pardoned, if I explain them in order to justify the frank language of this address.

When your representative, Dr. Chapin, asked me to be your speaker on this important anniversary, I declined. It is customary on birthdays to say only pleasant things, and this I knew I could not altogether do. I foresaw a struggle between courteous desire to follow a kindly custom and the duty to greatly use a great occasion. When Dr. Chapin, after consulting some of you, came back to say it was still your desire that I should speak, I reflected that men who could thus ask the criticism, which they knew must come without mercy, were well worth talking to. I said, at last, that I would address you to-day, but that it would be boldly and with no regard to persons. That was a momentary insanity; I have been sorry ever since.

You are on the dividing year of your first century of life. You look back with just pride as alienists on the merciful changes made for the better in the management of the chronic insane. It is to be feared that you also have cause to recall the fact that as compared with the splendid advance in surgery, in the medicine of the eye and the steady approach to precision all along our ardent line, the alienist has won in proportion little. This is partly due to the nature of the maladies with which you have to deal; but there are many other causes at work to retard the wholesome progress. Just that which is impairing the usefulness of the lesser specialties in medicine has been more gravely enfeebling your value, and retarding your development. I mean the tendency to isolation from the mass of the active profession. At first, as concerned the eye for instance, this separation seemed but too complete—the new terms, the methods, the instruments of the ophthalmologist were for a time absurdly unfamiliar. It is not so at present. The general practitioner has come again into touch of the oculist, and understands his terms and his methods. In fact, every sudden advance of a brigade of our great line for a time appears to break our ranks; but soon we get up to it and go on as before.

With you it has been different. You were the first of the specialists and you have never come back into line It is easy to see how this came about. You soon began to live apart, and you still do so. Your hospitals are not our hospitals; your ways are not our ways. You live out of range of critical shot; you are not preceded and followed in your ward work by clever rivals, or watched by able residents fresh with the learning of the schools.

I am strongly of opinion that the influences which for years led the general profession to the belief that no one could, or should, treat the insane except the special practitioner, have done us and you and many of our patients lasting wrong.

Standing here in the home of Rush, I cannot forget that he was an alienist and a general practitioner; nor can I cease to lament the day when the treatment of the insane passed too completely out of the hands of the profession at large, and into those of a group of physicians who constitute almost a sect apart from our more vitalized existence. What evil this has wrought, what harm it has done to us and to you I shall try to show. Why it has been so much more grave in its results here than in Europe is not clear to me, or would take too long to discuss.

I should, indeed, be easy enough in mind if I had only to criticise an uneducated public, ignorant legislators, and the boards which control our civic, state and endowed institutions. But I shall have frankly to reproach as to certain things many of those who still bear the absurd label of "medical superintendents." If any here think it pleasant to fire opinions into a crowd, not knowing who are hit, whether his shot finds out the right man, or only annoys the entirely efficient, I am not that man. Moreover, abrupt statements are apt to be needlessly annoying, and I have not time to be other than brief to abruptness.

But before I go on to the uncongenial task of being disagreeable, and, perhaps, ending with criticism which you may call ignorant, I would say a word.

I at first meant this address to be weighty with statistics and with carefully gathered knowledge of the way in which the medicine of the alien mind grew up in this country. After immense reading I gave it up, but it left with me the conviction that within ten or fifteen years things have been improving, and that within your own ranks are men who had early seen the need for much of what I urge to-day. Without this qualifying belief I should have hesitated still longer as to this ungracious work.

There were in this country in 1890, 120 public and some

40 private asylums; nor does this include insane wards of county alms houses, or those singular institutions known as sanitariums, which receive many insane and are, I fancy, little troubled by the lunacy commissioners. In 1889, the patients in these 160 hospitals numbered 91,152, and were treated at a cost of $10,692,000 over and above $2,209,000 spent that year in buildings.

The state and civic asylums are under boards appointed usually by governors of states, or mayors, sometimes with as much regard to politics as to quality of useful fitness. The great endowed asylums are ruled by self-constituted bodies, which in certain cases have the ponderous task of also managing a general city hospital.

Then there are the private asylums which have no boards and manage themselves, and are commercial enterprises. Over all, in many states, is the more or less efficient machinery of the lunacy commissions. Usually good enough as collectors of statistics and as historians, these bodies are, as to visits and accurate inspection in the higher sense, most plainly ineffective. Too often they are made up without one member who can be called an expert in neurological medicine. Is this vast trust so handled as to satisfy the intelligent conscience of my profession? I have read and thought about its every phase an inconceivable amount. I saw that here or there some one had shown what could be done in the face of preconception, traditional usage or want of means, and was so much ahead of his fellows as to excite wonder that such intelligent examples should lack efficient following. Yet, after all I thus learned of growth and thoughtful gains, it did seem to me that the sowers of good seed were sadly few, the progress strangely slow. When, indeed, I began to write what I had to urge, my charges appeared to me so grave as to require the expression of other opinions than those of a single thinker in order to give him the courage to speak them to the world. I, therefore, resolved to call a jury and use its decisions to modify or give force to my own.

The men before me see asylums from within. Some live on quietly. Some are vaguely dissatisfied. Some are half-hopelessly striving to better things, which only in part lie within their power to change. Outside, and of late years, your asylums are relentlessly watched by one of the ablest groups of men known to me, the neurologists and consultants of our cities. To thirty of these I addressed the following letter:

DEAR DOCTOR.—I have been asked to deliver, in May, the address on the occasion of the Fiftieth Anniversary of the Society of the Medical Superintendents of the Insane, now known under the name of the Medico-Psychological Society. I have consented with the clear understanding that I shall be free to represent the best professional opinion in the country to the gentlemen who are at the head of these institutions. I am told that I shall have full freedom. To enable me to carry out this plan I have addressed duplicates of this letter to a few of the leading American neurologists, and to certain consultants not neurologists. May I ask you to answer the following questions:

Do you think the present asylum management of the insane in America as good as it could be made?

What faults do you find with it?

If you had full freedom to change it what would you do?

I do not want a written treatise on the subject, but within a

reasonable time a reply of such brevity as will cover the ground for an expert.

Yours truly,

S. WEIR MITCHELL

The men I called to my aid are physicians accustomed, in recent days, to treat the insane. Some of them are familiar with asylums; most of them have contributed largely and originally to neuro-pathology, symptomalology and therapeutics. No man can afford to set quite aside the criticism of their replies. To sustain my position I print in an appendix their letters. They are severe, but not unkindly; nor do they fail to point out how largely you are trammelled by custom, lack of means, and above all, in some cases, (and this is saddest and most shameful of all), directly or indirectly by politics. [Appendix not included in this supplement because of space limitations.]

I have used, also, certain communications from able asylum officers, which I cannot print, and, also, I have had in the past letters from intelligent people, some of them doctors, who speak of their own experiences as patients in asylums, and make reflections thereon.

But it is the arraignment of the neurologist which ought incessantly to trouble you and the boards which you have to manage—for the management of managers is an important business. It is this outspoken discontent which ought to make you ask how far you, yourselves, are responsible. If we are right, neither States nor boards nor you are ardently living up to the highest standard of intelligent duty.

And now as to boards of managers.

You know too well, I fear, how state boards are generally constituted. There the mischief begins. They meet exceedingly variable intervals—some monthly, and some every third month. When once they have decreed a superintendent physician for the asylum his reports must largely guide them. I approach a delicate matter when I say that in some states the selection, both of these boards and the appointment and continuance in office of a physician superintendent, is said to be more or less a question of politics. I am told that this inconceivably shameful thing is past doubt. But to accept such office as a mere bit of party spoil! Can a man do that and be fit for the work? Let us hope it is all mere scandalous gossip, and turn from a too painful topic. Money changers in the temple! Ward politics at the bedside of the lunatic, How can one with patience even speak of it?

These boards have to learn duties and acquire knowledge common enough among neurologists. But what governor of a state comes to us and asks whom he shall appoint? That you depend for sympathy, intelligent help, and even your livelihood, on the continued good-will of bodies thus made up is a grave evil. It leads to this need to manage the manager, to want of decision, to rose-colored reports, to deference to potent trustees as to your minor appointments; or else these boards do not manage at all. The steward and physician run the concern. Meetings are rare; business is kept straight of course; and so we blunder along.

But, surely, the private or endowed asylums should be

better off. I think not. Their boards are self appointed, and are made up of very excellent, kindly, middle-aged clergymen, merchants, lawyers and the like. They fill their own vacancies as they please. I do not see why there should not be on these boards one or more physicians, and not old ones, either. Also, I should like to drop managers every ten years. and change committees as often as once a year.

The psychology of boards is, as yet, unstudied. It is not in the text-books. The best of them get wooden and lose capacity to change with ease. A man who is too self-critical is sure to lack enterprise, and a board is nothing if not critical. Even the feeble have this retarding power, and soon or late, the doubts and prejudices of the old cripple with splints of inertia affect the mindjoints of the fresh comers. All boards age rapidly, and acquire young the senile characteristics. They assimilate with difficulty and abhor change; meanwhile, they are dealing with an art and its assistive sciences which are changing at such a rate as taxes the industry and watchfulness of the best of us to keep in the van of their bewildering advance. All this, the boards which manage our hospitals rarely apprehend. That our art fails in the same ratio as our science falls behind, is not such a truth as the mental structure of boards can grasp; and hence half-equipped hospitals, and hence new hospitals built with small contribution from modern constructive art, the old stupidities in brick and stone repeated, as is happening even now as I write.

I sometimes think that it would be in our great cities, a wise thing to have any hospital staff say frankly what it thinks of the management back of it. Perhaps I had better pause here.

A managing board has committees, and these inspect their hospitals,—I really do not know how often. Such occasions used to greatly amuse a sometime patient of mine, convalescent from much drink in a great asylum. He was given a good deal of freedom, and his letters to me delineating a managerial inspection were really worth publication in the interests of human mirth. Once I, myself, saw a large part of such an inspection. I assure you it was interesting. The visit was, of course, expected. Is it in human nature not to get ready just a little? We walked all over the wards, we spoke kindly to a few amiable patients, we asked a reasonable number of obvious questions, we partook of a very good luncheon, praised everything, including the cook, received bouquets or grapes, and, after three hours, departed, having made an inspection! I thought it a neat little comedy; no one there suspected the audience of smiling not with, but at, the players. It seemed to please the superintendent and the managers, and, if I saw certain things which were not after my mind, I was not a manager and had no experience except of those ruthless inspections in the great war. A visit without warning, by night, or at a meal-hour, causing relentless blanks to be filled, a report to a despotic authority, and all with no least will, or wish, or reason to hide the truth.

It is certain that hospital inspections by managers are simply valueless. Every doctor laughs at them. Yet no one thinks these honest gentlemen either stupid or undutiful. They merely do not know their business, and do not know that they do not know. Yet to learn this work were easy.

Why not have blanks to tell them what to see? Why not condescend to learn? Why not drop in at a meal, at night? Really this whole thing is of incredible stupidity.

Corporations are said not to have souls; I sometimes think that this grouping of men with selection limited by creed, habit, or social caste, lessens the individual good sense, or kills its large use by the cumulative curse of critical doubt. I have seen hospitals that smelt and looked like second-class lodging-houses, and have found their managers serenely contented. What we want is a training-school for hospital managers. Perhaps some of you keep one. I wish you all success.

I do not know just how the boards of your special hospitals appoint a physician. I wish I thought our general city hospitals were governed as to appointments in some degree by the scientific record of the man. I would stand on that alone if I had to be limited to one form of knowledge of a candidate, and in any case it would influence me largely. In one hospital of this city, the medical staff nominates, and the board takes or rejects at will. There, too, the staff sit in the board, but do not vote. I consider this the approach to an ideal hospital management. It works perfectly.

I know clearly what a group of neurologists will do in the ideal days, when a board of humble-minded managers desires us to select a superintendent of the minds and bodies of men out of their poor wits. I fancy we shall ask first for large general hospital experience, for ample knowledge of psychology and pathology. Then we would want to know what books or papers on the insane the man had written, whether these were fresh with new thoughts, or made up of vague pilferings from better brains. We should wish him to have other qualities,—but of this again.

So much for your rulers—the hospital boards. They have much to learn, and those who appoint certain of them have still more to learn. I have dealt especially with these because I think their members do usually desire to do right, and know not how. Strangely enough, the best of boards are not always those of the endowed asylums, but the changing groups of the state boards. The permanent boards more readily acquire the contagious disease of hospital torpor. It is well known to us, and has no least excuse where money is abundant. I have seen it creep into quite young institutions, and have seen it cured only by very radical means. Also, it is strangely insidious. The price of security from hospital torpor, from the sclerosis of custom, is constant vigilance. This malady comes to one institution from a too wooden board; it comes to another from the inertness of doctors. Hospitals, good to-day, in a few years may become bad. I saw the worst hospital in this city pass quickly into the first rank; I have seen a hospital once first, drop to a second rate.

I have said the ailments of hospitals begin, as a rule, in the governing boards; they do not end there.

In our general hospitals there is a diffused medical authority, but yours is a monarchy more or less limited. And now, my next query is as to whether you, who thus govern and make reports and live amongst your armies of the insane, are, in all respects, doing what you should and might do. We have done with whip and chains and ill-usage, and having won this noble battle have we not rested too easily content with having made the condition of the insane more comfortable?

The question we here ask at starting is if you, who are so powerful within these alien camps, are really doing all that might be done without serious increase of expenditure? Frankly speaking, we do not believe that you are so working these hospitals as to keep treatment or scientific product on the front line of medical advance.

Where, we ask, are your annual reports of scientific study, of the psychology and pathology of your patients? They should be published apart. We commonly get as your contributions to science, odd little statements, reports of a case or two, a few useless pages of isolated post-mortem records, and these are sandwiched among incomprehensible statistics and farm balance-sheets; and this is too often your sole answer. Where, indeed, are your replies to the questions as to heredity, marriage, the mental disorders of races, the influence of malarial locations, of seasons, of great elevations, all the psychological riddles of a new land, a forming breed, never weary of quickening the pace, of inventing means of hurry—relentless workers? When I put such questions I am always met with the doleful reply. "We have no time; we want more money; we have not enough assistants." I am quite willing to admit that for the careful treatment of the possibly curable insane, none of you have enough help. I grant that, but it is not all. I could say the like of many a fertile man in this city. I can but partially admit this endless plea of overwork in extenuation of the charge of scientific unproductiveness; that serious symptom of a larger malady. Surely the immense and habitual hospital work among the sick which numberless city doctors do, their professional teaching, their clinics and societies, the endless cares, trusts, and social duties of a city life, do these make them fail of scientific productiveness? No, it is not time alone your people want. There is something defective besides number in your organizations. And as to this, what prevents your endowed suburban hospitals having any quantity of young resident physicians? It is only to choose with care and to feed them. There is much they can do, and be taught to do, which will relieve you, and set you free for the higher work we ask of you.

But if your own institution is unhappily connected with a general hospital, do not let it send you residents for the first three months of their two year term, as is done, I hear, in this city. Could there be a more useless and thoughtless way of giving these young men a knowledge of insanity?

And then as to your paid assistants. You need as aids men who, first of all, have had long training in a general hospital, and here, the choice, I suspect, is left largely to you. Ask your boards to have competitions for your permanent assistants. Insist on hospital training, knowledge of psychology, of neuropathology, and then demand of your people original reports or product of some kind. I find myself that nothing is so useful as original research to urge on my aids. But then you must lead or they will not go the way you would have them go. I should insist, were I you, that your aids spend daily some hours outside of your walls and have a long summer holiday. There have been some among your best who have insisted that incessant contact with mental imperfection is not a wholesome thing.

Want of competent original work is to my mind the worst symptom of torpor the asylums now present. Contrast the work you have done in the last three decades with what the little group of our own neurologists has done. To compare your annual output with the great English or German work were hardly a pleasant thing to do. Even in your own line, most of the text-books, many of the ablest papers are not asylum products. What is the matter? You have immense opportunities, and, seriously, we ask you experts, what have you taught us of these 91,000 insane whom you see or treat? You will point to certain books, some good work in this or that asylum, but, as we judge you, to no such amount of thoughtful output as your chances might lead us to expect.

There are other material failures by which we test as much of your work as we can see, and thence suspect the precision and general value of what we do not see. When we ask for your asylum notes of cases, or by some accident have occasion to look over your case books, we are too often surprised at the amazing lack of complete physical study of the insane, at the failure to see obvious lesions, at the want of thorough day by day study of the secretions in the newer cases, of blood-counts, temperatures, reflexes, the eye-ground, color-fields, all the minute examination with which we are so unrestingly busy. It is not thus in all your asylums, but you will see from the letters appended that I am not alone in this critical complaint. Not so many years ago in a certain asylum I could not get a stethoscope or an ophthalmoscope; and too often when we receive a patient, and write and ask for his hospital record it is such as would surprise, for meagreness, the resident of a city hospital. I had recently occasion to see the printed schedule guide to symptom notes in an asylum; it was oddly defective, had been ten years in use and would excite a smile from any of my clinical aids. If, as to all these defects, I am still told that they are due to lack of means, I make answer that our criticism applies as decisively to some of the amply endowed asylums as to those for the poor of the states.

A clever woman once said to me that only the rich did not get the worth of their money, and here it is true. Set aside the state hospitals for the while, and let us consider the others. Why have not more of you started training schools? This would at once enliven the air of the place and assist you to get good nurses. Can you get these at from twelve to eighteen dollars a month? No. But for nothing you can get them, because if you train nurses during two years, the second year the nurse is of real value and can be promoted. Some will stay on with you, and then, if you furnish nurses really trained to the care of the insane you can reward your best nurses with convalescent cases leaving your care and able to pay, as we pay outside, larger prices than you can give as wages. Try this, and see how it works. You will get better aids. Make your young men teach the nurses. There is nothing teaches the teacher like teaching. And let me helpfully insist that there is a real outside demand for nurses trained to intelligent care of the insane. I wanted a dozen this winter. The fact is your nurses are, as a rule, of an unfit and quite uneducated class. When one of them comes to me to take a case, or comes with a case, and I give her a careful schedule of the day, I find I have to teach what a pack means, and a drip sheet, and Swedish movements, and massage, and soon we part.

Indeed, we with difficulty understand how you get on in your work with the nurses you employ. It must make the individualization of treatment impossible. The thinking general practitioner knows that what he has to deal with is not a disease, but a disease plus a man. This is deeply true of insanity. Nowhere is it more needful to study the human soil in which the disorder exists. We think you too largely fail to do this, and we think such success impossible without educated nurses taught to observe and to handle the insane.

Have you people in your asylums trained to use massage? I see plenty of folks in your wards who need this potent blood-stiring tonic. In how many hospitals is there an electric room and a trained electrician? I wrote an asylum some time ago to ask for a statement of the electric reactions in a certain case. I was told in reply that the muscles "moved pretty well with a faradic battery!"

You will see in the appended letters that some of us think hydro-therapeutics of great value. How many hospitals are provided with the appliances for such treatment? How many of you employ it at all? How far are your nurses acquainted with its various forms of use? Much of that I here speak of can be obtained at slight cost. But when I read your reports (I have read many of late) I do not find an urgent, repeated demand for these obviously needed things. I find too comfortable assurance of satisfaction: too much stress on mere amusements; too little on rewarded work; too many signs of the contented calm born of isolation from the active, living struggle for intellectual light and air in which the best of us live.

The cloistral lives you lead give rise, we think to certain mental peculiarities. I could tell you how to mend them; I shall by and by. You hold to and teach certain opinions which we have long learned to lose. One is the superstition (almost is it that) to the effe[c]t that an asylum is in itself curative. You hear the regret in every report that patients are not sent soon enough, as if you had ways of curing which we have not. Upon my word, I think asylum life is deadly to the insane. Poverty, risk, fear, send you of true need many patients; many more are sent by people quite able to have their friends treated outside. They are placed in asylums because of the wide-spread belief you have so long, and, as we think, so unreasonably, fostered to the effect that there is some mysterious therapeutic influence to be found behind your walls and locked doors. We hold the reverse opinion, and think your hospitals are never to be used save as the last resource.

I have found some heads of asylums a trifle shy about discussing the question of the occasional use of mechanical restraint. There lingers a dislike to admit that it should never be used, as, we thank God, some of your best assistants earnestly believe. We think it a question settled past argument. Many years ago while using it I got a lesson never since forgotten. During the war, Drs. Morehouse, Keen and I, had always about eighty to one hundred epileptics in charge, and some insane. We employed at times the camisole, or straps, in protracted convulsions. I tried them once on myself a half-hour for a purpose needless to mention. Before ten minutes had gone I began to have a half frantic

sense of desire to fight for freedom. It was really very hard to conquer. Try it, and you will think long before you add to insanity this temptation to be violent.

We think, also, of your too constantly locked doors and barred windows, as being but reminder relics of that dismal system which we are pleased to think is gone forever. I presume that you have, through habit, lost the sense of jail and jailor which troubles me when I walk behind one of you and he unlocks door after door. Do you think it is not felt by some of your patients?

I know this is a hard question, much discussed. Grated windows and bolted doors may be more or less needed where, as in State asylums, insane hordes are in overcrowded dormitories, and attendants are absurdly few. But elsewhere, these irritating means might be used far less than they are if only you had more and better nurses. Many of you believe that these barriers do no harm; I incline to think you wrong. Here is what an able physician wrote years ago. I once printed his comments in a paper partly fictitious.

He writes: "I then felt what I suppose thousands have felt, the exasperation of these locked doors. Twice as I passed one I furtively tried the latch, and in all my weeks of confinement I never came near such a door without a wild desire to open it. If it were of any use to lock these doors all day, except to save attendants from the need to be watchful, I should not mention the matter, but the precaution is a foolish one, save in rare cases; and if a sane man wants to test his feeling in regard to it, let him get some one to lock him in a room—it may be one he does not care to leave for hours. The effect is strange. He becomes at once uneasy and speculative as to when he will be let out. The idea of loss of freedom annoys him."

It chanced, indeed, to me many years ago to be locked up for half a day in a room. I was at a hotel in New England and broke the key in locking the door. The bell brought no one; the windows looked nowhere on man. It was six hours, or more, before I got out. I think of that when I walk down your grim, conventional wards and see some poor fellow try a door and walk away. I know how he feels.

My asylum should have no exercise yards; no airing courts. More attendants? Yes, and as little as may be of this quasi-prison business. And æsthetically there is something to be said. Into one ward I sometimes see open the rooms of people of almost all social ranks. They meet more or less unrestrainedly in the common hall. Do you think the educated and well bred do not feel this; or, too, the absence of refined table settings, or the dreadful formality of walls and furniture? I have letters which complain of these things. One woman says, "I dare say I was queer enough, but neither my tastes nor my manners were cracked," and then she goes on to criticise with some amusement the table and its furniture.

I took a clever woman through an asylum of late; she had never seen one. She is not a sensational woman—far from it. She said to me, "Oh, I should go mad here if I were not so when I came. Why can't some one move the furniture about and make it look less sepulchral. And those parlors! I should like to be let loose there with a very little money and some women I know, How we would move things about."

I want also to say (and I am all this while speaking only

of hospitals for those who pay), that the monotony of diet, the plain food, is constantly spoken of in the letters I refer to. I suspect that it is too often a just complaint on the part, at least, of people of the refined class. A friend of mine in one of the great asylums wrote, when mending, "I have heard of the horrors of asylums. Let me assure you that although there is much here that is sad, nothing is half so tragic as the diet."

Of the feeling of distrust concerning the therapeutics of asylums now fast gaining ground in the mind of the general public I have said nothing. This lack of medical confidence is of recent growth. Once we spoke of asylums with respect; it is not so now. We, neurologists, think you have fallen behind us, and this opinion is gaining ground outside of our own ranks, and is, in part at least, your own fault. You quietly submit to having hospitals called asylums; you are labelled as medical superintendents, and some of you allow your managers to think you can be farmers, stewards, caterers, treasurers, business managers and physicians. You should urge in every report the stupid folly of this. Knowing what we do of the rate of the growth of medicine, does any man in his senses think that you can be even decently competent and have anything to do with outside business? You may be fair general practitioners in insanity, but productive neurologists of high class regarding disease of the mind organs as but a part of your work? No—I think not. That, you cannot be if you are also in business. It is a grave injustice to insist that you shall conduct a huge boarding house— what has been called a monastery of the mad—and keep yourselves honestly able to move with the growth of medicine, and to study your cases, or add anything of value to our store of knowledge. Some of you have, in a measure, shed this cumbersome coil of unprofessional business, but still declare yourselves overweighted with letters to write, people to see, and so much to do that it is clear either that you do need help and more assistants, or that you are cursed by that slow atrophy of the energizing faculties which is the very malaria of asylum life. Asylum life! There is despair in the name as there is in the idea.

And the title "superintendent." Of what? You have let the word go as concerns this society. Insist to your managers that you are physicians and no more. There may be something to dread in a label.

The many grave questions which remain I can do no more than lightly mention. Some I may but touch and leave as texts for thought. I have notes of six cases dismissed as cured from great endowed hospitals without one written word of warning or direction as to the work, the play, the diet, holidays or future of these people. When you find a case getting well, and let it go home or elsewhere, is it as common as this would seem to make it that you no further concern yourselves with it? I never had much evidence that the reverse is often done, and yet with some of us mere outside practitioners the future of our convalescent, or cured, cases is a matter of the most thoughtful care and of the most anxious solicitude, of long written instructions how to live so as to avoid relapses.

As to work for the chronic and convalescent insane, I never yet saw in America the hospital where all was done that can be done in this direction. These alien people are relatively capable of bribery. Tobacco, later hours, better diet, larger freedom, a little wage, the use or non use of certain privileged rooms, leave among women to wear this or that, putting some who shirk work with others who do work, the influence of example, all these helps may be more ingeniously varied than they are. But as long as you pay common nurses (whom, perhaps, you do well to describe as attendants), untaught and uninterested, to watch hordes of people, or to preside over men and women far better educated than those who watch them you will do little with this essential means,—work. I think there must be no effort to make this work pay. It is education we want. Moreover, if you can make the work interesting and productive, it will be best.

As I want this address to help you and to be read by laymen, I shall ask to have added a newspaper report of that noble object lesson seen at Wernersville, when one hundred and thirty insane were set to work in the open, guarded by no walls, and there did work which would amaze many a so-called superintendent. I wish the account could be scattered wide. It greatly affected me as I read it. I wish, as an object lesson, the good people of this city could have seen this merciful success where the insane were working out of doors. For then I would take them where, in the sadness of our city wards at Blockley, the insane, who have lost even the memory of hope, sit in rows, too dull to know despair, watched by attendants; silent, grewsome machines which eat and sleep, and sleep and eat. Once in the women's wards the bright cap and white aprons of the nurse of the training school were seen. She is there no longer. I should like to know why? It is condemnation enough to say that here are 1,100 insane, and that of these a small percentage are doing any work. This is not the fault of those in charge, or of any but the people of this great city. I dare not revile you for the motes and neglect the beam which makes us seem blind to the sin of this abominable wrong.

There is another function which you totally fail to fulfil, and this is by papers in lay journals to preach down the idea that insanity is always dangerous; to show what may be done in homes, or by boarding out the quiet insane, and to teach the needs of hospitals until you educate a public which never reads your reports, and is absurdly ignorant of what your patients need. Do you not see that what I need for every hospital is a certain noble discontent, a vitalizing headship, which shall be itself scientifically productive, and shall insist on this from the aids? Believe me, the best hospitals of any kind are those where the most precise scientific work is done. There the treatment becomes accurate, the results best. In our city hospitals, the physicians are continually changing service and there is no single head. With you, there is but one head, and this may, if the head possess brains, have the huge advantage that its owner can suggest, direct and encourage research, and by his personal work and enthusiasm keep his whole hospital toned up to the highest intellectual and moral health. It is not a mere well-worked, so-called model, institution which I want to see, where easily pleased managers come and go, and routine is perfect, and every one is satisfied, and the nice little reports describe the amusements, and the new dairy and the statistics are there, and we lament the death of our efficient manager,

Mr. Blank; the whole smug business as monotonously alike as are your asylum corridors.

Where, meanwhile, I repeat, are your careful scientific reports; where, the earnest note of indignant appeal to your boards and to the world without, which should help you and will not? Is this all nonsense? Not so. When you read the appended letters, you will see how constantly these men point out that it is the system which is most to blame, not you alone. My fear is that some of you would not change your organization if you could. My belief is, as to much beside that might be, and is not, that your lives are destructive of energy. You live alone, uncriticised, unquestioned, out of the healthy conflicts and honest rivalries which keep us up to the mark of the fullest possible competence. I hardly blame you. The whole asylum system is, in my opinion, wrong, and has been let to harden into organized shapes which are difficult to reform. How further it should change, I shall presently say; but until we have you all on our side, it will not change. Nor does it surprise me that some many are contented and ask no radical alterations. I think I should in time become but formally dutiful, if I lived all my days in any kind of hospital. When I go into my clinic or wards, I take with me the fresh air of the outer world, and this is what you want. You ought not to live and sleep in your hospitals at all; you ought to be in contact with the world of sane men, having consultations outside, seeing us and our societies. At least you should have in your wards weekly consultations from without. That, I think, would be a good prophylactic against the inertia fed by the amount of hopeless cases which surround you. I cannot see how with the lives you lead, it is possible for you to retain the wholesome balance of the mental and moral faculties.

There should, I think, be in America somewhere one large, perfected hospital for the possibly curable insane, and it should of need, include a home for the education and uplifting of the chronic and hopelessly insane.

Let me conclude with a sketch of my ideal hospital; I seem to see it as I write. It is near to a city and close to a railway. Its grounds, fenced in, not by walls, but by railings, vine covered and hidden by trees and shrubs, are amply acred, and include some forest and wide, cheerful gardens. Without are the farm and vegetable garden. I go in with my patient. We drive through an ample gate, ever wide open and watched. There is no loop-hole for the gate guard to look out of, no mysterious opening of barred doors. We enter an avenue among flowers and trees, out of view of the larger buildings. Shall we drive up to a formal hall and cold doric portico, and be met by a smileless janitor, and then wait in sad expectancy the long delayed coming of the doctor in one of your vast, melancholy, unsympathetic parlors? No. We pause amid thick shrubbery at the side door, which is like that of a private house. In a small room, as pretty as taste can make it, we are received by a well-dressed head nurse, neat in cap and apron—pleasant and kindly she shall be. My patient is then given a room, temporary quarters, in a special reception house, for it is part of my plan that this hospital shall be made up of grouped cottages, each with its family of ten or twelve, or less. In each is a head nurse and attendants. There are no bars, no locked doors. Apart stand smaller homes for those able to pay more. I want to get it as

near to the life of the outer world as I can. At a distance, hidden by trees, is the administration building, vine clad, I trust, and flanked by the wards for those who can pay little or nothing. There are no barred windows, and here are open doors, with attendants ready to say a kindly word to the too restless. I can see you smile. It has been tried, I believe, and has not been found impossible. Connected or not (better apart) are the library, reading rooms, billiard and amusement rooms, and gymnasium. In the grounds are tricycles and bicycles, etc., tennis, and croquet grounds of course. Also, further away, are the work shops, with tools, lathes, all the means needed, and, too, the school rooms, for how do your chronic insane differ from the little defective ones at Elwyn? Yours are, many of them, like these children. I would have the kindergarten methods, and modelling and patterning and embroidery, etc. Let those who will not work watch those who do; use the contagion of example.

My patient is not at once put in charge of a nurse. An assistant, male or female, a physician, is with him for three days or more (one of his own class or above it). He shall study the case, and quietly record its mental peculiarities. As the patient gets used to him, and less suspicious, he goes over him physically with extreme care. Then there is the report with the added statements on his certificate, every detail of life, business, habits. A consultation with the physician in charge follows, and a decision as to the mental, moral and physical needs of the case, and, above all, in every instance, a written schedule as to how it is desirable that the day be spent; all of this the nurse shall read: I mean all of the notes. Is this too much? We closely imitate it in our own hospitals and in our private work. Every week for the acute cases the nurse turns in her written report as part of her work. How far the patient has lived up to the schedule; how far not. It is added to the case, and the cases are kept as indexed cards, not in cumbrous books.

Of treatment I say no word. It would often include much that you do rarely use, and to which I have already alluded. You may have many means and many helps which we cannot employ except for the amply rich. Years ago I tried in vain to talk certain boards into having convalescent seaside homes, not farms near the hospital; I utterly failed. Now, this is coming, but not as yet is the need felt to have those homes where the alterative change of air is complete, as by the sea.

There is a steward for purchases and for care of farmgarden and grounds. The senior physician with no business cares, a trained neurologist, living in the city, spends two-thirds of his day in the hospital: he has only consultations in town. Then there are resident physicians in charge, who shall live in the house. On the female side it is a woman helped by women. After three to five years these aids should be transferred under a new and reasonable state system to another hospital; or, in an endowed hospital, changed yearly from one ward or group of patients to another. Here, alone, is rotation in office valuable. Under the chief are young physicians, internes who serve two years, and both classes compete to win these places, which are paid—as to the younger internes but modestly. One resident is a pathologist. There is a bath master; but in rotation a resident sees and becomes familiar with this service. We have, too, a skilled electrician. The nurses are taught massage, but there is one person who is, as to this, an expert. I would also have on the staff a city oculist and gynæcologist to be used on call, and above all, I would have once a week a long consulting visit from outside neurologists. For this visit the staff should select cases of doubt or difficulty, and this should be a serious and formal matter. The men chosen should be paid, and well paid, for I shall ask from them help in research and in the training of nurses. And as to these latter aids, they should have very little pay the first year, and more and more as they elect to stay upon receiving their diplomas after two years.

Again I wish to emphasize the fact that the nurse is by far the most important part of my organization. How can you hope for the best help from the class we usually see in your wards? I could surprise you a little with the dismay and disgust expressed as to these agents by refined and educated men and women in their letters to me. A few minutes a day make your visits, and the rest of the time, where there is an attendant, is too often spent by your patients in society little above that of the cook or maid.

One wing of my control building shall have a good library of medicine, a laboratory, rooms for pathological research, and also (as we have in the Infirmary here) a room for the study of such phenomena as reflexes, reaction times, with chronographs and the like.

And now, the life, the soul, the driving power, shall be in the physician-in charge. The training schools, the meetings for organizing combined or individual research shall have his eager care. He shall possess the ingenuity to point out paths untrodden by discovery, the energy to lead on these and to put life and vigor and sympathy into all the work. Above all, he must be gentle, refined and courteous and insist that good manners prevail. I have seen in asylum wards, and seen unrebuked, bits of discourtesy to a well-bred gentlewoman for which I would have dismissed a nurse on the spot.

On the rest of this great, and quite possible organization, of the rewards for scientific work, of the extra compensations, or the medals for nurses who show courage or have exceptional success I cannot speak; nor of much else besides.

A good deal of this cannot ever be had in your state hospitals, for incredible folly has put most of them remote from cities. But suppose some great souled man, or some State, decreed such a hospital as I have made a day dream of, would it not become radiant of useful example far and wide? I used to be hopeless that any board would ever rise to an intelligent apprehension of the splendid value of such a scheme. But already at Elwyn certain steps have been taken to secure outside counsel, help, and criticism, and I trust scientific use of the nine hundred defective children. The plan as yet lacks the essential element of pay, but perhaps this will come. Watch it and see how it works. The day dreams of the thoughtful sometimes materialize as practical working things, and the years will surely bring something like, or far better, than what I have sketched. If it will be created by the generosity of a man, or the educated demands of the Commonwealth, I do not know. But it will come.

And now, a word more. I accepted this ungracious post from honest sense of duty. I have said no word of dispraise or critical annoyance that I did not eminently dislike to say. I may be wrong as to some men and to some hospitals. It would be strange if it were not so. But let me add this on parting. One preaches to a congregation. It is impossible to select individuals for blame or praise. Try not to be merely hurt or disgusted by the verdicts of my fellow neurologists and myself. If what we have said causes only bitterness and leaves you in thought, action and purpose where it found you an hour ago, then I have assuredly failed as I do not want to fail and had better never have spoken. If it should happen, please God, that my words bear fruit of good I shall get more happiness out of this occasion than I ever thought could come out of most distasteful task of a varied life. If I have hurt or personally annoyed any man here to-day I am, believe me, sincerely sorry. Perhaps many of you who do not feel vexed may yet rest sure that I am largely wrong in my censure and my theories; but fifty years hence, when we must all have been swept away, another will possibly stand in my place and tell your history, and to him and the bountiful wisdom of time I leave it to be declared whether I was right or wrong.

I have been very long, and you as patient. I thank you.

SOME REMARKS ON THE ADDRESS DELIVERED TO THE AMERICAN MEDICO-PSYCHOLOGICAL ASSOCIATION, BY S. WEIR MITCHELL, M.D., MAY 16, 1894

By Walter Channing, M.D.

Private Hospital for Mental Diseases, Brookline, Massachusetts

Nearly every point taken up by Doctor Mitchell has in some form been discussed by those having the care of the insane, and given rise to very serious consideration. At every stage of progress of the association, there have been anxious and able men in its ranks, alive to the problems and duties of the hour. They have not sat blind-folded, or played puss-in-the-corner, or milked the cows. This is a veritable fact, strange and impossible as it may appear to those ignorant of insane-hospital history. They were given a high trust, which was to take and care for the most unfortunate, weak, miserable, and pitiable class in the community. Neglected and abused even by their own families, the insane had no place to lay their heads, until hospitals, built, organized, and managed by medical men, had arisen.

Fifty years ago, when Ray, Kirkbride, Stribling, Brigham, Earle and the others, formed the Association of Medical Superintendents, it was not a question of knee-jerk, or ankle-clonus, or reaction-time which confronted them, but how to house the then already large numbers of insane, who, as shown by Miss Dix, were suffering the tortures of the damned in alms-houses and in their own homes; and from that day to this the pressure has never relaxed for more accommodations. There are still thousands scattered through the country, kept in the vilest of alms-houses, still suffering tortures. If any one doubt these statements, I will give him proof in this State of Massachusetts. Or let him turn to the history of alms-houses in New York within very recent times.

How best and cheapest to provide for the wants of the insane in State institutions is still the first question, which it is the bounden duty of the association to consider. "How shall we humanely care for those wretched creatures which society tramples on?" Miss Dix asked all those years ago, and the medical superintendents of insane hospitals have been the ones who have courageously and efficiently answered her ever since.

A number of years ago, the writer, fired by youthful enthusiasm, conceived that it would be a noble purpose to enlarge the plan and scope of the association, and with a handful of others endeavored to have its name changed to the present one. It was urged that the time had come to leave building, and to give more time to the discussion of neurological and psychological subjects. The older men dis-

approved of such a change, and Doctor Nichols, a learned as well as a grave and dignified man, got up and said pompously that the superintendents were obliged to build, it was one of the most important things they had to do, and he believed they should come together and talk about the subjects that most interested them. And then the project fell flat.

At the time the writer was disappointed, but since then he has come to see better and better the true object of the association, which is to consider the practical management of insane hospitals and all subjects pertaining thereto. The medical superintendent, whatever he may wish to be, is essentially an executive officer, and if he is deficient in practical ability, though he might write a volume on the cerebral anatomy of a spider, would be of no value whatever. His real specialty is insane-hospital management. From force of circumstances he comes to know the insane as a mother knows her children, and gains a knowledge of them which no one can get who does not live with them. Such knowledge is peculiar and valuable in determining what the acts of the insane may mean, but whether it entitles a medical superintendent to be called a specialist, in a strictly scientific sense, is open to question. No man can do everything, and only in a very few cases are scientific and executive talent combined. Scientific men, put in charge of institutions, are apt to be failures, and the usual medical superintendent has little taste for science and can hardly give a proper medical twang to his annual report if he tries.

But why should he try? Why should not he and his confreres be free to come together and discuss any questions they please? The association is largely made up of able, efficient physicians of business instincts, a combination which makes them appreciate, as no other men ever have or can, the peculiar needs of the insane. They are not neurologists, or psychologists, and should not set out to be. Their work is one of the broadest humanity; namely, that of giving rest and succor to as many of a wretched and neglected class as a niggardly and ignorant public will allow, and their work will never be done until ever insane pauper is the ward of the State. Let them never be frightened, or deterred, or turned aside from this high purpose, however much they may be misunderstood by their well-wishers.

From his observation of insane hospital management, it

is the writer's opinion that the chief medical officer must always have charge of all departments of administration. Other systems have been tried, but they have not been an unqualified success, for the instant a layman takes his (the medical officer's) place, the patient loses his identity as such. He becomes one of a large number to be clothed and fed for as little as possible. The humane and sentimental relation existing between physicians and patient gradually becomes dimmed, and finally lost altogether. There is something in the training of the medical man which makes him a little different from what he would otherwise be, for he is more gentle, tolerant, patient, appreciative, and sympathetic in dealing with poor human nature. Call the medical superintendent "farmer," "steward," "caterer," "treasurer," or whatsoever name we choose, there still beats within his breast a heart not dead to the cry of suffering and distress.

So much then experience seems to prove; we must have a medical man to administer the hospital in all its branches. Can he do much more than this? Let us imagine putting a neurologist of reputation at the head of an existing hospital. Is he to carry it on in the interest of humanity or science first? He will answer that the two can be combined; he will have a business manager, and give up his time to purely medical work. Where will he get his business manager, and if he does get him, how will he know he is doing his duty both by the State and its wards? He must admit every patient he can, for their number is legion, and he must usually spend only a definite sum fixed by law. Where has he got his experience to guide him in these vital matters, for on their settlement his ultimate success must depend. The first requisite must be the mastery of all the details appertaining to these things, and this requires not laboratory or bed-side experiment, but study of every department. He need not say he keeps a boarding-house, but if he is faithful to his trust, on him rests the final responsibility for seeing that his charges are fed in the best possible way, at the least cost. Will he relegate the authority to the steward, saying he is too busy with tests of reaction-time in dementia, then when complaints begin to assert themselves, he will find he is no longer the head, but one of two, and his house will soon be divided against itself, with the usual result. He may make wonderful experiments, and have rare skill with electricity, and know something of massage, but once let the bread be sour, the sheets dirty, and the sewerage defective, and all his knowledge will not avail him. One thing is lacking, and that is executive capacity; he commands a ship which he does not know how to steer, and the sooner some one takes his place the better.

It is in the writer's opinion, as a rule, useless to expect that neurologists will make successful executive officers of insane hospitals, or that these executive officers will make successful neurologists, for each is working in a different field. Neither does he believe that even brilliant original work is any criterion whatever of efficient and thorough insane hospital work. On the contrary, with such contracted staffs of medical officers, as our hospitals usually possess, it might mean that the patients were being actually neglected. The point to consider is always, Are these unfortunates being considerately and properly cared for as individuals? And until this question can be answered in the affirmative, without hesitation, the original work must wait. Sometimes the writer has read reports of such work done, perhaps in an institution with nine hundred inmates, by one of the two assistant physicians. He could hardly understand how such elaborate investigations could be undertaken without infringing on the time belonging to those four hundred and fifty individuals under his care, and instead of judging of his capacity for the duties of his position by his published writings, he would have looked into the actual condition of those patients.

The attempt has been made to turn out original work in various insane hospitals in this country, but so far with very doubtful success. One striking example of such an attempt was that made at the State Insane Hospital at Utica early in the seventies. A skilled pathologist was employed, and he was fitted out with the best of apparatus at a large expense, and stimulated to do the best he knew how, and his results were widely published. But there was no lasting or even temporary effect. The whole thing was felt to be forced—a flash in the pan—and it gradually died of inanition. Such is one illustration of trying to introduce scientific research into hospital work. There have been others less mechanical, but have they had any far-reaching influence on the conduct of the institution? Supposing it be assumed that the Blockly Alms-house, which was a disgrace to civilization fifteen years ago, and is now again apparently, from what Doctor Mitchell says, should have a staff of three or four medical officers appointed to take charge of the 1,100 insane patients, and they should have a finely equipped "neuro-psycho-physiological laboratory" (let us call it) fitted up, and be set to work on lines of original investigation. If they actually take charge of the patients they must see them at least once daily, and many twice; and if the alms-house has ceased to be a disgrace, which we will pray for at no distant day, they must know that every one has a good, clean bed to sleep in; good, nourishing food to eat; clean clothing to wear; a neat place to stay in day and night; good ventilation and temperature in-doors, and fresh air and occupation. Medicine, electricity, massage, and bathing can be utilized, either before or after these things, according to one's scientific point of view. Notes must be made, of course, of many cases, and records written, and anxious friends informed by word of mouth or letter of the patient's progress.

When then, under these conditions, is the laboratory work to be done? "But they do it abroad," might be answered. "Well, then" we reply, "they must give their patients less individual attention than we are in the habit of giving them here, for if they actually attend to their medical duties, their time will be fully occupied." "But why should there not be internes to do the routine work?" might be the next question. At Blockly, of course, situated as it is, in a city, internes might be available, but most institutions are too remote from medical schools to be able to secure internes. Furthermore, a large part of the regular medical work must be done by the regular medical officers, if it is to be reliably and satisfactorily done for the public good. They may be supplemented by students, but can not relegate to them their responsibilities.

And here, perhaps, will be the place to consider the subject of visiting staffs for insane hospitals. One fatal objection to such a plan is the remoteness, just spoken of, from medical schools or large medical centers. No staff could be secured to spend several hours daily in a visit to distant points; so this plan would not work for most of the hospitals. For those easy of access, it would be an interesting and desirable experiment on many accounts. Expert neurologists and psychologists might compose the staff, and they could institute and carry forward investigations and experiments in the hospital laboratory, drawing, of course, their material from among the patients. The resident medical officers could continue to take the actual care of the inmates as before. The visiting staff would learn a good deal about insanity, and the resident staff would get an inkling of neurology and psychiatry, and thus the good of all would be advanced. Before the experiment failed, as it inevitably would after a while, the writer fears, two points would be brought out with convincing clearness. First, it would be found that the inmates of an insane hospital are largely under treatment because society can not care for them. The chief medical officer is their guardian, and they are his helpless children, not only to have their bodily ills relieved, but to be watched over and protected. The custodial care is quite unlike that pertaining to any other class of the community, and is both delicate and exacting. It requires great tact and discretion, and is a responsibility of no mean proportions to the conscientious physician. Second, it would be found that the therapeutics of neurology are not after all a novelty in well-managed hospitals, even to the point of the animal extracts. We have recently been told that these therapeutics are not efficacious in all cases in their own field, and they present the same short-comings in the insane hospital. The fact is that, while there have been splendid advances in the anatomy and physiology of nervous diseases, their treatment and cure is both unsatisfactory and baffling. It is highly probable that the day will come when simple suggestion will accomplish quite as much, if not more, in the cure of these diseases, than anything that is now done. Both hypnotism and mental healing promise to put regular therapeutics to the blush, if present indications can be relied on.

Doctor Mitchell conjures up, as many a hospital superintendent has done, a pleasing vision of an ideal hospital. He would have a cheerful entrance, with a broad, open gate (such as most hospitals now actually have), and he lingers upon the picture of a "well-dressed head nurse, neat in cap and apron," receiving the patient and himself in a small room. He loves, as we all do, this ideal, well-dressed head nurse. What a multitude of sins a cap and apron cover nowadays in a nurse! How many the writer has known of who were hard, cold, and unsympathetic, and totally unfitted for their calling, though trained in the best hospitals and wearing the whitest of caps and broadest of aprons! At times he has longed for the dowdy old woman in her black alpaca, with no cap, and little apron, a born nurse from her youth up, with tact, sympathy, and love in her heart! There are too many trained nurses, following the profession simply as a money-grubbing business, and deficient in all the qualities which make the true nurse. Some day there may be an examination of the heart as well as the head.

In going on to describe the general plan of his "ideal hospital," Doctor Mitchell speaks of cottages for ten, or twelve, and smaller homes for those able to pay more, and then wards near the administration building for those able to pay little or nothing. Of course such a plan as this is applicable to a well endowed incorporated hospital like Bloomingdale, or the Butler Hospital, but these are exceptional institutions, providing for a very small percentage of the insane, the immense bulk of whom go to the public hospitals. In the writer's opinion three grades of hospitals are to be considered, which are: Those providing for the pauper insane, or the public hospitals; those providing for the impoverished, middle, and upper classes, or the incorporated hospitals, and those providing for the affluent middle and upper classes, or the small hospitals, now private, but later perhaps in some instance to become incorporated. The system of classification of course varies in the different States, many of those belonging to the second class going to the public hospitals, and many of the affluent going to the incorporated institutions, but fundamentally the principle appears to be a correct one. It may at once be said it does not generally prevail at present, for the incorporated hospitals receive a large proportion of the affluent class, and the private hospitals make a very small showing as to numbers. The writer does not contest this point, he would only take the ground that incorporated hospitals of large size, meaning by that, those that accommodate more than fifty, should be essentially for the indigent members of the upper and middle classes. They certainly are founded on a philanthropic basis, and fail in accomplishing their highest purpose, if they are built and organized on a plan suited to the rich few, instead of the indigent many. Their motto should be the greatest good to the greatest number, and not a moderate amount of good to a moderate number. If this principle were rigidly adhered to, it is probable their per capita cost would be decreased, their accommodations extended, and many of the worthy, but poor upper and middle classes saved from association with the pauper insane in the public hospitals.

The demand for private institutions has steadily and rapidly increased during the last fifteen years, and they may now be said to be on trial in this country. No doubt the demand has in part risen from a desire to save the patient from going to a formal institution, and give him the advantage of "home treatment" in a modified form away from his home. To fulfill their purpose, they must be small, yet large enough to obtain the services of physicians of skill and experience. Ten is probably too small a number and fifty too large. The mean should fall between these limits. They should have the most diversified and plastic organization, with single houses for single patients, or houses for several, and every detail arranged for the comfort, convenience, and individualizing of the patient. Whether this class of institutions will continue to be, in the future, of a private character, is a matter which time will settle. If they are thoroughly and frequently inspected by a board of supervision, there need be no doubt that they are as well managed, as such facilities as they possess will allow, and just here a difficult question presents itself which can only be alluded to. Even a small number of patients require large grounds, good buildings, the best of food, skilled medical service, and nursing, and appliances for gymnastics, driving, diversified occupation, and amusement. To furnish these things properly requires a considerable amount of capital, and where is it to come from? The public are attracted by the idea of sending an insane person into a doctor's family to be treated, but if the doctor is an unsuccessful, shiftless, and unskilled member of the profession, he is hardly a desirable person to assume such responsibility. It is no doubt right that doctors should be allowed to take single patients into their families as boarders rather than patients, provided they are looked after by a competent authority, but when any one starts a private hospital, it should have certain definite and prescribed facilities, if it is to do justice to the patient and the public, and as has already been said, the cost is so large that few single individuals can furnish the requisite capital. As time goes on the requirements for obtaining licenses will be more and more rigid, and more of the small hospitals will be incorporated than at present.

In Doctor Mitchell's ideal hospital, as already mentioned, the administration building is to be flanked by the wards for those who pay little or nothing. Such an arrangement as this is a good illustration of a mistaken way of classifying patients in a hospital on a financial basis, instead of on the basis of disease. It would be a serious injustice to bring all kinds of patients, acute and chronic, noisy, quiet, or convalescent, together in a few wards, simply because they were poor. The superintendent's ideal plan is much better. There are very few of such wards, which are used for the more acute cases that properly can be classified together. Patients are retained in them (they often are called "infirmary wards"), only until they can be transferred to cottages, where they will come in contact with others in a similar condition of illness. Even in existing hospitals patients are necessarily, in severe cases, classified only on the basis of disease. In the ideal hospital there should be financial equality, so that it may live up to its highest function, which is to cure disease.

Doctor Mitchell's patient is not at once put in charge of a nurse. "An assistant male or female, a physician, is with him for three days or more (one of his class, or above it)." To carry out such a plan as this would require not only an ideal hospital, but also an ideal bank account. As the ideal we are considering is either a State or incorporated hospital, we must imagine from one to several patients being admitted daily; let us assume there is an average of two. These would require the constant services of six physicians. Unless we are to idealize the patients as well as the hospital, we should have a large majority of paupers, many of foreign birth or parentage, speaking only a foreign tongue; a large percentage of all would be chronic cases, already residents of other hospitals. Some would be quiet and depressed, others violent and homicidal. Many would refuse to utter a word, and others would rapidly develop delusions, if closely observed. In some a physical examination would lead to violence, and it might take weeks to bring it about. The very fact that the patient felt himself under the espionage of this superior being, would tend to develop suspicions and foster those already existing. The insane person, even when quite sick, still has a personality which is his own property,

and which he guards with a degree of his ordinary care and prudence, and he will not part with it, even if cajoled by the softest-tongued young or old doctor now in existence. It is reckoning somewhat without one's host, when one expects to get very far with a newly admitted patient, by putting him in the society of a physician for three days. A normal individual would divulge little under such circumstances, and an insane person might be quite as difficult a subject. Provided there were enough assistants willing, to undertake what would essentially be nurses' duties, and an institution rich enough to employ so many, it is probable that, with few exceptions, little would be gained over what could be accomplished by shorter periods of association. The writer naturally believes that medical records should be thorough and accurate, but also believes they can be made so without a prolonged period of forced association.

The ideal hospital, Doctor Mitchell says, should have (as most do) a steward for making purchases, a senior physician, a trained neurologist, passing two-thirds of his time in the hospital (which would generally be impossible on account of distance, as we have shown above), resident physicians in charge, paid internes, a pathologist, a bathmaster, a skilled electrician, an expert masseur, city oculists, gynæcologists, consulting neurologists, all well paid, used on the scale suggested. It is doubtful when so much expense can be incurred in one institution, but let it not be forgotten some of these officials already exist in insane hospitals. The bath-master is an unknown factor, and if he uses water as severely as it seems to be used abroad, it is to be hoped he will not make his advent for some time. Nevertheless in our insane hospitals, as in our general hospitals, we utilize water far too little, and we deserve to be criticised for not using it more.

There are various problems which Doctor Mitchell mentions or discusses, such as bolts and bars, mechanical restraint, open doors, etc., which have over and over again been considered by hospital medical officers, and they have come to wise conclusions, which are pretty generally acted upon. Mechanical restraint is reduced to a minimum in the best hospitals. Its total abolishment is not a justifiable procedure, and should the writer be told that in a large hospital it was never used, he would shrug his shoulders, and say to himself, "that is not the truth; in some way, some kind of restraint is used, however much it is denied." It is much more manly to assert that there are cases where it should and must be used, and such is the attitude of many of the best of American as well as English superintendents. They refuse to deny plain facts, in order to make a good showing. Anything is better than the horrible encounters which occur between patients and nurses employing so-called "manual restraint." Both may be injured bodily by such collisions, and patients are often made more irritable and violent, and nurses more brutal, and the harmony and good-feeling which should exist between them is destroyed for all time.

No doubt it is a painful thing for a well, rational person to have restraint placed upon him, but the wildly excited insane are not well and rational, and it is hardly fair to compare them together. The form of restraint makes a very great difference, and only certain kinds should be allowed. That restraint is not always repugnant to insane persons can be testified to by almost any hospital superintendent who probably has had patients come to him and ask to have it applied when feeling the premonitions of excitement. One patient of the writer's, who lived at home, and went about in society, occasionally had attacks of paroxysmal excitement and violence. At such times he would get his restraining apparatus himself, take it to his wife and beg her to put it on him. To him it not only possessed no terrors, but was a positive blessing, and not one in disguise by any means.

Of bolts and bars it may be said they grow less and less conspicuous in each new hospital, but in large institutions patients must in some way be securely kept, or the public would be up in arms immediately. Open doors are also admirable, and they also are increasing, but the increased watching they entail is often a source of extreme annoyance and irritation to the patient. One of the questions which occasions the conscientious superintendent the most solicitude is that of the personal liberty of his patients. He wishes to restrain them as little as possible, and with the least fric-

tion, and he has learned to open the doors, and leave off the bars in as far as he can do so with the best practical results. Give him buildings varied enough to properly classify his patients, and more doors will open at once.

There are other points considered by Doctor Mitchell, which the limits of this paper render it impossible to discuss. The attempt has been made to say something for the association by one who belongs to it, yet is hardly of it. This peculiar position allows him to understand and recognize the spirit of the work of its members and appreciate their virtues, while not blinding him on the other hand to their short-comings, which do not seem to him very glaring, and largely grow out of the peculiar relations which they bear to the public. The standard of hospital care set by the foremost members is a high one, perhaps quite as high, when looked at from all points, as that of Doctor Mitchell, and in the end will accomplish even greater results, because it has grown out of a practical acquaintance with the insane, covering, one might say, the last hundred years.

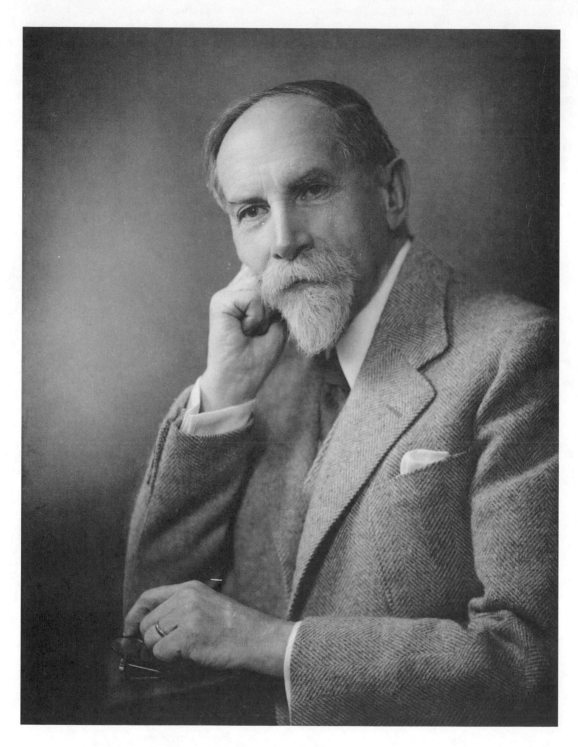

Adolf Meyer, M.D., 1866–1950

A Short Sketch of the Problems of Psychiatry

By Adolf Meyer, M.D.

*Assistant Physician to the Worcester Lunatic Hospital
and Docent of Psychiatry at Clark University, Worcester, Massachusetts*

Owing to the marvelous change of thought in this century we have learned that man is not so different from the rest of creation as was formerly thought. We are subject to the same laws of the universe with all other creatures. We are the outcome of a slow, gradual development of the living world, different from the rest in degree only. We all grow from fertilized egg-cells. Division of cell after cell takes place, and differentiation of cells; the egg, as it lives and grows to be a foetus, grows to be a moving, active being; action becomes more and more differentiated, in a measure, as the body differentiates itself, and we say that we recognize in the foetus and in the child a body and its function, the objects of anatomy and physiology. The infant goes on growing, and with the development of the brain gives evidence of what we call sentient or conscious life, a feature common to all higher animals at least, expressed in various motions and actions, and in man, more especially in his language, the most differentiated movements of expression. Thus we have three fields of observation in the higher animals—anatomy, physiology, and psychology; they study the respective sides of what developed from the one fertilized egg-cell, and with all that, there is nowhere a gap through which we might say life crept into the cell and, just as little, a gap through which mind might have crept in.[1] As I say, this holds for all higher animals, but owing to the slow and highly differentiated development of our brain, we reach a degree which makes us eminently gifted with the ability of seeing behind us a past to learn from, and before us stages of higher development, and, owing to this ability, we are under the moral obligation to aspire to an ideal more than any other living creature. All this develops from the fertilized ovum of a mother. The body and its mechanical and chemical functions, and the mental life associated with it, make out the biological unit, the person, as we would say in the case of a man. In this unit the development of the mind goes hand in hand with the anatomical and physiological development, not merely in a parallelism, but as a oneness with several aspects.

To make myself understood by a simile from inorganic nature (which has for centuries been able to get along without mystic spirits), I would refer you to a red-hot iron. That the iron is the same iron, whether it is hot or cold, gray, red, or white, nobody would doubt. But it undergoes changes by absorbing heat. It becomes hot—we feel this by the sense of temperature; it changes its color—we see this with our eyes; it becomes larger—we appreciate that with considerations on the ground of the sense of space. We know that the iron is one, but our senses are so organized that we recognize several aspects in the one iron; the heat is to be studied with the methods of the theory of heat, the color with the methods of optics, the expansion with the methods of measurement of space, and yet we never think a moment that anything but one iron is before us. In an analogous and more complicated way we see in the living person the body with its mechanical and chemical functions, and further, the mental aspect, and this one person is to be studied with methods of anatomy, physiology, and psychology.

The fundamental principle on which the psychiatry of to-day is built is undoubtedly this biological conception of man. From the purely materialistic conception of the middle of this century this biological view has developed which does better justice to our entire experience, not solving the ultimate problems, to be sure, but furnishing a rational working basis.

This genetic view of man is altogether borne out by the reverse process, the destruction. The clinical and pathological studies have furnished satisfactory evidence to the effect that the brain is the "bearer of mental activity," and that destruction of certain parts of the brain is identical with destruction of certain mental functions, or even more or less extended domains of mental life.

We must, on the ground of our present knowlege of physiology and of psychology, accept the statement that all mental activity must have its physiological side and its anatomical substratum in the forms of nervous mechanisms, combinations of cells, especially of the cerebral cortex. A disease of these cells and their processes means at the same time a *physiological* and a *psychological* disorder; destruction of these cells a destruction of *physiological* and *psychological*

Read before the Worcester District Medical Society, March 10, 1897.

1 This implies that the fertilized egg-cell as long as it lives is not purely "matter" but includes the elements of vital processes and among them of the physical processes, whatever they may be. What we see as "matter" is not more real than what we recognize as its physiological and psychical life. Materialism claims that we know matter to be the only real thing and everything else as an attribute of it. This view seems untenable; it is an undue exaggeration of the importance of our tactile senses which forces us unnecessarily into dualistic difficulties.

"function." Further, we can not conceive a disorder of the mind without a disorder of function of those cell mechanisms which embody that part of the mind.

This is, in a few words, the working hypothesis on which we approach the review of the problems of psychiatry today. I admit at the outset that the evidence for this view is far from being exhaustively worked out. The opportunities for detailed study are not very abundant. Especially in the hospitals for the insane satisfactory cases are rare. The best studies come from a few German clinics of psychiatry which are allowed to admit nervous cases as well as the insane, and from a few general hospitals of all countries where specialists get an opportunity to study patients with brain lesions, aphasia, etc. The only chance for such study is offered by defects of brain through traumatism or disease in *well educated*, intelligent patients, and these are just the cases which hardly ever reach the general hospital or the hospital for the insane, at least not often, at a time when they have the intellect necessary for these very difficult studies. Neurologists certainly describe the paralyses and various forms of aphasia, but usually not from a psychological point of view; just as if the mind were really something apart from the field of medicine, and not what we stated above, the only direct vital manifestation we get of the working of certain brain mechanisms. Brain lesions must be studied neurologically and psychologically; to study them one must know the problems of both neurology and psychology.

All life is reaction, either to stimuli of the outside world or of the various parts of the organism. We recognize death by the absolute absence of these reactions. In our mental life these reactions are pictured as if in a mirror. But not every reaction appears in this mirror, i.e., becomes conscious. Most of the reactions during sleep, all during epileptic fits, during syncope, remain unconscious, i.e., we do not remember having been aware of them and do not give any evidence of consciousness at the time. In our daily life, in walking and working, we heed many things without thinking of them. Further, many reactions take place in our mind which are not expressed. They take the form of "simple" thought. They seem, indeed, purely mental, and create the appearance on which the idea of mind independent from the body is built. Will this shake our biological conception? Hardly. We do not see direct evidences of the process of digestion, of action of sensory nerves, not even of the flowing of the blood on hasty examination. On the other hand the work of Mosso and others have shown us that accurate methods of observing changes of blood pressure, variation of the pupils, of respiration, in the rhythm of the heartbeat, give us physiological evidence of reactions which were formerly believed to be purely psychical. One might ask further, how it is that there are so many physiological reactions of which we are not conscious? Would not this rather speak for the independence of the mind? We find in normal man that a stimulus, in order to be noticed, must produce a sufficient change in the equilibrium to become conscious at all. Not all reactions become conscious, but largely those which mean a change in the relations between the whole individual and the outside world. In other words, the circle of consciousness is limited largely to those reactions which we say make up the personality.

In this lies the essence of the possibility of concentration of thought and reactions generally in the so-called mental realm. The greater part of our nervous system works automatically. Those nerve-cell mechanisms, however, which represent reactions of the individual as a whole, that is the personality, have a physiological and a psychological aspect. The extensive development of just these mechanisms subserving the personality is characteristic to man as compared to animals. I need hardly point out that what we say of mind has absolutely nothing to do with soul; soul is a concept which can not be an object of biology. If we give the concept "soul" a proper definition, the idea of its persistence and immortality meets absolutely no objection in biology; but our principles of biology say that a persistence of the *biological* phenomena "mind" is inconceivable without the coexistence and persistence of the living body.

With this we imply also that all mental reaction is one aspect of a process which must have its physiological aspect; and we must further claim that a purely psychical disorder, commonly called functional, is just as well a disorder of the life of the brain as any organic lesion; and although we have not learned yet to see the changes in the cells and their processes we must admit that a functional disorder can be just as serious, and is as actual, as an "organic" one.

The biological working hypothesis forces us at once to recognize a fact very important in the method of study of psychiatry. As long as the view of an independence of mind and body could be maintained, the alienist was allowed to work largely in the field of mental symptoms, with little care about the physiological or, rather, pathological condition of the physical side. These were the days when the professor of philosophy felt himself called upon to write on the diseases of the mind in preference to the physician, and when in a text-book on mental diseases you could hardly find the body mentioned. As a contrast the so-called somatic school was formed by physicians, and it lived in the form of materialism through the greater part of this century. We know now that we must attack the problem from the biological side, from the point of view of *mental* pathology and of *physiological* pathology; further, that we must not attack the two at points which are farthest apart, but where they touch each other most closely. Such complex mental phenomena as delusions and hallucinations are surely of practical importance, but not open to accurate methods, while the elementary psychical reactions, as voluntary movements, perception, choice of movements, and, within the range of ideation, the associations are accessible; we can study just in what way these elementary reactions are changed, whether they take place at all, or slowly or rapidly, with early signs of fatigue and exhaustion or long perseverance, normally or with certain characteristic modification, etc. On the physiological side we can test the simplest reactions, of the vasomotor and motor apparatus, up to the complex questions of nutrition and chemistry of metabolism. The working hypothesis is, however, not only essential in these lines which many of you would probably be little interested in, as too theoretical and remote from practice. I wish to make an attempt to show you how the general principle can be profitably carried into the heart of the practice.

We shall not speak of the pathology of complex special symptoms, such as delusions and hallucinations, but direct our attention to the principles according to which we make our specific groups of cases as representatives of specific pathological entities of abnormality.

The most common mental disorders are those of intoxication and fever delirium. In these we see plainly that the mental disease is purely symptomatic, so much so that fever delirium and acute intoxication, with alcohol or other poisons, is not usually looked upon as a mental disease. We look quite correctly on the cause of the fever and on the process of poisoning as the principal pathological feature. The same probably holds for a great number of mental diseases.

Just alcohol or the typhoid toxins show us how widely the symptoms of the mental disorder may vary with the same pathological process. An acute alcoholic intoxication acts quite differently on different men. The one becomes vivid, boisterous, jolly, exalted, with a feeling of huge mental and physical strength, even when the motor paralysis has set in; with this more or less irritability of character may crop out. Another person becomes rapidly stupid, dull, or depressed and emotional.

If the alcoholic intoxication is associated with gastritis and a changed metabolism acts on the weakened brain, besides the alcohol itself, we meet with a different picture—delirium tremens—usually with fear, excitement, and a great number of hallucinations; the feeling of being persecuted and in danger gradually vanishes with the attack. In a third form the change comes more slowly; during the slow deterioration of the brain, and under the demoralizing influence of the drinker's surroundings, a deep change of character takes place; the slow vitiation of the views of the drinker leads to a more orderly and better assimilated system of delusions of persecution (usually with hallucinations), and to a change of the personality. Even when the mind seems well rested and sober, the delusions of jealousy and persecution persist. They are not a simple toxic delirium, but a slowly acquired conviction.

Another instance of how the mental symptoms are largely symptomatic, and not the principal factor to go by in the consideration of insanity, is general paralysis. The etiology is so clearly worked out that it is difficult to-day to believe that it occurs on any other but a syphilitic basis. The work of Hirschl, Fournier, and others justifies us in defining it as a deterioration of the brain and mind under the influence of the change of metabolism, brought about by a syphilitic infection associated with excesses of any kind.

The common features are the progressive dementia, occurrence of motor symptoms, and the almost inevitably fatal termination. The ordinary mental symptoms, such as delusions of wealth, exaltation, are by no means essential, because they may be absent; hallucinations, which undoubtedly may occur, are certainly rare; sometimes the picture may be that of melancholia, sometimes of the old "mania of persecution," but whatever the special mental form be, on superficial inspection, the disease and its termination remains typical.

Considerations of this character show us that not so much a depression, or an exaltation, or delusion, or hallucination, make up the disease as a clinical entity, but that the whole course and the fundamental disorder underlying the mental manifestations decide the diagnosis, and with it the prognosis.

That mental symptom complex which we call hallucinatory confusion may occur in a fever delirium, in delirium tremens, and in almost any form of the so-called acute insanities. In itself it does not constitute a diagnosis; also what we call "mania" makes no diagnosis; it occurs in alcohol intoxication, in general paralysis, in the so-called simple psychoses. These symptomatic diagnoses are worth as much as a diagnosis of brain fever or lung fever, or cough, or albuminuria. If a diagnosis shall be more than a name, shall give an idea of the real condition and its probable course, we must resort to the general pathology of the organs affected, including symptomatology, but building it on rational principles.

We have seen that integrity of mental life presupposes integrity of the nervous system, at any rate of certain cell mechanisms of the forebrain. Mental pathology must, therefore, in order to be true, coincide in its broad frame with the pathology of these nervous mechanisms; there is one cause, a parallel evolution of the symptoms, and in the main one termination, or else we are not dealing with one disease.

We ask, therefore: What is the general pathology of the nervous system and what is the general pathology of the mental sphere? How far can we recognize the oneness, and where and why does uncertainty begin in the forms in which we are ignorant of the congruity?

From the time of the first evidence of the mental life in the child up to the time of death the nervous system goes through many phases of development and retrogression which we can not follow here in detail, each of which has its special weaknesses. You know that osteomyelitis occurs largely in the bones of a growing child and far less frequently in the adult; or that tuberculosis invades oftenest the glands, the bones and the meninges in children, the lungs oftener in the adult, or the chlorosis manifests itself largely in girls at puberty. In a similar way we recognize that certain pathological processes find different conditions in the brain.

In a general way the nervous system of a normal person may undergo the following disturbing influences at any age:

A. The nervous system as a whole.

1. Defective nutrition; the reception of an insufficient quantity of assimilated food into the circulation. This affects the brain little when it is at rest, but makes function dangerous.

2. Intoxications—by poisons introduced with the food or otherwise, or produced in the body, or by retention of waste products. Albu speaks of:

1) Auto-intoxications from the suppression or disturbance of the functions of an organ.

2) Auto-intoxications which occur from anomalies in general metabolism without any definite localization.

3) Auto-intoxications which are caused by the retention of the physiological products of metabolism in the different organs.

4) Auto-intoxication due to the overproduction of physiological and pathological products of the organism.

Between 3 and 4:

1. Auto-intoxications from the skin.
2. " " lungs.
3. " " kidneys.
4. " " supra-renals.
5. " " gastro-intestinal tract.
6. " " liver.
7. " " pancreas.
8. " " thyroid gland.

3. Insufficient, excessive, or abnormal function or practice (education), a very complex but most important element in the so-called constitutional derangements, such as constitutional overexcitability, leading to a morbid reaction, to quantitatively and qualitatively abnormal conditions.

B. More locally the following disturbances may come up:

1. Defective nutrition merely of a part may be due to a local disorder of circulation, such as occlusion of a blood-vessel by embolus or thrombosis, or by defective drainage of the venous blood and the lymph on account of pressure on veins and lymph canals, or of abnormal influences of gravity (stasis) when the circulation generally is weak. The result of local disorders of nutrition is a reaction which ranges between lack of the ordinary repair during rest, fatty degeneration of part of the elements, and, where nutrition is too much diminished, necrosis and decay of the essential tissues.

2. Local intoxications, including "inflammation," are usually of parasitic origin, and this implies that physical disorders are created beside the chemical intoxication—abscess formation, meningitis, etc. Moreover, we again mention here those general intoxications which affect just certain mechanisms of the nervous system, as anterior poliomyelitis, locomotor ataxia, general paralysis, etc.

3. Traumatic disorders, such as an actual cut or bruise, or bursting of a blood vessel, consist partly in the direct destruction of a number of nerve elements, partly in the interference with circulation, by tear of, or pressure upon, blood vessels. The result is paralysis of the destroyed and disturbed parts, and irritation or mere unbalancing of the remaining mechanisms. To some extent we are justified in putting here the formation of tumors, inasmuch as they act like traumatisms.

4. Overactivity of limited mechanisms is a further element. The cell elements will undergo the changes of fatigue to such an extent that recovery can only be obtained by prolonged rest. Writer's cramp might be taken as a type. Overactivity finds its cure in exhaustion and rest. It becomes serious through combination with defective nutrition, and especially with intoxications.

5. Finally, I mention as very important in our narrower field of psychiatry the perverted function, as perverted practice, imitation, and growth in abnormal directions. The most characteristic instance is the development of dominant ideas in cranks and in paranoia, a chronic phenomenon, and acute forms largely in the field of emotion, as the epidemics of religious mania so-called, hysterical outbreaks, epidemic chorea.

All these influences may work on the perfect "Anlage." In many cases, however, a number of data, which we call collectively hereditary predisposition, are to be held responsible for the readiness with which abnormalities are acquired. That certain forms of disease practically occur only on such a basis is a fairly well established fact. We must say, though, that a statement that heredity is present is by no means a pathological explanation. If we want to make any progress we must try to find out why heredity shows itself in some and not in other cases, and whether it is really necessary to consider heredity with the customary fatalism. There is another factor besides "heredity" which may modify the anlage so as to change the general constitution. This is the influence and residuals of previous diseases during foetal life, or childhood, or later. On careful study, many of the cases of "heredity" will perhaps be shown to have been under the influence of one or more of the above pathological factors during the years of growth.

Owing to the work of Dr. Cowles and of a number of European writers, the factor played by intoxications and auto-intoxication has more especially received attention. Lately Van Gieson has contributed a very noteworthy program of the work in this direction. But every one of the factors enumerated above must receive attention if we wish to remain in touch with the facts. The facts are furnished by clinical study, and clinical study must be the basis of all rational pathology. Post-mortem studies are certainly valuable; it seems, however that general pathology is about to grow out of the heaps of material gathered by pathological anatomy to its due position, slowly laying the foundation to all clinical study.

Time does not permit to enter upon the minute anatomical changes caused by all the causes mentioned, nor can we analyze here the data obtained by the psychological studies of Kraepelin and his pupils and others. I use the rest of the space allowed to show what prospects Kraepelin gives us in his excellent work concerning clinical psychiatry.

Kraepelin differs from all our American and English writers by insisting strongly enough on the fallacies in classifying the patients purely according to their mental symptoms. Not the mental symptom constitutes the disease, but the general pathological evolution of the symptoms, physical and mental. His principal division is into: *acquired psychoses* and *psychoses on the ground of a morbid disposition*; in other words, mental diseases for which we have a satisfactory cause, and a general pathological evolution, traceable to influences from the outside world (intoxications, infections), or to some definite abnormal condition of the organism—exhaustion, diseases of various organs, etc.; and mental diseases for which such a definite causation is not obvious, which are more properly constitutional.

Among the acquired psychoses we find—

I. Conditions of exhaustion. Usually characterized by a very acute or subacute delirium, or complete confusion (amentia), with a remarkable difficulty in understanding what is going on (disorder of apperception); certain forms of "puerperal" insanity belong to this group. Or a certain number of cases offer the symptom complex of so-called nervous prostration.

II. The conditions of intoxication as you meet them in

febrile delirium and infectious delirium generally, and also in the acute and chronic intoxications—alcoholism, morphinism, cocainism. To this group I would add the delirium accompanying multiple neuritis.

III. The third group embraces the disorders of metabolism, such as cretinism and myxoedema, which are a secondary consequence of disease of the thyroid gland; further, general paralysis, which must be traced to a previous syphilitic infection in the great majority, if not all, of the cases. And, finally, Kraepelin groups together those forms of acute psychoses which terminate almost invariably in so-called secondary dementia, as processes of mental deterioration, perhaps in connection with abnormalities in the sexual life. The chief types of this are dementia praecox, hebephrenia and katatonia, forms of insanity which are thrown together with mania and melancholia by most alienists, but are characterized from the start by signs of mental deterioration and fairly characteristic mental and physical symptoms.

IV. The fourth group consists in the case of psychoses accompanying gross lesions of the brain.

V. The last group of the acquired psychoses embraces the melancholia of the period of involution, and senile dementia.

The mental disorders on ground of a morbid constitution include imbecility and idiocy, psychopathic inferiority (constitutional depression and irritability, imperative concepts, and sexual perversion); further, the general neuroses, viz.: epilepsy, hysteria, and the neurosis of fear (constitutional neurasthenia). By far the most important group, however, is that of periodical insanity and paranoia.

You are familiar with the saying that whoever has been insane is liable to become insane again. A careful study of a great number of patients who had been discharged, and kept under observation for years after discharge, convinced Kraepelin that the majority of the cases of mania and melancholia of the older writers, which did not belong to psychoses classified as depending on exhaustion or intoxication, or as essential dementia, had such a tendency to recur without any apparent cause, and sometimes with great regularity, that they could well be compared with epilepsy. What we know as mania or depression would, therefore, not be a disease in itself, just as little as the attack of epilepsy is the disease itself; but the disorder would be a constitutional defect characterized by periodic conditions of disturbed metabolism, the chief symptom of which is the occasional epileptic attack, or the mania, or the depression. This is not without practical importance, both for the prognosis and for the problems of pathological study. Simple mania, eminently curable, is not such a harmless incident, but is the manifestation of a constitutional condition. It is impossible to give a clear statement of the status of this question in a few words. A demonstration of patients will be more suitable to convey an idea of the importance of this view.

Paranoia is a mental perversion of slow and gradual development, a chronic constitutional transformation of the personality. The disease has more than once not been recognized as a mental disease by the courts of this country; for instance, in the Guiteau and Prendergast trials, probably because the legal views of insanity have lost touch with the rapidly progressing psychiatry. Who could nowadays say with good conscience that the recognition of right and wrong excluded a diagnosis of insanity, and say that insanity was identical with absolute irresponsibility?

If I have succeeded in showing you that psychiatry *has* problems essentially medical, that we can not afford to disregard any side of the biological unit in the patient, but must use psychological as well as physiological and anatomical methods under the guidance of general pathology, and that on this basis progress has been made and will continue, I have solved the task I put before myself. You will understand what I mean by saying in conclusion that the customary pathological laboratory is not sufficient to meet the needs of the study of so-called mental diseases. The first and fundamental prerequisite is careful and broad clinical observation. This will necessarily lead to careful collection of histories, physical and psychical examinations with exact methods; for this purpose the means for clinical chemistry and clinical microscopy must be procured, and finally the laboratories will also be fitted so that post-mortem pathology can be carried on. Wherever they began at the wrong end, at post-mortem pathology, the results have been so meager that we have a right to urge strongly the need of clinical facilities.

I hope you will excuse me for trying your patience so long. There is something unsatisfactory in talking about diseases without being able to show patients and then deriving the statement from what everybody can see and verify. I conclude with the following statement:

The biological view of man offers a fruitful working hypothesis for medicine, especially for psychiatry.

A mental disease is a disorder of the person following the laws of general pathology like any other disease.

Mental symptoms do not constitute the disease exclusively, and are not safe guides for diagnosis without general pathological views taking into consideration all the aspects of a man.

The clinical study of psychiatry is the natural basis for the study of mental pathology.

THE ATTITUDE OF NEUROLOGISTS, PSYCHIATRISTS AND PSYCHOLOGISTS TOWARDS PSYCHOANALYSIS

By Abraham Myerson, M.D.

Professor of Neurology, Tufts University School of Medicine, Boston, Massachusetts

Psychoanalysis is one of the oldest systems of concepts and of therapeutics in modern medicine. The beginning of Freud's work in psychoanalysis is, in fact, contemporaneous with the introduction of diphtheria antitoxin. His first paper appeared in 1893 and von Behring's publications culminated in 1893, although they started in 1890. Before von Behring's introduction of diphtheria antitoxin, the diphtheric exudate was treated by a host of methods. With the introduction of antitoxin, the other forms of treatment disappeared, and only one method remained in the field of therapy, the injection of diphtheria antitoxin. Before its superior potency, haphazard empirical guess-work therapeutics suffered the fate that the clearly inferior technique always experiences when the superior one is introduced into the world. Natural selection operated at once, and only one therapeutic measure for the treatment of diphtheria has remained.

In the 45 years that have elapsed since psychoanalysis was born into the family of scientific work, the Wassermann reaction has been introduced (1906). Arsphenamine appeared upon the scene in 1910 as the primary basis for the modern treatment of syphilis. In 1907 Wagner von Jauregg brought into medicine the idea that heat in the form of fever was an important therapeutic tool. In 1922 the young Canadian, Banting, with his co-workers added to the armamentarium of medicine insulin to combat diabetes. Thirty-three years after Freud started his reign as the head of psychoanalysis a group of American scientists, Minot, Murphy and Whipple, completely changed the fate of people suffering from pernicious anemia by introducing liver extract as its main therapeutic avenue. In 1913 Schick published his first paper on the technique which bears his name, and thus started a campaign for the eradication of diphtheria, the value of which cannot be overestimated.

The skeptical, hard-boiled medical profession has completely accepted all these advances in diagnosis and therapy and without any real struggle. The general law of life has operated, namely, wherever a method has shown superior therapeutic power, it has won the day, just as in the field of transportation the horse and buggy gave way to the auto-mobile, and the mechanical methods of heating and cooling won over more primitive techniques. Results count, and where the results are clear-cut, the technique which brings them wins the day.

The psychoanalysts, when this is brought to their attention, have a ready answer which is primarily the same one that they use when a patient fails to get well and which is the most beautiful instrument for successful argumentation ever devised by man, namely, the medical profession has *resistance* based on prejudice, unconscious fear and anxiety, and a general distaste and dislike for the grim and remorseless truths initiated by analysis. True, there are many people to whom the sexual factors and unconscious basis of psychoanalysis are offensive in a prejudiced unthinking way. But after 40 years of social inoculation and when generations of medical men have grown up with active psychoanalysts writing, talking and working, the professional prejudice would have been broken down if results were overwhelmingly clear and valuable.

The present study did *not* start as an effort to answer the question, "How far do those people who might be assumed to know the field of nervous and mental diseases and who can be listed in a wider sense as professional students of the mind and its diseases accept psychoanalysis?" It started as a reaction against the very extreme statement of a psychoanalyst to the effect "that practically all informed scientists accept psychoanalysis." To see whether or not this was the case, a questionnaire was drawn up, which at first was sent rather haphazardly to many entitled to be called leaders in psychology, neurology and psychiatry. As the answers became interesting, the scope of the inquiry was extended, so that finally four questions comprising the questionnaire were sent to a group of leading psychologists connected with universities, to the officers and every third member of the American Neurological Association, to the officers and every tenth member of The American Psychiatric Association, and more or less haphazardly a group of psychoanalysts were canvassed on the assumption that their very membership in the psychoanalytic society necessitated only a small sample. Nevertheless, the proportion of psychoanalysts who were questioned was larger than the proportion questioned of members of The American Psychiatric Association, and in fact many of them had been questioned as members of the American Neurological and American Psychiatric Associations.

From the Division of Psychiatric Research, Boston State Hospital, Boston, Massachusetts, aided by grants from the Commonwealth of Massachusetts and the Rockefeller Foundation.

Beyond any doubt, the questions which were submitted are imperfect and do not permit of any complete answer. Many people pointed out the difficulties in their mind as they attempted to answer the questionnaire, and I have no hesitation in saying that the questionnaire could be improved and the whole technique of canvassing made more scientific. However, I have no intention of presenting a completely scientific answer to the question, "In how far has psychoanalysis been accepted and in how far do psychologists, neurologists and psychiatrists believe that important therapeutic results have been contributed by this technique," since this is impossible. Despite objections, most of the writers had no great difficulty in classifying themselves somewheres in the four categories or else placing themselves between one category and the succeeding one, and the results are interesting and important.

The first questionnaire sent out asked the recipient to classify himself in one of the following groups:

1. Those individuals who completely accept psychoanalysis.
2. Those who feel very favorably inclined towards it but do not wholly accept it and are, to a certain extent, skeptical.
3. Those who, in the main, tend to reject its tenets but feel that Freud has contributed indirectly to the human understanding.
4. Those who feel that his work has, on the whole, hindered the progress of the understanding of the mental diseases and the neuroses and reject him entirely.

The second questionnaire was modified somewhat and the recipients were asked to classify themselves as follows:

1. Those individuals who completely accept psychoanalysis. The term "completely" need not be used too literally. One may substitute "whole-heartedly" or "in general."
2. As above.
3. As above.
4. As above

The most serious objections came from psychoanalysts who protested that nobody could accept completely a technique or point of view. Nevertheless nearly all of them finally registered themselves in Group 1, to the effect that they did completely accept psychoanalysis, by which I infer that certainly they may have points of difference with Freud and the Freudian doctrine, but that on the whole they accept the leading tenets and are optimistic about the therapeutic results. Similarly, people who were on the whole not friendly to the psychoanalytic movement expressed themselves as balking at a complete rejection and insisted that they belonged between the attitudes expressed by Groups 3 and 4. Still others found the second attitude difficult to accept, and some asked me to leave out the word "very" from the phrase "very favorably."

The *first* position may be considered as the extreme of acceptance and friendliness, as well as of optimism, concerning therapeutic results, although this is not directly questioned. The *second* position represents friendliness, but is sufficiently divergent from acceptance to embrace the individual who is not eligible to membership in the American Psychoanalytic Association. It is the position of a man who has been profoundly influenced by the psychoanalytic movement, accepts a great many of its terms, believes in the unconscious, and usually agrees that a longer or shorter process of self-revelation on the part of the patient is desirable, but who is an eclectic in the treatment of the neuroses. The *third* position is one of rejection but not of marked unfriendliness; such people do not accept the psychoanalytic theories or use its technique. They believe in psychotherapeutics of other types and follow physiologic measures of treatment as well, but they acknowledge the value of Freud historically and indirectly. The *fourth* position represents a completely hostile attitude. Not only is it implied that the psychoanalytic procedures and doctrines are invalid, but that the movement as a whole has done harm to psychiatry and to the research by which the general understanding of mental states, both normal and pathologic, is furthered. It is obvious, of course, that there are intermediate positions, as will be seen. These were assumed by many of those questioned.

RESULTS

Of the 428 questionnaires sent, 307 individuals replied, which on the whole is a good percentage. Only inference can be made as to why the others did not reply. Some explanation of this reticence appears in answers made to a later questionnaire in which the individuals were asked to answer as follows:

1. I am willing to be quoted by name in respect to my attitude on psychoanalysis as evidenced in my reply to the questionnaire.
2. I am willing to be quoted but not by name or identification.
3. I do not wish to be quoted at all.

Of these, a considerable number did not want their names given or to be identified, while others stated they did not wish to be quoted at all. Obviously, there was to some extent a distaste for or fear of the controversy implied in the whole procedure, so that it appears at once that a great deal of emotion is involved in any study of the psychoanalytic movement in a way which would undoubtedly not be found in a similar study, for example, which would involve the treat of syphilis by arsphenamine or by fever therapy. This is confirmed by the fact that those who did not wish to be quoted belong mainly in the groups which, though friendly, do not completely accept and those which reject but are not unfriendly. The usual reasons why questionnaires are not answered probably also operated, because, first, there are persons who do not believe in questionnaires, and secondly, there are those who forget to answer.

POSITION OF MEMBERS
OF THE AMERICAN NEUROLOGICAL ASSOCIATION

Of the 97 members of the American Neurological Association who received questionnaires, 75 replied. These may be classed as follows: five belong in Group 1; eight classify themselves between 1 and 2; 23 stated they belong in Group 2; four classify themselves between Groups 2 and

3; 25 declared themselves to be in Group 3; three stated that between Groups 3 and 4 was a good enough allocation of their position; four totally rejected psychoanalysis and were hostile; three were definitely non-committal or equivocal.

In general (Chart 1), the American Neurological group shows a beautiful curve of replies, about an equal and small number who accept and completely reject; an equal number who are friendly and to a certain extent are linked up with the psychoanalytic movement as compared to those who are not unfriendly, but who reject psychoanalysis, conceding that Freud has contributed to the learning and procedures of psychiatry.

POSITION OF MEMBERS
OF THE AMERICAN PSYCHIATRIC ASSOCIATION

Of the 266 members of The American Psychiatric Association canvassed on the basis stated above, 179 replied. Twenty-five classed themselves in Group 1; 15 between Groups 1 and 2; 54 in Group 2; 32 between Groups 2 and 3; 39 in Group 3 rejecting; 8 belong between this group and total rejection; while there was none who completely rejected psychoanalysis as having had some value. Six were non-committal.

It will be seen that the members of The American Psychiatric Association accept psychoanalysis in greater degree than do the members of the American Neurological Association; that if we place Group 2 as the middle of the series of positions, the American Psychiatric as judged by these replies is about equally divided, there being 94 on the friendly and more or less acceptance side of the fence and 79 on the rejecting side of the barrier.

POSITION OF MEMBERS
OF THE AMERICAN PSYCHOANALYTIC ASSOCIATION

Of the members of the American Psychoanalytic Association, 28 replies were received to 36 questionnaires sent. Of this group, 16 were in Group 1; 4 between Groups 1 and 2; 3 in Group 2; and 5 were skeptical or non-committal.

As would be expected, this group is largely on the acceptance side, although without too great a slavish adherence to psychoanalysis. The most heated letters sent me came from individuals in this group. Some took me to task; some took the position of instruction in the art of questionnairing; and others even felt impelled to lay down the elementary laws of scientific thought and procedure.

MISCELLANEOUS GROUP

Of a miscellaneous group, made up mainly of important members of the American Psychological Association and some physiologists interested in psychological research, 25 replies were received to 29 questionnaires sent. Two accepted psychoanalysis; 5 belonged in Group 2; 6 placed themselves between Groups 2 and 3; 7 placed themselves

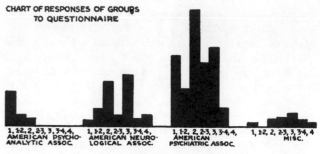

CHART OF RESPONSES OF GROUPS TO QUESTIONNAIRE

CHART I.

in Group 3; and 3 between Groups 3 and 4; 2 completely rejected and placed themselves in Group 4.

Thus, in this group of eminent men, having an almost 100 percent inclusion in Who's Who in Science and in America, the general attitude is more on the rejection side than on the acceptance, and goes a little further in the direction indicated by the position of the American Neurological Association.

CITATIONS

Many exceedingly interesting letters were received in answer to the questionnaire. Space does not permit the citation of all of these. I cite, therefore, a few from each group of those who have permitted citation.

Group 1

Those who placed themselves in Group 1 in my classification ranged in their answers from the statement made by Isador Coriat, "In reply to your inquiry, I place myself in category number one, namely, those individuals who completely accept psychoanalysis" to those who are less terse and more cautious.

For example, Lucile Dooley states, "I am in class 1, as completely accepting psychoanalysis, if by psychoanalysis is meant a valid *method* of investigating the human personality. I do not accept all its present formulations as final, nor, I believe, does its founder do this. Additions, revisions and corrections are hoped for and earnestly sought. As a valuable instrument for research, and in some cases for therapy, I accept it. Further, I believe that the method is not entirely replaceable by any other as yet discovered method. And for the one who would use it a personal analysis is as indispensable as is a high powered microscope for the bacteriologist." Her letter which ends by thanking me "for the opportunity of responding to the questionnaire and thus aiding in a valuable project" may be placed side by side with the letter of Smith Ely Jelliffe who writes as follows:

"By experience and study I would place myself in Group 1—just as if you asked do I believe 'completely in the concept of evolution.' 'Completely' is an intangible phrase for any growing body of experimental science, such as 'psychoanalysis,' or 'evolution' or similar large aspects of operational concepts. Questionnaires of this type do not mean much to me. I think they are usually very stupid. But 'chacun a son gout,' as the old lady said when she kissed the cow."

Group Between 1 and 2

Of those placing themselves between Groups 1 and 2, I cite Lawrence Kubie's letter as summarized by me and approved by him. Dr. Kubie, after a preliminary discussion as to the validity of the questionnaire, points out as follows: "For instance, I personally cannot accept either of your first two categories, although in a vague way they come nearer to my point of view than the other two. The first category is too blindly sectarian; the second one vague, muddled, and chicken-hearted in its ambivalence. Therefore, I think you need at least three more categories, to wit, 1) those who believe that the psychoanalytic technique, properly employed, uncovers significant dynamic psychological facts not obtainable in any other way at present; and 2) those who believe that the psychoanalytic technique, judiciously employed, can in certain cases secure therapeutic results not obtainable in any other way at present; and 3) those who believe that the basic principles of psychoanalytic theory are sound, however much they may disagree with any details of theory. (These basic principles could easily be formulated for your questionnaire to lessen still further its ambiguity.) I will classify myself under all three of these categories. I cannot, with any justice to my own convictions, classify myself under any of the four categories which your questionnaire would impose."

I have taken the liberty, however, of classifying Dr. Kubie between Groups 1 and 2. His characterization of the second point of view classifies a good many men of The American Psychiatric Association as "vague, muddled and chicken-hearted" in their reaction to psychoanalysis.

I cite Louis Casamajor: "I do not particularly like the four groups you make of people who react towards psychoanalysis. I feel that they are not near enough. Personally I stand somewhere between one and two; probably closer to one than to two. While I doubt if I 'completely accept psychoanalysis' yet I am sure that my feelings toward it are much more than 'favorably inclined.' If you should have to put me in either one group or the other I would prefer to be in group one."

William Malamud, who is in favor of the research, states, "It is somewhat difficult to fit my own reactions into any one of the four groups that you mention, but I would feel inclined to place myself somewhere between groups one and two. By this I mean that my attitude is that psychoanalysis has contributed a great deal of knowledge to the fields of psychopathology and psychotherapy. At the same time there are certain features both in the theoretical concepts and in some of the practical technique that leave me skeptical or appear to me superfluous."

Tracy J. Putnam writes as follows, "I feel that none of your categories exactly fits my attitude toward psychoanalysis, which might fall between 1 and 2. I certainly do not agree with all that Freud has to say and feel that some of his followers are of a low order. On the other hand, I do feel that Freud has made a tremendous and theoretical and practical advance in psychology and psychiatry. It seems to me that one can well compare psychoanalysis to neurological surgery. It has some brilliant successes to its credit, some gallant failures, some egregious mistakes and some charlatanism, but even the mistakes have contributed information, and it is inconceivable that we can ever do without it in the future."

Group 2

Of the men in this group, Karl M. Bowman answers as follows, "It is not easy to classify myself in the manner you have suggested, as I am perhaps somewhat ambivalent. I would say that I feel Freud has made many important and valuable contributions to psychoanalysis, and that there are many of his formulations which I would essentially accept. On the other hand, there are many of his other formulations with which I definitely disagree. Again, if the term is used as psychoanalysis, one might have many objections to the attitudes and opinions of a large number of the psychoanalysts of this country, without that being particularly a reflection on Freud himself. I would think that I fit most nearly under your second group, but I do not feel that this is quite an exact statement of my attitude. Number three would seem to me to give less credit to Freud than I would feel inclined to give."

A very cogent statement is that of Clarence O. Cheney, "I feel that it (psychoanalysis) has contributed a good deal to psychiatry but I am not by any means willing to accept all of the theories or conclusions that have been formulated by Freud and some of his disciples who, I feel, are inclined to reason from the particular to the general and oftentimes seem not to be able to use common sense. I regret also that not a few of them seem to be interested only in the psyche of the patient and not in the patient himself and in his living in and adjusting to a community. I think it does not help psychoanalysts either to see so many persons who are analysts unable to adjust themselves in their lives very well and who, in fact, at times seem infantile. I grant, of course, that psychoanalysis in itself should not be blamed for this. I feel that there may be many persons, including social workers and other professional groups, who have become instilled with the idea that psychoanalysis is necessary whereas they are using time that might be more profitably spent."

Stanley Cobb expresses the following point of view, "I should think on the list of attitudes toward psychoanalysis you could put me down as a number two. In fact, in almost anything that you ask me about, I think I would be a number two, because anybody who accepts anything whole is sure to be wrong. Therefore, I strive to remain a skeptic in all fields. I rather wish you had left out the word 'very.' Perhaps your paragraph would then express my attitude more exactly."

A typical attitude is expressed by Eugen Kahn, "Let me say that I seem to belong to your group two with some modification insofar as I feel favorably inclined towards Freudian analysis, cannot wholly accept all of it, and am skeptical to quite some degree."

Nolan D.C. Lewis takes the following position, "I usually think of psychoanalysis in terms of at least three of its aspects—first, a good deal of it exists as a body of doctrine, metapsychology or philosophy, if you will; second, another aspect is the application of the technique as a research method which can be used for the purpose of deeper dissection of mental content; and third, its psychotherapeutic possibilities. I still think there are certain types of cases that respond better to psychoanalysis if well done, by an expert, than to any other variety of psychotherapy. In other words, in some cases, it is the most valuable approach. I have never thought of psychoanalysis in terms of any possibility of its replacing psychiatry or that the terms psychoanalysis and psychiatry are in any way synonymous. It is only a part of the body of knowledge included in psychiatry, but I do believe that the method and findings justify additional clinical researches and evaluations."

While William L. Russell thinks he fits best in Group 2, he makes the following important statement in regard to those who should practise psychoanalysis, "I believe, however, that I should say that on the other side I believe that only those who are well qualified in general psychiatry should undertake to practise psychoanalysis. I am under the impression also that where psychoanalysis dominates in a psychiatric organization the young physicians entering the service do not get a proper foundation for a sound development in psychiatry. They become imbued with the idea that the main task is to work out a theoretical formulation on psychoanalytic lines of the problems presented by the patient. There is a tendency to neglect the more obvious factors in the understanding and the treatment of the patient. There is also a tendency to neglect the physical. In fact, Freud has written that a person does not need medical training to practise psychoanalysis successfully. This view is, of course, far from what we have been teaching and practising in psychiatry as a branch of medicine."

Israel Strauss feel favorably inclined towards psychoanalysis, but adds this sting to the tail of his remarks "but more skeptical of some of those who practise it."

Group Between 2 and 3

In this group particularly, a large number of individuals did not wish to be quoted either by name or at all.

One important psychiatrist of the elderly group, who does not wish to be quoted by name, states, "Indeed I am quite sure that I stand somewhere between the 2nd and 3rd (group). I certainly can credit psychoanalysis with more than those in your third group. Probably my chief difficulty lies in its direct therapeutic use, particularly in the practice of psychiatry. As far as I am able to observe, while it gives one an insight into mechanisms, it signally fails to produce beneficial results."

Group 3

Of this group, Gordon Holmes states, "I think you can place me in the third group, that is, I believe Freud has contributed to our understanding of the human mind, although I have never been convinced that many of his tenets are acceptable. I am also of the opinion that except in a small proportion of cases psychoanalysis has failed as a line of

treatment, and that in the hands of uncritical enthusiasts and of those without adequate experience of clinical work it has often produced more harm than good."

Selecting Group 3 in preference to the others, Samuel D. Ingham states, "I think it is probably true that my own conception of the motivation of human behavior may on the whole be better than it would have been if Freud had not written the Scenario of Psychoanalysis. I do feel that he has made important contributions to the understanding of human nature. I also feel that most of his would-be followers have been woefully misled. I am inclined, too, to think that enthusiasm in regard to a psychoanalytic viewpoint has tended to inhibit progress in psychology on the basis of a more strictly biological approach."

Andrew H. Woods' letter speaks for itself, "For your own interest I should say that the word psychoanalysis ought not be spelled with a capital P as if it were a new denomination or school of medicine. Taking all the florid literature produced by Freud, but added to enormously by his followers, perhaps it has to be considered as a new school of thought. I look upon the technique for re-discovering experiences that have emotional value, that is the technique of guided memory associations, as extremely valuable. It is, of course, nothing new, but has been organized into a much more useful form under Freud's stimulation. The careful study of dream symbolism and the symbolism of psychoneurosis appears to me another contribution of great value. The idea of catharsis is to me nothing more than confession and has always been useful. I feel sure that many of the so-called cures through psychoanalysis are nothing more than relief gained through Christian Science and other dramatic performances by self-confident operators."

Group Between 3 and 4

The following is an abstract of the letter of a very well known neurologist, who does not wish to be quoted by name, "I would say, offhand, that less than five per cent of the patients in my office were cases where the major causation of the condition was such as to include them in the Freudian group. By this I mean that the other ninety-five per cent of the cases were amenable to other forms of therapy, and the therapeutic results were to be obtained in a much shorter period of time and with more lasting effect. Of the five per cent of the cases, these were treated, and very successfully, with the Freudian technique . . . . . In reply to question four, I think that psychoanalysis has been the greatest block to the study and understanding of mental disease, and by this I mean insanity, that has happened since the time of Rush. All doctors in all institutions for the care of the insane that I have been in touch with in the United States were so saturated with the Freudian concept that real investigation of mental diseases was almost entirely excluded. There was some little work here and there but in an entirely unsympathetic atmosphere . . . . ." He ends up by stating, "From the standpoint of the professional psychoanalyst, I, not having been psychoanalyzed, have no right to the above opinions, and they are, therefore, of little or no value."

Since the above is a typical answer, I am not quoting further from the group standing between 3 and 4.

Group 4

The outstanding personality in this group is Bernard Sachs. He underlines Group 4, to wit, he is of those who feel that Freud's work has, on the whole, hindered the progress of the understanding of the mental diseases and the neuroses and *reject him entirely*. In a footnote he states, "Strongly for No. 4 with a little concession as to the introduction of a few useful concepts." Thus, he is willing to admit that Freud has indirectly and to a limited extent enriched human knowledge.

AUTHOR'S PERSONAL OPINION

I take it that the instigator of this questionnaire has a right to express himself more fully on the matter than any of his subjects, so that his "cultural compulsives," which is a polite phrase for prejudices, may directly appear. I also find it somewhat difficult to confine myself to the categories of classification. Roughly, I can state that I belong mainly in Group 3 with a flow towards Group 2 and an equal flow towards Group 4.

I am definitely of the opinion that Freud is a great man and entitled to be called one of the great men of his times. Greatness, I believe, does not reside in the truth or non-truth of what the great man believes, since the truth is an inaccessible ideal of human striving. The effect of Freud on his generation has been enormous and it is probably impossible for any contemporary to say whether that has been good or non-good, since these are viewed from the standpoint of the individual's trends, desires and wishes, being in the main subjective.

The concrete value of Freud's work seem to me to be as follows, and they are, in the main, indirect results of his work:

1) Freud has been one of the men who has taken the obscenity out of sex and made it possible to study its phenomena objectively. While he has had predecessors and co-workers, such as Krafft-Ebing, Moll, Havelock Ellis and others, no one has been so ruthless as he in the approach to the matter. Homosexuality, autoeroticism, and the various manifestations of heterosexuality have been emphasized as authentic and competing directions of human sexuality and have been brought fully to the social consciousness by his work and, to a lesser extent, by his followers.

2) He has emphasized struggle within the personality more emphatically and more candidly than any predecessor or contemporary. Inner struggle as such has been well recognized by the theologians, the philosophers, the psychiatrists, and is deeply imbedded in the consciousness of the average man. Whether his analysis of the struggle is the correct one or not, even those who reject his point of view have had to pay more attention to the details of human life and to the *concealed* human difficulties because of the pressure of his ideas and his work. Whether we agree or not as to the facts of his discovery, research into the human mind has been stimulated by his activities. In my opinion, this is an indirect result since I do not agree with the findings. All in all, therefore, this bold voyager into the realm of human attitudes and mental diseases has exercised a great influence directly useful in the opinion of his followers, indirectly of great value in the opinion of a humble psychiatrist who, nevertheless, rejects the authenticity of the phenomena described.

This rejection includes Freud's concept of the consciousness, of the censor, and of the sharp separation of unconscious processes from the conscious activities of the individual. I do not believe the unconscious is an organized personality or is a place where complexes, forgotten experiences, so to speak, roam around looking for chances to express themselves, by eluding the vigilant censor or the preconscious in neuroses, dreams, slips of the tongue or any of these phenomena. To me, the unconscious is the sum total of those drives, instincts and activities which the viscera would naturally bring into action. The social structure, through the forebrain, tries to limit by injunctions of morality, fitness and decorum the activities, let us say, of the male genitalia; but these organs and their linked-up glands and hormones do not often easily submit to culture, morality, decorum and fitness. The forbidden activities are called crime. The struggle between the visceral drives and the forebrain and society, which may be concealed or diverted, can easily be brought into consciousness and, in fact, is a component of the consciousness, whether acknowledged or not.

3) I reject entirely the so-called free association technique. I submit that you can take ten words of a time-table and get at any hidden struggle of the individual and reach as many mental situations and complexes as you can by the words of the dream. *In other words, the patent content of the dream has nothing to do with what is called its latent content or to the matter which is disclosed.*

Moreover, the associations *are conditioned* by the examination and study itself. A beautiful young psychoanalyst of the female sex would arouse other associations than the austere Freud would or could. The very fact that psychoanalytic doctrines have infiltrated the thinking of the community and the fact that the patient seeks a psychoanalyst alters the associations in a very significant manner.

4) The doctrine of infantile sexuality is completely against the facts of patent type. There are no sexual acts corresponding to the postulated sexual attitudes. Moreover, *the infant does not have hormones in his urine or has so little as to be almost negligible. Hormones appear in puberty in a great flood corresponding to the overt behavior.* Throughout the writings of Freud and his followers, *sensuality* is continually identified with *sexuality*, as in the classic statement made by Freud, that when one sees the infant after nursing at the breast, relaxing with satisfaction, it brings to mind and apparently is identical with the relaxed lover after a sexual relationship.

5) The whole concept of symbolism seems to me an exercise in ingenuity and without the slightest proof. Straight things, round things, enclosed things—all these are too common, too universal, in fact, to be symbols of the phallus, the lingham, the vagina, and any other part, male or female. Vigorous objects, like bulls and horses, can be symbols for everything under the sun, as well as the father. It is an arbitrary selection which makes them symbols in the

Freudian sense and gives them value accredited them by psychoanalysis.

The psychoanalysts have a very ingenious subterfuge for escaping criticism. So long as you have not been psychoanalyzed, you cannot judge the results of psychoanalysis. But I am not a surgeon and yet I can judge the results of surgery. I can tell when my patient has had a successful operation for brain tumor, even though I could not bore a hole straight in the skull. I can even judge when a chemical problem has been attacked properly, although I am no chemist. The general criteria of science can be utilized by a non-psychoanalyst with validity in judging both the analytic idealogy and its results.

And when one sees the analysts passing judgment on the quick and the dead with as complete assurance in the one case as in the other, one must come to the conclusion that a clinical psychoanalysis is largely superfluous. If one can speak as freely and as authoritatively of Leonardo da Vinci and of Moses as of a little four-year-old boy subjected to an analysis, then surely it is not necessary to do an analysis at all in the technical sense. By extending themselves too far, the psychoanalysts have proven quite clearly that their clinical technique is unnecessary.

When one runs across such biological absurdities as that the child is the symbol of the lost penis, and then sees mother love operating with vigor throughout the whole animal scale and realizes that the lioness probably has no particular complexes due to the operation of the super-ego, one can only reject the interpretation of human mother love as given by Freud and his followers . . . . .When one reads in Freud's "Discontents of Civilization" that woman has become the guardian of the hearth-fire because she is anatomically so constituted that she cannot put out the fire with a stream of urine, one wonders why there has been any acceptance of such doctrines.

And so on, and so on, and so on!

An omission of serious type is conspicuous throughout the work of Freud and his followers. The *present moment* and the *present situation* are entirely neglected as practically having no etiologic bearing. So far as Freud and his followers are concerned, all causation is entirely a matter of the very earliest period of life. The rest is of little significance. Moreover, one would never know from Freud that patients live in an economic world, have a struggle for existence; that the society in which they live is clumsily adapted to their individual needs and, in fact, often maladapted to the human being and his mental health. The long lag between sexual maturity and the legitimate and proper satisfaction of the sexual impulses would seem to me of huge importance, and the other strains of mankind are given, practically speaking, no weight or importance by him . . . . .The arduous preparation for life which we call education and which is often a crucifixion of all the natural desires of the child has no weight so far as psychoanalysis is concerned . . . . .The struggle to develop constant purposes in an organism which is built up around shifting polarities of expression and which is poorly designed for the coordinated life of civilization apparently has no importance . . . . .The strain of the competitive impulses and their effect on ego-evaluation, and this independently of any sexual relationship whatsoever, receives a bow of acknowledgement but nothing more. In a word, the important strains of existence, the discrepancies between the biologic nature of man and the social nature, and that independently of any unconsciousness, or sex, or what you will of complexes, is passed over almost disdainfully.

Psychoanalysis is reactionary. This sounds like "tu quoque" in a world where the psychoanalysts accuse the nonbelievers of just exactly this. Essentially analysis harks back to the ancient separation of mind and body, even though analysts continually give lip homage to the relationship of mind and body. But this is only lip homage. Practically, it is considered bad form and poor psychoanalysis if the patient with a neurosis under analysis gets sedatives for sleep, tonics for his appetite, exercises and physiotherapy to increase his muscular endurance and general sense of well-being. I do not know whether there is any ex cathedra prohibition of the care of the whole individual which is so important a part of present day medical belief, but in practice the psychoanalyst constantly operates as if the patient's complexes existed in a sort of physiological vacuum; as if somehow the analysis would be injured, if side by side with it the hygiene of the individual was changed so as to improve his general health, and if the well established procedures by which the body is made more vigorous would contaminate the purity of the psychoanalytic procedures. This is true reactionism. It is against the attitude of modern scientific thought, which states that the separation of mind and body is an artifact harking back to primitive and theological thought.

I state definitely that as a therapeutic system, psychoanalysis has failed to prove its worth. First of all, it has not conquered the field as is the case with any other successful therapeutic approach, as I have indicated in the first part of this paper. There is more reason to extol in the case of the psychoses the pharmacological measures and physiological stimulations than psychoanalysis. The neuroses are "cured" by Christian Science, osteopathy, chiropractice, nux vomica and bromides, benzedrine sulfate, change of scene, a blow on the head, and psychoanalysis, which probably means that none of these has yet established its real worth in the matter, and surely that psychoanalysis is no specific. Moreover, since many neuroses are self-limited, anyone who spends two years with a patient gets credit for the operation of nature.

Some Trends of Psychiatry

By Abraham Myerson, M.D.

Professor Emeritus, Tufts University School of Medicine, Boston, Massachusetts

Introduction

The many trends in modern psychiatry may, perforce, be brought into three great groups, and in the fore front of these movements are three great figures symbolizing and enhancing the form and power of our discipline. It is not sufficiently realized that Emil Kraepelin and Sigmund Freud were born in 1856, and that Ivan Petrovich Pavlov's birth was in 1849; and the fact that each lived to a vigorous old age gave them a long ascendancy, so that they founded powerful schools which, while theoretically complementary, were often at great odds with one another. Kraepelin's work quickly captured psychiatry, and although very vigorously attacked, his opponents generally worked within the framework of his classification. The ideas of Freud were slower to enter into the everyday thinking of psychiatry, but they finally succeeded in exercising a tremendous influence. Pavlov's work, primarily that of a great physiologist in an era rich in such workers, has only slowly become of moment in modern psychiatry, but points the way to the transformation of theory-ridden psychiatry into a field of experimental science.

Medical Psychiatry and the Kraepelinian Influence

Classification has it dangers. Galton once said that the natural groupings have discrete nuclei, but their peripheries overlap. Classification may link together the unlike, establish false boundaries, and give a satisfaction which is spurious because it diverts the mind from the contradictions of individual differences. But the existence of individual differences does not in itself invalidate group classifications. Every cat can legitimately claim individuality, but there is a perfectly good basis for the general term (or diagnosis) of "Cat." A distinguished American psychiatrist (1) has objected to the one-word classification of mental disease. There are some overlooked individual differences in the classification "schizophrenia," but this semantic deficiency applies to cases of pneumonia, tables, constellations, and undoubtedly to molecules, atoms and ions.

In fact, treatment has become practical and successful in other branches of medicine when general principles have pervailed which essentially disregard the individual's life history. Thus, the treatment of pneumonia by sulpha drugs cannot depend on the fact that *individuals* of *markedly different background* have acquired an infection; it depends on the *sameness of that infection*, although one must treat a child somewhat differently than his grandfather.

The mass of psychiatric disorders is here split up into three main groups, excluding from our consideration because of lack of space feeblemindedness, epilepsy—in which field great advances have been made both in essential physio-pathology and treatment (2)—and constitutional psychopathic inferiority. These are: 1) those diseases firmly established as essentially *somato-psychic* or of organic-physiologic origin; 2) the so-called functional mental diseases, which is really equivalent to the statement that cause and pathophysiology are not known; 3) the great and divergent groups unified under the term "neuroses," which in reality means those "mental" diseases which do not usually bring the sufferer to a custodial institution.

A few words about the *somatopsychoses* or the established organic diseases: These have been removed from the fused mass of insanity and placed into separate pigeonholes by dint of long-continued and successful work. The establishment of the various clinical forms of neurosyphilis, recognized as being different from the other organic diseases only in the yesterday of science, is a triumph of the collaborative modern scientific method, and welds together the names of Charcot (3), Fournier (4), Nissl (5), Alzheimer (6), Noguchi (7) and MacDonald (8)—its roster of heroes includes those neurologists who evolved the study of the reflexes (Erb (9) and Westphal (10)), of pupillary anomalies (Argyll-Robertson (11)), and of spinal fluid (Quincke (12), Nonne (13), Ayer (14), and many others). With the establishment of a cause, which has no fundamental dependence, so far as we really know, on individual constitution or individual psychology, and substantially is the invasion of the nervous system by the trepanoma pallida, therapeutics entered the field, due to Ehrlich (15) and Wagner von Jauregg (16), who gave the main directions to treatment.

But here, as elsewhere, prevention is greater than cure—neurosyphilis is declining because early syphilis is better treated. As the mores become civilized and theology ceases to meddle in matters of health, syphilis will be prevented and one field of psychiatry will disappear.

The aging of the population, due to the decreasing birth

From the Division of Psychiatric Research, Boston State Hospital, Boston, Mass., Aided by a Grant from the Commonwealth of Massachusetts.

rate and the advance in longevity, brings with it the distressing fact that more people, consequently, outlive their brains. Psychiatry will have to face this fact, since the real increase in mental diseases comes by the roads of senile dementia (17), with its placques, and cerebral arterio-sclerotic dementia, with its more direct cardio-vascular changes. That the lack of minerals in the brain may have some therapeutic implications is here hesitatingly set forth.

Triumphantly, the science of medicine has conquered, or points the road to conquest, of another great somatopsychic disease, pellagra. We may well be proud that Lombroso (18) was the first to regard this scourge as a disease of poverty and poor diet; we may well be grateful for that crusading work of Goldberger (19) and the United States Public Health Service which finally led to the establishment of pellagra as a deficiency disease, with a specific cure and a technique of prevention which needs *only* (sic) social intelligence and social good will.

But a kindred set of diseases, the alcoholic mental diseases, the result of the great drug addition of western civilization, is not being curbed in the least. Too much is said of individual psychology in the genesis of alcoholism and too little is said on such matters as racial-social custom and pressure (20). It is of obvious importance to explain why the depressed and harassed Irishman escapes by the route of alcoholism, whereas his equally depressed and harassed neighbor, a Jew, does not (21). The admixture of politics and finance with the sale of alcohol, the notion that somehow virility is measured by the quantity one can drink, point the way to social action and education in which the psychiatrist should play his social part, just as he play his scientific part in studying the effect of the lack of nicotinic acid in the cells of the cortex and the absence of thiamin in the integrity of the peripheral fibers.

Kraepelin and Functional Mental Disorders

Kraepelin (22) represents medical psychiatry, that is, the growth of classification, the development of the study of the mental diseases as clinical syndromes, with the establishment of nosology and prognosis, thus bringing the subject matter of psychiatry into the pattern of the other fields of medicine.

There have been classification systems from the earliest days of psychiatry: Hippocrates (23), Galen (23), the countless authors cited in Burton's *Anatomy of Melancholy* (24)—each had his classification. Benjamin Rush (25), Hack Tuke (26), Esquirol (27), Morel (28), Pinel (29), Spurzheim (30), Lombroso (31), Mendel (32)—to cite only a few—developed systems, some entirely based on *a priori* hypotheses, for example those of the earlier writers—Hippocrates, Galen, Paracelsus—and even including the founder of this society, Benjamin Rush, and others which approach more nearly the clinical descriptive analytic work, which reached its fruition in the work of Kraepelin. There were precursors of Kraepelin in the understanding that there was a cyclothymic disorder (33), the manifesta-

tions of which alternated between melancholia and mania. There were those who described the various phases of what later became dementia praecox. To cite one neglected paper, Farrar (34) gives an illuminating view of the evolution which led to Kraepelin. But nosological psychiatry, which had many precursors, dates from Kraepelin, and every classification system in use in every state hospital, the tool of diagnosis and prognosis for every practising psychiatrist, even those who decry his work, can be directly traced to his concepts and ideas.

Kraepelin was no mere classifier. He made psychological studies under Wundt, and he attempted to discover the central and underlying psychological basis for the diseases which he welded together in the widespreading syndromes of dementia praecox and manic-depressive insanity. It is also an error to believe that he thought the diagnosis of dementia praecox rested entirely upon deterioration and a fatalistic type of prognosis. In many of his lectures he points out that cases of dementia praecox make clinical recoveries, and he even uses that term. It is to his great credit that he viewed the mental diseases as clinical entities, having a beginning, a course and an end, and he struck a powerful blow to the *post hoc propter hoc* tradition of psychiatry. Thus he conceived of dementia praecox as usually starting early in life, hence the name; that through the paralysis of the will, which he considered to be the central psychological feature, there took place a final deterioration and splitting of personality, as well as apathy, catatonia, passive obedience, senseless negativism. That at one time he described eleven different forms of dementia praecox indicates the minuteness and keenness of his observations, although psychiatry has failed to find substantiation for so fine a division of an obscure disorder. His concept of an organic intoxication as etiological was linked with his emphasis on heredity and constitution as basic. In other words, he did not accept any fundamental etiological environmental circumstances, although he gave a place to the adversities of life as contributing factors.

Although Bleuler (35) added an "interpretive" feature to the study of the group of diseases unified under dementia praecox, although he painstakingly and, to me, often confusingly, divided the symptoms of what he called schizophrenia into primary and secondary groups, it can only be stated that the terms schizophrenia and dementia praecox are in reality used interchangeably in present day psychiatry. The same diseases, the same conditions, the same combination of symptoms are now called schizophrenia, which were called dementia praecox prior to his time. The analysis of the symptoms of the disease or group of diseases took on a different and important slant. Complexes, struggles within the personality, the Freudian ideas of a subconscious which battled, so to speak, with the conscious self, were woven into the pattern of schizophrenia. Autistic thinking was emphasized and many other phases of the Bleuler approach have left their impress, but he can only be regarded as far secondary to Kraepelin in his influence in psychiatry.[1]

Sharply set aside from dementia praecox or schizophrenia is the other great mental disease which Kraepelin unified

---

[1] It is interesting to note that scientific nomenclature finally by a long roundabout comes to mean the same as some long prevalent lay term. The word "crazy" comes from ceramics, meaning a split in the pot. So when a man is called crazy or schizophrenic, one really uses the same word.

under the term "manic-depressive psychosis," although the clinical insight of others had noted this polarity disease. No one doubts that there are cases which through life show an alternation between the syndrome characterized by mental and physical retardation, gloom, self-accusation and a general deflation of egotism, together with an absence of all desire and satisfaction, and a state almost exactly the opposite, which is manifested by increased physical and mental activity, elation, ideas of grandeur and importance, and inflated egoism in every direction, as well as the sharpening of desire and satisfaction.

The In-Between Syndromes

But the clinical patterns under which patients present themselves to the psychiatrist cannot be grouped under these two headings of dementia praecox, on the one hand, and manic-depressive psychosis, on the other. Many workers emphasized this difficulty and a procrustean technique had and still has to be followed to fit any particular syndrome, as presented by any patient, into the bed of schizophrenia or that of manic-depressive psychosis.

Adolf Meyer (36) is one of the outstanding opponents of too rigid a classification, and he introduced the terms "allied to dementia praecox" and "allied to manic-depressive psychosis" to cover up the difficulty. Later, with the introduction of the terms "schizoid" and "affective disorder," "schizo-affective states" (37) became the term which smoothly, although unsatisfactorily, bridges the gap between the classical case of schizophrenia and the unmistakable case of manic-depressive psychosis. Meyer stressed individual difference and, as stated in a previous paragraph, objected to any one-word classification of the mental diseases. He states quite eloquently and, to my mind, in one of the most fundamental of formulations, that "mind, like every other function, can demoralize and undermine itself and its organ and the entire biological economy, and to study the law of miscarriage of function in life is one of the conditions for any true advancement in psychopathology" (38).

There are essential difficulties which underlie every classification by psychological symptoms. In the first place, what one man may call "torpor and apathy," another man may call "depression," and so through the gamut of psychological signs. In the second place, a *common etiologic agent* may manifest itself *psychologically quite diversely* in differing individuals, and where that etiological agent is unknown, the greatest confusion may arise. Thus, under the influence of alcohol, one man may become talkative, euphoric and present the picture of something resembling the manic state. Another may be depressed, self-accusatory, lachrymose and superficially, at least, resemble melancholia. Another may become belligerent, sadistic, brutal and may murder or ravish; while still another may become the very embodiment of the milk of human kindness, giving away all he has, loving others with a zeal that is embarrassing and even disgusting. Did we not know the common etiological agent of alcohol was present, we might easily classify these reactions as different mental diseases.

Ernesto Lugaro (39), in my opinion one of the most brilliant of modern psychiatrists, stated that he could not make a real classification because he doubted the validity of a purely symptomatic one and not enough is known of etiology and pathology to make a classification on that basis. In this I think he was entirely correct. Whatever classifications we have at present must do until that happy day arrives when we have measurable, objective, physiological-chemical, physical reactions and tests.

To make a few minor points. There is still a separation between involutional melancholia and the manic-depressive states in most classifications. Dreyfus (40) challenged this division long ago, and, in my opinion, established the identity of the classical involutional melancholia with the depressions seen earlier in life and diagnosed as depressive phases of manic-depressive psychosis. In recent years there have appeared therapeutic tests which at least hint at the common basis. *The two diseases best treated by metrazol and electric shock are involutional melancholia and the depressive phase of manic-depressive psychosis* (41).

The establishment by Kraepelin of paranoia (22) (later paraphrenia) as a separate syndrome can, I think, be challenged. There *is* a group in which there is a classical evolution in the two directions of grandiosity and persecution without any impairment of intelligence or without the appearance of hallucinations. But there is a merging of such cases, which are relatively few, through a series of intermediate states, with the paranoid psychoses which occur as part of schizophrenia.

Individual Psychopathology, Especially Psychoanalysis

Running parallel in time with the general and classificatory work is that which is individual and analytic, devotes its attention to the individual state and the individual life history, and which tends on the whole to disregard classification, although generally speaking it works within the nosological boundaries. Eminent workers in all the important cultural countries of western civilization have labored assiduously and written voluminously in the latter part of the 19th century and within our own times, on individual psychopathology. This work, although it reaches its peak with that of Freud, owes much to somewhat lesser lights. Prince (42) and Sidis (43) in America, Jung (44) and Adler (45) in the Germanic tongues (although neither was an "echt" German), Janet (46), Déjérine (47), and many other analyzed the individual case, sought to isolate mechanisms, emphasized struggle and conflict, spoke of consciousness, subconsciousness, coconsciousness, and developed their own systems of psychopathology. But either these spring from Freud, as in the case of Jung and Adler, or else they become completely overshadowed by Freud, although I believe that Janet, particularly, is entitled to a great place in the history of psychopathology.

Freud's ideas have not only strongly influenced psychiatry, but have permeated into the thinking, literature and art of our day. The language has been enriched or at least amplified by many potent words. One of his greatest contributions was that, together with such writers as Krafft-Ebing (48) and Havelock Ellis (49), he helped destroy the concept of obscenity as it damns some of the most important functions and organs of man. Sex has become a topic to be discussed anywhere and everywhere and this, I think, is a notable advance in the history of human thought, since one of the stumbling blocks to human progress has been the shame and obscurantism, as well as the mystery, which have covered over the sexual life of the human being. Sex has been taken from the mores, theology and law and brought into the fields of physiology, psychology, sociology and medicine. Freud emphasized, as no one else has ever dared to do, the conflict that ranges within the human being between the socially permissible feelings, thoughts, and acts, and those which are socially prohibited and condemned, but which, nevertheless, are primitive and important as native biological drives and activities. He built up a technique called psychoanalysis, and with this tool, which is fundamentally based on the analysis of dreams by the free association method, an enormous structure of psychopathology has been erected. The sexual difficulties of man have been systematized and given the leading place, if not the only place, in the genesis of many of the neuroses and the psychoses. Incidentally, it may be stated that Freud believed that many of the neuroses rested on a physical basis and were not analyzable or treatable by psychoanalysis (50). He and his followers extended the concepts of psychoanalysis into fields other than psychiatric, including the creation of such characters as Lady MacBeth (51) and the structure of society. Some of the analysts have analyzed multiple sclerosis, pneumonia, pernicious anemia, and every other disease of importance, and found psychoanalytic trends which finally lead to the conclusion that disease is a self-punishing wish-fulfillment and thus a seeking for death (52).

This is not the place to enter into an elaborate discussion of the accomplishments of psychoanalysis. I have expressed myself rather freely on this matter in other writings (88), but wish merely to state at this point that *had Freud sought for the least accessible and the least reliable psychological phenomenon, and the one in which any certainty of results of study could be least expected,* he would have selected what he did—the dream. The free association method has been adversely criticized by so many that I forbear to say more than this—that the term "free" must be used entirely relatively, since every examiner and every setting condition the type of associations that come to the surface (53).

To speak of lesser influences, Jung's work became mystical. His concept of introversion and extraversion is valuable, but not conclusive as to clinical syndromes. Adler, I believe, contributed something of great importance in his concept of the inferiority complex, although his analysis of its origin does not seem to me to be at all conclusive. What I think he was really describing was a striking phase of anxiety and the understanding of anxiety will some day lead to the roots of many of the manifestations of mental disease (54).

No matter what the value of psychoanalysis may be in the treatment of the neuroses, it has been of no value whatsoever in the treatment of schizophrenia, manic-depressive psychosis, or any of the so-called major mental diseases. I think this is a statement with which any candid psychoanalyst will agree. In fact, it is a very sad reflection for the psychiatrist of whatever school, when he realizes that the most effective means in the treatment of psychoses have mainly come from non-psychiatrists. The treatment of syphilis by the arsenical drugs gives us most of whatever success we have in the treatment of general paresis, although Wagner von Jauregg (16), a psychiatrist, introduced hyperthermia. The rationale of the treatment of the alcoholic diseases originates in the realm of biochemistry, nutrition and experimental physiology (21). And whatever the final verdict on the therapeutic value of the shock treatments will be, which at present are the only means of remarkably—even if temporarily—changing the mental state in schizophrenia and in the depressive psychoses, this form of therapy originated with Sakel (55), who was not then a psychiatrist, although Meduna (56) and the Italians, Bini (57) and Cerletti (58), who followed Sakel, are psychiatrists.

CONSTITUTION AND HEREDITY

Infiltrating into all this labor of classification and individual study have been the results of another major effort—the attempt to find in physical constitution and heredity the bases for the development of the functional mental diseases. Again this work goes back to the father of medicine, Hippocrates, with his four humours and his physical types. Constitution was also emphasized by Paracelsus. Lotze (59) gave a classic description which bears re-reading even in these days. Raymond Pearl (60) makes a statement which, I think, it is essential to keep in mind—that constitution is no unalterable hereditary character, although heredity plays an important part in its evolution. But external events may alter constitution. Thus an infection alters, constitutionally, the immunity of the individual (61). Thus, encephalitis profoundly alters the constellation of reactions which may be expected from the individual, and Adolph Meyer (62) stressed that alteration in personality which follows trauma and which has since then been called the post-traumatic constitution. We are not, therefore, committed to a hereditary basis of constitution. We can seek for environmental causation, even though we grant that most of the particular individual experience plays no rôle or a minor one in determining the onset of mental sickness. *We may properly believe that the social structure by its fantastic demands, excitations and inhibitions changes normal to abnormal constitution.*

The main influence in psychiatry, so far as constitution is concerned, is that of Kretschmer (63). To his division of body forms into pyknic, leptosomic and athletic types, he added a revolutionary relationship to mental disease of the pyknic body form to cyclothymic temperament, and thus, the liability to the alternating manic-depressive psychosis; and of the leptosomic body (the asthenic, as it is often called) to the schizophrenic temperament; and finally, that the nuclear groups of schizophrenia arise from the athletic body form. But Kretschmer goes further and says it is quite possible to classify normal personalities into two main groups of cyclothymes and schizothymes, which in a general way correspond to the pyknic—asthenic division. This clearcut and nuclear relationship stimulated much research and many conflicting conclusions. Of the difficulties which at once appear is, at what age is a man's bodily type to be classified? (A distinguished American critic stated that in his youth he was asthenic, later on he was athletic, and finally he became pyknic.) Kretschmer obviously did not take into account many other factors of importance, such as race, occupation, state of nutrition, etc., in analyzing his results, all these being important. Furthermore, only relatively few bodily types are definitely pyknic, asthenic or athletic, and the range of intermediate types is so confusing as to make it almost impossible to get any agreement on the classification of many individual cases.

For a discussion of the literature on this important matter, the reader is referred to the monograph of P. deQ. Cabot (64). The psychologists have not, as a whole, accepted the relationship of these body forms to normal type (65), and in general there has been a gradual *disregard* for the Kretschmer postulates and findings, although his terms have remained on the tongues of psychiatrists.

Much as my personal bias would lead me to accept Kretschmer's postulates, my rather skeptical point of view is as follows. The human being is essentially a mosaic of qualities, due to the Mendelian laws of inheritance, and so a man may have a very athletic pair of shoulders and a quite asthenic pair of legs. He may be pyknic so far as his face is concerned and possess an athletic torso. One sees very thin women with very large legs, and broad-shouldered men with defective asthenic jaws. Further, there is just as much of the mosaic in human personality, and rarely is there even an outward consistency and harmony. A man may be of a gigantic whole in his scientific and philosophic activities, like Bacon, and be a venial seeker of bribes in his more personal life. He may write loftily of the struggles of the human being and be a petty pretty-woman lover, like Goethe, or he may stir men's souls by sublime music and engage in trivial struggles for money and prestige, like Beethoven. Thus any separation of human beings into schizoid and cyclothymic or any dichotomy or triad or quartet of qualities has to be supplemented by so many in-between forms that the differentiation becomes quite hazy.

Nor have the classifications of bodily types by other workers helped us much. It is probably not in such crude matters as total or gross bodily form that we are to seek for the differentiating bodily structures which determine the liability of the individual to one mental disease or another. The constitutional vulnerability, which certainly seems to exist, will, I think, be found to rest in mechanisms too refined for our present day instrumentation. We may have to await that day when the analysis of emanating electric currents, the closer studies of chemical interchange, the rapidly evolving knowledge of the structures and chemistry of the brain and body will give us the illumination we seek.

Certain American workers (66) have quite logically approached the problem of the pre-psychotic personality from the social-psychological angle, rather than from the study of the corporeal types. Of these Hoch (67) developed the outstanding concept of the so-called "shut-in" personalities as basic for the development of dementia praecox. He describes the shut-in personality as "reticent, seclusive, (they) cannot adapt themselves to situations, are hard to influ-

ence, sensitive and stubborn (passively); they do not unburden their minds and have a tendency to live in a world of fancy." Hoch also speaks of the over-systematic, finicky individual of shallow emotion with abnormal insistence on precision and day-dreaming. This incubation period of personality alteration proceeds dynamically in some cases to dementia praecox; in other cases the individual remains odd and peculiar but may not reach the stage of an active psychosis.

Jelliffe (68) added to this concept in his study of predementia praecox. Meyer described all this as a lack of sense for the real, a tendency towards the mystical, fantastic, and probably also other factors of habit-deterioration, based largely on a psycho-biological trend towards evasion of situations and unhealthy biological adjustment (38).

The difficulty stressed by those other writers (69) who did not confirm Hoch's findings is the fact that the term "shut-in" means only a retreated personality. It is obvious that such a retreat may take place on many grounds, as fear of others, hatred for one's fellows, lack of interest, inferiority feeling, and so forth. Thus, the term "shut-in" depicts a *result* rather than an exclusive personality type.

I will briefly discuss one of the most important subjects in the field of psychiatry—the relationship of the mental diseases to heredity. Elsewhere I have summarized the world's literature on this subject (70). The polymorphic theory of the heredity of the mental diseases, sponsored by Esquirol (27) and Morel (71) and brought to its great climax by Lombroso (72), gave way to a study of the inheritance of the individual diseases, as classification appeared, and the laws of Mendel were transferred from the consideration of the characters of the pod of the pea to the explanation of the inheritance of the complex, obscure and poorly defined mental diseases. Although polymorphism has disappeared, no Mendelian laws of the inheritance of the psychoses have been validated, in spite of the valiant attempts made in those earlier enthusiastic days when it seemed possible to many to equate in nice mathematics the intricacies of the mental diseases. A concept that has not received the attention it deserves was given the name "blastophoria" by August Forel (73). Briefly defined, it states that the cells which transmit hereditary characters, like all other cells of the body, may become "sick" and transmit sick traits for several generations, and so there is a sick hereditary process. There is much evidence for this and kindred phenomena, for example, phenocopy (74), by which mutations are artificially produced which mimic hereditary characters. These theories of the origin of the mental diseases constitute my working hypothesis.

In truth, the separation of heredity and environment (75) is a fine example of the incorrigible tendency of the human being to make natural phenomena as separate, as dichotomic, as the abstract words used to delimit them. Since the mental diseases are amongst the most common afflictions of man, and the mind of man is probably the most easily disturbed of all human functions, whatever family group is studied long and intensively enough shows mental disease, and its denial means little or nothing. There are no negative family histories so far as mental disease is concerned, if one includes in the term "family" three generations in direct line and the collaterals extending to grand-aunts and uncles and first and second cousins. Schizophrenia, manic-depressive psychosis, and the kindred states occur in a sprinkle everywhere. In some unfortunate families the sprinkle changes to a shower, and we then speak of heredity.

A Personal Point of View

There is, I think, an essential psychopathological difference which has not been, so far as I know, emphasized or given weight, between the manic-depressive states and schizophrenia or dementia praecox. The typical reactions of schizophrenia relate to the attitude of the individual to The Others, and can be fairly called social anxiety and retreat. The averted gaze, the extreme passivity and the senseless resistance, the peculiar handshake on which Kraepelin laid so much emphasis, the feeling of reference, the delusion of persecution, the sense of being influenced and influencing, the depersonalization itself, all these are *social* reactions, based on an inadequacy of the individual to meet his fellows with ease, certainty and the maintenance of the feeling of self. And if sex has its hormones and its chemicals of activation and direction, it may well be that the social drives and directives also have their endocrinology and physiology.

The symptoms of manic-depressive psychosis are mainly related to the individual's feeling of well-being or the reverse, his good or bad estimate of himself based on his mood; and one can view all that happens in any clear-cut case in the light of a hypothesis which assumes that a disharmony in the shape of a plus or minus activity in the emotional and drive-creating mechanisms of the body exists.

The Neuroses and Thus, Pavlov

To attempt to bring into a limited discussion the vast field of the neuroses is a task doomed to failure in either completeness or even in essentials. Hysteria has been known and studied from time immemorial, and the classical studies of Charcot (21, 76) and the school of Nancy (77) gave incentive and direction to Janet (46) and Freud (78). Beard (79) gave the first coordinated approach to neurasthenia, Janet evolved the term psychasthenia with its complex and manifold implications and obscurities, and Freud, though his work has made it necessary for all psychiatrists to dig beneath the expressed into the reticent areas of the Self, has not succeeded in making psychoanalysis a therapeutic tool of real consequence, nor have we reached through his labors a proven psychopathology. Like Alexander the Great, his posthumous empire is rapidly splitting into hostile encampments. Meanwhile there arise new and magical names. Psychosomatics (80), which starts from the highly original basis that mental states affect the body, which is only as old as medicine itself, is rapidly burying, though unintentionally, consciousness and unconsciousness; complexes, Id, Ego and Superego in an avalanche of facts; and workers everywhere, whether they give or do not give homage to Freud, are delving (81) into the physiology of the neuroses and the direct effect of the emotions. And on the war fronts of the world (82), the shattered men who have succumbed to the devastations of anxiety, the dissociations of hysteria, and the void of amnesia are treated—sensibly, and in correspondence with a technique that knows not the subtleties of metaphor and symbols, but rests heavily on quiet, rest, reassurance, and a therapeutics which spares not those chemical shock absorbers, the sedatives, particularly sodium amytal. In the treatment of the acute war neuroses, an ounce of this barbiturate is worth a few tons of psychological analysis.

Moebius said somewhere that the "Urschleim of mental disease is the neurosis." Every important writer in psychiatry has noted the transition from what are called the neuroses to the psychoses. The distinction in many cases seems to be a matter of degree rather than of kind. Thus, if a man's fear of disease is governed by insight, he has a neurosis; but if his hypochondriasis reaches the stage where he develops somatic delusions, he has a psychosis. In other words, hypochondriasis in the one case is neurosis, and in the other psychosis, which is as if a lung infiltrated by tuberculosis but maintaining its integrity of function presented a different disease than that in which tuberculosis cause cavitation and destruction of function. Many recurrent neurasthenic states are merely mild forms of manic-depressive psychosis.

Everyone has seen the social-psychosomatic beginnings of schizophrenia (84). Anxiety states may come and go and never reach beyond the border of insight and control, and so remain neuroses. Then at the involutional period, the recurring attack first reaches grave proportions. Delusions appear for the first time, and lo, the neurosis becomes involutional melancholia. This is an absurdity from the nosological and from any relevant and coherent scientific point of view. The term psychosis is nowadays used, practically, as the equivalent of insanity. It ought to be discarded just as was the term insanity. We might then expect to speak of a neurasthenic state which, in certain phases, left the main functions of the personality intact, but in its evolution might invade the personality to the point of needing commitment. One often sees a patient discharged from a mental hospital with the diagnosis, No Psychosis, although the patient clearly has a mild manic-depressive condition. But since committability is out of the question, the term psychosis, in the opinion of the hospital authorities, cannot be used, since this *implies* committability.

The general idea of mind and body unity is as old as Plato; its application to the problems of human diseases is as recent as the brilliant work of Wolf and Wolff (85) on the creation of ulcers. The most important and most promising work on the experimental genesis of mental sickness we owe to the great Pavlov (86), to whom I now do homage because I believe that one good experiment is worth a dozen subtle theories piled dubiously and uncertainly. The technique evolved in Pavlov's conditioned reflex studies had as its most important outcome the artificial creation in animals of all kinds of mental states comparable to the depressive and anxiety states of man. The frustration of inherent and conditioned reactions, confusion in the choice of competing stimuli, and the artificial nature of the laboratory life lead to fatigue, restlessness, gastrointestinal disturbance, sexually ineffective conduct, insomnia and that destruction of desire and satisfaction, which in the case of man I have called anhedonia (83); and the afflicted dog, cat and sheep act and look as neurotic as any human beings. That this is a great milestone will be at once apparent to any experienced psychiatrist.

It is because I believe that in the closer study of the so-called neuroses we shall find the clue to the understanding and treatment of the major mental diseases that I acclaim the work of Pavlov and his pupils (87) as even greater in its significance and value to psychiatry than that of any other single man and his followers. Except for the verbal manifestations of human disease, one sees in the dog, the cat and the sheep the psychosomatic disorder of the neurasthenic, the suspicion and hostility of the paranoid, the aboulia and anhedonia of the psychasthenic, the psychomotor inertia of depression, and the retreat into the passivity and negativism of the schizophrenic . . . . Gradually gaining in momentum, experimental psychiatry is now a great reality and the prime basis for any biological science, namely, the controlled experiment, now appears as the hope of those who look beyond classification of the vaguely known, and analysis by means of metaphor and symbols, to a real science of psychiatry.

Epilogue. History has the deplorable habit of making ridiculous the acuity and discernment of the contemporaneous historian. I have the uneasy notion that when the history of psychiatry is written for the one hundred fiftieth anniversary of the American Psychiatric Association, the end of the era of therapeutic defeatism will be found to date from the time of the introduction of the shock treatments, and that the advent of these queer and rather barbaric additions to the "gentle" art of healing will mark the beginning of a real and much better therapeutics, which will in its turn lead to a new and better classification and a completer understanding. I think it quite likely that certain contemporary great names and theories will become curiosities, and that relatively new people, let us say, Sakel and Meduna, and Bini and Cerletti will have become the great of their era. And whatever the value of psychosurgery will turn out to be, its advent will also be hailed as a boldly conceived attack upon the problems of psychiatry (89).

BIBLIOGRAPHY

1. Meyer, Adolf. Fundamental concepts of dementia praecox. Brit. Med Jour., p. 757, Sept. 29, 1906.
2. Gibbs, F.A., Gibbs, E.L., and Lennox, W.G. The electroencephalogram in diagnosis and in localization of epileptic seizures. Arch. Neurol. and Psychiat., 36: 1225, 1936.
3. Charcot, J.M. OEuvres Complètes in 9 vols. Paris, 1885-1890.
——. The faith cure. New Review, Jan 1893.
——. La foi qui guérit. Arch. de Neur., Jan. 1893.
Charcot, J.M., and Richer, P. Contribution à L'étude de l'hypnotisme chez les hystériques, du phénomène de l'hyperexcitabilité neuro-musculaire. Arch. de Neur., 1881, 2.
4. Fournier, H. Syphilis secondaire tardive. Paris. 1906.
5. Nissl. Centralbl. f. Nervenheilk., 1904, s. 171. Histologische und histopathologische Arbeiten, etc. Herausgegeben von Nissl, Bd. i, 1904.
6. Alzheimer, A. Histologische Studien zur Differential Diagnose des Progressiven Paralyse. Hist. und Histopath. Arbeiten, 1904.
7. Noguchi. Serum diagnosis of syphilis. J.B. Lippincott Co., 1910.

Noguchi and Moore. Demonstrations of spiroschaeta pallida in brain cases of general paralysis. J. Exper. Med., 17:232, 1913.
8. MacDonald, C.A., and Taylor, E.W. Herpes zoster oticus. Arch. Neurol. and Psychiat., 25:601, 1931.
9. Erb. Die Krankheiten der peripheren-cerebrospinalen Nerven. Leipzig, F.C.W. Vogel, 1876.
——. Krankheiten des Rückenmarks und des verlängerten Marks. Leipzig, F.C.W. Vogel, 1878.
10. Westphal. Einige Beobachtungen bei der Salvarsanbehandlung im Garnisonlazarett Windhuk, Deutsch-Südwestafrika. Mün. 1912. In: Abhandl. über Salvarsan. Ehrlic, v.2.
11. Argyll-Robertson, P. Four cases of spinal myosis; with remarks on the action of light on the pupils. Edinb. Med. J., Dec 1869 and Feb. 1870.
12. Quincke. Korrespondenzblatt für Schweizer Arzte XII. Zur Kasuistik der Visceralsyphilis. Drei Fälle von Hirnsyphilis. Dtsch. Arch. f. Klin. Med., Bd. 77.
13. Nonne, Max. Syphilis of the nervous system.
14. Ayer, J.B., and Solomon, H.C. Examination of cerebrospinal fluid from different loci. The Human Cerebrospinal Fluid. Hoeber., 4:84, 1924.
15. Ehrlich, P. Abhandlungen über Salvarsan (Ehrlich-Hata-Präparat 606 gegen Syphilis). Gesammelt und mit einem Vorwort und Schlussbemerkungen herausgegeben Mün., 1911.
16. Jauregg, Wagner v. Mechanism of action of infection and fever therapy. Klin. Wschr., 15:481, 1935.
——.Treatment of general paresis by inoculation of malaria. J. Nerv. and Ment. Dis., 55:369, 1935.
——. Malaria therapy of general paresis and syphilitic infections of the nervous system. Rev. Neurol., 36:889, 1929.
17. Cowdry, E.V., Ed. Problems of ageing. 2d. ed. Baltimore, Williams & Wilkins Co., 1924.
18. Lombroso, C. Die Lehre von der Pellagra. Ätiologische, Klinische and Prophylaktische Untersuchungen. Unter Mitwirkung des Verfassers Deutsch herausgegeben von Hans Kurella. Berlin, 1898.
19. Goldberger, J. Relation of diet to pellagra. J.A.M A., 1617, June 3, 1992.
20. Emerson, H.W., Ed. Alcohol and man. The Macmillan Co., London, 1933.
21. Bloomberg, W. Treatment of chronic alcoholism with amphetamine (benzedrine) sulfate. New Eng. J. Med., 217:611, 1937.
Dayton, N.A. New facts on mental disorders. A study of 89,190 cases. Springfield, Ill.: C. C. Thomas Co., 1940.
Fleming, R. A psychiatric concept of acute alcoholic intoxication. Am. J. Psychiat., 92:89, 1935.
Jolliffe, N., Bowman, K. M., Roseblum, L.A., Fein, H.D. Nicotinic acid deficiency encephalopathy. J.A.M.A., 114:307, 1940.
Kirby, G.H. A study in race psychopathology. N.Y. State Hosp. Bull., New Series, 1:663, 1908.
Meyer, A. On parenchymatous systemic degenerations mainly in the central nervous system. Brain, 24:47, 1901.
Minot, G.R., Strauss, M.B., and Cobb, S. Alcoholic polyneuritis; dietary deficiency as a factor in its production. New Eng. J. Med., 208:1244, 1933.
Myerson, A. Alcohol. A study of social ambivalence. Quart. J. of Studies on Alco., 1:1, June, 1940.
Shattuck, G.C. The relation of beri-beri to poly-neuritis (Avitaminosis). Am. J. Trop. Med., 8:539, 1928.
Shimazono, J. B-Avitaminosis und Beri-beri. Er gebn. d. inn. Med. u. Kinderh., 39:1, 1931.
Spies, T.D., and DeWolf, H.F. Observations on the etiological relationship of severe alcoholism to pellagra. Am. J. Med. Sc., 186: 521, 1933.
Tillotson, K.J., and Fleming, R. Personality and sociologic factors in the prognosis and treatment of chronic alcoholism. New Eng. J. Med., 217:611, Oct. 1937.
Wechsler, I.S. Unrecognized cases of deficiency polyneuritis (avitaminosis). The Med. J. and Rec., 121:441, 1930.
22. Kraepelin, Emil. Psychiatrie. Leipzig, 1913.
——. Lectures on clinical psychiatry. Auth. trans., Rev. and Ed., T. Johnstone. New York, William Wood & Co., 1904.
——. Manic-depressive insanity and paranoia. Trans. by M. Barclay. Edinburgh, E. & S. Livingstone, 1921.
——. Dementia praecox and paraphrenia. Trans. by M. Barclay. Edinburgh, E. and S. Livingstone, 1919.
23. Whitwell, J.R. Historical notes on psychiatry. (Early times to end of the 16th century) Philadelphia, P. Blakiston's Son & Co., Inc., 1937.

24. Burton, Richard. Anatomy of melancholy. London, Chatto & Windus, 1907.

25. Rush, Benj. Medical Inquiries and Observations upon the Diseases of the Mind. Philadelphia, John Grigg, 1830.

26. Tuke, D.H., and Bucknill, J.C. A manual of psychological medicine, containing the lunacy laws, the nosology, the etiology, and treatment of insanity. With an appendix of cases. Philadelphia, Lindsay and Blakiston, 1874, 3d ed.

27. Esquirol, E. Mental maladies. A treatise on insanity. Trans. by E.M. Hunt. Philadelphia, Lea & Blanchard, 1845.

28. Morel, B.A. Traité des maladies mentales. Paris, Librairie Victor Masson, 1860.

29. Pinel, Ph. Traité medico-philosophique sur l'aliénation mentale. Paris, J. Ant. Brosson, 1809.

30. Spurzheim, J.G. Observations on the deranged manifestations of the mind, or insanity. London, Baldwin, Cradock, and Joy, 1817.

31. Lombroso, C. Le nuovo conquiste della psichiatria. ed. 2. Torino, J. Vigliardi, 1887.

32. Mendel, E. Leitfäden der psychiatrie für studirende der medicin. Stuttgart, Ferdinand Enke, 1902.

33. Burrows, S.A. Commentaries on the causes, forms, symptoms and treatment of insanity. 252. London, 1828.

34. Farrar, C.B. Some origins in psychiatry. Am. J. Insan., 64:3, Jan., 1908; 65:1, July, 1908; 66:2, Oct. 1909.

35. Bleuler, Eugen. Textbook of psychiatry. Trans. by Dr. A.A. Brill, New York, The Macmillan Co., 1903.

36. Meyer, A. An attempt at analysis of the neurotic constitution. Am. J. Psychol., 14:90, 1903.

37. Schizophrenia (dementia praecox). Assoc. for Research in Nerv. and Ment. Dis., Vol. V., 1925. New York, Paul B. Hoeber, Inc.

Schizophrenia (dementia praecox). Assoc. for Research in Nerv. and Ment. Dis., Vol. X., 1931. Baltimore: Williams and Wilkins Co.

Manic-depressive psychosis. Assoc. for Research in Nerv. and Ment. Dis., Vol. XI., 1931. Baltimore, Williams and Wilkins Co.

38. Meyer, A. Fundamental concepts of dementia praecox. Brit. Med. J., 757, Sept. 29, 1906.

39. Lugaro, Ernesto. Modern problems in Psychiatry. Trans. by D. Orr and R.G. Rows. Manchester, University Press, 1909.

40. Dreyfus, G.L. Die melancholie, ein zustandsbild des manischdepressiven irreseins. Jena, Gustave Fischer, 1907.

41. Fitzgerald, O.W.S. Experiences in the treatment of depressive states by electrically induced convulsions. J. Ment. Sci., 89:73, Jan. 1943.

Gonda, W.E. Treatment of mental disorders with electrically induced convulsions. Dis. Nerv. Sys., 2:3, March 1941.

Lowenbach, Hans. Electric shock treatment of mental disorders. N. Caro. Med. J., 4:4, April 1943.

Myserson, A. Experience with electric-shock therapy in mental disease. New Eng. J. Med., 224: 1081, 1941.

Nussbaum, Kurt. Observations on electric shock treatment. Psychiat. Quat., 17:327, April 1943.

42. Prince, Morton. The dissociation of a personality. New York, Longman, Green & Co., 1913.

——. Association neuroses. J. Nerv and Ment. Dis., May 1891.

43. Sidis, Boris. The causation and treatment of psychopathic disorders. Boston, Richard G. Badger, 1916.

——. Symptomatology, psychognosis and diagnosis of psychopathic diseases. Boston, Richard G. Badger, 1914.

44. Jung, C. G. Über die psychologie der dementia praecox. Halle a S., Carl Marhold, 1907.

——. Collected papers on abnormal psychology. Auth. Trans. by C.E. Long. 2d ed., New York, Moffat, Yard and Co., 1917.

45. Adler, Alfred. The neurotic constitution. Outlines of a comparative individualistic psychology and psychotherapy. Auth. Trans.: B. Glueck and J.E. Lind. New York, Moffat, Yard and Co., 1921.

46. Janet, Pierre. La médecine psychologique. Paris, Ernest Flammarion, 1923.

——. Neuroses and psychoses. In A Psychiatric Milestone. Bloomingdale Hospital Cent., 1821-1921, printed by the Society of the New York Hosp., pp. 119-246, 1921.

——. Psychological healing. A historical and clinical study. Trans. by E. and C. Paul. New York, Macmillan Co., 1925.

47. Dejerine and Gauchler. Psychoneuroses and psychotherapy. Trans. by S.E. Jelliffe. Ed. 2, Philadelphia, 1913.

48. Krafft-Ebing, R.v. Lehrbuch der psychiatrie. Auf klinischer grundlage für praktische ärzte und studirende. Vierte theilweise umgearbeitete auflage. Stüttgart, Ferdinand Enke, 1890.

49. Ellis, Havelock. Studies in the psychology of sex. 1900-1928.

50. Freud, S. Autobiography. Transl. by James Strachey. New York, W.W. Norton & Co., Inc., pp. 46-47, 1935.

51. Coriat, I.H. The hysteria of Lady Macbeth. New York, Moffat, Yard & Co., 1912.

52. Menninger, K.A. Organic suicide. Bull. of the Menninger Clin., 1:5, May 1937.

53. Jastrow, J. The house that Freud built. New York, Greenberg, 1932.

Zilboorg, G., and Henry, G.W. A history of medical psychology. New York, W.W. Norton & Co., Inc., 1941.

54. Myerson, A. The social anxiety neurosis—Its possible relationship to schizophrenia (To be published.)

55. Sakel. Zur entstehung der medikamentösen schocktherapie der schizophrenie. Wien. med. Wschr., 1937, 87:1108.

56. Meduna. Die Knovulsionstherapie der schizophrenie. Psychiat. neur. Wschr., 1935, 37: 317.

57. Bini. L. Experimental researches on epileptic attacks induced by electric current. Am. J. Psychiat. (supp.), 94: 172, 1938.

58. Cerletti, U., and Bini, L. L'ettroschock. Arch. gen. di. neurol., psichiat. e psicoanal, 19:266, 1938.

59. Lotze, Hermann. Microcosmus. New York, Scribner and Welford, 1886.

60. Pearl, Raymond. Constitution and health. London, Kegan Paul, Trench, Trübner and Co., Ltd., 1933.

——. The experimental modification of germ cells. J. Exper. Zool., 22:125, 1917.

61. Draper, George. Human constitution. A consideration of its relationship to disease. W.B. Saunders Co., Philadelphia, 1924.

62. Meyer, A. Anatomical facts and clinical varieties of traumatic insanity. Am. J. Insan., 60:373, 1904.

63. Kretschmer, Ernest. Textbook of Medical Psychology. London, Oxford Univ. Pres., 1934.

——. Heredity and constitution in the etiology of psychiatric disorders. Brit. Med. J., 2:403, 1937.

64. Cabot, P.S. de Q. The relationship between characteristics of personality and physique in adolescents. Genetic Psych. Mono., 1938, 20:3.

65. Stockard, C. The physical basis of personality. New York, W.W. Norton & Co., 1931.

Bauer, J. Vorlesungen über allgemeine konstitutions and vererbunglehre. Springer, 1921.

66. Campbell, Macfie. Modern concepts of dementia praecox. Rev. of Neur. and Psychiat., Vol 7. 1909.

Bolton, J. Amentia and dementia. A clinicopathological study. J. Ment. Sci., 53:223, 1907.

Kahn. Potentiality for change in personality. Am. J. Psychiat., 12:3, 1932.

67. Hoch, A. Constitutional factors in the dementia praecox group. Rev. Neur. and Psychiat., 8:463, 1910.

——. A study of mental make-up in the functional psychoses. J. Nerv. and Ment. Dis., 36:230, April 1909.

68. Jelliffe, S.E. Predementia praecox; the hereditary and constitutional factors of the dementia praecox make-up. J. Nerv. and Ment. Dis., 38: Jan. 1911.

69. Bowman, K. Study of pre-psychotic personality in certain psychoses. Am. J. Orthopsychiat., 4:473, Oct. 1934.

70. Myerson, A. The inheritance of mental diseases. Baltimore, Williams & Wilkins Co., 1925.

——. Chairman, Eugenical sterilization. A reorientation of the problem. The Comm. of the Am. Neur. Assoc. for the investigation of eugenical sterilization. New York, The Macmillan Co., 1936.

71. Morel. Traite des dégénerescences physiques, morales et intellectuelles de l'espèce humaine. Paris, 1860.

72. Lombroso, C. Men of genius. London, Walter Scott, 1891.

73. Forel, A. Alkohol und keimzellen. Munch. Med. Wschr., 58:2596, 1911.

——. Abstinenz oder mässigkeit, Grenzfragen Nerv-und Seelenlebens, H. 74, 1910.

74. Goldschmidt, R. "Progressive heredity" and "anticipation." J. Hered., 29:140, 1938.

75. Jennings, H.S. Biological basis of human nature. New York, W.W. Norton & Co., 1930.

76. Charcot, J.M. Lecons sur l'hystérie chez l'homme. Prog. med., May 2, 1885.

77. Richer, Paul. Etudes Cliniques sur l'Hystéro-Epilepsie ou Grande Hystérie. Paris, A. Delahaye et E. Lecrosnier, 1881.

78. Freud, Sigmund. Collected papers, Trans. by J. Riviere. The International Psychoanalytic Press. New York, London, Paris. In four volumes, 1924. (It is futile to cite any one publication. The reader is referred to the collected papers, to the books in which psychoanalytic theory is developed, to the interesting little monograph called his "Autobiography," and to the psychoanalytic literature in general, as well as Zilboorg's History (53).)

79. Beard, G. Practical treatise on nervous exhaustion. 1880.

——. American Nervousness. New York, G.P. Putnam's Sons, 1881.

80. Dunlap, K. Elements of scientific psychology. St. Louis, 1922.

Masserman, J.H. Behavior and neurosis. An experimental psychoanalytic approach to psychobiologic principles. Chicago, University Press, 1943.

Myerson, A. Psychosomatic disorders. War. Med., 1:404, 1941.

Shilder, P. The somatic basis of the neurosis. J. Nerv. and Ment. Dis., 70:502, 1929.

Weiss, E., and English, O.S. Psychosomatic medicine. The clinical application of psychopathology to general medical problems. Philadelphia and London, W.B. Saunders Co., 1943. (An excellent bibliography.)

81. Cobb, S. The diagnosis of neurasthenia. Practitioner, Ap., 1913.

——. Neurasthenia, its causes and treatment. Practitioner, Aug. 1915.

——. Manual of neurasthenia, New York, 1920. Dunbar, F. Emotions and Bodily Disease. 2nd ed. Columbia University Press, 1938.

Finesinger, J.E., Sutherland, G.F., and McGuire, F.F. The positive conditional salivary reflex in psychoneurotic patients. Am. J. Psychiat., 99:61, 1942.

Macfarlane, D.A. The rôle of kinesthesis in maze learning. University of California Publ. Psychol., 4:227, 1930.

82. Ebaugh, F.G., and Johnson, G.S. The literature on military psychiatry since 1938. Am. J. Med. Sci., 201:6, 1941.

Pegge, G. Psychiatric casualties in London, September, 1940. Brit. Med. J., p. 553, Oct. 26. 1940.

Sargent, W. Treatment of war neuroses. Lancet, 240:107, 1941.

——. Modified insulin therapy in war neuroses. Lancet, 241:212, Aug. 1941.

Wilson, H. War strain. Its manifestations and treatment. The Institute of Living Abstracts. Brit. War Psych., 20:25.

The Psychiatric Toll of Warfare. Fortune, 27:141, Dec. 1943.

83. Myerson, A. Anhedonia. Am. J. of Psychiat., 79:1, July, 1922.

84. Bleuler. Primäre und sekundäre symptome der schizophrenie. Ztschr. f. d. ges. Neurol. u. Psychiat., 124:607, 1930.

Meyer, A. The relation of psychogenic disorders to deterioration. J. Nerv. and Ment. Dis., 34:113, 1907.

85. Wolf, S., and Wolff, H.G. Gastric mucosa, "gastritis," and ulcer. Am J. Digestive Dis., 10: 23, Jan. 1943.

86. Pavlov. I.P. Conditioned reflexes; an investigation of the physical activities of the cerebral cortex. Trans. by G.V. Anrep. London, Oxford University Press, 1927.

——. Lectures on conditioned reflexes. New York, International Publishers, 1928.

——. Neuroses in man and animals. J.A. M.A., 99:1012, 1932.

——. Experimentally produced neurosis and its cure in the weak nervous type. Acta psychiat. et neurol., 8:123, 1933.

——. Essai d'une interprétation physiologique de la paranoia et de la névrose obsessionnelle. Encephalé, 30:881, 1935.

——. Conditioned reflexes and psychiatry. New York, International Publishers, 1941.

87. Cook. S.W. The production of "experimental neuroses" in the white rat. Psychosom. Med., 1:293, April 1939.

Damrau, F. Experimentally induced neuroses in guinea pigs. Med. Rec., April 1940.

Dimmick, F.L., Ludlow, N., and Whiteman, A. A study of "experimental neurosis" in cats. J. Compar. Psychol., 28:39, 1939.

Gantt, W.H. The origin and development of nervous disturbances experimentally produced. Am. J. Psychiat., 98: 475, 1942.

Liddell, H.S., Sutherland, G.F., Parmenter, R., and Bayne, T.L. A study of the conditioned reflex method for producing experimental neurosis. Am. J. Physiol., 116:95, 1936.

88. Myerson, A. The attitude of neurologists, psychiatrists and psychologists towards psychoanalysis. Am. J. Psychiat., 96:3, Nov. 1939 [reprinted in this sesquicentennial anniversary supplement of the *Journal*].

89. Freeman, W., and Watts, J.W. Psycho-surgery. Intelligence emotion and social behavior following prefrontal lobotomy for mental disorders. Springfield, Ill., Baltimore, Charles C. Thomas, 1942.

Moniz, E. Les possibilités de la chirurgie dans le traitement de certaines psychoses, Lisboa méd. 13:141-151, March 1936.

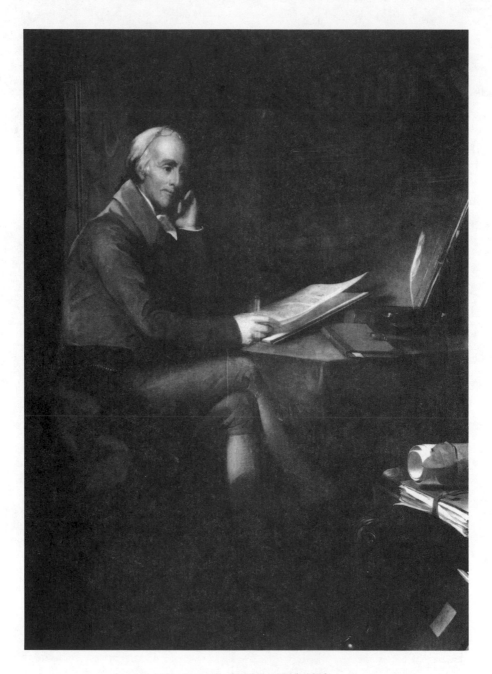

Benjamin Rush, M.D., 1745–1813
"The Father of American Psychiatry"

Benjamin Rush and American Psychiatry

By Clifford B. Farr, M.D.

Psychiatrist, Institute of Pennsylvania Hospital, Philadelphia

PART I

THE BASIS FOR HIS TRADITIONAL POSITION
AS PATRON OF THE AMERICAN PSYCHIATRIC ASSOCIATION

Probably no man in American medicine has been, and continues to be, more frequently commemorated in medical literature than Dr. Benjamin Rush. The reasons for this are sufficiently obvious, since the beginning of his medical career coincided with the birth pains of this Republic and he himself was one of a few enthusiastic spirits who, from the first, advocated independence.[1] The same radical spirit which inspired his politics urged him on to medical and social reforms and innovations, while his multifarious interests and versatile talents (typical of the leaders of that age) led him to explore many, at that time, untrodden paths. He was, strictly speaking, not a medical pioneer, for he and his contemporaries were the product of one hundred and fifty years of Colonial medicine and even in psychiatry Thomas Bond had inspired the foundation of the Pennsylvania Hospital (partly, if not mainly, with a view to the care of "lunaticks") before Rush had reached school age. Nevertheless, Rush stands out as the Founder of our national school of medicine by virtue of his teaching (his pupils numbered approximately three thousand), his voluminous publications, and his longevity (for he survived the Revolution by thirty years).

His schoolmate, John Morgan, actual founder of the first medical school (in the narrower sense) barely survived the Colonial period (1789). Rush introduced new ideas and novel practices into general medicine and into almost all its branches, and gave psychiatry preeminence in his teaching and writing. His medical interests included balneology, climatology, epidemiology, gerontology, ethics of the profession, military and legal medicine, physio- and occupational-therapy, and he is hailed as a pioneer by obstetricians, pediatricians (Ruhräh), tuberculosis specialists, veterinarians, etc. He dabbled in anthropology, ethnology, psychology and sociology. In the latter field he tackled all five forms of what Southard later called "The Kingdom of Evils"[2] (Morbi, Errores, Vitia, Litigia, Penuriae) with reforming zeal.

He was a founder of the American Anti-Slavery Society and a consistent advocate of the social rights of freedmen. He initiated the anti-alcoholic crusade in 1783 and for this reason the W.C.T.U., a century later, erected a commemorative tablet in front of his tomb in Christ Church Cemetery in Philadelphia. He also advocated establishments for the cure of alcoholism, a measure even yet inadequately realized. In penology he worked for prison reform and the abolition of cruel and unusual punishments, including the death penalty. In education (like H.G. Wells in our day) he deprecated the study of the classics, and urged advanced study for women. In both instances, being in advance of his times, he merely succeeded in arousing prejudices. He was active in promoting the establishment of public schools (one of his fruitful efforts), and suggested a national university for training public servants (an unfulfilled dream). He actually was one of the founders of Dickinson College, and his services to medical teaching are well known. In the latter field his influence was in some respects equivocal. His own lectures were brilliant and inspiring but imposed the paralysing idea of "principles" on the medicine of the succeeding generation which tended to discourage unbiassed observation and experiment; he also, despite or because of his own long apprenticeship, advocated a short medical course as sufficient, in view of the relatively few facts to be taught and the ability to *deduce* details from principles.[3] Possibly, in this instance, he also felt the need of furnishing an adequate number of American trained physicians for the rapidly expanding young nation.

This incomplete list of his medical and scientific activities may be supplemented by reference to his pioneer efforts as a teacher of chemistry and physiology, and to his numerous publications on most of the above mentioned topics. (He wrote the first American textbook on chemistry.) He also, as will be mentioned later, edited several medical classics. It is only natural in view of his many-sided interests that some of his contributions, aside from any defects due to personal bias, are not very profound; for he would never allow himself to be stumped. The following quotation from a student's note-book[4] is illuminating: "In all controversial points I feel a diffidence; but lest silence should be con-

---

1 Holmes, O.W. Medical Essays. Riverside Press, Boston, 1889. (Currents and counter-currents in medical science, 1860.) P. 180 "If we come to our own country, who can fail to recognize that B.R., the most conspicuous of American Physicians, was the intellectual offspring of the movement which produced the Revolution. 'The same hand,' says one of his biographers, 'which subscribed to the declaration of the political independence of these States, accomplished their emancipation from medical systems formed in foreign countries, and wholly unsuitable to the state of disease in America.'"
2 Southard, E.E., and Jarrett, Mary C. The Kingdom of Evils. Macmillan, New York, 1922.
3 In a sense Rush's idea is still valuable; *e.g.*, Barcroft in a recent (1938) book on Physiological Function says "Now the student is given principles," formerly "he was only given facts."

strued into cowardice, I will risk an opinion." Again—Dr. Holmes (*l.c.*, I, p. 192) "Dr. Rush must have been a charming teacher, as he was an admirable man. He was observing, rather than a sound observer; eminently observing, curious, even, about all manner of things."

In this survey of his activities, his ten years immersion in public affairs,[5] detrimental as he felt it was to his medical practice, must not be forgotten. Sincere advocate of the rights of the underprivileged, perhaps in part a reflection of his work among the poor, and convinced republican, he was an early and assiduous pamphleteer (under assumed names) for independence, and incited others, and particularly Thomas Paine, to more ambitious attempts (*e.g.*, the booklet: "Common Sense"). His passion for anonymity, partly motivated by fear of injuring his practice, was later to get him into difficulties with Washington. He was a member of the Continental Congress (1776), an organizer on its behalf of war time industries, and a Signer of the Declaration of Independence. He was active in securing the adoption of the National Constitution both in state and nation, and later in life in reforming the Constitution of Pennsylvania. He was surgeon of the Pennsylvania Navy and later Surgeon General of the Middle Department of the Continental Army. The latter position involved him, as well as Morgan, in a controversy with Shippen because of the latter's alleged maladministration. In his last years, long after his retirement from active political life, he became (by appointment of President Adams) Director of the Mint. It is of interest that one of Rush's sons, Richard, whose biography has recently been published,[6] followed the law, went into political and diplomatic life and held almost every appointive office in the gift of a President, in five or six successive administrations. Three sons continued his medical interests. One of the latter, James, endowed the Ridgway Library (Philadelphia Library Company), which now houses the Rush archives.

Rush has long been considered the peculiar Patron Saint of American psychiatry and his scholarly angular visage adorns the banner, stationery and occasionally the annual buttons of this Association.[7] The actual value of his contribution to our specialty, in spite of the multiplicity of biographical articles, has seldom been weighed, and even then too much emphasis has been laid on his treatise of 1812 (*v.i.*), the more reasoned parts of which are entirely obsolete, and too little on his actual practice and teaching. A true estimate of his place in American psychiatry will depend on an analysis of his heritage (political and religious), his education, his environment, his talents, his character and achievements. His personality was complex and compound of incongruous elements. The hundredth anniversary of the Association seems an appropriate time to attempt such an estimate.

But before going further it will be well to refer to the sources, primary and secondary, including in the latter category many of the brief biographical sketches, most of which are laudatory, some equivocal, and a few frankly antagonistic.

In this age of the popular biography, romantic, candid, witty or even sardonic, for which Maurois, Ludwig and Strachey have set the pattern, only two extended biographies, those of Good[8] and Goodman,[9] have appeared, the former dealing mainly with his services to education; neither of them by physicians. Both are adequate and conscientious performances, but lack the qualities above mentioned, which might have illuminated some of the obscure phases of his career and enlivened the narratives. Both biographies have complete, critical bibliographies, which are extremely useful. Rush's own Memorial (a) with extracts from his Common Place Book (b),[10] his Selected Letters,[11] and his Collected Works[12] are the best and most available original sources in print, and the ones upon which I have mainly depended. The Philadelphia Library Company in its Ridgway building has an extensive file of his voluminous notes and correspondence and miscellaneous private papers. The Library of the College of Physicians contains all or almost all his medical writings, many series of notes taken by his students, as well as other data. Other Philadelphia institutions, including the Pennsylvania Hospital and the University of Pennsylvania, house valuable original material.

The minor biographies of Rush have a remarkable similarity and are probably all based on his own Memorial (*l.c.*, 10(a)). That of Packard[13] has been called the most authoritative; that of Mills[14] gives the best account of his psychiatric accomplishments.[15] Mills includes a chronological chart of his life to which readers may be referred. This will

---

4 Library of College of Physicians (Griffith, 1797)

5 He was involved, off and on, for twenty years. After the organization of the government his sympathies were with the "Republicans."

6 Powell, J.H. Richard Rush, Republican Diplomat. Univ. of Penna. Press, Phila. 1942.

7 Proceedings of Am. Psychiat. Assoc., June 2, 1921. Dr. Brush moved that the button with picture of "our psychiatric progenitor" . . . . "be adopted as the emblem of the Association." Unanimously carried. Am. J. Psychiat., 78:259, 1921-22. This "picture" is the Haines' engraving (1805), *ibid.*, 106-107. The Sully portrait, spectacles on brow, is more usual.

8 Good, H.G., Ph.D. Benjamin Rush & his Service to American Education, Bluffton, Ohio, Am. Educator Co., 1918.

9 Goodman, N.G. Benjamin Rush, Physician & Citizen, Univ. of Penna. Press, Phila., 1934.

10 A Memorial—of Dr. Benjamin Rush—written by himself (a)—*also* extracts from his Commonplace Book (b)—etc. Published privately—by L.A. Biddle, Lanorie, 1905. (Subsequently referred to as 10(a) or 10(b).)

Note.—The collections of Alexander Biddle, descendant of Rush, who died in 1898, were sold in New York in May, Oct. and Nov., 1943. The MS. of the "Memorial" was acquired by the American Philosophical Society.

11 Benjamin Rush Old Family Letters—Series A & B.-Privately printed for Alexander Biddle, Phila., 1902, contain correspondence with wife Julia, and with John Adams respectively.

12 Rush, Benjamin. Medical Inquiries and Observations, 2nd Ed., 4 vols. Conrad, Phila., 1805.

Essays, Literary, Moral and Philosophical, 2nd Ed. Bradford, Phila., 1806.

Introductory Lectures to courses—on Institutes and Practice of Medicine, (also) two lectures on the pleasures of the senses and of the mind. Bradford & Innskeep, Phila., 1811.

Medical Inquiries and Observations on Diseases of the Mind, Kimber and Richardson, Phila., 1812 (other Editions: 1818, '27, '30, '35).

The great variety of topics treated can only be appreciated by reading the subjects of the inquiries, essays and lectures—too numerous to cite here.

13 Dict. of Am. Med. Biog., Kelly & Burrage, pp. 1066-69 (Rush, B., by Packard, F.R.).

14 Mills, Chas. K., Benjamin Rush & American Psychiatry, Medico-Legal J., 4:238-273, 1886-7.

15 Dr. J.H. Lloyd was a stout defender of Rush's psychiatric record.

allow me to discuss his character and achievements, untrammelled by time sequences.

PART II

RUSH'S CHARACTER AND ATTAINMENTS—HIS POSITION AS PHYSICIAN AND SCIENTIST—FORMATIVE INFLUENCES

Rush's attitude as a thinker and man of science was more profoundly influenced by his family tradition and ideology and by his upbringing than was that of many of his great contemporaries and associates, of whom I might cite Franklin, Priestley and Jefferson and, by the same token, less by the rationalistic spirit of the age (eighteenth century). He was pious in the old Roman sense, in his reverence for his ancestors, as exemplified in a genuinely sentimental letter to John Adams (l.c., 10(a)). This concerns a visit to his birthplace at Byberry[16] near Philadelphia, whither his immigrant ancestor, late in life, had come in 1683 to share Penn's Holy Experiment after having, in youth, fought valiantly under Cromwell, as a troop captain, against royal pretensions; in the end in vain. This ancestor and succeeding generations (Rush was fifth in line) were "pious folk"—mostly "Quakers and Baptists," farmers, and later also gunsmiths. The "dissenting" spirit characterized Rush early in life, though he was actually baptized in the Anglican communion (Christ Church), but the political ideals of his ancestor lay latent in his mind (aside from a brief explosion at the time of the stamp acts) until aroused by a fellow student at Edinburgh, who shared a similar Cromwellian tradition. From that moment he was a convinced republican (l.c., 10(a)). One of the most thrilling moments of his life was his visit to the aged William Cromwell, who remembered clearly his great uncle Richard, son and successor of the Protector Oliver. Thus two generations spanned the interval from the beginning of the Commonwealth to the onset of the American Revolution! It was characteristic of the cautious Rush, that he did not disclose his convictions, at this time, to an unsympathetic world. I might interpolate that in his subsequent life there was always a certain ambivalence between his desire for the approval and support of the conventional and well-to-do classes, to whom he was more and more drawn by common tastes and pursuits (and with whom his family became assimilated), and his championship of novel and radical ideas, ideas which antagonized pet prejudices and endangered material interests. Revolutionary politics, subversive medical doctrines, antislavery and antialcoholic activities, army (medical) reform and similar crusades earned him more bitter enemies than his personal charm, friendliness and broad culture could gain him friends. In combat he was impatient of delay, denunciatory (yet supersensitive), rigid, uncompromising, and in at least one instance sardonic. Thus, in his controversy with the College of Physicians over the yellow fever epidemic of 1793, he coupled his resignation with the presentation of the works of Sydenham, his authority on this topic. Nevertheless, he insisted that he never cherished any personal enmity and it is a fact that some of those whom he had denounced most bitterly in the heat of controversy called him to attend them in their last illnesses, e.g., Provost Smith, Professor Joseph Woodhouse and even Edward Shippen, Jr. Nevertheless, he did not forget and paid them left-handed tributes in his diary. The following examples are from his journal (l.c., 10(b), 192) 1808, July 11, "died—aged seventy-two years, Dr. William Shippen"—"He had talents but which from disuse became weak"—"He was to indolent to write, to read and even to think"—"with the stock of knowledge he acquired when young"—he maintained some rank "especially as a teacher of Anatomy, in which he was eloquent, luminous, and pleasing"—"I attended him in his last illness." (Ibid., p. 195):1805, June 5, Notes death of Dr. James Woodhouse whom he attended and gives an account of his character. "He was a neat experimenter but was adverse from principles [Italics mine.] in chemistry"—"His lectures contained nothing but facts" [Italics mine.]—"a rude infidel"—"manners gross and vulgar"—"He was my pupil"—"I procured him his professorship." He was "ungrateful"—"the most indecent" among my enemies but "I never resented his behavior." "He spoke ill of everybody" was "intemperate for several years"—"He scouted the utility of medicine upon all occasions." A letter to Adams written in 1812 (l.c., 9, p. 126) lumps all these latent hates in a striking paragraph:

> I thank God my destiny in the world of spirits to which I am hastening is not to be determined by slave holders, old tories, Latin and Greek schoolmasters, Judges who defend Capital punishment, Philadelphian physicians, persecuting Clergymen nor yet by General Washington. All of whom I have offended only by attempting to lessen the misery and ignorance of my fellow men.

I may explain that Rush, justifiably disturbed by the abuses in the medical department, which Washington (then at Valley Forge), engrossed with overwhelming difficulties, and characteristically loyal to his subordinate Shippen, did nothing to correct, wrote a compromising but unsigned letter to his friend Patrick Henry. Governor Henry turned the letter over to Washington who, recognizing the handwriting, was never afterwards able to reconcile Rush's secret denunciations with "his suave and ingratiating" manner towards him. For Washington's character was as simple and straightforward as Rush's was complex and devious. Outwardly they remained on friendly terms. Rush could never forgive himself for his indiscretion, nor Washington for not absolving him from blame. He subsequently went to great pains to have passages in this letter expunged from Marshall's Life of Washington, as a result a half page of stars!

It is curious that in his catalogue of hates he does not mention William Cobbett who under the pseudonym of Peter Porcupine satirized his treatment of the yellow fever unmercifully in a Philadelphia newspaper and subsequently in special publications such as The Rush Light.[17] Perhaps

---

16 The home farm, sold by Benjamin's father when he moved his family to Philadelphia, still stands in large part unaltered. See frontispiece of Goodman's biography (l.c., 9). It is not far from the Philadelphia State Hospital, locally known as Byberry.
17 Clark, M.E. Peter Porcupine in America. Dissert., Univ. of Penna., Philadelphia, 1939.

Rush's chagrin was in this instance salved by damages of $5,000 which he obtained from the offender in 1797. Cobbett's satire dealt with medical matters[18] but had a political motive, as his *Federalist* employers wished to discredit a well known Democrat. Cobbett was later to become England's best known political pamphleteer ("Political Register" and "Rural Rides"), a master of the language of invective.

As I have said his religious and ethical ideas were fixed at an early date. His father died when the boy was six and his strong minded, deeply religious mother not only supported the family, but provided Benjamin and his brother Jacob (subsequently a member of the Supreme Court of Pennsylvania) with a sound classical and religious education at the Nottingham (now West Nottingham) Academy in Maryland. This Presbyterian school had recently been established by her brother-in-law, the Rev. Samuel Finley, an enlightened educator, who afterwards became the President of the College of New Jersey (Princeton). This basic training was supplemented by several terms at Princeton where he completed his rather narrow academic education, in which, however, ethics and Calvinistic theology, had not been overlooked, before he was sixteen. Rush remained deeply religious throughout life, but his denominational ties were always light, and were severed and reunited, because of passing antagonisms or changing opinions. At Princeton he learned to note down in a book striking passages from his reading, to which he later added comments on men and events, as well as original ideas and observations. This Commonplace Book as he called it was meticulously kept for the remainder of his life, and, with other notes, was the foundation for many of his papers. His motto was "*Studium sine Calamo Somnium*"; rendered by J.C. Wilson: "To study without the pen is to dream."[19] Alluding to the same note-taking habit Rush said: "Ideas, whether acquired from books or by reflection, produce a plethora of the mind which can only be removed by depletion from the pen or tongue" (*ibid.*) (a reference of course to his favorite form of therapy).

On graduation Rush, at first inclined to study law, was advised by Finley to avoid the "temptations of the bar" and to study "Physick" instead. He therefore apprenticed himself to the severe, but just, Dr. John Redman and "continued constantly in [his] master's family and shop," keeping the accounts, "preparing and compounding medicines, visiting the sick and performing many little offices of a nurse to them" (*l.c.*, 10(a)). He attended lectures by Shippen and Morgan (just launching the medical school) and "was admitted to see the practice of five other physicians," besides Redman's own, in the Pennsylvania Hospital. His association with this hospital continued with intermissions for fifty years. His spare time was devoted to the study of Hippocrates (whom he translated at this time), Sydenham and Boerhaave (Van Swieten). He took no recreation except his favorite alternation of writing and reading, and missed

only eleven days in five and a half years. Here was confirmed his habit of untiring industry and devotion to professional duties during working hours and his utilization of free periods for study, meditation and writing, which characterized the balance of his life. He and Redman remained devoted friends till the latter's death at an advanced age, only five years before Rush's own. Lest we receive too grim an impression we must recollect that he was later a pioneer in emphasizing the value of exercise for the maintenance or restoration of health. He made an elaborate therapeutic classification of exercises, even including the game of golf, which he had observed in Scotland. His favorite exercise was horseback riding, which preference was possibly motivated by its usefulness in his practice. In old age he derived much pleasure from his farm ("Sydenham") in the suburbs (now Fifteenth and Columbia Avenue), subsequently the favorite residence of his widow (died, 1848) and of his son Richard (died, 1859).

At Edinburgh, where he studied from November 1766 to September 1768, he was a favorite student of Cullen and had exceptional contacts with Scotch theologians, historians and philosophers—including Witherspoon, Robertson and Hume. (Incidentally, after others had failed, he was able to persuade Witherspoon to accept the presidency of "Princeton," a side light on the serious character of the youth.) He became thoroughly indoctrinated with the Scotch gift, undoubtedly a natural product of Calvinism, of reasoning from a few well established truths, principles or facts and by their aid deducing needed details, or testing new observations. This Aristotelian rather than Baconian method simplified medicine, in itself a valuable service, and helped to clear away a mass of classical and mediaeval dross as well as some gold. It is not the usual method of modern science. Rush's master, Cullen,[20] was a brilliant clinician and reasoner, and at a time when the anatomy and physiology of the cerebrum was scarcely known, correctly deduced the coordinating function of the brain from the then but recently differentiated functions of the sensory and motor nerves. Cullen, as well as Boerhaave earlier, and Rush and others later, erected elaborate systems of medicine, based on principles or dogmas, which were at best half-truths. Homeopathy is the only system of this sort which has persisted, even in name, to our own day. Rush, in his preface to the American edition of Sydenham[21] condemned his favorite hero's distrust of general principles, and his dependence on observation alone, in modern eyes his greatest merits. Incidentally, Sydenham's bizarre theory of epidemics ("constitution of the year") was Rush's greatest stumbling block. (Introductory lectures, *l.c.* (12), p. 45.) In addition, Rush felt it necessary to carry a theological load, as if the "Deity" required his assistance against the pretensions of the profane goddess Truth.

All these masters—Sydenham, Boerhaave, Cullen and Rush—were noted for their keen clinical observation, their

18 Examples from Cobbett: "Dr. Death"; Rush's "Samson of Medicine" (Mercury) "slew more Americans than even Samson slew of the Philistines"; "Master Sangrado."
19 Wilson, J.C. Address at College of Physicians of Phila. on Centennial anniversary of the death of Benjamin Rush. Wilson had given the address at the unveiling of the statue of Rush, which stands in the grounds of the Naval Museum of Hygiene in Washington, D.C. The base bears the above motto. J.A.M.A., XLII:1601-6,1904.
20 Cullen. First Lines of the Practice of Physick, Am. Ed. edited by Rush. Steiner & Cist, Phila., 1781, 83 (2 vols).
21 Sydenham, Thos., M.D. Acute & Chronic Diseases, with Notes by Benjamin Rush, M.D., Kite, Phila., 1809.

therapeutic common sense (except when misled by "principles"), their sympathy and understanding and for their devotion to the poor;[22] the three last named in addition for their clinical teaching.

After he took up practice Rush championed the system of Cullen (l.c.,20) as against the prevailing tradition of Boerhaave, and later on when that had become the accepted practice, introduced his own system, in both instances antagonizing the majority of the profession. I need hardly say that he believed that the cause of diseases of the mind was seated in the blood vessels and that antimony, blood-letting and mercury were the sovereign remedies. The Nineteenth Century exaggerated the harm that Rush had done, by his advocacy of venesection, for this after all formed but a small part of his therapeutic armament, which was minutely concerned with diet, rest, exercise, hydrotherapy, occupation, diversion and travel. The Twentieth Century cannot stress the dangers of bleeding quite so feelingly, when every debutante is offering her pint of blood every six months or oftener, while single patients receive as many as seventeen quarts of plasma in the same space of time (newspaper), nor complain of his drastic methods, when patients are given huge doses of novel specifics and sedatives or are convulsed with metrazol.

But to return to our topic. Modern scientific medicine, like science in general, depends upon the collection, and evaluation by statistical methods, of a multiplicity of observations or experiments, and after comparison, on the construction of plausible hypotheses to assist in their interpretation, and in the prediction and discovery of further facts. Even well established theories are always to be held suspect and subject to revision. Deductive logic plays a necessary but subsidiary role. Of all this Rush was practically, if not theoretically, ignorant. To use a phrase of Huxley he was a useful "Hod carrier of Science,"[23] but contributed little to scientific theory (medical or other), though he fancied this was his special province. It must be admitted in extenuation that our scientific age has also had its "decalogues" and dogmas. According to Garrison[24] Rush stated that "medicine is my wife and science my mistress" to which Dr. O.W. Holmes added the caustic comment: "I do not think that this breach of the seventh commandment can be shown to have been of advantage to the legitimate owner of his affections."

While much of Rush's training and experience tended to depth of conviction, coupled with narrowness and rigidity, he was nevertheless exposed throughout life to many humanizing, broadening influences which contended for the mastery in his character. Even in Scotland, religion, though rigid, had created the middle classes and given them their political importance, and the capacity to think and act for themselves (Froude); and at the period of Rush's residence advanced thinkers like Hume were coming to the front. In

London with the aid of Franklin and West, his contacts were not limited to medical men—such as William Hunter, Hewson and Fothergill (to mention a few still remembered), but included artists, actors and literary men, to many of whom he was introduced by West;[25] and philosophers, scientists, and politicians, both in London and Paris, for whom Franklin was responsible. He dined with Johnson, Goldsmith, Wilkes (who entertained at Newgate!), Garrick (even saw the latter act, not without scruples!), met Hume and Gibbon and admired Burke at a distance. Franklin gave him letters to similar notables in Paris of whom I might instance Diderot, the encyclopedist, and Mirabeau, later the leader of the first state of the French Revolution. He only knew of Voltaire and Rousseau at second hand but generally speaking he was little influenced by the sceptical philosophy and sentimental democracy of the period, though he later paid lip service to Rousseau's ideas as embodied in the Declaration of Independence.[26]

During his residence abroad he acquired a speaking knowledge of French, a reading knowledge of Italian and German, and brushed up his Latin, in which he wrote his Thesis. These unusual social and educational opportunities gave him that familiarity with polite society, and that immense fund of information on every topic, which afterwards made him such a charming host and interesting teacher. In later life his young wife, who came of a family of social prominence in New Jersey, ably seconded this side of his life.

After his return to America and his prompt appointment as professor of chemistry in the new medical school he was of course intimately acquainted with all the medical men of the day, though often at odds with them. He was one of the founders of the College of Physicians (he later set up a rival society) and for thirty years visiting physician to the Pennsylvania Hospital, where his psychiatric experience was gained. He was an influential member of the American Philosophical Society which brought him a large circle of scientific friends, including Joseph Priestley and David Rittenhouse, with both of whom he had much in common. His political activities placed him on familiar terms with delegates from all the Colonies and many like John Adams became life-long friends and correspondents. He was particularly intimate with the Pennsylvania and New Jersey patriots including Dickinson, Miflin, Wilson, Clymer, Witherspoon and Stockton (his father-in-law) and in advanced life used to talk them over with the aged Charles Thompson, secretary of successive Congresses. They knew of many scandals and frailties among their old associates but as Thompson told Rush (l.c., 10(a)): "Let the world admire the supposed wisdom and valor of our great men. Perhaps they may adopt the qualities that have been ascribed to them and thus good may be done. I shall not undeceive future generations." In Thomas Paine, who came to Philadelphia in 1775, he found an able coadjutor in the cause of

---

22 Rush founded the Philadelphia Dispensary for the Poor (now amalgamated with the Pennsylvania Hospital), the first of its kind in the Colonies. He estimated that he had not been paid for more than one-fifth of the labor of his life.
23 Robinson, V. Myth of Benj. Rush. Med. Rev. of Rev., 35:621-24, 1929, does not grant him even this distinction: "Volumes"-"and not one page of scientific value."
24 Garrison, F.H. History of Medicine. Phila., 1929.
25 A portrait of this period is attributed to West.
26 Adams writing to Rush: "The Declaration of Independence I always consider a theatrical show. Jefferson ran away with * * * all the glory of it." Evening Bulletin, Phila., Oct. 13 (A.P.), 1943.

Independence but he abhorred his later association with the Paris Convention and his anti-religious views. At the time of Paine's death he noted in his diary: (*l.c.*, 10(b)—195-7) June 5, 1809 "Thomas Paine died at New York—He wrote his Common Sense at my request. I gave it its name. He possessed a wonderful talent of writing to the tempers and feelings of the public."—"Intemperate and"—"debauched in private life"—"his vanity" was conspicuous.— "His Age of Reason probably perverted more persons from the Christian faith than any book that ever was written." He quotes with approval a newspaper estimate which recognized Paine's past influence on the "wonderful events [of the] present age" but adds "the faculties of an angel were connected with the dispositions of a fiend,"—he was a "traitor to his Country and his God."

PART III

RUSH AS PSYCHIATRIST

Rush's reputation as a psychiatrist has often been ascribed mainly to his book on "The Diseases of the Mind" (*l.c.*,12) published a year before his death "in compliance with the solicitations of the author's pupils," and some have felt that this was a modest foretaste of the present day insistence on formal psychiatric instruction. That the latter is a gross understatement is easily proved by a study of the notebooks of his pupils at the University of Pennsylvania, many of which are preserved at the Library of College of Physicians of Philadelphia and elsewhere. There is also a manuscript, in Rush's own handwriting,[27] which is evidently of much earlier date than his text-book. It is in lecture form and consists of general considerations on the "faculties" of the mind, etc., treated in much greater detail than in the book itself and comprising a discussion of the theories of Gall. It includes a consideration of the metaphysics of mind; the immaterial and the material views, as well as the orthodox view championed by Rush. This manuscript had been extensively revised from time to time. It is chiefly interesting because of its introduction in which Rush Stresses the importance of "Disease of the Mind." The following extracts are from the introduction:—

> This part of our course, gentlemen, should command your closest attention, and that for the following reasons:
> "1. The knowledge of the human mind is the most *important* branch of all the sciences." . . . . After elaborating this theme, he makes the following dogmatic statement!
> "2. The history of the faculties and operations of the human mind is the most *certain* of all kinds of knowledge. It consists of facts only. It relates to feelings and actions which take place within ourselves, and in which it is not possible for us to be deceived." . . . . And this of phrenology! . . . .
> "3. It is an intelligible science . . . . ."
> "4. It is the most useful of all the sciences . . . . . To a physician it is useful in an eminent degree, for the diseases of the mind are as certainly objects of medicine as those of the body . . . .

> But there are other advantages to be derived from a knowledge of the component parts and operations of the mind by a physician. He may draw many active and useful remedies from this source, for the cure of diseases which belong exclusively to the body . . . . ."
> " . . . . I am not singular in introducing the history of the human mind into a course of physiology. It has been done by Dr. Boerhaave, Dr. Haller and by their successors in that branch of medicine in all the Universities of Europe."

This manuscript which originally extended to 475 pages has an index which proves that it was an exposition of the popular psychology ("physiology of the brain") of the day with references to phrenology (Gall and Spurtzheim). It formed a part of Rush's course on the Institutes of Medicine. In addition [h]e prefaced his course on the Practice of Medicine with somewhat similar general observations, and in the section on neurology considered the significance of general symptoms: headache, vertigo, insomnia and the like. Finally he devoted several lectures to mental diseases proper. These points are brought out in the students notes[28] to which I will now refer.

The earliest notes which I have found (Alison, 1771) are scanty, little more than prescriptions, *e.g.*, for epilepsy.

Griffith's notes (1797-98) Vol. II were evidently on the Institutes of Medicine and contain an interesting discussion of the mental peculiarities of men and women. Although one of the early advocates of higher education for women, his comparison is not flattering to "the sex" except as to "refinement," "taste" and "sensitivity." In all, some 20 pages are devoted to these topics.

Darlington's notes, taken from Rush's lectures on the Theory and Practice of Physick, include eight lectures (88th to the 95th—Feb. 24 to March 4, 1803) on Diseases of the Mind. He devoted 17 closely written pages to this division of the subject. These lectures cover substantially the same ground as those taken later by Mitchell in 1809 to 1811, and already correspond closely to the text-book (1812) in nomenclature.

In 1803-4 Darlington added notes on ten psychological lectures, five on the Senses, and five on The Mental Faculties, etc. Both volumes bear the warning of Rush: "Let no man enter the *Temple* of medicine who is not acquainted with the pulse."

The most complete notes are by Thos. D. Mitchell (1809-11). This same Mitchell some ten years later read a paper before the Philadelphia Medical Society in vindication of Rush against charges of misrepresentation and even deliberate falsehood which had been raised against him during the yellow fever epidemic of 1793. Contrary to the lecturer's expectations not a voice was raised to impugn "the moral character or purity of motives of the deceased physician" and he adds "No citizen" (of Philadelphia) "ever enjoyed a fairer reputation than Dr. Rush." The discussers, however, did strongly object to Rush's opinions on the uselessness of "the dead languages as part of a medical education." But to return to the notes. These two volumes of notes are prefaced by three metrical eulogies of Rush which

---

27 Lectures upon the mind. Original manuscript in library of the College of Physicians of Philadelphia.
28 A considerable number of note books by students of Rush from 1771 till his death have been preserved at the College of Physicians and other Philadelphia libraries.

leave nothing unsaid. I quote a single couplet from each of them. 1) "Lo! where he comes with robes of science drest, The fire of genius glowing in his breast"; 2) "Chant his works in sweetest lays, Raise him high to honor's throne"; 3) "Thy fame shall burn, when dazzling lights expire, And unborn ages feel the glowing fire."

Volume I (Mitchell) contains among other considerations brief generalities on the psychology and therapeutics of mental disease. Volume II devotes nearly 100 pages of beautifully written notes to diseases of the mind alone, in addition to much material in the section of functional nervous diseases in which hysteria is included. To illustrate the relatively full treatment given to mental disease it may be worth noting that the previous hundred pages of notes cover: diabetes, the liver and gall-bladder, the spleen, hemorrhoids, ophthalmia, cystitis and other causes of obscure febrile reactions,[29] apoplexy, palsy, paraplegia, hemicrania, hysteria, dyspepsia, epilepsy, asthma, angina pectoris, etc.

There is another set of notes of about the same time (1810) by Joseph G. Shippen, 60 pages of which are devoted to mental diseases, out of a total of 396. Under the head of manicula (manalgia?) there is an excellent description of catatonic stupor, more explicit than in the textbook itself.

Other sets of notes are similar, including one entitled: The Essence of Dr. Rush's Lectures, from notes taken in the winter of 1815 and 1816 (he died in 1813). Evidently Rush's successor used the lectures as a text, feeling that they could not be improved upon. This shows the authority which Rush had acquired and retained and at the same time may account in part for the period of stagnation which followed.

I have cited these notes at some length to prove that Rush considered diseases of the mind as the most important topic in the practice of medicine, and devoted a correspondingly large proportion of his teaching to their exposition. Also he stressed the mental aspects of other diseases in the various sections devoted to their consideration. In the following century this point of view was neglected and even the recent revival of interest in the psychiatric aspects of disease has not brought us back to relatively the same level. In fact this would not be desirable when we consider the immense mass of factual material in the domain of somatic medicine, which has accumulated in the century and a half since he initiated his courses. At the risk of depreciating our hero one might add that Rush's practical opportunities were vastly greater in psychiatry, which is so little dependent on instrumentation and laboratory aids, than in general medicine where he had to depend mainly on history inspection and palpation (and that mainly of the pulse!).

Finally we must give some consideration to Rush's "Medical Inquiries and Observations upon Diseases of the Mind" (l.c., 12) of which five editions, substantially unaltered, appeared between 1812 and 1835 as well as translations into various languages. In his journal at the end of February 1812 (l.c., 10(b), 212) we read: "This day I finished my lectures—I have reason to believe my pupils were satisfied—For this favor I desire to be thankful to that Being who alone gives favor in the eyes of men." Under date of

October 27 (ibid., p. 273) Rush says: "This evening corrected the last proof sheet of my Inquiries." Again in Chapter I of his book he writes: "In entering upon the subject of the following Inquiries and Observations, I feel as if I were about to tread upon consecrated ground." This is followed by an invocation to the Deity. On page 45 we read, "Let not religion be blamed for these cases of insanity" (re: delusions of guilt, etc.); on page 97: "Blessed science!" (referring to bleeding, emetics, purges, reduced diet, etc.) "Which thus extends its friendly empire [over] the minds of the children of men"; on page 273 et seq. he treats "Of Derangements in the Principle of Faith." Having disposed of this pious aspect of his work, which appears throughout and was characteristic of the religious people of the period but not of the votaries of French philosophy like Jefferson, we can turn to the more serious features of the volume, which according to Mills had no rival in America till Spitzka's work appeared seventy years later.

Rush's discussion of the faculties of the mind, and of proximate, remote, exciting and predisposing causes is interesting and, aside from his fixed opinion (p. 17) "that the cause of madness is seated primarily in the blood-vessels of the brain," contains many sound observations, consonant with the best ideas of the time, some of them still valid. If he fell into more errors than the practically contemporary Haslam and Pinel, it is because these authors, and particularly the former restricted themselves to clinical and pathological observations, and avoided theories. By his theorizing he "exposed a larger surface" to criticism—to paraphrase a phrase he uses in quite another connection. Unlike most contemporary (I exclude the authors just mentioned) and earlier writers on psychiatry, Rush did not support his opinions by a multitude of Greek and Latin quotations but did refer to some seventy-five, mainly recent, medical writers—repeatedly to Cullen, Coxe, Heberden, Haslam, Pinel. He also utilized numerous literary allusions and quotations. A touch of modernity is added to his work by his reference to a dozen investigations made at his suggestion by his assistants (eight or nine) at the Pennsylvania Hospital. "The Inquiries," in turn, was widely quoted by later authors, thus Esquirol (Pinel's successor and the greatest European authority in the first half of the nineteenth century) refers to this work repeatedly in his famous treatise.[30]

Rush avoided entirely the late eighteenth century attempt to classify diseases, including mental diseases, under the fallacious idea that they were species, and might be arranged in orders and genera, after the manner of Linnaeus, like plants and animals. Instead he adopted a clinical classification with names mostly of his own invention. For example he uses the term "tristimania" to designate hypochondriasis and rejects Cullen's use of the term melancholia. His clinical description of tristimania indicates that the more severe cases were instances of involutional psychosis or of agitated depression with somatic delusions. Indeed he told the students in his lectures that hypochondriasis and melancholia were only different grades of the same disease (Mitchell). This is a distinction that frequently offers difficulties at the present day. His

---

29 Rush recognized diseased teeth as causative factors in arthritis, etc.
30 Des Maladies Mentales (2 vols.). Baillière, Paris, 1838.

"amenomania" characterized by pleasant delusions is a mixed group which could hardly have been split up in his day, though Haslam, according to Solomon, had already described cases which were clearly paresis (*e.g.*, case XV, 2nd Ed.). "Manicula" is described as a reduced form of mania (*i.e.*, hypomania), while "manalgia" designated instances of general torpor of mind and body: taciturnity, downcast looks, neglect of dress and person, indifference and insensibility, beneath which he nevertheless sensed emotion. Sometimes these patients assumed a fixed position, bent forward like a statue, drooled saliva. He stresses chronicity, ten to fifty years. Other categories are "demence," "derangement of will" (psychopathic personality) and "fatuity." His descriptions merit careful study but his nomenclature has not survived. Instead the profession adopted the modest classification of Pinel upon which foundation his successor Esquirol, and the latter's pupils and colleagues erected the superstructure of modern psychiatry; later simplified, synthesized and crystallized by the German school.

The book is especially notable for the wisdom of its *general therapy*, excluding the depleting measures necessitated by his theories (as already mentioned) and occasional vagaries such as the "tranquilizer" and the "gyrater." In the treatment of the various types of mental illness almost every measure now used in mental hospitals and in psychiatric practice is recommended. These include, carefully classified exercises, occupational therapy, productive work, reading, music, diversion, travel, hydrotherapy and balneotherapy and even malarial therapy, a far from complete list. He also stressed the importance of the physicians' and attendants' attitude towards patients: dignity, truthfulness, sincerity, respect, sympathy, etc. I would like to go into detail but space forbids. I will quote one passage at length, which hints at a form of therapy even at present too little employed. He writes (*l.c.*, 12, 241-4):[31]

I cannot conclude this part of the subject of these Inquiries, without lamenting the want of some person of prudence and intelligence in all public receptacles of mad people, who should live constantly with them, and have the exclusive direction of their minds. His business should be, to divert them from conversing upon all the subjects upon which they had been deranged, to tell them pleasant stories, to read to them select passages from entertaining books, and to oblige them to read to him; to superintend their labours of body and mind; to preside at the table at which they take their meals, to protect them from rudeness and insults from their keepers, to walk and ride with them, to partake with them in their amusements, and to regulate the nature and measure of their punishments (*sic*). Such a person would do more good to mad people in one month, than the visits or the accidental company, of the patient's friends would do in a year. But further. We naturally imitate the manners, and gradually acquire the temper of persons with whom we live, provided they are objects of our respect and affection. this has been observed in husbands and wives who have lived long and happily together, and even in servants, who are strongly attached to their masters and mistresses. Similar effects might be expected from the constant presence of a person, such as has been described with mad people, independently of his

performing for them any of the services that have been mentioned. We render a limb that has been broken, and bent, straight, only by keeping it in one place by the pressure of splints and bandages. In like manner, by keeping the eyes and ears of mad people under the constant impressions of the countenance, gestures and conversation of a man of a sound understanding, and correct conduct, we should create a pressure nearly as mechanical upon their minds, that could not fail of having a powerful influence, in conjunction with other remedies, in bringing their shattered and crooked thoughts into their original and natural order.

At the present day such a paragon could not be found, his functions are shared by trained nurses, social and occupational workers, music teachers, librarians, athletic instructors, junior physicians, etc., without entirely covering the field. Possibly well educated, broad-minded, versatile, tolerant and withal discreet lay volunteers could be found to afford the desired background of normality, to discover the patient's traits and tastes, and the best means of developing and gratifying them. The employment of theological students in hospital work is a step in this direction—it would have pleased Rush!

Many apt phrases might also be quoted, such as (*l.c.*, 12, 114) "Tory rot and the protection fever"; (p. 246) "The willow weeps" says the poet "but cannot feel; the torpid manic feels, but cannot weep"; (p.286) "Two knocks to open the memory." Also pregnant passages such as: "In like manner, depression of mind may be induced by causes that are forgotten, or by the presence of objects which revive the sensation of distress with which it was at one time associated, but without reviving the cause of it in the memory."

The preceding summary and citations, while inadequate, are sufficient, with what has gone before, to establish Rush's place as a great teacher and practitioner of psychiatry. His contributions to nosology and symptomatology were useful; his specific therapies, deduced from a fallacious theory of causation, were harmful in their day and are now forgotten. Pliny Earle,[32] in an effort to destroy the last traces of Rush's teaching in regard to venesection, felt it necessary to publish one of the most elaborate and well documented articles ever to appear in the Journal of the Association, a high testimonial to Rush's persisting authority. As a scientist Rush does not rank high though he observed and published a multitude of facts which are the raw material of science. At other times his observations were superficial and his interpretation based on preconceived ideas. He is credited with the description of at least one new disease, cholera infantum. He employed his assistants on problems of clinical research, mostly of a statistical type; the principle was excellent, the matter for the most part trivial.

SUMMARY AND CONCLUSIONS

Rush was a complex character; his fundamental trends: conscientiousness, methodical industry, religious and reforming zeal, logical but dogmatic reasoning, humanitari-

---

31 In his journal (*l.c.* 10 (a), 191, 1801, January 4) he presented this matter to the Managers and Physicians of the Pennsylvania Hospital in identical form. I do not know the outcome.
32 Pliny Earle. Bloodletting in Mental Disorders. Am. J. of Insanity, X: 387-405, April 1854.

anism, republicanism, are clearly the product of his ancestry and early education. His culture and widely diversified interests, his charm, suavity, friendliness, were in part the result of his unusually rich associations with the leaders of Scotland, England, France and the Colonies. Among his faults were pride, an eye to posterity, irritability, sensitivity,[33] loss of judgment and of a sense of proportion in the heat of conflict. To some of his contemporaries the odd mingling of these characteristics made him appear hypocritical, but he can be cleared of this charge. He acquired a host of enemies, but the enmity was usually limited to the occasion. His admirers were legion, *e.g.*, practically all of the medical profession in South Carolina, and his intimacies were numerous, close and long enduring, including men like John Adams (another man who never minced words), Priestley and Rittenhouse. His position as a humanitarian and philanthropist has been sufficiently emphasized, as has also his political importance. Finally his position as psychiatrist and scientist has been amply indicated.

---

[33] His medical and political rivals were not the only ones who suffered from his sensitivity and irritability. The following selections are from his diary (*l.c.* 10(b), p. 210—1811, Sept. 13 (after he failed to receive letters by packet from his son and daughter who had gone abroad):

"The distress I have felt in being thus disappointed, neglected and ungratefully treated by two children upon whom I have lavished acts of paternal kindness has been to me very great. It has prevented me from sleeping and impaired by health, Lord lay not this conduct to their charge."

(*Ibid.*, p. 211—1811 Nov. 23) "My son Richard Rush was appointed Comptroller of the United States, and to my great astonishment and distress" accepted the position in spite of my suasions. "Oh, my son, my son Richard, may you never be made to feel in the unkindness of a son the misery you have inflicted on me by this rash conduct." He regarded this acceptance as a "degradation," and "dishonorable" to his son's understanding, yet as we have seen it was the opening to a career of statesmanship and diplomacy, quite as distinguished, as his own in medicine and psychiatry.

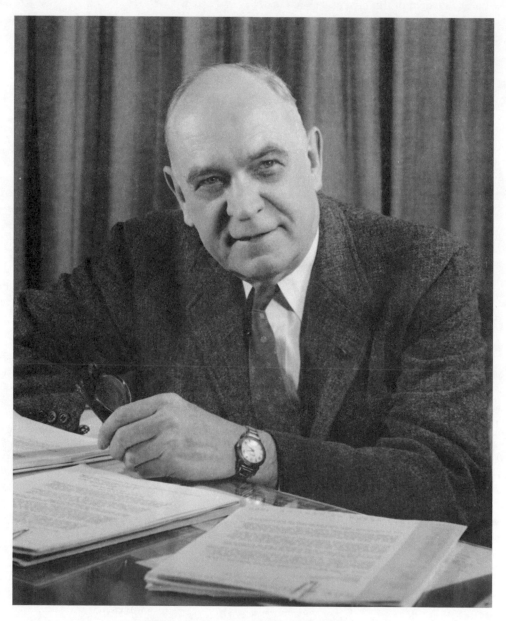

William C. Menninger, M.D., 1899–1966

September 1947

The Rôle of Psychiatry in the World Today

By William C. Menninger, M.D.

*Professor of Psychiatry, The Menninger Foundation School of Psychiatry
and the University of Kansas Medical School, Topeka, Kansas*

To formulate the rôle of psychiatry in the world today is a challenging task and a formidable one. In attempting to do so, one is handicapped by the limitations of his own experience—his experience in psychiatry and his experience in the world. It becomes a matter of a personal point of view as to the rôle psychiatry could or should play. Not only does such a formulation suffer through limitation of individual experience but it will be colored by one's optimism or pessimism, by one's confidence or lack of faith in psychiatry as well as in the topsy-turvy world of today.

For one who has great faith in the potential contributions of psychiatry, this assigned title tends to stimulate expansive phantasies. Perhaps we should limit our discussion to the western world, and even there the influence of or the knowledge about psychiatry is ultra-microscopic. Certainly few, if any of us, have enough information even to make assumptions about the rôle of psychiatry in much of the world. We must recognize that great geographical areas containing millions of people have never heard of psychiatry. We should be humble when we consider that among the 400,000,000 people of China, there are probably not 10 physicians with any training in our specialty. The ratio for the continent of Africa is probably even less. But in these days of internationalism, when our country has finally accepted some types of responsibility for other parts of the globe, should not we in psychiatry be alert to the international trend?

My own conception of the rôle of psychiatry even in our immediate world, this North American continent, includes an immense program. Merely to attempt to define it is disquieting because of the responsibility it implies for each one of us. My impression is that many psychiatrists may be disturbed by a consideration of our potential responsibilities in those broad areas that are less well known or unfamiliar to us. There are very few, if any, of us who are not already heavily taxed. Any additional burden is a threat to our personal equilibrium, the more so if that burden requires change or innovations. For many of us, it is more comfortable to remain in our secluded cloisters or our ivory towers where we can continue treating some of the increasing number of patients who are coming to us. But a comparison of the present rôle with the potential rôle of psychiatry should call for reconsideration of our priorities for the investment of our very limited manpower.

Psychiatry is a medical science but of necessity it is also a social science. The psychiatrist more than the physician in any other of the medical disciplines must concern himself with the social situation of his patients. In no other specialty is there the routine necessity of considering the environmental background and the modification of that environment and the personal relationships involved. Of necessity then the psychiatrist must be concerned with our social units—the family, the community, the state. In the ordinary practice of civilian psychiatry the average specialist rarely becomes involved personally in this direction. He may make recommendations to a patient or to his family for certain changes. Occasionally, through the aid of a psychiatric social worker, he may be instrumental in making environmental changes. There have been excursions by a few of our number into the social fields of criminology, penology and industry. On the other hand, by necessity and without choice, psychiatry in the army had to function literally in the field rather than being limited merely to treatment in the hospital or office. The situation demanded our services in selection, classification and assignment, concern for morale, preventive measures, correctional institutions, and criminology, as well as in treatment.

As a background in formulating the rôle of psychiatry today it may be helpful to face frankly our position in 1941 when we were catapulted into the world crisis. Despite our lessons in World War I and the great increase in our fund of knowledge in the following 25 years, we were as unprepared at the beginning of World War II as we had been in 1917. Psychiatry was far from being generally accepted by those in military authority or even by many of our own medical confrères. Not only did we lack standing but we lacked plans. We suffered along with all of medicine in having no voice in high councils. We were lacking in medical statesmanship. Three years ago Alan Gregg told us kindly, but bluntly, that we lacked an organized front and that our inarticulateness was essentially self-destructive. These facts were painfully apparent to some of us during our experience in the war.

Further, we lacked tested knowledge—knowledge about selection methods, about placement, about treatment and, above all, about prevention. Many of our number did not even know the functions or the potential contributions of our co-workers, the psychiatric social worker and the clinical psychologist. Finally, psychiatry was sorely lacking in acceptance and understanding by the public. Through much of the war we fought ignorance, prejudice and misconception on every side.

We gained attention from the military command in part, and perhaps in large part, because of excessive loss of manpower from the armed forces on account of personality difficulties. Nearly 2,000,000 men were rejected for psychiatric disorders at the draft level and over 500,000 men were discharged from the army alone for personality disorders. With the navy discharges, this figure was considerably over 600,000. We were called upon to explain this loss and to take prompt measures to reduce it. Through necessity again we were obligated much further than the traditional rôle of the psychiatrist in diagnosis and treatment of the sick individual. I hope we have learned some valuable lessons. For most of us who had the privilege of experience in the service, our horizons as to the responsibility of psychiatry have been immensely broadened.

The World Today

It is difficult, if not impossible, to classify the human activity of warfare in psychiatric terms. Such pathological outpouring of aggression and destructiveness well might be regarded as a psychosis. The overt outlet of killing which the shooting war provided is over but one would need the utmost optimism to regard our present world status as any stage of convalescence. Nationally and internationally, our relationships are marked with tension, mistrust, suspicion and selfishness. We cannot be unaware of the physical and emotional suffering that affects the majority of people in the world today, even though that suffering occurs thousands of miles from us. Our advances in physical science, as represented by the atom bomb and television, have progressed so much farther than our social advances that our very existence is dangerously threatened. We have learned how to eliminate space and to annihilate people but we still lag far behind in learning how to get along with each other.

During the war we had frequent occasions to contrast the psychiatrist's job in civilian life with his job in combat. In civilian life he attempted to understand and treat the abnormal reactions of persons to normal situations. In military life he attempted to understand and treat the normal reactions to an abnormal situation. One might seriously question if our world condition does not now place many of us in a continuously abnormal situation to which we are having normal reactions, even though these by all previous standards are pathological. To such a turbulent world, one might legitimately ask, what is a normal reaction?

If one turns the microscope on the world close at home we find evidence of many different types of man's maladjustment. Let us start with the family. It is apparent that major changes are taking place in its organization and structure. The tremendous number of rejections for military

service and the large number of psychiatric discharges from the army made us feel that something must be radically wrong in the early experience and development of a large segment of American youth. The present status of the family has been described as at a crisis, and unless the trend is changed it has been forecast that the family as we have known it will disintegrate by the end of the century. As evidence for this are the facts that 44% of our families have no children and an additional 22% have only one child.[1] In 1945 there was one divorce for every two marriages in urban areas and one divorce for every three marriages in the country at large. In figures the divorces increased from approximately 250,000 in 1937 to over 500,000 in 1945.[2] Before the war approximately 11,000,000 women worked outside the home; 2½ million more wanted or needed work. In March 1944, there were over 16,000,000 at work away from home, 7,000,000 of whom were married.[3]

There would be one hundred percent agreement among psychiatrists that the healthy development of the child depends on an early home situation which provides affection, good example and security. These figures given above show that homes in increasing numbers fail to provide such conditions. These figures do not include the unknown toll exacted by the war in the temporary separation and disruption of millions of American—and world—families. The institution of the family must be the object of serious study by all who claim to be interested in mental health.

We can turn our microscope from the family to many other areas of man's maladjustment. It is variously estimated that the total cost of crime in America is between 10 and 18 billion dollars a year.[4] This is more than six times as much as we spend for public education. Our overflowing penitentiaries, reformatories and jails cost us over $100,000,000 a year to operate. The Federal Bureau of Investigation reported[5] that the crimes in 1946 broke all records for the last decade, with more than a million and a half committed during the year. This was an increase of 120,000 over the previous year. Approximately 120,000 juveniles passed through the courts in 1945.[6] That the behavior represented in crime and delinquency is evidence of maladjustment is another point on which there would be nearly one hundred percent agreement among psychiatrists.

One is forced to assume that most of our citizens, including psychiatrists, have a total blind spot for the atrocious conditions which exist in our penitentiaries, reformatories and jails. This is in spite of the fact that many of us feel that there should be little distinction between the psychiatric hospital and the reformatory. Both should be institutions for the examination, treatment—and in some instances permanent detention—of individuals with behavior ineptitudes, distorted personalities, social maladjustment and sick minds.

In addition to delinquency and crime, there are still other evidences of mass maladjustment. Mores and standards are giving way in other directions. There is no doubt that non-

1 Editorial, Life Magazine, March 24, 1947.
2 Jenkinson, B. L. Marriage and Divorce in the United States: 1937-1945. Vital Statistics, Special Reports V. 23, No. 9, Sept. 10, 1946.
3 A Woman's Place Is—Where? Talk It Over, published by National Institute of Social Relations, Washington, D.C. Series G-107, 1946.
4 Morris, A. Criminology, New York: Longmans, Green & Co., 1938, p. 20.
5 Press Release, Mar. 5, 1947.
6 Juvenile Court Statistics for 1944-45. U. S. Children's Bureau of Federal Security Agency, Washington, D.C.

marital sexual relations have greatly increased. There can be no vital statistics on this point but we do know that the cases of venereal disease reported for the first time in the continental United States indicated that the number of cases of gonorrhea doubled between 1941 and 1946, from 191,000 to 367,000.[7] Someone has been brave enough to estimate that alcoholism costs $750,000,000 annually and is steadily on the increase.[8] We in America can hardly be proud of the fact that 4.5% of all men examined in the draft were mentally deficient. Nearly 4% of our population in 1940 had no schooling and 2½ times this number had less than 4 years of schooling.[9]

Quite apart from these direct evidences of maladjustment in our midst is an equally long list of our situations and attitudes and practices that are producing great stress and unhappiness for millions of Americans. Theoretically psychiatrists can limit themselves to diagnosis and treatment of patients in offices and hospitals isolated from community life. They can, and some do, ignore the social problems which bring their patients to them. Some do so because they are too busy with their patient load. Others do so because they feel impotent to effect any change or do not even know how to approach these larger problems. These problems are probably solvable, and with a united front psychiatry might study and offer some constructive solutions. These might not be effective; they might not even be received. Nevertheless, some of us would feel that we had at least accepted a responsibility in actively attacking these so-called social neuroses which are such real threats to our patients, our families, and ourselves.

Number one among all of the social neuroses in America today is the wide-spread prejudice and discrimination against persons because of race or color or religion. Bigoted intolerance, the thesis of "white supremacy," anti-Semitic prejudices, discriminatory practices, hostile attitudes toward Catholicism and Protestantism are all present in varying degrees in every section of America. Canadians are keenly aware of the potential dynamite in the French-Canadian problem. As psychiatrists we are not only aware of these prejudices and resentments as seen in our patients, but we have an opportunity to learn much about their dynamics and therefore their significance. As a group, have we no constructive steps to recommend in the reduction of this problem?

As psychiatrists, certainly we are aware of the effect on mental health of forced unemployment. It is variously estimated that 60 to 80% of unemployed persons manifest definite signs of mental ill health. In a majority of instances the father appears to be a failure in the eyes of his wife, his children, his friends and the community, often even to himself. Most tragic is the effect on the children. Unemployment becomes then a mental health problem which always affects two generations. The problems of unemployment

have received little attention from psychiatrists, except as we have seen them in occasional non-paying patients. Our psychiatric social workers are much more familiar with the effects of mental health on the family group. Is it not another area where studied psychiatric advice should be formulated, with the hope that the state and federal authorities might give us a hearing?

None of us can be unaware of the unhappiness and distress caused by the housing shortage which makes it impossible for so many of our veterans and former war workers to have a home or to find suitable accommodation in which to live. In 1946 we built approximately 500,000 homes but we needed 3,200,000.[10] The resulting dislocation, crowding and family friction added together compound an enormous emotional cost.

One can go on with the list almost indefinitely—strikes and their concomitant economic loss to the family and to the community; the 350,000 persons who are permanently disabled each year as a result of accidents;[11] our systems of political graft and private racketeering that exist in so many states and communities. Last but not least, no thoughtful person can be unaware of the anxiety and the insecurity caused by our tenuous international relations.

One might inquire, what have all of these to do with psychiatry? As a group of scientific experts who are interested in and concerned with the way men think and feel and behave, it is only logical to assume that these social ills might be among our very special concerns.

PSYCHIATRY'S RÔLE AS IT IS TODAY

Surrounded as we are with these many evidences of man's maladjustment and unhappiness in the world today, we ought to examine the rôle of psychiatry as it exists at the moment. What has it done? What is it doing? What is its status in relation to the world? Again, of necessity, we must confine our survey to the United States.

Within The American Psychiatric Association, we have approximately 4000 members from the United States and Canada. There are, perhaps, an additional thousand physicians now in training in this field. A little over 60% of this group are devoting their full efforts to the treatment of some 625,000 patients in state and federal institutions. These physicians are responsible for the patients in 38% of all hospital beds in the United States[12] at a direct cost of about $300,000,000 a year. However, there have been various estimates[13] that we need between 10,000 and 14,000 trained psychiatrists at the present moment. Dr. Paul Hawley[14] indicated that he could use all of the first class psychiatrists now available in the United States to meet current needs with the Veterans Administration. Dr. Daniel Blain has indicated that he has about 600 now on duty but needs three

---

7 Figures obtained from U.S. Public Health Service, 1946.
8 Bowman, K.M. Presidential Address. Am. J. Psychiat., 103:1-17, July 1946.
9 Bureau of Census. Series P-10, No. 8, Apr. 23, 1942.
10 Wanted—A Home. Talk It Over, published by National Institute of Social Relations, Washington, D. C. Series G-103, 1946.
11 Rusk, H. A. The Forgotten Casualty: The Disabled Civilian. New York Times Magazine May 12, 1940.
12 Based on figures given in the Hospital number of the J.A.M.A. 130: 1073, Apr. 20, 1946
13 Felix, R. H. Annual Meeting of Mass. Soc. for Mental Hygiene, Jan. 24, 1946; Rennie, T. A. C.: Ment. Hygiene 29:644-690, Oct. 1945
14 Hawley, P.R. Neuropsychiatric Problems of the Veterans Administration. Milit. Surg. 99:759-762, Dec. 1946.

times that many and within 12 years will need seven times that many. All of these will be required for the direct treatment of patients. Very roughly, we have about one-tenth of our current personnel needs in clinical psychology, psychiatric social work and less than this in psychiatric nursing.

Many of us believe that most of the minor psychiatric problems could and should be cared for by the general practitioner and specialists in other fields of medicine. However, in the army I was repeatedly impressed by the fact that only a small percentage of medical officers had enough psychiatric knowledge to carry out any psychiatric treatment. Despite the astounding figures of incidence of emotional illnesses, our medical schools are still allotting an average of 4% of their total curriculum hours to the teaching of psychiatry. In no medical school is it classed along with anatomy and physiology and pathology as a basic subject.

Psychiatry has made halting steps into the area of public health. In 5 of our states we have a psychiatrist in the department of health. In 7 others we have a mental hygiene program under some separate unit or division within the state. In an additional 5, psychiatry functions under the Department of Public Welfare. It must be acknowledged, however, that in none of these has psychiatry made more than a start. In very few of them are any efforts directed towards the prevention of mental ill health. Nearly two-thirds of our states have no psychiatric program other than that of the state hospitals.

We must frankly face our group responsibility for the practice of psychiatry in the state hospitals. From my point of view, the recent exposure of situations in certain of these has been very worthwhile. It would be my hope that such exposures be aggressively continued until such time as the public conscience is awakened. But we in psychiatry can hardly remain indifferent or passive for we are not blameless. We are faced with the paradox that in many states there are excellent psychiatric departments in a university. Within a few miles is a state hospital which can provide only one physician to 300 or 400 patients, perhaps has no graduate nurses and most likely no trained psychiatric social workers or clinical psychologists. Until recently, these institutions have personified psychiatry in America. They still are the embodiment of our specialty in the eyes of the public. How can the public respect us and have confidence in us when we are silent in the face of these conditions?

Going further into the inspection of our own realm, we must clarify our concepts of clinical psychiatric entities so that we may have a better understanding of our diagnostic nomenclature. We should have no illusions that our own confusion is not sensed and capitalized upon by our medical confrères. It also adds to their misunderstanding about our field. Our inability to agree on various concepts is not nearly as important as the fact that we do not have sufficient knowledge on which to come to an agreement.

Psychiatry has made some excursions into some of our social problems though, unfortunately, they are very limited. Although it has been 30 years since a psychiatrist first interested himself in the mental hygiene of industry, at present we still have less than a dozen full time workers in

this field. Although Healy, White and Adler pioneered in fields of delinquency and criminology nearly 40 years ago, we have only 10 adult criminal courts with psychiatric service and probably considerably less than 100 psychiatrists practicing in criminal institutions. We have made real progress in the provision of psychiatric assistance to juvenile courts but unfortunately in the great majority of these, this service is limited to providing a diagnosis and no treatment.

Psychiatry has made a little greater inroad into the field of academic education. This has not been so much because psychiatrists have taken the initiative in this direction as because the intelligent educators have sought the help of mental hygiene. It is encouraging to see the increasing number of colleges and high schools in which mental hygiene consultation service is available. There is an increasing number of universities and colleges which are providing courses in mental hygiene for their students. However, the number of institutions with such a service is still a small minority of the total.

THE RÔLE OF PSYCHIATRY IN THE FUTURE

When we look at the status of psychiatry today we find that it is acutely lacking in personnel. It is lacking in tested knowledge. It has given minimal attention or study to social problems or their possible solutions. By force of circumstances it has been so busy attempting to treat patients, in many instances merely caring for them, that there has been little time for consideration of preventive measures. The same factors have limited its permeation into the general practice of medicine. Unfortunately, many of us within the ranks of psychiatry have worn blinders which were forced upon us by our daily load. Our vision has been restricted and unless forced to do so, we have taken little or no time to consider our greater responsibility for the troubles of the world in which we live.

As I have said, anyone who presumes to formulate the rôle of psychiatry in the world today can do so only in terms of the limitation of his vision. Also I have indicated my opinion that organized psychiatry has the responsibility for outlining its goals. This could happen only if many of us are willing to crystallize our own thoughts in this direction. For whatever value they may have I wish to indicate my opinions as to the rôle that psychiatry should play in the world.

Our greatest immediate need is for trained personnel— psychiatrists, clinical psychologists, psychiatric social workers and psychiatric nurses. There is no greater nor more important contribution to be made by any individual in our membership than to be engaged in the training of personnel. We must recognize that this job of training comes near to being a sacred trust. If we expect to have psychiatrists who are competent to handle the increasingly complicated problems confronting all of us, they need an intensive, integrated, well planned training. From personal experience I know that there are numerous so-called residencies, many of which are on the "approved list," that provide little training other than what the man can dig out for himself. Good training must be on a broad base. In addition to the knowledge about the structure and function of the personality, this training ought to provide the psychiatrist with a knowledge of his co-workers in social work, psychology, nursing, occupational therapy, and how to use their skills. It ought to provide some information relative to the relations of psychiatry to our world—in religion, politics, literature, art. Certainly it should introduce the student to the social issues and problems of the day. The need for the training of personnel has number one priority in psychiatry at the moment.

Next to personnel, an extensive broadening of our body of tested knowledge is most needed in our field. We know very little about the "normal" personality or why it is or is not normal. We cannot adequately define a psychoneurosis. We have minimal data on why one set of organs is picked out in preference to another in the development of the neurotic reaction. We have only the vaguest knowledge of the cause of schizophrenia. If we are to apply ourselves to social problems, every avenue leading to any one of these should be classified as research. Research, like teaching, is a specialized job requiring unusual abilities and long training. At the present moment we have a piteously small number of full-time research workers in the whole field of psychiatry.

Psychiatrists will always have a major responsibility for the treatment of mental illness. There are many areas within this field which need to be greatly perfected, by the development of shorter and more effective methods of treatment. We need to think through with the clinical psychologists and psychiatric social workers their contribution to psychotherapy and then provide the training for them. We need to develop far more extensively than we have to date our milieu treatment within the hospital. For the most part we still lack specificity in our prescriptions for occupation, education, recreation, industry and all of their variations of reading, art, music, horticulture and many other activities. Most of us have only meager knowledge about remedial reading, speech training, and the applications of psychiatric principles in physical rehabilitation.

In this area of treatment, we in psychiatry share with all medicine, a current and perhaps recurrent crisis in providing the best medical care of veterans. Under Generals Bradley and Hawley, a remarkable system of treatment with highest standards has been organized in the Veterans Administration. Along with current congressional economy measures, this medical service has suffered, and faces potential regression to a pre-war status. Reductions in appropriations and personnel in the face of an increasing patient load inevitably will lower morale, impair service and provoke resignations of medical and allied professional personnel. It is imperative that we in psychiatry, along with all real friends of disabled veterans, point out to the public and Congress immediately the certain results of such cuts in appropriations. If Congress wishes to provide only mediocre medical care, it is its decision. We in medicine, however, must make it clear that to reduce finances, personnel, consultants, teaching programs, and travel for supervisors will drastically reduce the gains that have been made for the sick veteran.

As a step toward meeting the great treatment need, we must place a high priority on the integration of psychiatry with the rest of medicine, particularly in the curriculum of the medical school. It is entirely our responsibility to recommend and direct how psychiatry itself should be taught. It is also our responsibility that psychiatric principles should permeate the teaching of all medicine, and that a helpful body of usable knowledge should be made available to all physicians.

Our Association needs to be organized so that it permits and stimulates every member to make a contribution towards the solution of the problems facing psychiatry today. We can hardly expect progress when certain of our committees meet only once, if at all, during the course of a year. Even then there may be no obligation or finances to initiate studies or surveys or research into the problems for which they are nominally responsible.

This prompts me to mention briefly the organization of The Group for the Advancement of Psychiatry. As was evidenced at the meeting a year ago, some of us felt dissatisfied with the progress of psychiatry, were impatient with our own limitations, and with our lack of opportunity to sit down and think and work together on problems that seemed vital to all of us. At that time some of us verbalized this mutual feeling but felt that we were not justified in merely criticizing or being impatient. We concluded that we should find ways and means to promote some group thinking and surveys and study. The result was an informal, very loosely organized conference group which, with the financial aid of the Commonwealth Fund, held a three day conference last fall and will shortly hold a second one. We organized in small working committees, every member of which was required to be a worker. We agreed to sacrifice in time and money to a considerable extent in order to study such problems as the needs of state hospitals, medical education, contacts with lay groups, preventive psychiatry, psychiatric social work, treatment and other subjects. At present there are 15 different committees each with specific responsibility. We limited the participants to members of this Association. In no sense was our action meant as a revolution or a secession or a competition with this Association. It was originally and still is our hope that the aims and methods and work of the Group might become an integral part of this Association. It seemed to me a year ago, and equally so today, that every member of our American Psychiatric Association capable of doing so should be contributing to the development and leadership of psychiatry beyond his daily work.

One of the essential rôles of psychiatry must lie in the field of prevention of mental ill health. If we continue to confine ourselves to treatment only, it is inconceivable that we could ever meet the obligation. Not until we have learned effectively to prevent mental illness can we begin to discharge our responsibility. Psychiatry in the war started on the basis that treatment was the sole province and responsibility of the psychiatrist. We learned by experience, however, that our greatest contribution should have been in the field of prevention. This involved putting psychiatrists into the field to live with the soldiers, thus learning their problems, attempting to modify their stresses and develop their supports. Only there could they advise leaders effectively about immediate factors that affected mental health. It would seem that psychiatry's great opportunity is to work similarly in the fields of academic education, public health, recreation, delinquency and industry.

Our lessons in preventive psychiatry from the army emphasized three major factors in maintaining mental health. The first, and most important, was that quality of leadership was a cause of or prevented mental ill health. We learned that the development of positive rational attitudes towards the job to be done, *i.e.*, conscious motivation—could be a great aid to the doing of that job. Unquestionably, "good" motivation was an important factor in maintaining mental health, and "poor" motivation was followed by an increase in the number of psychiatric casualties. The development of an identification with a group which permitted a sense of pride, and provided comparative security, satisfaction and unity of purpose was extremely important to mental health. It was apparent that these elementary lessons which applied to the maintenance of an individual's mental health in the army, could apply in the family, the group, the community and the nation. One of the chief aims of preventive psychiatry should be the continued attempt to educate parents and all leaders as to the importance of developing mature persons, in line with the challenge that Brock Chisholm gave us in his William Alanson White lectures.

Preventive psychiatry must concern itself with the cause and alleviation of mental illness—neuroses, psychoses, the character defects. It must find ways to reduce the many symptoms of social ills enumerated earlier—delinquency, crime, divorce, illiteracy, mental deficiency. It should certainly concern itself with forced unemployment, prejudices, discrimination, strikes, accidents.

Psychiatry should place a high priority in its efforts to provide the "average" person with psychiatric information he can apply to his own problems. As I have tried to indicate previously, the great number of psychiatric casualties during the war called attention to the need for public education in the field of mental hygiene. The public wants this education. If adequately given it could be very helpful. Very possibly it may increase the number of patients who seek help from a psychiatrist just as a campaign about cancer or tuberculosis increases the number of patients who go to doctors about these problems. The aim of such public education, however, certainly should be to provide the average man with a better understanding of his own mental health, how to fortify it, how to improve it.

We in psychiatry in America must become more international in our interests and work with psychiatrists abroad. Some years ago, an international mental hygiene organization was formed and plans are on foot to revive it. The American Psychoanalytic Association has always been a part of the International Psychoanalytic Association. With the increasing necessity for a world point of view today, we should have a vital part in any international psychiatric effort, through the United Nations Health Committee as well as an international psychiatric organization.

Through the foresight of Dr. Frank Fremont-Smith of the Josiah Macy, Jr. Foundation, we have as our guest at this meeting Dr. J. R. Rees of London who is here to solicit our interest in an international congress of psychiatry in England next year. It is my impression that our best contribution to the United Nations Health Organization might be made through an international psychiatric organization.

To accomplish all of these aims may appear an impossible assignment. They can be approached only if every individual member of the organization is willing to contribute. It is essential that the organization provide ways for him to make his contribution. In addition, however, such a program for psychiatry calls for immense support through public understanding and financial backing.

The most immediate and concrete encouragement for the further development of psychiatry has come through the National Mental Health Act, sponsored by the United States Public Health Service. From this source a considerable sum of money will be available immediately, with a promise of a much larger amount in the coming years.

Over the years, the National Committee for Mental Hygiene has given leadership in providing a better understanding of mental health in the national scene. The recently formed National Mental Health Foundation is championing the needs of our state hospitals, and particularly the improvement of the status of the ward attendant. We in the Menninger Foundation are devoting ourselves to an all out effort in training and research. All of us in psychiatry are in great debt to the several general Foundations which have done so much for us, and express the hope for their continued support.

This section of the program of this convention is under the auspices of the most recently organized group for the support of psychiatry—The Psychiatric Foundation. It has long been recognized that to give leadership in our field, our own Association needed far more financial support than could be obtained from membership dues. With this need as a stimulus, a small group of our members, through the personal work of Austin Davies, launched the Psychiatric Foundation. It is my fervent hope that its development will be supported and hastened in order to permit it to launch whatever program is agreed upon by The American Psychiatric Association.

This we must make clear to the public and to the profession—all the efforts of the various Foundations are cooperative attacks on the immense problems ahead; none of these varied enterprises is in competition with the others.

CONCLUSIONS

We all look with pride on the phenomenal victories of preventive medicine. No longer is the world cursed with smallpox or cholera or yellow fever or typhoid. World epidemics of these diseases are no more. Is there any hope that medicine, through its Cinderella, psychiatry, can step forward to offer its therapeutic effort to a world so full of unhappiness and maladjustment and varying degrees of social disintegration? Can our intensive study of the individual lead us to a better understanding of his environment, of the social forces that affect his life? And can this understanding, if made available to the right leaders be helpful in alleviating these social ills? Perhaps some psychiatrists might answer this in the negative. My own strong conviction is that psychiatry *can* help.

Some of my confrères who will answer in the negative may do so because of a misconception that this program may be an attempt to over-sell psychiatry. My contention has always been that one cannot over-sell the value of a tested product except in terms of ability to deliver. In outlining this program I have had no intention of selling psychiatry except to ourselves. I feel strongly that we are not now in a position even to deliver much of the available information that we might assemble. It has been my intention to direct our thought to a wider horizon and to urge acceptance of our responsibility for contributing what understanding and therapy we can for the problems of unhappiness and maladjustment that exist in the world today. To do this we must greatly increase our trained personnel. We must extend our frontiers of knowledge. We need to crystallize our goals. Our organization should require that groups of us survey specific problems, collect data about these, apply our knowledge to them, and produce a program of action. We need to develop more medical statesmanship, so that our findings and recommendations can be presented to leaders in high councils in many fields of activity. Can we and should we undertake this? We can no longer evade a decision on the matter.

CURRENT TRENDS IN GERMAN PSYCHIATRY

By Prof. Kurt Schneider

Editor's Note [Dr. Clarence B. Farrar].—Professor Kurt Schneider, Director of the Psychiatric and Neurological Clinic, University of Heidelberg, in response to our request for a statement of the main trends in the psychiatric field in postwar Germany kindly contributed a report of which the following is a translation.

Much research activity is again going on in the German psychiatric and neurological clinics—nearly all of which are now, significantly, called "neurological clinics"—and in the few research centers having similar objectives. Most of this work is in the fields of neurology, histopathology of the brain, serology, brain physiology, and has little or no relation to psychiatry proper. Clinical studies of psychic disorders and somatic investigations directly connected therewith are seldom encountered.

Herewith are presented briefly the main trends of German psychiatry today.

1. Brain localization studies are still the principal objective of Kleist, such studies naturally not being limited to brain histopathology. Because of the practical difficulties in carrying forward his main line of investigation Kleist is turning more to purely clinical studies.

2. Physiological psychiatry, seeking the causes of the (endogenic) psychoses in pathophysiological findings, is unfortunately hardly represented at all. None of the few investigators previously occupied with initiating such studies is still so engaged.

3. Kretschmer is consistently following up his constitution [Konstitutionswissenschaftliche] psychiatry, also into the physiological field. He has many followers. This approach seems to offer clear and illuminating possibilities for the mastery of the question of the endogenic psychoses. In this connection should be mentioned also the genealogical branch; but it must be said that genealogical investigations, formerly carried to such exaggerated dimensions, have not yet been vigorously resumed.

4. Psychopathology, by which term we would designate psychiatry in the narrow sense, is little cultivated. We distinguish the following subgroups:

(a) The conceptual-descriptive [begrifflich-beschreibende], i.e., clinical in the narrow sense. This viewpoint has become less common, although it is represented by Gruhle and the writer as well. The new edition of Jaspers' *General Psychopathology* attracted the widest attention but will hardly have great influence, since the book, although uniquely ingenious, betrays the lack of recent clinical experience.

(b) Related is a strongly logical-phenomenological trend that is again becoming manifest, but which because of its difficult intelligibility will not become common property among psychiatrists.

(c) German psychiatry continues of one mind in excluding psychogenetic, or more strictly speaking psychoanalytic, psychiatry, insofar as the causation of the psychoses is concerned. It makes use of such interpretation to some extent in investigating the conflict reactions ("neuroses," a term that I reject).

(d) Existence-analytic [daseinsanalytische] psychiatry (Binswanger, Storch) is scarcely represented in Germany and is not here regarded as an avenue for empirical research.

(e) Of good prospect although not yet possible to set forth fully is a functional-analytical psychopathology of which Carl Schneider was an exponent. From related viewpoint Conrad is carrying on investigations in the sequelæ of brain injures.

These are some of the types of research in Germany today. That all are more or less closely related is obvious, likewise that many fields inevitably overlap.

A word about therapy. In the conflict reactions, as has been mentioned, various analytical methods are more or less used. The endogenic psychoses are mainly treated by the different shock therapies, electroshock being far in the lead. Insulin was scarcely available until recently. Opinions as to the results of shock therapy are, on the average, much less optimistic than in America. We have had hardly any experience with lobotomy. There is great reluctance to undertake this operation and a pretty general tendency to reject it on grounds of principle. Penicillin treatment of the luetic psychoses has been tried here and there—and only very recently—encouraged by the lectures of E. Straus in the summer, 1948, which were received with the greatest appreciation and interest.

REMINISCENCES: 1938 AND SINCE

By John Romano, M.D.

Professor of Psychiatry Emeritus, University of Rochester, Rochester, New York

The author cites significant changes in the conduct of the psychiatric profession between the fourth and ninth decades of this century. Determinants of the changes included the impact of World War II, the National Mental Health Act of 1946, the evolution of multiple modes of psychotherapy, the move from a system of involuntary incarceration and treatment in public institutions to a voluntaristic and pluralistic system, the provision of public and private insurance support for office, outpatient, and inpatient psychiatric care, the resurgence of psychopharmacology, and the pursuit of research in biological and psychosocial fields. The social goals of the profession are also discussed.

On the afternoon of June 7, 1938, during the 94th annual meeting of the American Psychiatric Association (APA), which took place in the Fairmont Hotel in San Francisco, I read a paper on studies of schizophrenic patients. I had spent a considerable part of my third year as a Commonwealth Fellow in Psychiatry at the Colorado Psychopathic Hospital in Denver conducting a follow-up study of schizophrenic patients admitted earlier to that hospital. The title of the paper was "Prognosis in Schizophrenia: A Preliminary Report"(1). My coauthor was Franklin J. Ebaugh, then Professor and Chairman of the Department of Psychiatry at the University of Colorado School of Medicine and Director of the Psychopathic Hospital.

As this was my first experience of reading a paper before such an audience, I was somewhat anxious and, regrettably, my anxiety was not lessened by the behavior of the chairman of the session, Richard H. Hutchings, President-Elect of APA. In introducing me and reading the title of the paper, Hutchings had inadvertently turned to the wrong page of the program; he introduced me as Dr. Violet Bathgate and the title of the talk as "Birth Histories in Superior and Inferior Children." When I approached Dr. Hutchings to tell him that I was not Violet Bathgate and that the title of my talk was not "Birth Histories in Superior and Inferior Children," he looked at me over his half-lenses and in a kindly, avuncular manner said, "It's OK, son, you'll be all right in a few minutes." After I had introduced myself and my title, someone turned on a very loud air conditioner in the room where I was speaking, and a number of persons in the back of the room asked me to speak louder, which I did. About halfway through my 15-minute presentation, the air

conditioner was suddenly turned off, whereupon Dr. Hutchings came over and said to me, "Son, no need to shout." That was my baptism under fire, or should I say, under freon—my first presentation before a national, professional body. The effect of this experience is evidenced in the fact that 51 years later I still speak in subdued tones.

That year, 1938, was the first time APA had held its annual meeting in California. In 1911, the meeting had been in Denver, but it had never been held further west. The total registration for the 1938 meeting was 1,076, of whom 284 were members. The total membership of the Association in 1938 was cited as 1,880 (2). I became a member in 1939, together with my friends and colleagues Henry W. Brosin and Jack R. Ewalt and many others.

As far as I know, all the activities of the 94th annual meeting took place in the Fairmont Hotel; perhaps a few events took place at the neighboring hotel, the Mark Hopkins. Most of the younger members and nonmembers could not afford to stay at these posh hotels and found reasonably antiseptic, if not aseptic, lodging in rooms in small hotels at the foot of the hill.

May I remind you of the times? The 1930s were called "the decade of the lean years." Notable changes took place in the role of the federal government in employment, in the multiplication of alphabet agencies, in the increasing strife between management and labor, and in the rise of demagoguery. I realize now, but certainly did not in 1938 during the annual meeting, that in the entire program there seemed to be no mention or discussion of the remarkable changes which were taking place in our government, nor of crime, poverty, labor relations, or demagoguery. Similarly, before Pearl Harbor, our profession, like the nation at large, had remained relatively indifferent to, if not uninformed about, the European situation (3).

And what of our professional and scientific concerns? Earlier in the century (in 1918), Wagner von Jauregg had

Adapted from a special lecture presented at the 142nd annual meeting of the American Psychiatric Association, San Francisco, May 6-11, 1989. Received May 23, 1989; revision received Oct. 11, 1989; accepted Nov. 1, 1989. From the Department of Psychiatry, University of Rochester.

introduced malaria treatment in general paresis (4), and Klaesi had used prolonged narcosis treatment as early as 1922 (5), but it was a decade later that the major thrust of physical treatment took place, initiated by Sakel in 1936 with hypoglycemic coma treatment (6) and by von Meduna in 1938 with pharmacological convulsive therapy (7). Electroshock therapy was demonstrated by Cerletti and Bini in 1938 (8), and in 1936 Moniz, in cooperation with Lima, reported on a surgical approach to the treatment of psychosis (9). In a parallel instance, Elvehjam et al. in 1938 showed that nicotinic acid could cure black tongue in a pellagra-like disease of dogs (10). Shortly thereafter, nicotinic acid proved effective in the therapy of clinical pellagra. Quite predictably, during the 94th annual meeting there were a number of papers concerning the use of Metrazol and insulin in the treatment of schizophrenic patients, as well as papers on the effects of malaria treatment of CNS syphilis. As yet there was no mention of the surgical approach to the treatment of psychosis reported by Moniz in 1936, nor were there papers on the use of nicotinic acid in the therapy of clinical pellagra. These came later.

I remember vividly the excitement and promise that attended these ventures in the physical treatments of that day, and later it occurred to me that our expectations may have been similar to those of clinicians who worked with psychotic patients following the demonstration by Noguchi and Moore in 1913 of Treponema pallidum in the brains of paretic patients, thus substantiating a physical basis for madness; subsequently the fever treatment was introduced. At long last, we then thought there appeared to be a physical basis for mental disease, and many believed that shock treatments and lobotomy supported the idea of a physical basis for the enigma of schizophrenia. Nebulous neurophysiologic notions emerged from these empiric approaches and were considered the theoretical basis for action, but none was convincing.

In a short time (with the addition of penicillin), two of the major psychotic illnesses, namely, syphilis and pellagra, were treated or eliminated by chemical means. Impressive, too, were the remarkable benefits obtained through the use of ECT in psychotic depressed patients. These gains supported the use of physical methods. However, the use of Metrazol and insulin in the treatment of schizophrenic patients did not fulfill our high expectations, and the risk with insulin was considerable.

Since the 1930s, the magnitude, as well as the rate, of change in the form and content of our profession has been unparalleled in our history. The psychiatrist's almost exclusive engagement in the study and treatment of patients in a mandatory, involuntary, intramural detention unit changed to care of patients in multiple sites outside the hospital. Understandably, this led to considerable confusion in the modern psychiatrist as to his or her professional role: Who am I? What knowledge and which skills will I need in my professional work? Who will be my patients and with whom do I share responsibility for the care of the sick? Earlier, I wrote, "There is as yet no satisfactory unitary concept which encompasses human behavior in biological, psychological, and social terms. We have yet to acquire a full and proper language to deal with the whole of man in his soci-

ety. We have withdrawn into secluded apartments in our Tower of Babel and at times speak to each other in tongues. But this has been so since the beginning, and I would expect it to be so for some time to come" (11).

As a participant observer, I shall draw attention to what I believe were significant factors that brought about this change. The experience in World War II—the screening of draftees for the Selective Service system and the increasing concern about environmental factors that precipitated neuropsychiatric problems in military personnel—supported the belief that environmental stress played a major role in the etiology of mental maladjustment. The war experience also emphasized the magnitude of mental distress in our society and led the profession to consider, perhaps for the first time, that our objectives must include those of primary prevention. These matters were later reflected in the community mental health movement, which insisted that psychiatrists become informed about and socially and politically active in reducing poverty, population increase, and racial discrimination and in improving education, employment, and housing.

Few would disagree with the judgment that the National Mental Health Act passed by the 79th Congress in 1946 was the single most influential factor in producing change. For the first time in our national history, the law provided generous financial support for both psychiatric education and research. Its immediate influence was that of increasing the number of psychiatric residents in training and initiating programs for the pursuit of new knowledge. It was my privilege to have served as a founding member of the National Mental Health Council and as chairman of its first research study section. My memory remains vivid of the first meeting of the council on Aug. 15, 1946, in the American Red Cross building in Washington, D.C., with Surgeon-General Thomas Parran presiding. You can well imagine the excitement, the hope, and the aspirations of those of us newly entrusted with federal funds to promote research, patient care, and education programs for psychiatrists, psychologists, social workers, and nurses. The National Mental Health Act, followed by the Hill-Burton law enabling the building of psychiatric units in general hospitals, stimulated the creation and development of departments of psychiatry in our medical schools, the teaching of psychiatry to all medical students, the establishment of residency programs, and the initiation of research activities. One must remember that in the 1930s and as late as the mid-1940s, the few university departments of psychiatry that existed at all were staffed by one or two part-time faculty members. The active, full-time faculty at Yale in 1934 was three in number. In the spring of 1989, the department was one of the largest in the Yale School of Medicine, with 92 full-time faculty members and 90 residents-in-training. During my professional life, from the early 1930s to date, there has been an increase of psychiatrists from fewer than two per 100,000 persons to about 14 per 100,000.

The increase in the number of psychiatrists led to considerable diversity in their function and practice. Unlike 50 years ago when the few psychiatrists who existed served almost exclusively in public and private mental hospitals, today's psychiatrists are found in community, private, and group practice; in clinics and general hospital settings, including those for children and adolescents; in schools, courts, and government agencies; on the faculties of our medical schools and schools of social work; on radio and TV educational programs; and at the National Institute of Mental Health (NIMH).

Before World War II psychiatry had no Rockfeller Institute to groom its young professors as was the case in medicine and physiology. We had to wait until 1946 before NIMH became a reality. Our professional models in the past were the hospital administrator, later the clinician, teacher, and scholar, and then the psychoanalytic psychotherapist-practitioner. Not until the early 1950s was the Career Investigator Fellowship program established by NIMH, with the hope that a new model of psychiatrist-scientific investigator would be created and fostered (12).

On my return to active clinical research after many years as department chairman, I noted with dismay that only a small number of clinical investigators were psychiatrists. Few senior professional workers have direct contact with a research subject or patient, such contact being made principally by junior professionals or by technicians. The basic problem with this is, again, the crucial necessity of obtaining an informed, sensitive, and precise appraisal of the subjects who will provide the primary data.

Further, I have been overwhelmed by the vast number of rating scales and wonder whether our reaching for reliability has lessened validity. I learned that my concern in this matter is shared by another. Prof. D. Bobon of the University of Liège, Belgium, has said, "Quantification of psychopathology with the help of psychiatric rating scales has reached the point of no return; there is no research in psychiatry without a search for its clinical significance and no research on this clinical significance without rating scales. But there is a dramatic need for an increase in the number and quality of projects not only with rating scales but on rating scales. At present, there exist too many such scales and not enough research on their validity versus limitations, which could become the field of a fruitful collaboration between psychiatrists and clinical psychologists" (13).

Another factor that brought about change in our profession was the impact of psychoanalytic psychology. I have drawn attention to the impact of psychoanalysis on psychiatry in the United States as contrasted with Europe, which, in turn, led to a wider polarization of the belief systems of American psychiatrists as compared with those of our European colleagues. We have championed the psychosocial model of behavior, at times to the detriment of the genetic, biological model, and this has led us, quite predictably, to respond to a considerably broader variety of people in distress. Many psychotherapists in private practice are concerned principally with neurotic middle-class patients. However, the nature of the neurotic distress we treat has changed from symptom distress or symptom neurosis to character neurosis. This, in turn, has expanded to our responding to the needs of those who are unhappy, troubled, alienated, lonely, and afflicted with the malaise and anomie of our time. Psychotherapy, formerly a province of psychiatrists and psychoanalysts, is now practiced by clinical psychologists, social workers, nurses, clergymen,

and a large group of paraprofessionals. A host of psychotherapeutic modes have emerged from analytically oriented therapy, behavior therapy, humanistic therapy, and transpersonal therapy. Nonpsychiatric professionals and paraprofessionals far outnumber psychiatric psychotherapists. At the moment, much if not most of psychotherapy is being conducted by the nonpsychiatric groups (14).

Psychoanalytic psychology helped me understand the significance of the life story narration and, in particular, the natural history of disease when attention was focused on the sequence of forgotten as well as remembered events. The predominant concept in the life history narration is that the organism carries past experience as long as life endures. Psychoanalytic psychology, with its concepts of transference and countertransference, deepened my understanding of the physician-patient relationship. It led to awareness of the universal experience of anxiety and of the regressive, maladaptive behavior that occurs in response to illness—the repression and denial—as well as the mastery (14).

Although there were beginnings in the 1930s of certain types of limited community services (for example, we helped to establish outpost clinics in western Colorado for triage, diagnostic study, first-aid treatment, and referral), the community mental health movement emerged early in 1954 when New York State enacted its community mental health services legislation. It is difficult to specify the determinants, but it is generally believed that two developments, more than any others, both of which occurred in the early 1950s, revolutionized the field. One was the introduction of rauwolfia and the phenothiazines, which contributed to the effective treatment and symptomatic management of many severely psychotic patients. These drugs also made possible a reduction in the duration of hospital stays and increased the percentage of patients discharged from hospitals after acute episodes. These achievements made deinstitutionalization possible. The second development was that new psychosocial methods of treatment, together with the introduction of hospital milieu treatment of schizophrenic patients, initially introduced by Maxwell Jones, appeared in Great Britain and were later brought to the United States. As mentioned earlier, these and other factors led to a major shift from almost total reliance on a system of involuntary incarceration and treatment in public institutions to a voluntaristic and pluralistic system. Regrettably, the initial phases of this movement were launched without adequate systematic experiment and trial, and as a result many chronic psychotic patients, who had long been institutionalized and who lacked or had lost social skills, were catapulted into the community without adequate means for their care. We learned that chronic illness is not a myth, nor is it necessarily a result of neglect, and it cannot be removed by sweeping it under the rug of ill-prepared facilities.

Parallel with the development of the community mental health movement has been the almost exponential growth of self-help/mutual-aid groups. In this century social changes have diminished the traditional support of the nuclear family, and today mutual-aid groups develop when families and/or professional services no longer meet the needs of a great number of persons. These groups are based not on residence or kinship but on their members' shared conditions and experiences. They may supplement or complement the help, support, and information once provided only by natural or professional assistance. Since the founding of Alcoholics Anonymous in 1935, it is estimated that mutual-help groups now serve more than 15 million persons in the United States and Canada (15).

As I mentioned earlier, the introduction of drugs, and practicing psychiatrists' prescribing them for daily use by their patients, has returned psychiatrists to their biological heritage and grown attention to neurobiological as well as motivational models as determinants of illness. This has led to a more balanced view of psychopathology as explicable not only in the paradigmatic terms of psychological conflict but also in terms of deficit. The daily use of medication requires physical as well as psychological screening of patients, and psychiatrists have had to become familiar with certain laboratory methods to help them gauge drug dosage and avoid complications. This trend has been called neo-Kraepelinian and is characterized by serious consideration of genetic factors, greater diagnostic precision in noting signs and symptoms of disease, charting of the natural course of illness, and follow-up studies of the effect of intervention on prognosis. In short, the psychiatrist has again become a doctor. What has been disappointing is the indiscriminate prescribing of medication by psychiatrists who are hesitant to learn more about the correct use of drugs and the hazards of their abuse.

In the past several years, several brain imaging techniques have become available. A recent review of these techniques as they apply to psychiatry (16) included those used to evaluate brain structure (computed tomography and magnetic resonance imaging), techniques to assess functional activity (measurement of regional cerebral blood flow, single photon emission computed tomography), and positron emission tomography. These techniques have been used to map brain structure and function in normal human beings. They have also enlarged our knowledge of the pathophysiology of mental illnesses. The long-term promise of brain imaging is still to be established (16).

As I have already noted, the National Mental Health Act made possible funds for the appointment of psychiatric faculties in our medical schools, one of the functions of which was the teaching of psychiatry to medical students. Major emphasis in our teaching was placed on the concepts of health and disease, those of growth and development, and those of the social matrix of the patient and his or her family. We were concerned with the psychology of illness, convalescence, and disability, the relationships between brain and mind and those between mind and body, and the phenomena basic to the idiosyncratic human interaction between patient and physician. It was our expectation, which I believe was fulfilled, that students would have ample opportunity to learn, through personal experience in their clinical assignments, about those events which would enable them to discipline their capacity for human intimacy, a basic ingredient in the preparation of clinicians for their task.

One major theme of my professional life has been and remains the education of medical students. I have been dis-

tressed by the changes in the university medical centers where teaching has been diminished and neglected. I am not alone in my concern.

In a critique (12), I remarked about the downgrading of the teaching of psychiatry to medical students. Some years ago, as I went about the country, I found very few department chairmen or senior professorial staff members working intimately with medical students. Part-time faculties appeared to be harassed in their hurried visits to their patients. Much of the teaching was relegated to residents and junior staff members without adequate models for them to emulate and with negligible reward systems. In the same critique I pointed out that students perceived the concern of psychiatrists about the definition of their professional role, I wrote,

> When the student comes to these floors, unlike the other clinical services, he finds that most of the staff are not in uniform. He finds them in open shirts, loose gypsy blouses, hip-hugging jeans, wooden shoes, Indian beads, and an abundance of hair. There are nurses, nursing assistants, nurse practitioners, nurse clinicians, assistant clinicians, psychiatric technicians, social workers, social work assistants, mental health aides, program coordinators, psychology students, primary therapists, secondary therapists, behavior therapists, occupational therapists, recreational therapists, physical therapists, family and group therapists, mental health information service clerks, junior psychiatric faculty, senior psychiatric faculty (not many of these), full-time (less of these), part-time (often in a hurry), sometime, one-time, and regrettably, most of them never on time. From time to time, from out of the medical mist emerges a silent white-coated person with a stethoscope, who conducts a physical examination of the patient, records such illegibly on the chart burgeoning with check mark forms, and leaves almost as quietly as he came. We brought them, all of them, to our floors in our evangelical egalitarianism. Most patients are now called clients and soon may be called penitents. Small wonder the medical student asks, "Who is the doctor, and what does he do?" (12)

Is it any better now?

Our residency programs have changed, too. Initially, they were quite informal and apprentice-like, based on the graduate training of interns and residents in medicine at the Johns Hopkins Hospital at the turn of the century. With the increased number of residents, programs became more formal, more structured, more didactic, and less personal and there was an expanded set of clinical assignments. In several programs opportunities were provided for engagement in ongoing research in the department or in research based on the resident's own ideas. In general, the content of the teaching program was pluralistic in that it was concerned with the determinants of behavior from genetic, biological, psychological, and interpersonal factors—all of this in a developmental time sense of phases of growth.

Obviously, there were considerable variations on a theme. Some programs were fairly monistic in their espousal of psychoanalytic or behavioral theory points of view. Others gave lip service to psychological and social matters while emphasizing genetic and biological factors. In general, the curriculum reflected the beliefs, experiences, and prejudices of the senior faculty. There was somewhat of an estrangement between neurology and psychology, and only in the past two decades has there been a more viable relationship with pharmacology.

On May 16, 1894, at the 50th annual meeting of our Association (then called the American Medico-Psychological Association) held in Philadelphia, Silas Weir Mitchell, distinguished American physician, neurologist, and author, gave the major address of the meeting. Perceptive and relentless was his critique of our profession at that time. He drew attention to the isolation, geographical and intellectual, of psychiatrists from the rest of medicine. He deplored the "multiplicity of the nonmedical duties of most medical superintendents" and stressed the importance to staff morale of original scientific work in the asylums of that day. He was troubled by the dearth of nurses and attendants trained properly to care for the insane and by the inadequate use of work as a means of therapy and education. He criticized the lack of attention to patients' needs at the time of their return to ordinary civilian life (17).

Fifty years later, at the centenary meeting of APA in Philadelphia in May 1944, Alan Gregg, Director for the Medical Sciences of the Rockefeller Foundation in New York City, presented his critique of psychiatry. Gregg was neither a psychiatrist nor a neurologist but, because of his long experience with support for medical education and research, served well as a flying buttress to the profession, a support from without. Gregg referred to Mitchell's talk 50 years before and pointed out that Mitchell's remarks were confined almost exclusively to the institutional aspects of the care of the insane, which was the major occupation of the psychiatrist in the 1890s. Gregg remarked that between the 50th and 100th anniversaries of the Association, it and the profession at large had added to their memberships persons who practiced psychiatry in their offices and in the wards of general hospitals, in schools and in guidance clinics, as well as mental hospitals. Obviously, the profession had achieved a far wider range of interests, training, and capacities than was characteristic of psychiatry in 1894. In 1944, Gregg's formulation of our major limitations was, "You were badly recruited, you are isolated from medicine, you are overburdened, and you are too inarticulate and long-suffering to secure redress from the public of some of the handicaps from which you and your patients suffer" (18).

In his concluding remarks, Gregg said,

> Before the two hundredth anniversary of this Association [which will take place in the year 2044], psychiatry will find great extensions of its content and of its obligations. There will be applications far beyond your offices and your hospitals of the further knowledge you will gain, applications not only to patients with functional and organic disease, but to the human relations of normal people—in politics, national and international, between races, between capital and labor, in government, in family life, in education, in every form of human relationship, whether between individuals or between groups. You will be concerned with optimum performance of human beings as civilized creatures.(18)

We shall have to wait 55 years for the 200th anniversary of APA. In 5 years we will celebrate the sesquicentennial anniversary. Just as Silas Weir Mitchell's remarks nearly 100 years ago were concerned principally with the institutional life of the psychiatrist, Gregg 45 years ago drew attention to the beginning diversity of psychiatrists' roles in practice and was principally critical of our poor recruitment, which stemmed from inadequate and uninspired teaching of psychiatry to medical students and limited opportunities for career resident training. He also emphasized our continuing isolation from medicine and our inarticulateness in drawing attention to the handicaps that we and our patients suffer.

It is unlikely that I shall be present at the bicentennial meeting in 2044, and I am not sure that I will be able to be with you 5 years from now at the sesquicentennial. This gives me license to add my critique of our profession to those expressed by our esteemed predecessors. I am surely aware of the hazards of such an undertaking, particularly after learning of the short essay that a little boy wrote on Socrates: "Socrates was the father of and the greatest of philosophers. Socrates taught Plato, and Plato taught Aristotle. Socrates told all the people all their faults. They poisoned him."

In the substance of this paper, I have drawn attention to several of our shortcomings and areas of neglect. In spite of the exponential increase in our numbers and the wide range of our practice, we continue to be neglectful of chronic psychotic patients and alcohol- and drug-addicted, criminal, retarded, and aged patients—particularly, as I said earlier, when they are poor or black or both. Our uncritical acceptance of psychoanalytic psychology, both in theory and in practice, led to overly psychological explanations of human behavior to the detriment of the genetic and biological model. At the moment, this movement is being reversed, as pointed out by our colleague Leon Eisenberg, who remarked that we have changed from being brainless to becoming mindless (19).

Many scholars in the field, including practicing psychoanalysts, believe that psychoanalysis is in the doldrums. One such analyst stated, "There are signs of diminished vigor, of a dulling of its thrust, and of a muting of its influence. One wonders if these intimations are part of a natural history of all vital movements and represent only a momentary pause in development and preparation for new growth or whether it is an incipient senescence, a wearing down of vigor prior to death, or a warning sign of a major malignancy that threatens to cut off its contribution in mid-life" (20).

In their book *Cognitive Science and Psychoanalysis* (21), Kenneth Colby and Robert Stoller review the work of Grünbaum, Farrell, Spence, Wallerstein, Popper, and Ricoeur. More important to Colby and Stoller than the earlier critiques of the scientific basis of psychoanalysis based on hermeneutics, the tally argument, and falsifiability is their argument that psychoanalysis is not a science, as it does not have an adequate database. It lacks replicable data.

Earlier, I commented briefly on the community mental health movement and regretted that the movement was launched with inadequate systematic experiment and trial. As a result, many chronic psychotic patients who had long been institutionalized were released into the community without adequate means for their care.

May I remind you of Alan Gregg's prediction that in a century from the date of his address, in the year 2044, psychiatry would find great extensions of its content and of its obligations, namely, in politics, in national and international affairs, and "in every form of human relationship, whether between individuals or between groups" (18). We have come midway to the time of Gregg's prediction, but I know of no significant evidence at the moment of any advance in any areas about which he spoke. I question seriously whether we shall be more successful 50 years from now. Unless we undertake major changes in the preparation of the psychiatrists of tomorrow, how can they be sufficiently versed in economics, political science, and sociology to help us in our primary concern with men and women in situations of personal distress? We have, as yet, no clear definitions of public health and social and political roles to guide the preparation of those who may assume these new responsibilities. We have erred in promising not one but many rose gardens in response to society's insistent demands that we reduce crime, delinquency, drug abuse, and alcoholism.

I have read with interest and admiration most of Barbara Tuchman's historical books, particularly *The March of Folly* (22). In this book she illuminates four decision turning points in history—four instances of folly: the Trojan War, papal misrule during the Renaissance, the actions of George III during the American Revolution, and the war in Vietnam. Folly may be defined as foolishness, lack of good sense and understanding, lack of foresight. All of us, as individuals and as groups, have committed our share of follies. Let me share with you my thoughts about two events in our professional history that I believe would meet Barbara Tuchman's definition of folly. On July 24, 1964, 1 month after Barry Goldwater received the Republican nomination, *Fact* magazine sent a questionnaire to all the nation's 12,356 psychiatrists asking, "Do you believe Barry Goldwater is psychologically fit to serve us as president of the United States?" The names of psychiatrists were supplied by the American Medical Association (23). Of the 12,356 psychiatrists who were sent questionnaires, 2,417 (20%) responded. Of these, 571 said they did not know enough about Goldwater to answer the question, 657 said they thought Goldwater was psychologically fit, and 1,189 said he was not. In my view, this resulted in a considerable blow to the dignity of our profession. Imagine our problem in trying to explain to our students, house staff, and colleagues the behavior of almost 15% of the professional population who judged the fitness of a person without seeing him, much less studying him, and thus violated all principles of professional decorum and confidentiality.

Another event that in my view meets the definition of folly was the elimination of the internship. In late December 1969, directors of residency training programs in psychiatry were notified, "Effective July 1, 1970, the American Board of Psychiatry and Neurology will not require the completion of an internship as one of its requirements for eligibility" (24). A similar recommendation was submitted (on Oct. 31, 1969) by the APA Committee on Medical Education to its parent body (24). I was asked by Francis Braceland, then editor of the *American Journal of Psychiatry*,

to comment on this action, and I wrote a detailed statement, published in May 1970 in the *Journal*, entitled "The Elimination of the Internship—An Act of Regression" (24). What was most distressing was that even though professional bodies such as the American Association of Chairmen of Departments of Psychiatry were and are deeply concerned, no attempt was made to obtain empirical data or to propose discussion and debate of the issues in a scholarly and systematic manner. In my concluding remarks I indicated that "the elimination of the internship year as a minimal requirement, together with a shortening of the residency period, will seriously impair the education of the psychiatrist. The contribution of the psychiatrist as physician is different from those made to the field by our professional colleagues in psychology, social work, nursing, and social science . . . To reduce the dimensions of the role of the psychiatrist as physician would seriously impair his contributions as practitioner, teacher, scholar, and investigator. It is a degradation of quality" (24).

Marc Hollender, a colleague and friend, is currently preparing the history of the American Board of Psychiatry and Neurology (M. Hollender, personal communication, March 1989). In this report he details in chapter and verse the events that preceded the decision to eliminate the internship, as well as several actions taken since then. In my mind, the Board, as well as the APA committee, acted foolishly and was unduly influenced by the Millis report (24), which, I believe, made questionable recommendations. To add to the folly of the decision, this regressive act was occurring while the profession was being revived by a renaissance of interest in matters biological.

I suppose one could add other instances of folly in psychiatry, for example, the widespread use of lobotomy, but as Elliot S. Valenstein has recorded in a scholarly book, *Great and Desperate Cures*, the lobotomy movement emerged more from desperation than from foolishness (25). In the late 1940s and early 1950s, the mutilating brain operation known as lobotomy (or more generally, psychosurgery) was performed on tens of thousands of patients. One cannot overestimate the despair felt by psychiatrists, nurses, and families of patients in dealing day in and day out, at times for years, with patients who were assaultive, suicidal, homicidal, and overactive, conditions which at times led to exhaustion and death. In the United States, lobotomy was militantly and vigorously promoted by Walter Freeman, who traveled coast to coast to undertake this operation on disturbed patients in hospitals for the chronically insane. Truly, a sad chapter in our history.

And now, what of the present day? We have fulfilled our expectations in producing an increase of psychiatrists. (The increase in the number of psychologists, social workers, and counselors is two to four times the increase in the number of psychiatrists). We did introduce psychology and the social sciences into the matrix of the medical schools. We established psychiatric units in general hospitals and promoted research in biological as well as psychological and social fields. This took place at NIMH and in many university departments. We took part in the exponential increase in psychotherapeutic modes that allowed us and, increasingly, other professionals and paraprofessionals to respond not only to the needs of traditional neurotic patients but, more broadly, to those who are unhappy, troubled, alienated, lonely, and affected with the malaise and anomie of our time. We have separated homosexuality from the concept of disease, and with the proper use of psychotropic drugs, including the remarkably useful lithium, we have improved our treatment of acutely psychotic patients. We have lost the demented patients and others with organic brain disease to the neurologists because of our negligent attention to biological matters. Our liaison ventures with our sister clinical departments have not survived well, and family medicine seems to disregard our contributions. We have helped to increase public awareness of the prevalence and magnitude of mental illness but have bungled our move to care for chronic psychotic patients in the community. Our love-hate relationship with the press, Hollywood, radio, and television has remained fairly constant. The degradation of the teaching of our medical students and residents cannot be attributed solely to our profession, as it is part and parcel of major changes in the world of medicine today.

Obviously, we have much to do, particularly in the study and care of the abandoned and neglected, the chronic schizophrenic patient, the alcoholic, the criminal, the addict, the retarded, and the aged. Are we doing as much as we can and should in caring for AIDS patients and their families? Do we not have responsibility to participate in the diagnosis of AIDS and in support of the patient, the patient's family, and health care workers? Could we not give more support to the self-help groups and to community enterprises? Most important of all is the need for the continued and vigorous support of research in all the fields, relevant to our concern.

At the beginning of this essay, I remarked briefly about the events of the fourth decade of this century, the 1930s, "the decade of the lean years." And now, 50 years later, we are ending the ninth decade of the century. I leave it to you to judge what progress we have made in terms of crime, violence, poverty, racism, education, housing and the homeless, environmental pollution, and the fact that 37 million of us have no health insurance. I leave it to you, too, to judge to what degree our annual professional program reflects the problems of the day. While I am fully aware that the good old days were never that good, it seems to me that we suffer from a deficiency disease. I think there is marked evidence of a deficiency of outrage. I do not think we are sufficiently outraged when we consider how pervasive are venality, corruption, and ineptness in law, medicine, science, government, religion, commerce, Wall Street, education. Are there not sufficient reasons to be outraged? Perhaps the magnitude of this behavior is such that we have become benumbed and anesthetized or feel powerless to do anything about it.

In closing, I had intended to salute and pay tribute to those from whom I learned. I am afraid if I were to cite them, I could not do justice to them. Let me conclude by saying what I have said before; namely, I have learned most from my students and my patients (26).

And now, those of you with intact episodic short-term memory may join me in saying, Good night, Violet Bathgate—wherever you are.

REFERENCES

1. Romano J, Ebaugh FG: Prognosis in schizophrenia: a preliminary report. Am J Psychiatry 1938; 95:583–596
2. American Psychiatric Association, proceedings of the ninety-fourth annual meeting, June 6–10, 1938. Am J Psychiatry 1938; 95: 421–486
3. This Fabulous Century, 1930–1940, Time-Life Books, vol 4. New York, Time, Inc, 1969
4. Wagner von Jauregg J: Die Einvirkung der Malaria auf die Progressive Paralyse. Psychiatrisch-Neurologische Wochenschrift 1918; 20:132–134
5. Klaesi J: Uber die therapeutische Anwendtung der "Dauernarkose" mittels Somnifen bei Schizophrenen. Zeitschrift für die Gesamte Neurologie und Psychiatrie 1922; 74:557–592
6. Sakel M: Zur Methodik der Hypoglykamieve-handlung von Psychosen. Wien Klin Wochenschr 1936; 49:1278–1282 [reprinted in translation in this sesquicentennial anniversary supplement of the Journal]
7. von Meduna L: General discussion of the cardiazol therapy. Am J Psychiatry 1938; 94(May suppl):40–50
8. Cerletti U, Bini L: L'elletroshock. Archivio Generale di Neurologia, Psichiatria, e Psicoanalisi 1938; 19:266–268
9. Moniz E: Tentatives opératories dans le traitement de certaines psychoses. Paris, Masson, 1936 [reprinted in translation in this sesquicentennial anniversary supplement of the Journal]
10. Elvehjam CA, Madden RJ, Strong FM, et al: Isolation and identification of the anti-black tongue factor. J Biol Chem 1938; 123:137–149
11. Romano J: On the teaching of psychiatry to medical students: does it have to get worse before it gets better? Psychosom Med 1980; 42(1, suppl):103–111
12. Romano J: Requiem or reveille: psychiatry's choice, Thomas W Salmon Lecture. Bull NY Acad Med 1977; 53:787–805
13. Bobon D: Psychiatric rating scales: a breakthrough or a breakdown? (abstract). Psychiatric Bulletin (RC of Psychiatrists) 1988; 12(suppl 1):3
14. Romano J: On becoming a psychiatrist: 1934–1942. JAMA 1989; 261:2240–2243
15. Romano J: How do we transmit the humanistic factors in the practice of medicine? in Medical Education for the 21st Century. Edited by Warren JV, Trzebiatowski GL. Columbus, Ohio State University College of Medicine, 1985
16. Andreasen NC: Brain imaging: applications in psychiatry. Science 1988; 239:1381–1388
17. Mitchell SW: Address before the fiftieth annual meeting of the American Medico-Psychological Association, held in Philadelphia, May 16th, 1894. J Nerv Ment Dis 1894; 21:413–437 [reprinted in this sesquicentennial anniversary supplement of the Journal]
18. Gregg A: A critique of psychiatry. Am J Psychiatry 1944; 101:285–291
19. Eisenberg L: Mindlessness and brainlessness in psychiatry. Br J Psychiatry 1986; 148:497–508
20. Holzman PS: The future of psychoanalysis and its institutes. Psychoanal Q 1976; 45:250–273
21. Colby KM, Stoller RJ: Cognitive Science and Psychoanalysis. Hillsdale, NJ, Lawrence Erlbaum Associates, 1988
22. Tuchman BW: The March of Folly: From Troy to Vietnam. New York, Alfred A Knopf, 1984
23. Ginzburg R: Goldwater: the man and the menace. Fact 1964; 1(5):3–22
24. Romano J: The elimination of the internship—an act of regression. Am J Psychiatry 1970; 126:1565–1576
25. Valenstein ES: Great and Desperate Cures. New York, Basic Books, 1986
26. Romano J: On those from whom we learn. Calif Med 1972; 117:72–75

INTRODUCTION

The period in American psychiatry covered by these papers on clinical description encompassed major swings of the pendulum between psychosocial and biological explanations of mental illness. In the early part of the nineteenth century, Moral Treatment was introduced into the United States from the York Retreat in England as an enlightened reform, an alternative to the warehousing of the mentally ill that had preceded it. The underlying premise of Moral Treatment was the educability of psychiatric patients. The hospital was reconceptualized as a "reparenting" experience, to retrain and correct presumed developmental deficits. These reforms vastly humanized psychiatric care.

With impetus from crusaders such as Dorothea Dix, many state mental hospitals were built in the nineteenth century, replacing the dilapidated jails in which many of the mentally ill languished. However, by the latter part of the century these hospitals had become overcrowded, inundated with severely ill patients, and treatment was increasingly replaced by confinement. Earle's paper signals the breakdown of the myth of curability—he noted that in many reports the same patients had "recovered" numerous times. This ushered in an era of descriptive psychiatry, emphasizing genetic contributions to mental illness. Indeed, fears about an influx of immigrants at high genetic risk for mental illness were the basis for many of our immigration laws, first enacted in the early part of the twentieth century. Interest in psychiatry shifted to more objective description and neurobiological conjecture, heavily influenced by Kraepelin.

In the twentieth century, the pendulum began to shift in a developmental and psychosocial direction again, with work reflecting description of the internal subjective and interpersonal phenomenology of mental illness. American psychiatry was heavily influenced by Freud and his disciples and began again to explore the meaning of mental illness to the patient, family, and friends. Thus, Sullivan describes what it feels like to be with a schizophrenic patient, and Kanner discerns meaning in the utterances of autistic children. Lindemann provides us with the obverse of psychobiology—the biopsychology of trauma, or effects of physical events on the mind.

This era of clinical description is rich if inconsistent. It draws from the British tradition of empiricism in evaluating outcome as well as from European objective clinical description on the one hand and theoretical metapsychology on the other. American psychiatry is moving again in a Kraepelinian direction, emphasizing precise objective description (DSM-III and DSM-IV) and biological underpinnings of mental illness (the Decade of the Brain). However, the evidence of the past 150 years of clinical description suggests that our birthright as a profession is in discovering, describing, and treating the disorders of the mind as well as the brain and impairments of intrapsychic cognition and affect as well as disordered interpersonal relationships. Some of the most original American contributions to psychiatry have involved exploring the intrapsychic meaning and interpersonal implications of psychopathology as well as describing neurobiological dysfunction. Clinical description is rich and varied precisely because it attempts to depict complex mind/brain phenomena. Our history of accomplishment in this task suggests that the future of clinical description will continue to be similarly rich and varied.

Hegel said that the great lesson of history is that people are ignorant of history. One reads the past 150 years of research and writing in American psychiatry with both anxiety and awe. The anxiety stems from recognition of the foolish mistakes our forebears made, leading to uncomfortable reveries about our descendants' reactions in reading our work 150 years from now. The awe comes from those moments of recognition, when one can see the wisdom of our predecessors and their almost uncanny ability to describe clearly, analyze problems, and reach conclusions that have stood the test of time remarkably well. This is especially noteworthy in the field of clinical description, which was at the heart of forming the discipline of psychiatry and was conducted with an elegance and precision that would shame much modern writing. Indeed, as our attention has turned to neurobiological mechanisms and psychopharmacological and psychotherapeutic treatments, emphasis on clear and gripping clinical description has taken a back seat, and we are the poorer for it. The richness of clinical description in the articles in this section only serves to underscore that we have as much to learn from the past as the future.

Amariah Brigham was the first editor of *The American Journal of Insanity*. He was a remarkably thoughtful, clear, and compassionate writer. In his article, Brigham describes insanity incisively as *"a chronic disease of the brain, producing either derangement of the intellectual faculties, or prolonged change of the feelings, affections, and habits of an individual."* This is not bad for 1844. With surgical skill and considerable diplomacy, Brigham distinguishes psychiatry from Satanism. Sensitive to religious sensibilities, he adopts a dualist position—the brain can be diseased but not the mind: "By such, insanity is regarded as a disease of the body, and few at the present time, suppose the mind itself is ever diseased. The immaterial and immortal mind is, of itself, incapable of disease and decay." He cites, as an example, a man with hemiparesis whose mental faculties were perfectly clear: "The brain is the instrument which the mind uses in this life, to manifest itself, and like all other parts of our bodies, is liable to disease, and when diseased, is often incapable of manifesting harmoniously and perfectly the powers of the mind." He goes on to postulate, incorrectly, that the outer portion of the brain is associated with mental function and the inner portion with voluntary motor control.

Interestingly, in exploring the causation of insanity, Brigham provides us with two cases of pathological bereavement, both involving the traumatic loss of a child. He describes reenactments of the traumatic loss in one case and an apparent psychotic delusion of the existence of the dead child in the other.

In describing personality change after head trauma, Brigham underscores the compassionate side of psychiatric description and diagnosis: "Such cases teach us to be cautious and tolerant in instances where change of character and misconduct are connected as to time, with injury or disease of the head, or even with general ill health."

Indeed, pathological compassion is described as the result of a severe head wound: "He was disposed to give away all that he had, and finally was placed in a Lunatic Asylum in consequence of the trouble which he made in his endeavors to benefit others and relieve suffering." While there is something sadly ironic about this, the poor man may have suffered from posttraumatic stress disorder.

Brigham points out that brain disease may impair not only intellectual capacities but moral, emotional, and relational abilities as well. He is thus parsing diseases and providing the ground for more precise and specific classification. The description of the mental disorder of Napoleon's general seems like a well-described case of mania, perhaps induced by syphilis, since after his manic activities he became paralytic and died.

Brigham also addresses the issue of moral insanity and legal exculpation, defending the concept on the one hand and pointing out on the other how well such disorders may be hidden in a legal setting. For all of this rich description, the article also has a free-wheeling nature that clearly would not pass muster in a current issue of the journal.

James Kiernan calls for a greater rigor in classification and a linking of clinical symptoms, etiology, and pathological anatomy, attacking colleagues for producing "sublime monuments to the scientific use of the imagination." At the same time he indulges in a bit of his own, linking masturbation to catatonia and catatonia to political activism, "the conduct of the chronic revolutionist." Reading Case II is also disturbing—"W.H.G., aged 26; colored, laborer, married, intemperate and syphilitic," who apparently suffered a seizure and then became depressed leading to hospitalization. He "passed into a cataleptoid condition, from which he emerged one morning; said he 'was equal to any white man,' and spoke very precisely." One can only hope that this was considered to be evidence of recovery rather than disease.

In turning from description to the problem of causation, Kiernan takes an important step, using a well-described case series. He takes apart the roles of physical illness and psychic trauma and documents the presence of either physical illness or a family history of disease. He observes a high prevalence of physical illness and alcoholism.

Lest the reader get too excited about Kiernan's prescience, however, he also notes that 22 of the 30 patients "admitted the practice of masturbation." It should be noted that masturbation was generally regarded as a disease by physicians in the nineteenth century, so psychiatrists were not alone in attributing pathological significance to it. Strange as Kiernan's attribution of recent depression to sexual activity may be, there is an odd reverberation in the paper of psychodynamic things to come. In 1877, he wrote, "A depression is produced during semi-lucid periods by the evident contradiction between the duties of religion and the strong sexual desires, which often control the conduct." This is a forerunner to Freud's description of the dynamic unconscious, the battle between superego and id (1).

Kiernan goes on to describe the evidence to support the idea of tuberculous meningitis as an etiological factor in catatonia. He is also sophisticated enough to propose a stress-diathesis model in which neurobiological damage makes the patient more vulnerable to stress, rather than attributing all of the pathology either to biological or psychosocial damage.

The precision in describing what may be a case of thyroid-induced psychosis is not matched by similar sophistication in describing social support: "If the case be a boy, and he has a doting, foolish mother, removal from her should be the first step in the treatment, as her sympathy would undo all otherwise beneficial measures."

However, at times the writing is irresistible: "Two ministers of this organization believed they had received, during a cataleptoid condition, a command from God to kill a certain man and raise him from the dead. The former they succeeded in doing, but in the latter they failed."

Pliny Earle, superintendent of the asylum in Northampton, Massachusetts, was a towering figure in nineteenth-century American psychiatry, notable for his unblinking honesty in evaluating the effects of treatment. A statement in his opening paragraph is a monument to clear-eyed scientific modesty: "Nature yields in a measurable extent to the conceptions, the devices, the ministrations, and the administrations of human skill, but, as if to mock them in the end, and to demonstrate the retention of her inherent supremacy, she at length establishes a position and defies their power."

He applies this humbling lesson to a piercing analysis of recovery rates in asylums in Great Britain and the United States. He notes trenchantly that widely cited recovery rates based on analysis of only a few hundred cases are twice as high as those from several studies based on tens of thousands of cases. Sophisticated statistical analyses are not necessary: the numbers speak for themselves. Furthermore, he has the unblinking honesty to point out that recovery rates in American hospitals are even lower than those from Great Britain.

Earle cannot resist sarcasm in describing some variation in reported results but must be admired for listing his own hospital as having among the lowest recovery rates. He goes on to document a declining rate of recovery over time, likely a reflection of the fact that, as Moral Treatment was on the wane, asylums became the repositories of more and more seriously impaired individuals.

Earle gets to the heart of the problem of inflated claims of recovery. In Pennsylvania, the same patient could be listed as recovered many times, since recoveries were classified as "cases." In his own data in Massachusetts, Earle counted people. Any person "recovered" more than once obviously could not be counted as a recovered patient. He explains that is why his recovery rate is lower. Earle's paper is a model of clarity of thought and scientific integrity. His modesty is a source of pride in psychiatric writing and research.

The article by Anton Boisen is noteworthy in a number of ways. Published in 1926, it reveals that the influence of psychodynamic thinking is broad-based, relying on Jung and Janet as well as Freud. Furthermore, there is a strong phenomenological influence as well. Boisen selects cases that illustrate the potential for personal growth in mental illness. Indeed, his orientation is remarkably existential, focusing on themes of meaning, death, and isolation that are the core issues in existential philosophy and psychotherapy (2). In addition, he addresses concerns that became the domain of ego psychology and other schools of psychoanalysis—the will to power and "the desire for self-realization." This is very similar to Mowrer's concept of self-actualization.

The caricature-like description of a "self-educated negro minister" who was "trying to compensate for a sense of inferiority which was both personal and racial," however, leaves no doubt that psychiatry has, at times, both reflected and perpetuated distasteful social norms.

Boisen's description of hypnosis is remarkably astute. He identifies it with the narrowing of attention, an observation not widely understood then but generally accepted now (3). He draws a useful analogy between induced hypnotic states and those which arise in shamanism, religious trance, or severe life stress. This recognition of an underlying mental mechanism that can be involved in positive reorganization as well as cognitive disorganization represents a remarkably contemporary point of view.

Despite this, there are some mistakes in the paper as well. Boisen's description of transference is woefully superficial. Although it is not clear by the end of the article that mental disorder has commonly resulted in personal growth, the theoretical breadth of the article in its attempt to get at the personal meaning of mental illness makes it important.

Harry Stack Sullivan, founder of the Interpersonal School of psychiatry, was a towering figure in twentieth century American psychiatry. He contributed one of the few genuinely American developments in the largely European school of psychoanalysis. In his paper he applies interpersonal theory to the onset of schizophrenia, contributing the important observation that a heterosexual impasse often triggers a first schizophrenic break.

Like Boisen, Sullivan tackles the problem of meaning, considering intention as important as behavior. Indeed, Sullivan cites Boisen's paper approvingly. He contrasts, in an interesting way, defense mechanisms that may have some adaptive value to the processes of depression and anxiety: "both of which are not only maladjustive but also methods which present no real attack upon the troublesome situation; as such, they may be regarded as a means of 'standing still' before a problem."

Sullivan combines a penetrating description of the internal mental state of the schizophrenic patient with a description of what it is like to be with one: "Pure depression is practically a standstill of adjustment, the schizophrenic depression is most unhappy struggle. Instead of literal or figurative sitting still, these people are striving to cut themselves off from painful stimuli." The interpersonal components of the resolution of symptoms do not escape Sullivan's withering attention: "There may be a fragile reorganization prone to relapse under fresh difficulties. Of grave portent, however, is the readjustment by paranoid processes. If it succeeds, we have a persistent paranoid state with more or less of schizophrenic residue (paraphrenias of Kraepelin). If it fails, we have an unhappy jumble of schizophrenic projections, any hopeful aspect of which is lost through the destructive hateful attitude of the patient."

Sullivan is especially good at describing not only the patient's feelings and intentions but those of the therapist in response to the patient, true to his emphasis on the interpersonal. He provides a phenomenology of interpersonal interaction as a reflection of individual psychopathology.

Adolf Meyer was the most prominent American psychiatrist of the early part of this century. His thinking was integrative, encompassing psychosocial as well as neurobiological components of psychiatry. His memorial piece for Kraepelin is notable for its dignified and balanced view of Kraepelin's contribution. Meyer expresses high regard for Kraepelin's devotion to precise description, his use of prognosis in making a diagnosis, and his fascination with the neurobiological underpinnings of mental disorder. At the same time, he parts company with the European master in his lack of interest in "constitutional background" as well as his movement from the degenerative prognosis to the pronouncement of a "metabolism disorder." Meyer notes correctly that the neuropathology of dementia praecox was never as clearly defined as that of general paresis.

Meyer engages in some interesting clinical description of Kraepelin, noting that the master of objective description treated himself as an object as well, not feeling the need to reflect on the development of his own thinking but, rather, writing each new edition of his *Psychopathology* as though it were the first, without a history.

J. Kasanin, author of the classic work, *Language and Thought in Schizophrenia* (4), takes pains to differentiate American clinical description from the Kraepelinian model predominant in Europe. He acknowledges that such precise description is crucial for developing a science of psychiatry. Kasanin notes that Meyer's contribution represented typical American optimism, emphasizing the adaptive resources of the patient that could be mobilized psychotherapeutically to bring the patient into remission. From the point of view of the Kraepelinian model, the main useful information about the patient was the description of the disorder and its prognosis, whereas Kasanin, Meyer, Sullivan, and others in America attempted to describe what the disorder meant to the patient and what the patient's early life experience, reaction to the disorder, and social support contributed to getting beyond or modifying the disorder itself.

Clearly, a willingness to integrate psychodynamic thinking infused this approach to psychiatric phenomenology. At times, however, it led to some of the least successful aspects of it, such as the preoccupation, seen throughout these papers, with masturbation as a sign of conflict over sexuality leading to psychosis. However, Kasanin's scope is broader than that. His case descriptions emphasize social and interpersonal factors that may indeed have influenced the time and type of psychotic decompensation. Examples include heterosexual impasses and failures at work. Kasanin's detailed and historically oriented descriptions provide a clear picture of the social context in which these psychotic episodes occurred and also underscore the subjective discomfort that accompanies psychosis. This is reminiscent of Freud's keen observation that psychotic symptoms could be understood as an attempt at restitution, a response to abrupt disruption of contact with the world. Thus, a reorganization of perception, while frightening, as in paranoid persecutory delusions, was at least understandable (5). This notion of paranoid psychosis may seem archaic, but it is quite compatible with more modern biological theories of thought disorder. Whatever the disruption in processing of perception and memory, the delusions and hallucinations can be understood as an attempt to restore some degree of orderliness to this disrupted information processing.

The reader is struck as well by the uniformly good outcome of these cases, which is rather surprising, and also by the distinct possibility that some of them, most notably the last case, may involve bipolar psychosis rather than schizophrenia, as well as the schizoaffective disorders that Kasanin is describing for the first time. His observations are important in noting an interaction between cognitive and affective psychotic disorders. He points out that this group is distinct from the relentlessly progressive dementia praecox described by Kraepelin.

Lindemann's classic paper is a model of synthetic clinical description. A pioneer in the study of grief and bereavement, Lindemann read to the Centenary meeting of the American Psychiatric Association the results of his study of 101 bereaved individuals, many of whom had lost loved ones in the tragic Cocoanut Grove nightclub fire in Boston. These few pages contain a well-described forerunner of the current DSM-IV diagnoses of acute and posttraumatic stress disorder. Lindemann clearly describes the intrusive and avoidant components of the response to traumatic stress along with the numbing, "disconcerting loss of warmth in relationship to other people" and hyperarousal components, irritability, and restlessness. He describes well the impaired concentration and guilty rumination seen in traumatic stress victims. Thus, the major elements of our current nosology for the response to trauma are captured in this paper.

Lindemann also describes phenomenology among the bereaved that is dissociative in nature: individuals who "go through all the motions of living" but without feelings, "stilted, robot-like." Indeed, Lindemann was among the first to recognize the negative symptoms of posttraumatic stress disorder, warning that those who appear to be doing unusually well after a traumatic loss may in fact be doing the worst, and he describes several. One young man who was initially thought to be doing quite well despite the death of his wife was in fact overwhelmed with guilt and jumped to his death from his hospital room. Lindemann also recognized the role that previous traumatic stress and bereavement can play in complicating the symptoms.

That would certainly be enough for an excellent paper, but Lindemann goes on to define "grief work" as the psychological means of coming to terms with the enormity of loss, enabling one to move on and form new relationships. Lindemann observes astutely that one of the major obstacles to performing the grief work is the associated emotional distress. Lindemann notes that when individuals were willing to deal with traumatic memories they experienced relief and a reduction in the numbing of affect. Indeed, his description of the management of grief is a remarkably concise and current view of the psychotherapy of traumatic stress. It involves the expression and management of strong emotion, dealing with guilt, and integrating the loss: finding "an acceptable formulation of his future relationship to the deceased" and "the acquisition of new patterns of conduct." Another thing that makes Lindemann's paper current is that he is conscious of a need for time-limited psychotherapy: "All this can be done in eight to ten interviews."

Lindemann's paper is thus remarkably prescient, providing an astute description of the response to traumatic loss, identifying all of the major categories of acute and posttraumatic stress disorder symptoms, distinguishing between the normal and necessary process of grieving and pathological depression on the one hand and absence of reaction on the other, and providing concise guidelines for the effective psychotherapy of bereavement. This paper is as salient and useful today as it was 50 years ago.

Kanner, in his classical paper on early infantile autism, provides a brilliant explication of the subjective meaning underlying the apparently nonsensical utterances of such children. He provides example after example of how understanding the child's history can help the careful investigator to decipher the meaning to the child of his or her utterances. Here we see psychiatry at its best, at once describing clearly psychopathological phenomena and advocating for those afflicted. Kanner clearly likes and respects these children whom he studies so carefully, and he puts himself in the role of translator as well as diagnostician. He thus manages to be objective without being reductionistic, using description to help the reader empathize rather than merely categorize. The rules of language construction that he deduces anticipate, by decades, the rules of linguistics and memory developed by modern cognitive psychologists.

These American psychiatrists succeeded in being both objective and empathic, describing psychopathology while evincing concern for the people who typified the syndromes. They were deeply influenced by a succession of European traditions: Kraepelin's precise objective description with its emphasis on prognosis in making diagnosis, as well as Freud's metapsychology and interest in the past history as having an etiological role in various kinds of psychopathology. The former relied on the future in establishing a diagnosis, the latter on the past. These writers also drew on the European phenomenological tradition in examining the problem of meaning and its distortions in mental illness. In addition, there is a dose of British antitheoretical empiricism, especially in Earle's and Kiernan's articles. Many of these writers borrowed from and integrated important aspects of European psychiatric description, nosology, and phenomenology, but in their commitment to learning from their patients and to careful observation and description, they supplemented rather than submitted to the European theories that influenced them. Sullivan and Meyer in particular explored the interpersonal and social domain of psychiatric illness, thereby enriching the breadth of clinical description and broadening our understanding of the causation and effects of psychiatric disease. Lindemann's paper is a striking example of this, describing beautifully the personal impact of interpersonal loss.

In reading these papers spanning more than a century, one senses psychiatric intelligence struggling with intangible problems that seem to defy description. They demonstrate the use of keen observation and large numbers of cases to force obscure illnesses to reveal their secrets, both psychosocial and neurobiological. Although many of these papers contain mistakes and biases based on social prejudices of their time, they are remarkable not only for their lucid clinical description but also for providing a profile of 150 years of American psychiatrists struggling to understand, describe, place in context, and think through the meaning of mental illness.

REFERENCES

1. Freud S: The ego and the id (1923), in Complete Psychological Works, standard ed, vol 19. London, Hogarth Press, 1961
2. Yalom ID: Existential Psychotherapy. New York, Basic Books, 1980
3. Spiegel H, Spiegel D: Trance and Treatment: Clinical Uses of Hypnosis. New York, Basic Books, 1978
4. Kasanin J: Language and Thought in Schizophrenia (1946). Berkeley, University of California Press, 1994
5. Freud S: Psycho-analytic notes on an autobiographical account of a case of paranoia (dementia paranoides) (1912 [1911]), in Complete Psychological Works, standard ed, vol 12. London, Hogarth Press, 1958

DAVID SPIEGEL, M.D.

DEFINITION OF INSANITY—NATURE OF THE DISEASE

By Amariah Brigham, M.D.

Superintendent, New York State Lunatic Asylum, Utica, New York

By Insanity is generally understood some disorder of the faculties of the mind. This is a correct statement, so far as it goes; but it does not define the disease with sufficient accuracy, as it is applicable to the delirium of fever, inflammation of the brain, and other diseases which are distinct from insanity.

Insanity, says Webster's Dictionary, is "derangement of the intellect." This is not merely too limited a definition, but an incorrect one, for in some varieties of insanity, as Prichard remarks, "the intellectual faculties appear to have sustained little or no injury, while the disorder is manifested principally or alone, in the state of the feelings, temper or habits."

We consider insanity, *a chronic disease of the brain, producing either derangement of the intellectual faculties, or prolonged change of the feelings, affections, and habits of an individual.*

In all cases it is a disease of the brain, though the disease of this organ may be secondary, and the consequence of a primary disease of the stomach, liver, or some other part of the body; or it may arise from too great exertion and excitement of the mental powers or feelings; but still insanity never results unless the brain itself becomes affected.

In former times, insanity was attributed to the agency of the devil, and the insane were supposed to be *possessed* by demons. Something of this opinion is still prevalent, and it appears to have been embraced by our Pilgrim Fathers.

Cotton Mather, in his life of William Thompson, thus remarks:—"*Satan*, who had been after an extraordinary manner irritated by the evangelic labors of this holy man, obtained the liberty to *sift* him; and hence, after this worthy man had served the Lord Jesus Christ, in the church of our New English *Braintree*, he fell into that *Balneum diaboli*, a black *melancholy*, which for divers years almost wholly disabled him for the exercise of his ministry."

Still we find this learned and good man saw the connection between the diseased mind and bodily disease, as he thus observes: "There is no experienced minister of the gospel, who hath not in the cases of *tempted souls*, often had this experience, that the ill cases of their distempered *bodies* are the frequent occasion and original of their *temptations*. There are many men, who in the very constitution of their *bodies*, do afford a *bed*, wherein busy and bloody *devils*, have a sort of lodging provided for them. The *mass of blood* in them, is disordered with some fiery *acid*, and their *brains* or *bowels* have some juices or ferments, or vapors about them, which are most unhappy engines for *devils* to work upon

their souls withal. The vitiated humors, in many persons, yield the *steams*, whereunto *Satan* does insinuate himself, till he has gained a sort of *possession* in them, or at least, an opportunity to shoot into the mind, as many *fiery darts*, as may cause a sad life unto them; yea, 'tis well if *self-murder* be not the sad end, into which these hurried people are thus precipitated. *New England*, a country where *splenetic* maladies are prevailing and pernicious, perhaps above any other, hath afforded numberless instances of even *pious people*, who have contracted those *melancholy indispositions*, which have unhinged them from all service or comfort; yea, not a few persons have been hurried thereby to lay *violent hands* upon themselves at the last. These are among the *unsearchable judgments* of God!"

We believe, however, that such opinions are no longer embraced by intelligent persons, who have paid much attention to insanity. By such, insanity is regarded as a disease of the body, and few at the present time, suppose the mind itself is ever diseased. The immaterial and immortal mind is, of itself, incapable of disease and decay. To say otherwise, is to advocate the doctrine of the materialists, that the mind, like our bodily powers, is material, and can change, decay, and die. On this subject, the truth appears to be, that the brain is the instrument which the mind uses in this life, to manifest itself, and like all other parts of our bodies, is liable to disease, and when diseased, is often incapable of manifesting harmoniously and perfectly the powers of the mind.

Insanity then, is the result of diseased brain; just as dyspepsia or indigestion is the result of disordered stomach; but it is only one of the results or consequences of a disease of this organ. The brain may be diseased without causing insanity; for although we say, and say truly, that the brain is the organ of the mind, yet certain portions of the brain are not directly concerned in the manifestation of the mental powers, but have other duties to perform. Certain parts of the brain confer on us the power of voluntary motion, but these portions are distinct from those connected with the mental faculties. Hence, we sometimes see, though rarely I admit, individuals paralytic, and unable to move, from disease of the brain, whose minds are not at all, or but very little disturbed. In such cases there is some disease of the brain, but of a part not concerned in the manifestation of the mental powers. We recently saw an aged gentleman, who had been, for several weeks, paralytic on one side, whose mind was not obviously affected. He died, and on examining his brain, a portion of the interior of one half of the brain was found much diseased, while the outer part was apparently in a healthy state.

From such cases, and numerous other observations, we are quite sure that the outer part of the brain is connected with the mental powers, and the inner portion with voluntary motion. These parts of the brain differ in color and structure. The outer is a greyish red color, and different from every other part of the system, while the inner part is beautifully white and resembles the nerves.

Again, the brain appears to be a double organ, or it is divided into halves, or hemispheres of like form and function, and therefore, though one side or one half of the brain may be affected, the powers of the mind may still be manifested by the other.

We may say then, that insanity is an effect of a disease of only a part of the brain—the outer or grey part. In most cases, insanity is the consequence of very slight disease, of a small part of the brain. If it was not so, the disease would soon terminate in death—for severe and extensive disease of the brain soon terminates in death. We see, however, numerous instances of insane persons, living many years, and apparently enjoying good health. We have seen several persons who have been deranged 40 and even 50 years, during which time they enjoyed in other respects, good health. On examining the brain after death, in such old cases of insanity, but little disease of this organ is often found, though a little, we believe may always be found; sometimes only an unusual hardness of the outer portion, but in so delicate an organ as the brain this is sufficient to derange its functions, just as a little disorder of the eye or ear, though not sufficient to affect the health, will disorder hearing and vision.

It is as if, in some very complicated and delicate instrument, as a watch for instance, some slight alteration of its machinery should disturb, but not stop its action.

Thus we occasionally find that violent mental emotions—a great trial of the affections—suddenly to derange the action of the brain, and cause insanity for life, without materially affecting the system in other respects. Esquirol relates the case of a young lady, who for several years expected to marry a person to whom she was engaged, and much attached. He finally deserted her and married another, on hearing of which she immediately became deranged, and for years remained in this condition, rejecting the attention of all other men, and constantly talking of her former lover, whom she still loved.

In this Asylum is an interesting patient, who became deranged suddenly, three years since, in consequence of the murder of her son. Her whole time and thoughts since that period, have been engrossed in searching and calling for her son, whom she believes to be concealed in the building, or beneath the furniture. Thus she lives in hopes of soon seeing him.

Garrick used to say that he owed his success in acting King Lear, from having seen the case of a worthy man in London, who, when playing with his only child at a window, accidentally let it fall upon the pavement beneath. The poor father remained at the window, screaming with agony, until the neighbors delivered the child to him dead.

He instantly became insane, and from that moment never recovered his understanding, but passed the remainder of his days in going to the window, and there playing in fancy with his child, then dropping it, and bursting into tears, and for awhile filling the house with his shrieks, when he would become calm, sit down in a pensive mood, with his eyes fixed for a long time on one object. Garrick was often present at this scene of misery, and "thus it was," he said, "I learned to imitate madness."

Sometimes, however, a severe trial of the feelings and affections produces death.

This is not merely the assertion of poets and novelists. Esquirol mentions the case of a young lady of Lyons, in France, who was engaged to be married to a young man of the same place. Circumstances suddenly occurred which determined the parents to prevent their marriage, and the young man was sent away. Immediately on learning this she became deranged. After five days spent in vain efforts to relieve her, the parents, to prevent her death, had the young man recalled, but it was too late—she died in his arms.

In such cases, and we could cite many, death does not occur from apoplexy, nor from the exhaustion following long-continued and great excitement, but from the want of sleep; the grief is too overwhelming for "poppy or mandragora, or all the drowsy syrups of the world," to medicine to repose.

Such was the sudden insanity and death of Haidee, described by Byron, and so true to nature and so beautifully, that we transcribe it.

> "The last sight which she saw was Juan's gore,
> And he himself o'ermaster'd and cut down;
> His blood was running on the very floor
> Where late he trod, her beautiful, her own;
> Thus much she view'd an instant, and no more,—
> Her struggles ceased with one convulsive groan.
>
> Days lay she in that state unchanged, though chill,
> With nothing livid, still her lips were red;
> She had no pulse, but death seem'd absent still;
> No hideous sign proclaim'd her surely dead.
>
> At last a slave bethought her of a harp;
> The harper came, and tuned his instrument;
> At the first notes, irregular and sharp,
> On him her flashing eyes a moment bent,
> Then to the wall she turn'd, as if to warp
> Her thoughts from sorrow through her heart re-sent,
> And he began a long, low island song
> Of ancient days, ere tyranny grew strong.
>
> Anon her thin, wan fingers beat the wall
> In time to his old tune; he changed the theme,
> And sung of love—the fierce name struck through all
> Her recollection; on her flashed the dream
> Of what she was, and is, if ye could call
> To be so being; in a gushing stream
> The tears rush'd forth from her o'erclouded brain,
> Like mountain mists at length dissolved in rain.
>
> Short solace, vain relief!—thought came too quick,
> And whirl'd her brain to madness; she arose
> As one who ne'er had dwelt among the sick,

And flew at all she met, as on her foes;
But no one ever heard her speak or shriek,
Although her paroxysm drew towards its close.
Hers was a frenzy which disdain'd to rave,
Even when they smote her, in the hope to save.

Food she refused, and raiment; no pretence
Avail'd for either; neither change of place,
Nor time, nor skill, nor remedy, *could give her
Senses to sleep*—the power seemed gone forever.

Twelve days and nights she wither'd thus; at last,
Without a groan, or sigh, or glance, to show
A parting pang, the spirit from her pass'd.

A little injury of the brain—a slight blow on the head, has often caused insanity, and changed the whole moral character—usually for the worse, sometimes for the better. We have known a most exemplary and pious lady—a most excellent wife and mother, whose mind had been highly cultivated—transformed by a little injury of the head, into one of the most violent and vulgar beings we ever saw, and yet the intellectual powers were not very much disturbed. For a considerable time she continued to take good care of her family, so far as related to household duties, but her love of reading, of attending church, and all affection for her family and neighbors was gone, and she became so violent that her friends were obliged to place her in a Lunatic Asylum. The celebrated Dr. Parry refers to a case in which, to use his own words, "an accidental blow on the head perverted all the best principles of the human mind, and changed a pious Christian to a drunkard and abandoned felon."

Such cases teach us to be cautious and tolerant in instances where change of character and misconduct are connected as to time, with injury or disease of the head, or even with general ill health.

Now and then an injury of the head seems to improve the intellect, and even the moral character. Instances of the former are not very uncommon. The disease or injury of the brain appears to give more energy and activity to some of the mental faculties. This we often see in the delirium of fever. The following very curious case was related to Mr. Tuke, of the Retreat for the Insane near York, England:

"A young woman, who was employed as a domestic servant by the father of the relater, when he was a boy, became insane, and at length sunk into a state of perfect idiocy. In this condition she remained for many years, when she was attacked by a typhus fever; and my friend, having then practiced some time, attended her. He was surprised to observe, as the fever advanced, a development of the mental powers. During that period of the fever, when others were delirious, this patient was entirely rational. She recognized, in the face of her medical attendant, the son of her old master, whom she had known so many years before; and she related many circumstances respecting this family, and others, which had happened to herself in earlier days. But, alas! it was only the gleam of reason; as the fever abated, clouds again enveloped the mind; she sunk into her former deplorable state, and remained in it until her death, which happened a few years afterwards."

Numerous cases are on record where a blow on the head by depressing a portion of the skull has caused the loss of speech, memory, and of all the mental faculties for many months; but which were restored on trephining and raising the depressed bone.

As we have said, sometimes the moral character is improved by injury or disease of the head. Dr. Cox, in his *Practical Observations on Insanity*, relates such cases. We sometimes see the same results from severe illness. Most experienced physicians must have noticed striking and permanent changes of character produced by disease. The insanity of some persons consists merely in a little exaltation of some one or more of the mental faculties—of self-esteem, love approbation, cautiousness, benevolence, &c.

A man received a severe wound on the upper part of his head, after which his mind became some affected, especially as related to his benevolent feelings, which were perpetually active towards man and beast. He was disposed to give away all that he had, and finally was placed in a Lunatic Asylum in consequence of the trouble which he made in his endeavors to benefit others and relieve suffering. Whenever he saw any cattle in a poor pasture, he would invariably remove them to a better; and whenever he heard of a destructive fire or shipwreck, he would hasten even to a great distance to endeavor to afford relief.

Among the insane in Lunatic Asylums, we sometimes see not only exhibitions of strength, mechanical and musical skill, powers of language, &c., far superior to what the same individuals ever exhibited when sane, but also a remarkable increase and energy of some of the best feelings and impulses of our nature, prompting them to deeds of self-sacrifice and benevolence, which remind us of the somewhat insane but ever memorable act of Grace Darling—

"Whose deeds will live
A theme for angels, when they celebrate
The high-souled virtues which forgetful earth
Hath witnessed."

In such instances, fear and every selfish feeling appears to be lost or overcome by the intensity of the benevolent impulse.

From the preceding remarks we see that insanity is often but an effect of a slight injury or disease of a part of the brain, and in many cases only a few of the faculties of the mind are disordered. From this we infer that the brain is not a single organ, but a congeries of organs, as maintained by the illustrious Gall and his celebrated successors Spurzheim and Combe. Thus each mental faculty has an especial organ, and therefore certain faculties may be disordered by disease of the brain, while others are not affected; a fact every day observed in Lunatic Asylums, but which we know not how to explain if we believe the brain to be a single organ.

We very rarely find the whole mind destroyed or disordered in insanity, except in cases of long continuance, or of unusual severity. A majority of patients in Lunatic Asylums have considerable mind left undisturbed, and some of them conduct with propriety, and converse rationally most of the time, and on all but a few subjects.

We have seen an individual who believed that he directed the planets and caused the sun to shine and the rain to descend when he chose, yet he was a man of much intelligence and conversed rationally on other subjects, and was remarkable for gentleness of manner and amiability of disposition.

We could cite very many cases nearly similar, and to those who have frequently visited this Asylum, we can appeal for the verification of the statement—that patients decidedly insane on one or more subjects, still manifest acute and vigorous minds, and appear to be sane on others.

Having seen that insanity consists in the derangement of one or more of the faculties of the mind produced by disease of only a part of the brain, we conclude that there is no one faculty of the human mind but may become disordered. If, therefore, we actually knew what mental faculties mankind possess, we might then know all the various forms of insanity, all the varieties of mental aberration to which these faculties are liable. But we do not know. Philosophers have ever disagreed as to the number of the faculties of the mind, and even as to what constitutes a faculty.

We shall not however particularise their views, but briefly allude to the constitution of the human mind, appealing to common observation for the correctness of what we assert on this subject.

In contemplating the phenomena of mind, we can not fail to perceive the variety of its faculties, and that there is an obvious general division of them into intellectual and moral, the latter comprehending the propensities and impulses.

These faculties, both the intellectual and moral, are originally possessed by all, and are alike dependent upon a healthy state of the brain for their proper manifestation. In some they are far more active and energetic than in others, owing in most cases we believe to original formation of the brain, and in others to education. That the intellectual faculties can be greatly improved by cultivation every one knows, and by many, too many we fear, this is regarded the most important and sole object of education,—as if the moral powers, the propensities, and impulses, were not a part of the mind, and not capable of improvement.

But however important the cultivation of the intellect may be, it certainly is not more so than the cultivation and improvement of the moral powers. We do not wish to undervalue the intellect, or discourage efforts for its improvement, but we wish that all might realise the superiority of our moral nature over intellect itself.

The intellectual faculties are but a part of our mental powers, and contribute but little in fact towards forming what we call the *character* of an individual. We call to mind our acquaintances and notice that their characters are very different, but this difference does not arise from the difference in their intellectual faculties, but in their moral powers. That one man knows more of the Greek language or mathematics, or has more knowledge of commercial or political affairs or of some mechanical art, or has the ability to acquire knowledge of many subjects faster than another, does not cause the difference we perceive in what we denominate the character. The character is determined by the moral faculties or propensities, by the affections, benevo-

lence, love, selfishness, avarice, &c. The difference in the activity and energy of these, create the differences we see in the characters of men; these constitute the man himself, or the *soul* of man, while the intellectual faculties are but instruments to administer to the wants and demands of the propensities.

Without these propensities or moral faculties, the intellectual powers would not be exerted at all, or but feebly. The stimulus or urgency of the impulses of our moral nature, of benevolence, love, avarice, &c., impel men to action—to gratify these the human race have forever toiled.

Now it is to these important faculties, the propensities of our moral nature, that we wish to call particular attention. Not merely to the importance of their early cultivation and improvement, but to the fact that they as often become deranged as the intellectual. They as truly use the brain for manifesting themselves; consequently when certain parts of the brain become diseased, they become deranged, and not unfrequently without the intellectual powers being noticeably disturbed. A man's natural benevolence or propensity to acquire, or to love, may become deranged from disease of the brain as truly as his powers of comparing, reasoning, &c.

Yet evident as this is from Physiology and Pathology, and from daily observation in Lunatic Hospitals, it is a fact, and an alarming fact, that when disease causes derangement of the moral faculties, and changes the character and conduct of an individual, he is not deemed insane, provided the intellectual powers are not obviously disordered.

It may be said that such a person has reason still left to guide him, as is evidenced by his ability to converse rationally on many subjects, and even to reason well against the very crime that he commits. All this may be true, and yet the person may not be accountable, for although reason is given to prevent us from doing evil, it can not be expected to resist a diseased and excited impulse.

Let not this be applied to crimes committed during voluntary intoxication, for though when thus intoxicated a man may be momentarily insane, yet it is voluntary insanity produced by gross misconduct, of which no one can avail himself to escape the legal consequences of crime. Still in such cases the crime must be the immediate result of intoxication, and while it lasts, to make a man accountable, as has been decided by Judge Story and other legal authorities. If committed afterwards during *delirium tremens* induced by intoxication, he must be acquitted on the ground of insanity, as he can not be held accountable for the immorality of the cause of his insanity, a disease which he can not successfully feign or voluntarily induce.

The disbelief in a kind of insanity that does not disturb the intellect, arises perhaps from the common phraseology, that the affections, passions, and moral qualities, have their seat in the *heart* and not in the brain, and therefore are not likely to be disordered by disease of the latter organ. But in fact the orderly manifestation of our moral faculties, our affections, and intellectual powers, are alike dependent on the healthy state of the brain. *The heart has nothing to do with either.*

We wish to repeat, that there is no faculty of the mind but may become deranged by disease of the brain. Disease of one part of this organ may cause the derangement of some of the intellectual faculties, while disease in another part may not disturb the intellect, but derange the moral powers or propensities. Thus we see blows on the head and wounds of the brain, sometimes destroy only one or two of the intellectual faculties, such as the memory of words, or the memory of places, and at other times to effect an entire change of the moral character.

But while the injury that affects the intellect is acknowledged to cause insanity, the injury that changes the moral character is not supposed to have this effect. The subject of the former is considered an object of concern and pity, while the latter is considered a depraved and wicked being deserving of punishment. Numerous cases have fallen under our observation, where a great change in the moral character occurred and lasted a year or two, and then the intellect became affected. This change of character was noticed and lamented, but those thus affected were not considered insane until the intellect itself became involved; while in fact they were insane from the first.

We wish all to be assured that a sudden and great change of character, of the temper and disposition, following disease or injury of the head, although the intellect is not disturbed, is an alarming symptom; it is often the precursor of intellectual derangement, and if not early attended to, is apt to terminate in incurable madness.

Within a few days we have seen two cases of insanity, both said to be quite recent, but on inquiring particularly of their friends, we found that they had noticed a striking change of character for several months before they thought of insanity. In one the change was from being naturally very generous and benevolent, to the opposite extreme of selfishness, and as they expressed it, of stinginess. In the other, the change was from great mildness and amiability of disposition, to that of extreme irascibility and moroseness. Now these persons were not deemed insane until their intellects were disturbed; but we regard the previous change of character as truly the consequence of disease of the brain as the disturbance of the intellect, and this is now the opinion of their friends.

Derangement of the intellectual faculties seldom occasions much dispute—every one easily recognizes it—but not so with derangement of the moral powers. Most persons have seen individuals who are crazy, and consider themselves qualified to judge whether a person is deranged or not, yet on inquiry we find that nearly all expect irrational and incoherent talk from those that are deranged, or wild and unnatural looks, or raving and violent conduct. Their opinions respecting insanity are derived from having seen *raving maniacs*, and not from observation in Lunatic Asylums; for in the latter may be found many whose insanity consists in derangement of the affections and moral powers, and not in disturbance of the intellect.

Owing to such limited and erroneous views respecting insanity, many persons are not disposed to believe in a kind of mental disorder that may impel men to commit crimes, unless such individuals exhibit derangement of the intellect, or conduct in a manner that they have been accustomed to see deranged persons conduct.

But notwithstanding this common opinion regarding insanity, it is a well established truth, that there is a form of insanity, now called by many *moral insanity*, arising from disease of the brain, which may impel men to commit great crimes, while the intellect is not deranged, but overwhelmed and silenced by the domination of a disordered impulse.

Sometimes insanity seems to arise from some defect of the organs of sense, from change in the nerves of sensation. It is said that in those who are troubled with hallucinations of sight or of hearing, some disease of the nerves of the eye or ear is found. Still, in such cases there must be in addition some defect in the power of comparison, or insanity would not result. Comparison is one of the most important of the faculties of the mind, and the one most liable to be affected in insanity, or in any disease of the brain, as in headache for instance.

Disorder of the nerves of sensation may also lead to insane ideas and conduct. Some have believed themselves converted into inanimate substances. One man thought himself changed into a teapot, another into a barrel which was rolled along the street, and another into a town-pump to which no rest was given day nor night.

Mr. Connolly, in his work on Insanity, tells of a respectable merchant in London who fancied himself metamorphosed into a seven shilling piece, and who took the precaution of going round to those with whom he had dealings, requesting of them as a particular favor, that if his wife should present him in payment they would not give change for him.

In all these cases—for they all admit we think, of one explanation—there was some affection of the nerves of sensation, and also some disorder of the faculty of comparison.

In some cases of mental disorder, there seems to be almost complete annihilation of sensation. This is the case with those who believe themselves dead; they feel not, and fully believe that they have ceased to exist, yet such persons will often talk rationally on other subjects. Most of their mental faculties are in perfect condition, and sometimes by exciting some of the most predominating impulses or passions, such persons are cured.

One of the Princes of the Bourbon family of France, imagined himself dead, and refused to eat. To prevent his dying of starvation, two persons were introduced to him, in the character of illustrious dead like himself, and they invited him after some conversation respecting the world of shades to dine with another distinguished but deceased person the Marshal Turenne.

The Prince accepted this very polite invitation, and made a very hearty dinner; and every day, while this delusion continued, in order to induce him to eat, it was necessary to invite him to the table of some ghost of high rank and reputation.

Dr. Mead relates, that an *old bell ringer* at Oxford University, imagined himself dead, and ordered the bell to be rung, as was usual on the occurrence of a death at that place. The bell *was* rung, but in a most awkward and unusual manner; the old ringer could not bear this, and leaped from his bed, and hastened to the belfry to show how it should be rung; he then returned to his room that he might die in a proper way, but the exercise and passion proved so beneficial that his delusion was broken up, and he soon recovered.

As I have already mentioned, some persons decidedly insane on some subjects, exhibit greater intellectual power on others during their mental derangement, than when they are sane. The following is an instance.

A general in the French army, who had the entire confidence of Napoleon, and who had been directed by him to superintend some immense military preparations at Boulogne, became much fatigued by his duties, which exposed him most of the day to the hot sun. Suddenly he quitted the work, and accompanied by one of his aids, set off for Paris, announcing on his way that he was the bearer of a treaty of peace with England. He traveled with great rapidity, not allowing himself time to eat, and paid postillions largely to hasten his speed. Arriving at Paris, the public funds rose from this news of the treaty. Not finding Napoleon at the Palace of the Tuilleries, he hastened to St. Cloud, and, in disordered dress, penetrated to the apartment of the Emperor, and announced to him what he alone, of all whom the general had met, knew to be incorrect. In fact, Napoleon was the first to discover his insanity, and committed him immediately to the care of physicians.

The insanity of the general continued through the summer, during which time he wrote comedies and plays which were much admired, and he also conceived or invented an improvement in firearms, and begged to have permission to visit a founder, in order to have a *model* made from drawings he had himself prepared. His physician reluctantly yielded to his request, on his giving his word of honor that he would not go elsewhere. He went and returned, and eight days afterwards went again and found the model completed, and then gave orders for 50,000 *models* to be made. This order for 50,000 models was the only symptom of insanity that he exhibited during the whole affair. He soon however, became worse, then paralytic, and died insane. But the efforts of his diseased mind have survived him; his writings are still read and admired, and his invention was soon found to be quite an improvement, and has since been adopted in the French armies.

In some cases of insanity, the faculties of the mind are so acute, that it is exceedingly difficult for a stranger to detect the mental aberration. The late Lord Erskine, in his speech in defense of Hadfield, for shooting at the King at Drury Lane Theatre, in order to demonstrate how cunning and acute in reasoning insane persons frequently are, and consequently how difficult it sometimes is to discover their insanity, referred to the following cases, which we quote in his own words:

"I well remember, (indeed I never can forget it,) that since the noble and learned judge has presided in this Court, I examined for the greater part of a day, in this very place, an unfortunate gentleman who had indicted a most affectionate brother, together with the keeper of a mad-house at Hoxton, for having imprisoned him as a lunatic, whilst, according to his evidence, he was in his perfect senses. I was, unfortunately, not instructed in what his lunacy consisted, although my instructions left me no doubt of the fact; but, not having the clue, he completely foiled me in every attempt to expose his infirmity. You may believe that I left no means unemployed which long experience dictated, but without the smallest effect. The day was wasted, and the prosecutor, by the most affecting history of unmerited suffering, appeared to the judge and jury, and to a humane Eng-

lish audience, as the victim of the most wanton and barbarous oppression. At last Dr. Sims came into Court, who had been prevented by business, from an earlier attendance, and whose name, by the bye, I observe to-day in the list of the witnesses for the crown. From Dr. Sims I soon learned that the very man whom I had been above an hour examining, and with every possible effort which counsel are so much in the habit of exerting, believed himself to be *the Lord and Saviour of mankind,* not merely *at the time of his confinement,* which was alone necessary for my defense, *but during the whole time that he had been triumphing over every attempt to surprise him in the concealment of his disease.* I then affected to lament the indecency of my ignorant examination, when he expressed his forgiveness, and said with the utmost gravity and emphasis, in the face of the whole Court, "I AM THE CHRIST;" and so the cause ended. Gentlemen, this is not the only instance of the power of concealing this malady; I could consume the day if I were to enumerate them; but there is one so extremely remarkable, that I cannot help stating it.

"Being engaged to attend the assizes at Chester, upon a question of lunacy, and having been told that there had been a memorable case tried before Lord Mansfield in this place, I was anxious to procure a report of it, and from that great man himself (who within these walls, will ever be reverenced, being then retired in his extreme old age, to his seat near London, in my own neighborhood) I obtained the following account of it. 'A man of the name of Wood,' said Lord Mansfield, 'had indicted Dr. Monro, for keeping him as a prisoner (I believe in the same mad-house at Hoxton) when he was sane. He underwent the most severe examination by the defendant's counsel, without exposing his complaint; but Dr. Battye, having come upon the bench by me, and having desired me to ask him what was become of the PRINCESS whom he had corresponded with in cherry-juice, he showed in a moment what he was. He answered that there was nothing at all in that, because, having been (as every body knew) imprisoned in a high tower, and being debarred the use of ink, he had no other means of correspondence but by writing his letters in cherry-juice, and throwing them into a river which surrounded the tower, where the Princess received them in a boat. There existed, of course, no tower, no imprisonment, no writing in cherry-juice, no river, no boat; but the whole the inveterate phantom of a morbid imagination. I immediately,' continued Lord Mansfield, 'directed Dr. Monro to be acquitted; but this man, Wood, being a merchant, in Philpot Lane, and having been carried through the city in his way to the mad-house, he indicted Dr. Monro over again, for the trespass and imprisonment *in London,* knowing that he had lost his cause by speaking of the Princess at Westminster; and such,' said Lord Mansfield, 'is the extraordinary subtlety and cunning of madmen, that when he was cross-examined on the trial in London, as he had successfully been before, in order to expose his madness, all the ingenuity of the bar, and all the authority of the Court, could not make him say a single syllable upon that topic which had put an end to the indictment before, although he still had the same indelible impression upon his mind, as he signified to those who were near him; but conscious that the delusion had occasioned his defeat at Westminster, he obstinately persisted in holding it back. This evidence at Westminster was then proved against him by the short-hand writer.'"

In a future number we shall resume the subject of this article, and we beg our readers to keep in view the statements advanced in this, as we purpose to refer to them in connection with the Medical Jurisprudence of Insanity, and in explanation of some cases of *moral insanity* that have much embarrassed both physicians and jurists.

KATATONIA, A CLINICAL FORM OF INSANITY

By James G. Kiernan, M.D.

Of the New York City Asylum for the Insane, Ward's Island

One of the disputed points in the history of insanity is classification. Single symptoms, causes or modes of manifestation are taken to signify distinct types of disease. Some writers and some medical superintendents of asylums in their reports go beyond this even, for they give diseases, apparently evolved from their internal consciousness, which are neither acute, nor chronic, have no aetiology, pathology nor mode of manifestation, but stand alone, sublime monuments to the scientific use of the imagination.

The principle laid down by Voisin in his "Clinical Pictures of Insanity," that classification to be rational, must be founded on the logical association of the clinical symptoms, the aetiology, and the pathological anatomy is the only one, as yet offered that is justifiable on any ground, than that of mere hypothesis. Such a principle may give rise, without doubt, to many new divisions of insanity, but even then they can scarcely be more numerous and more unwieldy than the divisions of the much lauded system of Skae. This principle has been independently adopted by a German observer, who is engaged in clinical researches similar to those of the French psychiatrist, Doctor Kahlbaum, Medical Superintendent of the Private Asylum at Gorlitz, Prussia, to whose observations are due the recognition and clinical demarcation of the subject of this paper.

The first volume of his recently published work, is devoted to consideration of the forms of disease in question. He claims that the distinguishing characteristic is an irregularity, or as he phrases it an insanity of tension, mental and muscular, whence the name Katatonia. His conclusions (which have received the approval of Meynert, Westphal and Von Krafft Ebing,) are that Katatonia is a distinct form of insanity having its own clinical history. Maudsley under the insanity of pubescence, and Bucknill and Tuke under choreomania, have noticed some of the individual symptoms, but have drawn no conclusions therefrom. The first symptom is like that noticed in the inception of other forms of insanity, a change in the temper of the individual. It presents at times well marked motions of a rhythmical character, always under control of the will. In this respect, while bearing some resemblance to, it is very distinct from chorea.

Another characteristic, but one which is not noticeable, unless the case be observed from the inception to the close, is its cyclical character, maniacal, melancholic and cataleptoidal conditions alternating, with more or less imperfect

convulsive attacks; there are also pathetic delusions of grandeur, and a tendency to act and talk theatrically. Erotic manifestations of some kind frequently occur, and, as is usual under such circumstances, the patient's ideas have a religious tinge. At any stage, as in other nervous diseases, remissions, or as is claimed, but I think erroneously, by Kahlbaum, complete recovery may occur. If the case is to end unfavorably, periods of excitement and stupidity recur, with more and more frequency, and the patient dies, with terminal dementia. The clinical history is best illustrated by the following cases.

CASE I.—T.R., age 36, policeman, single, common school education, intemperate, as were also his parents. The patient had been a masturbator, and had indulged in sexual excess. He was at first melancholic, subsequently maniacal, but recovering therefrom became what his fellow-policemen called "stuck up." His temper changed from good humor to irascibility, and asylum treatment was at length rendered necessary. He was admitted to the New York City Asylum for the Insane, March 17, 1873. A week previous he had gone to church, but soon returned, saying he had been followed by "droves" of dogs. He was a tall, powerful, good humored man, and though he asserted he would not commit suicide he had cut off the tip of his ear in an attempt of this kind. He was somewhat subdued in manner, and had hallucinations of sight and hearing. The day previous to admission he was affected with a spasm of the muscles of the extremities. Five days after admission he manifested delusion that he had committed a great crime, and refused food, but said: "This is not a penance for the crime." He required artificial feeding for three days, took food voluntarily on the fourth, and again refused it on the fifth day. A period of excitement then occurred, and he became the subject of hallucinations, differing from those he had on admission. After treatment a short time with opium and hyoscyamus he grew quiet and took food voluntarily, but very suspiciously. In about a week after, a spasm of the muscles of the neck, followed by slight unconsciousness and slumber, occurred, the pupils dilating widely, and so remaining for a few days. Two weeks after, he had very sluggish movements of the lower extremities, bearing a suspicious resemblance to functional paraplegia, but this was really an *incomplete* cataleptoid condition, involving also the muscles of the neck and upper extremities. The patient opened his mouth, and performed other simple actions of that nature; these, however, were not ideational, but sensori-motor acts, as his attention to the subject was nil, and he was in a peculiar emotional state. That all the mental faculties were not in abeyance was shown by the fact that he involuntarily raised his hands in an attitude of supplication, or as an acknowledgment of a favor just received. His pupils responded to light, and the organic functions were performed as usual. This condition continued for three days with very little

Read before the New York Neurological Society, April 2, 1877.

change, except that when asked to perform a simple action the request would be obeyed, and the action continued indefinitely in an automatic way.

Five days after the beginning of the condition just mentioned, the patient had a rapid, feeble pulse the beats of which ran into each other and did not correspond with the heart's action, which, though rapid, was otherwise normal. His eyelids and lower extremities soon became oedematous and the cataleptoid condition disappeared. The heart's action grew more irregular, the first sound being alone audible, and accompanied with a loud, blowing murmur heard at the base. Pulse one hundred and thirty-two and more rapid in the neck than at the wrist; respirations were increased, the lungs and temperature being normal. The heart's action soon returned to its normal condition, and the murmur disappeared. The treatment was directed to the alimentary canal only. The patient then became entirely unconscious as to his surroundings, though taking food and performing other actions, involving only the organic functions, normally, and so continued for about a week. He then began to have tonic contractions of the muscular system, followed by the lessening of the oedema which finally disappeared. The cataleptoid condition then returned and was accompanied by considerable waxy mobility. Two days after, his muscles were extremely rigid, and he remained apparently unconscious for sometime. One morning he suddenly spoke and being asked his reason for not speaking before said, "They told me not to," and when asked who told him not to, replied "God and others," and began to weep.

The following day he had a return of the cataleptoid condition in which he remained for some time. These alternations continued for three months, when he became suddenly violent, tore off a bar from the window and tried to make his escape. This excitement continued three days, the patient then passing again into the cataleptoid condition, on emerging from which he was markedly dignified, and very formal in conversation. This manner of speaking and acting continued for three months. He then had another cataleptoid relapse, succeeded by an attack of melancholia attonita. Then followed a condition during which his pupils at first contracted and then dilated; his left hand contracted firmly, and from it a quivering motion extended over the left side, and gradually involved the entire body. The irregularities of circulation formerly observed once more appeared, and as before went away without special treatment.

Melancholia attonita became the predominant condition, accompanied however, by increased susceptibility to external influences. This remained four months, and was followed by a cataleptoid condition with much waxy mobility. While in this state he was found to be developing phthisis. The disease ran a rapid, somewhat irregular course, terminating life July 22, 1875, twenty-six months after his admission to the Institution.

The details of the post mortem were as follows: Thoracic cavity; lungs the seat of tubercles, some undergoing softening, others calcification; remains of old adhesions in the pleurae. Heart, normal. Abdominal cavity; the liver was slightly cirrhotic; kidneys, normal; the mesenteric glands tuberculous, and undergoing same changes as the lungs; spleen congested and somewhat enlarged; the intestines somewhat congested and inflamed. Head-scalp thick; cranium normal, with the dura mater adhering to it in patches. There were firm coagula in the veins and sinuses. The arachnoid, especially over the fissure of Sylvius, was very opaque; the pontico-chiasmal lamina were very dense, and a pseudo-membrane was formed beneath. There was dullness of the membrane of moderate character between cerebellum and medulla oblongata. Epithelial granulations present in a rudimentary condition, pia mater removable from cortex except over frontal lobe. Cortex pale, a decided sinking of the surface of certain gyri below neighboring convolutions. There was a fusion of the opposite sides of the anterior cornua of the lateral ventricles. Cysts of choroid plexus were also present.

The first peculiarity noticeable in this case is its cyclical character. The tendency to act and speak theatrically is not so prominent. While this peculiarity has perchance attracted the attention of many alienists, it has been regarded as a curious fact, and dismissed to the limbo of unrecorded observations. Most of the peculiarities of the insane, have their correlations in the actions of the sane, and this forms no exception to the rule. The tendency of the paretic to wander, with his proclivity for arson, have their parallels in the conduct of the chronic revolutionist, and the prominent mental symptom of "katatonia," "verbigeration" as Kahlbaum calls it, finds its analogue in the chronic stump speaker. It is a peculiarity likely to attract attention from its occurrence in the comparatively ignorant, and with other prominent symptoms is well illustrated in the following cases.

CASE II.—W.H.G., aged 26; colored, laborer, married, intemperate and syphilitic. Mother had been insane, but recovered. The patient one day while at work fell down suddenly, and his face and arms began to twitch; from this he soon recovered, but in two months became much depressed, and was placed in the City Lunatic Asylum, where he soon became maniacal and violent, which condition was followed by a period of depression with hallucinations. He suddenly refused to eat, and soon after passed into a cataleptoid condition, from which he emerged one morning; said he "was equal to any white man," and spoke very precisely. He was afterwards taken out of the Asylum by his wife, and December 11, 1871, two months after this was readmitted, and after having remained two months was discharged improved. He was readmitted during 1874, then in a condition of melancholia attonita, out of which he gradually passed. When speaking he always observed great precision, and if he supposed the expression used was not correct he would alter it until he found one that might with propriety be substituted for it. He remained in this condition till July of that year, and was again discharged. He was readmitted March, 1875. Held his head up in a very consequential way, and prefaced every reply to a question by the phrase, "I do not doubt but what." What is your name? "I do not doubt but what it is William Henry G." How old are you? "I do not doubt but what I was born in the year 1838, so my mother said." Where were you born? "I do not doubt but what I was born in some part of the world." What part? "I do not doubt but what I do not know what part." His memory was somewhat deficient but not materially so, as he remembered that he was there before, that he went out on a furlough, and the physician's name. He was well built and comparatively strong, and while speaking wrinkled his face very much; this was somewhat of a sensori-motor act, and under the stimulus of some emotion, at variance with his "verbigeration," disappeared. Patient retained his peculiar manner of speaking and acting, but grew less inclined to walk about, would remain for hours in an upright position, staring straight ahead at vacancy. He manifested moderate erotic desires.

CASE III.—P.D.; Irish; aged 28, of intemperate habits, unmarried, of very ordinary education. The attack of insanity was preceded by dizziness. He entered the Asylum in a condition of melancholia approaching catalepsy. He brightened up somewhat in a few days, but was averse to conversation. About a week after admission he suddenly became communicative, said he had wasted time and opportunities, had led a loose life, and was now suffering the pangs of remorse. Excessive drinking and the loss of near friends were the causes he assigned for the present attack, of the nature of which he was quite conscious. He had then apparently no delusion, and was coherent. This mental condition continued for two months; there was no delusion present, and the mental tone was that of depression. Every idea expressed had that tinge. He said: "I have suffered blank disappointment in life. Men whom I expected were just and honest have been found wanting." He declared at the same time, with strong emphasis, that he had had no disappointment of the affections, as his ideas did not run in that channel. When asked to give the loss of friends that he had suffered in detail, said, "A host of tender emotions are thus raised that had better be quieted." The abstract sentiments were regarded by him as more sacred than the affections. The peculiar sensibility of the brain to depressing influences was undoubtedly heightened in his case, but not so much as to prevent a pleasureable feeling when excited by other emotions. He was very formal in conversation, and though his condition would not in a man of culture necessarily be morbid, yet in his case it was, because of its spontaneous origin, and of its being purely subjective. His proud semi-dignified, semi-melancholic expression, varied by an irregular play of the muscles concerned, was a fair index of his mental condition, for he was unable to give the bond of association between the tender emotions and the causes exciting them. His treatment consisted in hyoscyamus, cannabis indica and whiskey. About a month after the commencement of this treatment, the patient said he had found food for thought and wisdom, in the stability of the Christian religion, but dreaded events would go wrong in the future. When asked "what events" could give only his probable failure to obtain work. He remained a week in this state, then refused food and passed into a cataleptoid condition, with incomplete waxy mobility and irregular movements of the fingers. This lasted a week, he then spoke a few words, but continued to decline food, refusing to explain his action. He required artificial feeding for two days, then took food voluntarily and spoke freely; said, "that he was the son of a Portuguese noble, who had gone to discover the source of the Nile, and who was interested in literary pursuits, having written Virgil." Symptoms of phthisis made their appearance, and the patient being placed under tonic treatment improved somewhat. A month after cataleptoid conditions alternated with maniacal attacks, which were accompanied by hallucinations of sight. The patient died of phthisis a year after the first appearance of the symptoms. In this case the speech-making tendency was well marked, and, from the imperfect training received by the patient in early life, was very noticeable. This symptom, with a tendency to the use of peculiarly formed words, observed in one of Kahlbaum's cases, is to be found in a greater degree in the following case.

CASE IV.—J.E., aged 26; single, moulding-maker, fair education, intemperate. Admitted to the New York City Asylum for the Insane, September 23, 1874. Five weeks previously had been arrested for intemperance, which caused him to become very much depressed. After his release went on a spree, and while intoxicated fell down a cellar, striking on the back of his head. Shortly after this said that he heard voices threatening him; that everything was turning round. In obedience to these hallucinations he cut his throat, fortunately avoiding any important vessel, and causing only a flesh wound. On admission the patient seemed to have considerable difficulty in talking, opened and shut his mouth as if speaking, but did not utter a sound. He stared at everything with a very contemptuous expression. On the following day he spoke freely, but without any apparent difficulty, and said that he had attempted suicide because he heard voices threatening him. This communicativeness lasted only a short time, and was then replaced by the condition present on admission. Two days after he appeared to realize his condition, and said that intemperance and

the injury to the head were the chief causes of his mental trouble, which he recognized. For a fortnight he remained much the same. He had a defective remembrance of events in the immediate past, and exhibited a tendency to repeat a question several times, in a confused manner, before answering it. A week after this he cleared up markedly; said he had masturbated from the age of fifteen, and had drank as many as thirty glasses of beer a day. The confused appearance and defective memory returned, and were accompanied by considerable depression. In a fortnight the condition of the patient was the same as at the time of his admission. Five days after he said he saw blood on everything he looked at. In the course of a month he became very stupid, took off and put on his clothes purposelessly, and at length passed into a cataleptoid condition with waxy mobility, but offered very slight resistance to any attempt at movement. Artificial feeding was required for two days. He then took food voluntarily, spoke occasionally, but showed much confusion of ideas. A month after he had improved very much, and expressed a desire to go out and attend to his affairs, but had no recollection of his late condition, and the circulation in the extremities was very sluggish. He continued to improve, but was not considered recovered, when six months after, his friends, against the advice of Dr. Macdonald, the medical superintendent, removed him from the asylum. He was brought back in six days, and then said "that his father was a witch and his mother also, she having poisoned his food and bewitched the house, causing what he is unable otherwise to account for, the occasional stopping of the house clock on the mantlepiece." He had at times returns of the cataleptoid condition, with maniacal alternations, followed by a tendency to express the contrary of any proposition that might be made. These statements were intermingled with diatribes against the other patients, and expressions indicating a belief in his own importance. He made gestures sometimes indicative of devotion, but more frequently of contempt. Soon after the appearance of the last mentioned symptoms, he spoke in German about religious matters, but gradually changed to remarks about a girl he had seduced. Three days after he became maniacal, relapsing in two weeks into a cataleptoid condition, followed by rhythmic movements of the fingers. He now began to speak (in English,) and said, "I am Arminius and have swallowed J.E." He was very consequential, resisted any intrusion on a fancied privilege, and once knocked down a fellow-patient for sitting on the same bench with him. A period of excitement then appeared, followed by a relapse into the cataleptoid condition. On emerging from this, the rhythmic motions once more appeared, followed by incessant talking in German, implying that his family descent was noble, and making a semi-demand, semi-appeal for the regard due him on this account. A succession of the same phenomena as before then occurred, but the increased talking was in no known language. It was however, articulate, and he made many attempts at oratorical display. The patient still remains in this condition.

In the four cases thus far given there is a family likeness, modified it must be confessed, by surrounding circumstances, but such as to leave no doubt that they belong to the same clinical type. Thirty cases have come under observation having the same irregularity of mental association and cyclical character. One of the cases came to the asylum at the time of and apparently through the excitement of the Moody-Sankey revival. On examination of the case, however, it appeared that the father had died from phthisis; the mother also had the disease, and the patient himself had had meningitis at the age of ten, that he became insane therefrom, but recovered within a year and remained in mental health for seven years after. The fact of this case occurring during religious excitement is not peculiar, as that has been assigned as the exciting cause in many instances.

All the forms of religious belief have furnished cases of this kind, and they have even occurred during a polytheistic reaction from Christianity. Kahlbaum claims that the disease is very rare. My own conclusion from the facts coming under observation is that while the statement is apparently true, in reality the cases are frequent, but pass unrecognized.

Many cases are discharged from an asylum during a remission and are lost sight of, but return or enter other institutions with peculiarities that puzzle the medical attendant in classification. Such has been the experience with a few cases discharged at this stage, preceding my connection with the City Asylum, and which subsequently returned. The peculiarities of these cases are so frequently described in connection with the insanity of pubescence and menstruation, that there is little doubt that the disease, though not so frequent as general paresis, is entitled to a distinct place as a form of insanity so far as frequency of occurrence gives any right to the same.

Causation is always an obscure, and very frequently a disputed point in the history of insanity. It is set forth at great length in asylum reports, but he who expects to derive positive information on the subject from the statements therein contained, will be frequently disappointed. Either the mental or the physical influence is ignored, or both are so combined as to lead to erroneous deductions. Forbes Winslow's ten thousand cases of insanity in the United States caused by spiritualism is a recent example, and has been much commented upon. The only way to arrive at any definite conclusion is to take such facts as are given concerning the patient's ancestry, habits, age, education, civil condition, mental peculiarities, surrounding circumstances, the presence or absence of physical disease and of traumatic influences, and then to deduce the logical relation of cause and effect.

Examination of the thirty cases coming under observation, in accordance with this principle, shows that in ten cases, one of the parents was phthisical; in three, the father was phthisical and a paternal uncle died of hydrocephalus; in two, the mother died of phthisis and a maternal uncle died of hydrocephalus; in four, the father was intemperate; in five, syphilitic; in two, a maternal first cousin had been insane; in one case the mother, and in another an aunt was idiotic. Twenty of the thirty cases were intemperate, three took stimulants moderately, and seven were abstinent. Twenty-six of the thirty cases were below the age of thirty; eighteen had received the ordinary common-school education, four a high-school, two a liberal, and six the ordinary education amounting to an ability to read and write. Twenty-five were single, and five married. Twenty-two admitted the practice of masturbation; of these thirteen were in addition addicted to sexual excess, as also were three of the remaining eight. Twenty were religiously inclined; three were opposed to religion, not however, from a disbelief in doctrine, though they lived in defiance of its moral code; the remainder came under the head of what the religious press call indifferentists.

Fifteen of the thirty cases were somewhat quiet and reserved, four were jovial and pleasure loving, and of the remainder little definite information could be obtained. Concerning ten it was ascertained that they had been, what was called by their parents and relations, very studious, the study consisting in the perusal of works of fiction, sensational and biographical. The patients in three cases were in good circumstances; in ten belonged to the lower middle class, while the rest were from the lower class; in three cases the patient had in early life meningitis; in fifteen there was some evidence of scrofulous disease; in ten no history of preceding nervous or other chronic disease could be obtained. Of the thirty, all but one gave a history of rheumatism, and that was not articular, but muscular. Four had received injuries to the skull which, however, were said to be of a slight character.

The first deduction following from the facts already given, is that the inheritance of a scrofulous diathesis acts as a great predisposing cause, a conclusion borne out by the pathology of the disease. Age appears also to act as a predisposing cause. The influence of stimulants either as an exciting or predisposing cause, seems limited; the most logical conclusion being that since the proportion of those abstaining from stimulants is relatively greater in this than in the other forms of insanity, therefore the influence of alcoholic stimulants is antagonistic, rather than favorable to the production of the disease; in forming this conclusion, however, the prevalence of intoxication among the class from which many of the patients are derived, is taken into consideration. The influence of education can best be seen in its effects, rather than its amount, it being in most cases regarded by the patients, not as an end, but as a means toward an end; in short a property entitling the possessor to certain privileges. These effects of education led to depression on the part of our patient, because of his not receiving the consideration which he conceived its possession entailed. The determination of the influence of masturbation, and whether it is not an effect, is a question that requires some discrimination to decide. The practice, however, aided in reducing the already diminished vitality of the patient, and therefore, in adding to the existing depression.

Most probably masturbation was to some extent an outcome of the general morbid condition of the nervous system, and aided in increasing this. The influence of sexual excess was of a like nature, as the disease occurred at a period when the sexual passion was in process of development. Religious excitement like the sexual element, with which it is in close alliance, was both an effect and a cause. In individual cases coming under observation, there have been two phases, first, the patient's excessive devotion results in claims to extraordinary religious privileges; secondly, a depression is produced during semi-lucid periods by the evident contradiction between the duties of religion and the strong sexual desires, which often control the conduct. The influence of the literature usually perused by this class of patients, is very obvious from its effect on normal minds, leading to a luxurious day-dreaming propensity, and a disinclination to active exertion whether mental or physical. On a morbid condition like this, peculiarly suited for the reception of such impressions, the result must be much intensified, for what in the normal condition would simply be a day dream, in the disease, is converted into a delusion.

The influence of surrounding circumstances is perhaps nowhere stronger than in the United States. On the one hand examples of self-made men are held up as incentives to effort for high positions, while on the other the absence of wealth is regarded as a strong evidence of incapacity. Traumatic causes appeared in these cases to have had a slight influence in modifying, rather than producing the disease, which had existed before the beginning of their action. One of these cases has already been cited. The most frequent predisposing cause, as already stated, was the inheritance of a scrofulous diathesis; the other influences acted often as exciting causes, though at times they only increased the predisposition to the disease. That an acute form of disease directly traceable to the inheritance of a scrofulous diathesis, resembles katatonia very much in its general features is shown in the following case, from the *Virginia Medical Monthly*, September, 1876.

A young man 17 years of age, exhibited symptoms of mental aberration, consisting in an inordinate loquacity, a[nd] talking maudlingly on a great variety of subjects without pursuing one continuous train of thought. He was not insensible, and when spoken to, answered quite rationally, but immediately relapsed into the condition of incessant talking. The patient being sleepless, hydrate of chloral and bromide of potassium were given with good effect. About the end of this first week of illness he became very obstinate, but still answered rationally. During the second week he grew worse, bowels became constipated, and he had a temperature of 101 to 101½, a pulse of 120 to 140, with exacerbations in the evening. He soon began to show depression, accompanied with paralysis. Soon after there was a febrile reaction, a temperature of 102, a pulse of 120. His head was somewhat retracted; he was violent and impatient of restraint. Both pupils were normal and he was totally unconscious. By the end of the second week he was still unconscious and the pupils were widely dilated, head still retracted and very much emaciation present. At the close of the third week his pulse was 70, temperature 98° and the patient was rational. One child of the family died from acute, and one from chronic hydrocephalus, and another was, at time of the illness of our patient suffering from tubercle of the peritoneum.

This case resembles in many respects those already given, but the vagueness of the terms used show the reporter to be a poor psychological, although a good clinical observer and pathologist. These views as to the influence of heredity are likely to raise a disputed question, which will be considered under pathology. The post-mortems given by Kahlbaum show evidences of a healed up hydrocephalus and a basilar meningitis, which, the post-mortems I have made, confirm. Meynert's deduction from Kahlbaum's cases, is that the disease has been preceded by a patho-meningeal process, located at the base of the brain, and over the fissure of Sylvius. My own opinion from the cases examined is, that the disease has been most frequently preceded, during infancy, by a basilar meningeal process of a tuberculous character. In a patho-psychological aspect the localization of the process would be over the base of the brain, in the fourth ventricle, and over the fissure of Sylvius. According to Dr. O. Schultze, the motor symptoms in basilar meningitis, are due

to an acute spinal affection, occurring at the same time as the cerebral affection. Leyden maintains that tubercular, spinal and cerebro-spinal meningitis, the existence of which has been but little suspected, is certainly possible, and indeed, highly probable. Magnan, Lionville, Hayem and Schultze, all agree that this affection is very frequently present. Schultze concludes that the stiffness occurring in the course of so-called basilar meningitis, with the contractions of the muscles supplied by the spinal nerves, do not have their origin in the brain, but are due to the affection attacking the spinal cord; that these symptoms occur on account of the progression of the inflammatory process from the membranes by means of the vessels, to the nerve bundles; and hence, partly from the inflammatory irritation of the nerve bundles themselves, and partly on account of the irritation of the spinal cord in which myelitic changes are found. As has already been hinted at, one point raised by the pathology, is the question of recovery from tubercular meningeal processes.

From the post-mortem already given, and from others coming under observation, my opinion is that tubercular meningeal processes are more frequently recovered from than is generally supposed; that in reality many of the cases of so-called hydrocephaloid disease are really hydrocephalus. This inference is further sustained by a somewhat limited, though conclusive experience with children. I have seen four cases recover and two die, the symptoms in all being in no way distinguishable from those given as characteristic of hydrocephalus. One case which died, and one of the recoveries belonged to the same family, in which there was a strongly marked tubercular taint, as was also the case in another family which came under observation. It may be said that no post-mortem of a case of hydrocephaloid has shown that the lesions of it and hydrocephalus are identical. This argument is apparently a good one, and at first sight seems strongly against the position taken, but as all cases that die with certain symptoms are considered hydrocephalus, and all who recover hydrocephaloid, though they may have the same symptoms, the value of the post-mortem argument is rather doubtful.

These views regarding recovery from tubercular meningitis have, to a certain extent, the support of Hasse, one of the best authorities on the subject. Though the pathology shows that tubercular meningitis may be recovered from, still the brain is not restored to its normal condition, but is so far damaged as to yield when a strain is applied. The patient, of whose spinal cord and brain this microscopical examination was made, was thirty years of age; intemperate, of ordinary education. He made well marked rhythmical motions, had maniacal and incomplete cataleptoid alternations, followed by theatrical talking. His spinal cord, as will afterwards appear, showed changes which would seem at first sight to confirm the opinions of Lionville, Magnan and Schultze, but in reality are opposed to the conclusions of these observers, being, not as might be surmised, a cause, but an effect of the cataleptoid alternations. The disease had existed at least two years, and the patient died from tubercular enteritis.

Post-mortem.—Body emaciated, cadaveric rigidity well marked; lungs, seat of tuberculous deposit; heart, normal;

tubercle of the intestines and peritoneum; spleen, congested; kidneys, normal; liver, cirrhotic; head, dolichocephalic; scalp, thin; cranium, thick and not adherent to the dura-mater, which was normal. Sub-arachnoid space filled with a number of brownish flakes of a gelatinous consistency; most of these drained away with the cerebro-spinal fluid, but a few were quite firmly adherent to the underlying pia-mater; minute blackish or dark brown grains were disseminated through these, probably exudative products.(?) Arachnoid of base, pontico-chiasmal lamina, perfectly healthy, clear, and transparent; cerebello-medullary lamina, opaque, with whitish, dense bands. Sylvian fissure, slightly opaque. Pia-mater along the larger, and in some instances along the finer vessels, minute pale yellowish, whitish, and reddish bodies were found, supposed to be tuberculous. In the Sylvian fossa itself, over the island of Reil there was a fusion of the leptomeninges.

Blood vessels. A whitish spot, measuring one and one-half inches in every direction, existed on the under surface of the basilar arachnoid; the large veins were filled with dark continuous coagula, or with chains of whitish connected thrombi, such as occur in the ultimate agony, when prolonged in exhaustive diseases. The fine network of vessels was injected, and this condition was especially well marked over the island of Reil. Convolutions, few, simple and typical. The white substance of the centrum ovale of Vieussens, of the pedunculi, cerebellum, ganglia and tegmentum, as well as of the medulla and pons, showed numerous punctae vasculosae, all of a strikingly venous character; in every direction the veins, and these alone, were filled with blood. This was also true of the cortex, and was nowhere better pronounced than in the gyri-operti of the island of Reil. The claustrum which I have never before seen the seat of any marked injection, was filled with distended venous channels and puncta venosa. The grey ganglia at the base of the fourth ventricle, which depend for their color on the degree and kind of injection, as well as on the pigmentation of their cellular elements, appeared semi-transparent and cerulean in tent. Spinal cord; membranes healthy, no deviation from the normal standard; cord itself decidedly anaemic. Ventricles; a mucoid substance covered the parts at the base of these cavities, particularly well marked at the calamus scriptorious of the fourth ventricle. Over the stria cornua of the left side, the ground glass appearance was visible; this passed gradually into the mucoid substance on either side. Dilatation of the posterior cornua of the lateral ventricles existed, this extended backwards, and there was adhesion of the walls, so extensive on the left side as to cause the complete separation of the apex of the posterior horn from the body of the ventricle, giving it the appearance of a cyst in the occipital lobe. There was a beautiful venous injection of the ventricular lining.

It may be said in passing, that Meynert, two years before Kahlbaum, described katatonia, called by him a peculiar form of melancholia attonita, as "characterized by a series of fluxionary excitations, toned down by co-existent cerebral pressure, microscopic exudations, ventricular dropsy, and (perhaps) premature ossification of the sutures. From these would result forced and theatrical activities on the part of the patient. The convulsive state indicates the control of the irritative factors; the cataleptoid condition, the triumph of the depressing factors. The ideas of grandeur, following upon stupor, are the results of ideas previously caused by fluxionary conditions."

As the microscopical examination is perhaps the first as yet made in this class of cases, it was of importance that the observations should be under the supervision of one accustomed, not only to observe, but also to interpret observations. For this reason, and also because of great advantage derived from two observers working at the same time, the result obtained may, in a great measure, be attributed to the kind assistance and supervision of Dr. Spitzka. They are certainly of a nature to throw some light on the clinical manifestations of the disease.

The mucoid matter on the floor of the fourth ventricle was found to consist of an accumulation of round cells, not surpassing a red blood corpuscle in diameter, some nucleated, others not; all were perfectly colorless. Interspersed among them were larger elements, identical in every respect with white blood corpuscles.

Isolated bodies of an oblong shape with a distinct nucleus and pellucid protoplasm were noticed. All these were imbedded in a granular mass which showed a formation of imperfect fibrils. The arachnoid exudation consisted of the same matters together with a fair proportion of red corpuscles, large flakes of pigment and round spheres of a protean nature. The pia-mater of the convexity exhibited numerous small nodules, most of which were molecular, others calcareous, and a few contained large and small polynucleated cells; these nodules were periadventitial and hardly visible to the naked eye. The cortical substance of the island of Reil showed a marked increase of the nuclei of the neuroglia. The ganglionic cells, both pyramidal and fusiform were normally contoured, processes well developed; protoplasm healthy, in some cases diffusely pigmented, and nucleus round and clear. Free lymphoid bodies were accumulated in the pericellular spaces in prodigious numbers, in one instance, no less than twenty-three of these cells could be distinguished clustering around one pyramidal nerve-cell of the third layer. Frequently the nerve-cell was altogether hidden from view by such cell groups. In this respect the island of Reil presented marked regional differences. It was found that areas varying from a line to an inch in diameter were the seat of this appearance, while a similar, larger or smaller adjoining area was either less involved, or perfectly normal in this respect. The transition from the affected to the healthy areas was sudden.

The coats of all the vessels were entirely healthy, presenting no deviations from the appearance of cerebral vessels in sane subjects. The arteries were empty, the veins and many capillary districts filled with blood corpuscles; these latter were individually distinct, not compressed or fused by crowding as has been described to be the case in the stasis accompanying general paresis.[1] This engorgement was most marked in those areas, in which the accumulation of lymphoid bodies was farthest advanced. The periadventitial

---

[1] Spitzka "Patho-Psychology of Progressive Paresis."

space was filled with similar bodies, in the case of the vessels referred to. The same appearances in a lesser degree were noticed in the operculum, and the convolutions bordering the anterior part of the great longitudinal fissure. The remainder of the cortex cerebri appeared perfectly healthy. The accumulation of lymphoid bodies was still more marked in the nucleus lenticularis, than in the claustrum and island of Reil. The cerebellum, olivary bodies, nuclei of the cranial nerves, corpus striatum, thalamus and corpora quadrigemina, presented no deviations from the normal standard.

Spinal Cord; the nerve-cells of the grey cornua were perfectly healthy, a delicate granular material filled the dilated pericellular spaces; central canal open. The white columns showed everywhere an increase in the number and thickness of the connective tissue septa, and of Fronemann's cells. With this the medullary sheaths had undergone a slight degree of atrophy, while many axis cylinders were hypertrophic.

These conditions were most marked in the anterolateral columns of the cervical portions of the cord, although the posterior were not free from it, here it was limited to the peripheral portion, and a small area at the base of the posterior intermediate sulcus. The anterior pyramids of the medulla oblongata exhibited the same change as the spinal cord.

CONCLUSIONS

1. The pia-mater presented signs of an old tubercular process which had become latent.

2. The encephalon was the seat of a passive venous engorgement, which had been of long standing. No mechanical obstruction to the venous outflow could be found as the cause of this engorgement, and we must therefore suppose it to have depended on vaso-motor anomalies.

3. The gelatinous exudation of the arachnoid and piamater can not be considered an inflammatory product, but rather as a simple filtration of molecular matter and blood discs through the walls of the distended venous channels.

4. The accumulation of lymphoid bodies per diapedesis around the ganglionic cells was, in like manner, the result of the vascular stagnation. The fact that certain cortical areas were more severely affected than others, is to be attributed to peculiarities in the distribution of certain venous channels.

5. This accumulation of lymphoid bodies, of whose identity with blood corpuscles, both red and white, particularly the former, I am fully convinced occurs to such an extent only in one other cerebral condition, namely, that which accompanies the severer forms of typhus fever. The similarity between the pathological appearances of the cerebral cortex in katatonia and typhus is truly striking; the chief difference is that while in the former, certain parts of the cortex are, chiefly, if not exclusively, affected, in the latter the whole encephalon is involved equally. It should not be forgotten that a few of these bodies, one or two in the pericellular space of one out of from twelve to a hundred pyramids, occur in health, but so rarely that they have to be sought for, and are not, as in this pathological condition, so numerous as to actually conceal the nerve-cells from view. In a lesser degree such an increase of the lymphoid bodies takes place in many forms of insanity associated with atrophy; their origin here is however different, as has been explained on another occasion.

6. No destruction or degeneration of the essential nervous elements, the cells and fibres, was to be found, for no importance can be attached to the diffuse pigmentation of a few of the pyramidal cells, as many subjects who have never manifested any symptoms of mental alienation, show the same condition.

7. The condition of the spinal cord and anterior pyramids, is to be considered as a mild grade of sclerosis, approximating senile sclerosis in character. In a patient of this age, such a change is unquestionably pathological. I am inclined to consider it as a degeneration due in part to malnutrition, and partly to disuse of the motor tracts, in consequence of the long continued and oft repeated cataleptoid conditions. In this it offers a parallel to Charcot's "sclerose laterale," as found in an old case of hysteric contracture, where the connective tissue hyperplasia, was not the cause of the contracture, but the result of the consequent long continued disuse of the motor periphery. If future autopsies should reveal the same appearances, I should have no hesitation in pronouncing the characteristic pathological conditions to be an inertia of the vaso-motor centers, whose consecutive injurious effects were concentrated on the parts lying at the depth of, and around the fissure of Sylvius. Every other lesion is to be considered as secondary or accidental.

Vaso-motor anomalies, as have been illustrated in some of the cases, do occur in the course of the disease, and are quite prominent features in its clinical history. It is probable, however, that the exudation on the floor of the fourth ventricle exerted an influence in the production of these anomalies.

The symptomatic forms of insanity—mania, melancholia, etc., may be confounded with katatonia, since they all occur in the course of the disease. A differential diagnosis is, however, scarcely necessary here, the result being the same, as regards prognosis, as in the chronic cases.

Insanity of pubescence bears some resemblance to katatonia, but does not partake of the cyclical character of the latter disease, nor is there, unless complicated with epilepsy or chorea, any convulsive element about it. The delusions of the form of insanity occurring at pubescence are very vague, partaking rather of the character of those found in paresis, more particularly in the mental enfeeblement, the extremely stupid disregard of all conflicting circumstances, and the absence of any explanation; those of katatonia, on the other hand, are rather intellectual, and do not vary so indefinitely.

The katatoniac is consequential, but his dignity is not so obtrusively asserted as is the case in insanity of pubescence; the former likes to be left alone, the latter pushes himself forward. There is more or less simulation in both, as there is with most cases of insanity, but the victim of pubescent insanity grows indignant if detected, the katatoniac considers the detection a good joke.

It would appear at first sight that hysteria resembles katatonia so much, as to defy differential diagnosis. Excepting, however, cases in which there is mutual complication, the two are very distinct. The hysteric takes such care of herself as to avoid injury; the katatoniac frequently exhibits a blind recklessness of consequences. The hysteric requires sympathy for the continuation of her symptoms; the katatoniac would perform rhythmical motions in the darkest corner, and when entirely alone.

The form of nervous disease known as hystero-epilepsy[2] resembles markedly, in some symptoms, katatonia, but the general history of the disease is very different, and on this alone, rather than isolated symptoms, can a differential diagnosis be founded. Despite the apparent diversity, the delusions of grandeur may raise a suspicion of paresis, but the wide difference of physical symptoms will soon dissipate any doubt on the subject. Chorea complicating insanity may cause the confusion of it and katatonia, but the control of the motions found in the latter disease, and the cyclical phenomena will prevent a long continuance of the confusion. Multiple cerebral sclerosis is a form of disease that in some cases can only be diagnosticated from katatonia by the antecedent history, especially when accompanied with paresis.

The prognosis according to Kahlbaum is good; as far as my experience goes bad. Three cases only out of thirty having recovered, and of the permanence of the recovery of two of these I have my doubts. These contrasted opinions are not so contradictory as they seem, for though many, perhaps very many, of Kahlbaum's recoveries were remissions lost sight of, still his patients were in very different circumstances from mine, and were not compelled to re-enter the world during a remission with a damaged brain and endure the struggle for existence, under much the same adverse circumstances that led to their being placed under asylum treatment. The presence of a tubercular meningeal process need not militate against a favorable prognosis. However, taking everything into consideration, the prognosis should be guarded, not only as regards recovery, but as regards life, since katatonia *per se* is a disease causing death, and in addition the tendency to phthisis has to be taken into consideration.

The duration of the disease is from two to five years, depending on the hygienic surroundings and treatment of somatic affections. The treatment of katatonia is divisible into medicinal and moral. The medicinal treatment should be, in a great measure regulated by the symptoms, and should be of a tonic character, as the katatoniac is always more or less debilitated. The motor disturbance points to the use of conium. Alcoholic stimulants have had at times what could be nothing less than a food value, and have aided in sustaining the diminished vitality of the patient. Stimulant enemata have been occasionally of service and frequently prevented the return of a cataleptoid condition. The vasomotor anomalies seem to indicate the use of nitrite of amyl. I have tried this remedy, but not sufficiently long to speak decidedly of its beneficial effects, although satisfied

that it is of value. Three cases have certainly improved under its use, and it has caused a pleasurable feeling in all cases of katatonia where it has been given. One of the cases already cited showed an increased tendency to active exertion and a less theatrical tinge to his words and actions. The case in which an immediate effect was best shown is the following.

CASE V.—E.S., age 26; clerk, American, unmarried, temperate in the use of alcoholic stimulants, no hereditary taint ascertainable, although the father and mother died young. During the year 1874, an enlargement on the patient's neck which seems to have been of the thyroid gland, gradually disappeared, after which an alteration was noticed in his temper which changed from good humor to moroseness; he then became much depressed but soon grew maniacal, passed into a cataleptoid condition, during which he claimed to have an interview with the Deity; he was, on emerging from it, very precise and formal in conversation, and made rhythmical motions with his fingers. These conditions alternated with semi-lucid intervals marked by a morbid religious tendency. Three years after the first appearance of the symptoms, asylum treatment was rendered necessary by his violence. He was admitted March 23d, 1877, to the New York City Asylum for the Insane, was rather blank, but dignified in expression and in poor physical health. He had had, just previous to admission, the delusion that his nerves were all gone, but when admitted was unable to continue a conversation for three minutes, without passing into a very complete cataleptoid condition. Three days after admission he was placed under amyl nitrite; in the course of an hour he became quite vivacious, danced a jig, insisted on indulging in boxing, talked clearly and connectedly, said that he had been very lazy and disinclined to do anything for his own support. He showed no trace of any delusion, and had no further returns of the cataleptoid condition for two days, when the treatment with amyl was suspended. In the course of the afternoon subsequent to its discontinuance, he had a pr[o]longed cataleptoid relapse, followed by the same phenomena that marked him on admission. Treatment with amyl was again resumed on the following day, since which time he has had no returns of the cataleptoid condition, although he once attempted to feign it, to avoid being bathed. He now has the delusion that he is to live forever, but is clearer in its expression, although somewhat vague as to details. He gives as a reason why he is to live forever, that he is "all nerve." This privilege has been granted by the Deity to him as a special favor. The other cases did not show as immediate improvement, although one who had been in a cataleptoid condition for three months before the administration of amyl, now walks around and talks freely. What the ultimate result will be from this treatment, can not of course be stated, but I hope at the least for a prolongation of the patient's life, and that the correction of vaso-motor irregularities will, if long continued, tend to produce a healthy tone in the circulation, though the effects are, for the time being, temporary in character.

Moral treatment, of course, in a great measure, resolves itself into the consideration of the question of asylum treatment. This is of advantage, as it affords a means of isolation from friends, always the most disturbing influence in treatment. Change of scene and travel, under charge of a sensible, educated man, not a pedant, would benefit many, as it would enlarge the patient's ideas and stimulate him to a healthy tone of mind—in short, stir him up. If the case be a boy, and he has a doting, foolish mother, removal from

---

2 Hammond: "Diseases of the Nervous System."

her should be the first step in the treatment, as her sympathy would undo all otherwise beneficial measures; a remark that applies with equal if not greater force in the case of a wife and husband.

Balls and musical entertainments of a purely sensuous nature should be avoided, and all things of an intellectually stimulating nature brought as much as possible in contact with the patient. Faradization of the muscles of the chest, as a prophylactic against tubercle, is one means of treating probable somatic complications, to be recommended. The general treatment by tonics, etc., is of course, indicated in this and all other atonic physical conditions occurring during an attack of insanity. The preferable method of artificial feeding, often required in cases of katatonia, is by means of a Davidson's syringe, the use of which is unattended with the danger that accompanies the use of the elastic but stiff tube of a stomach pump, or the misadventures that follow the clumsy funnel method of feeding. From the irregularity of the symptoms, which set at defiance the dicta of the forensic psychologist, it would seem as if the disease could easily be feigned. Apart, however, from the probability of a criminal being so keen an observer as to attempt feigning so complicated an affection, one symptom could scarcely be feigned with even the slightest probability of success, namely, the cataleptoid condition. The failure in the simulation of this symptom, with a close examination of his antecedent history, would soon detect any attempt of this kind. The crimes that a katatoniac would be likely to commit are murder, arson and rape. The murder in obedience to an hallucination, the arson for a similar cause, while the rape would be an expression of his excited erotic condition.

If these crimes, however, were committed during a remission, the patient should be held responsible as he would for the time being, be capable of acting logically on any conclusion arrived at in a logical manner. An instance where a form of disease somewhat similar, and perhaps, were sufficient history on the point obtainable, katatonia itself, has been brought under cognizance of law. This occurred in a fanatical religious organization in Germany. Two ministers of this organization believed they had received, during a cataleptoid condition, a command from God to kill a certain man and raise him from the dead. The former they succeeded in doing, but in the latter they failed. In this case which illustrates the circumstances under which crime might be committed by a katatoniac, the accused were declared irresponsible. Any person, however, who has been acquitted on these grounds should be immediately sequestrated for the safety of the public.

Kahlbaum claims that katatonia can occur, and has occurred in epidemic form in France and Sweden. In this opinion he has the support of Bouchut, (Wien Wochenschrift, No. 43, 1861,) and Remak, (Med. Cent. Z. t. g. No. 87, 1864,) who believe in a nervous contagion causing diseases of the mind. Parallelism is a good thing, but may be carried too far, as it would seem to have been in this case. There is no proof of the existence of any contagion, and so long as these phenomena can be explained in accordance with the general clinical history of nervous diseases, there is no need of assuming its existence. Influences ordinarily producing insanity in persons predisposed to mental disease, may cause a number of cases to appear at one time, but never to the extent of, or with the uniformity in symptoms characteristic of a so-called epidemic. And this uniformity is the suspicious point in the hypothesis of patho-mental epidemics, but is one that admits of a very rational explanation on other grounds than contagion.

Most probably the greatest number of victims in a so-called katatonia epidemic, were cases of morbid impulse, simulating through a craving for notoriety, a few instances of katatonia that had occurred. It is a curious fact, however, that many of these epidemics, so-called, have occurred in regions subject to scrofulous affections. Mental epidemics have always a half truth in them, and half truths are extremely captivating to a certain class of minds, as a foundation for extravagant theories; but it is needless to say there is no reason to believe that a psychical influence, which resembles in action the contagion of ordinary physical disease, is aught more than a figment of the imagination that serves "to point a moral or adorn a tale" for some enthusiastic alienists of a rhetorical turn of mind.

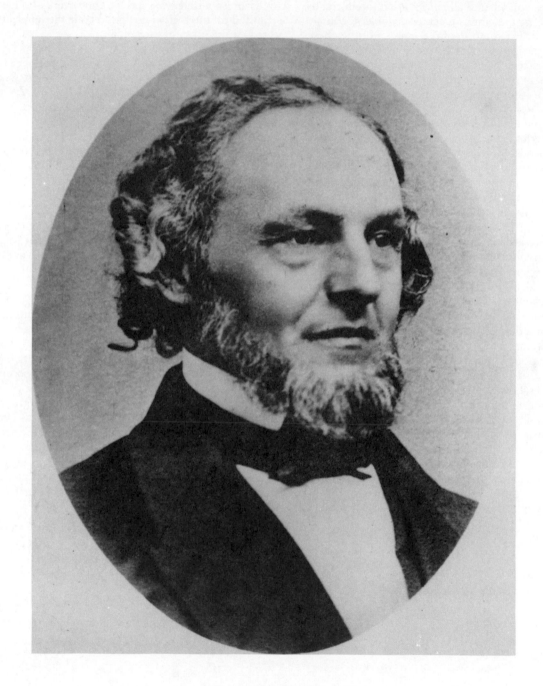

Pliny Earle, M.D., 1809–1892

THE CURABILITY OF INSANITY

A Statistical Study

By Pliny Earle, M.D.

Superintendent of the State Lunatic Hospital at Northampton, Massachusetts

Notwithstanding the manifold triumphs of medicine, of surgery, and of other sciences and arts, there are inexorable limits to their achievements and their power of achievement. Nature yields in a measurable extent to the conceptions, the devices, the ministrations, and the administrations of human skill, but, as if to mock them in the end, and to demonstrate the retention of her inherent supremacy, she at length establishes a position and defies their power. These are trite truths, so trite, indeed, that the mention of them is an apparent superfluity: and yet they answer my purpose as an introduction, and are not wholly inappropriate at the beginning of a paper in which their truthfulness receives another illustration.

Nowhere are these truths more conspicuous, than in the sphere of the enterprises to overcome the disabilities of what are termed the defective classes of mankind—defective from imperfections either congenital or acquired. It is, indeed, perhaps true that, in the treatment of the blind, in the attempt to obtain a substitute for the eye and thus open an avenue of perception to the imprisoned brain, although nothing has been discovered which is, by very far, a full equivalent of the perfect natural organ, the success has equalled the expectation. But in reference to some of the other classes this is not true; and the hopes and confident anticipations awakened in the public mind, in the comparatively early periods of the modern endeavors at improvement, have been doomed to at least a partial disappointment.

Some forty years ago, when the efforts of Dr. Guggenbühl, in Switzerland, to elevate the idiot from his congenital degradation had been imitated in other parts of Europe, the world of philanthropy and the world of thought were startled by the announcement of a certain degree of success; and this, in the minds of the people, was magnified to such an extent as to give the general impression, that idiocy is so far amenable to culture that the great mass of its subjects can be raised nearly to a level with the average of the race. But, after the experience of a sufficient number of years to furnish a reliable test, it is found that, although partial imbeciles are susceptible of a degree of elevation in a ratio

inverse to the degree of mental defection, and although, with the inclusion of the idiot, the advantages acquired are more than sufficient to vindicate the enterprise, yet the congenital idiot is essentially the congenital idiot still.

The history of the instruction of deaf mutes in vocal language is similar, in these respects, to that of the attempts to redeem the idiot from his infirmity. Surprising results were attained in some instances, and public opinion, taking its shape and tone from these, leaped to the conclusion that, although deafness might continue, permanent mutism was soon to become a thing of the past. Experience has not yet shown that a majority of deaf-mutes are susceptible of satisfactory instruction and achievement in this method of intercommunication.

A similar exaltation of belief and of expectation has occurred in the specialty in which we are engaged; and, unfortunately, a similar disappointment has awaited all who had become interested in the subject, whether in the profession or among the people at large.

It is proposed, in this paper, to show, by the collocation of statistics, the actual results of treatment at a large number of institutions, both foreign and domestic, bringing our knowledge of such general results to a later date than that contained in any former statistical essay.

RECOVERIES AT BRITISH ASYLUMS

It will be remembered that the reports of many, if not most, of the British asylums, contain a table, originally designed by Dr. Thurnam, in which the admissions, discharges, recoveries and deaths of patients are classified according to the duration of the insanity.

These classes are as follows:—

1st. First attack, and within three months, on admission.

2d. First attack, above three and within twelve months, on admission.

3d. Not first attack, and within twelve months, on admission.

4th. First attack or not, but of more than twelve months, on admission.

5th. Congenital and unknown.

This is a well conceived and useful table for its intended purpose; and, if prepared with sufficient care and discrimi-

---

Read before the Association of Medical Superintendents of American Institutions for the Insane, on retiring from office as its President, at Saratoga, N.Y., June 16, 1885.

TABLE I. Cases of Less Than Twelve Months, at Twenty-Three British Asylums

| Asylums | Years Inclusive | Cases of First Attack, With Duration | | | | | | | | | Not First Attack | | |
| | | Under Three Months | | | Three to Twelve Months | | | Total Under Twelve Months | | | Not Over Twelve Months | | |
		Adm.	Recov'd	Per ct. of Recover's	Adm.	Recov'd	Per ct. of Recover's	Adm.	Recov'd	Per ct. of Recover's	Adm.	Recov'd	Per ct. of Recover's
Somerset and Bath	1877–82	499	189	37.88	166	80	48.19	665	269	40.45	320	148	46.25
Devizes	1877–82	289	120	41.52	109	20	18.35	398	140	35.18	198	80	40.40
Abergavenny	1877–82	285	141	49.47	102	24	23.53	387	165	42.64	167	101	60.48
Carmarthen	1877–82	108	57	52.78	50	16	32.00	158	73	46.20	79	37	46.84
Derby County	1877–82	397	180	45.34	112	41	36.61	509	221	43.42	225	128	56.89
Hereford	1878–83	121	66	54.55	62	23	37.10	183	89	48.63	108	56	51.85
South Yorkshire	1877–82	1,251	565	45.16	214	55	25.70	1,465	620	42.32	693	335	48.34
Prestwich	1877–82	1,203	671	55.78	243	63	25.93	1,446	734	50.76	541	319	58.96
Lancaster	1877–82	654	393	60.09	344	90	26.16	998	483	48.40	444	309	69.59
Warwick County	1878–83	228	124	54.39	116	31	26.72	344	155	45.06	111	63	56.76
Edinburgh Roy	1878–83	755	381	50.46	298	98	32.89	1,053	479	45.49	673	381	56.61
Belfast	1877–82	444	234	52.70	147	49	33.33	591	283	47.88	112	74	66.07
Retreat, York	1876–80	40	20	50.00	21	9	42.86	61	29	47.54	36	13	36.11
Gartnavel	1875–79	541	227	41.96	126	22	17.46	667	249	37.33	235	108	45.96
Cambridge and Ely	1877–81	213	85	39.90	58	9	15.51	271	94	34.69	76	40	52.63
Barming Heath	1877–80	553	259	46.84	183	54	29.50	736	313	42.53	302	195	64.57
City of London	1880–82	62	27	43.55	28	10	35.71	90	37	41.11	44	28	63.64
Berrywood	1878–80	181	71	39.23	58	28	48.28	239	99	41.42	102	39	38.23
Worcester	1879–81	169	81	47.93	73	15	20.55	242	96	39.67	113	82	72.57
Nottingham	1877–79	119	54	45.38	31	12	38.71	150	66	44.00	44	19	43.18
Beverly	1876–78	87	44	50.57	23	2	8.69	110	46	41.82	42	20	47.62
Crichton	1877–79	47	25	53.19	14	4	28.57	61	29	47.54	30	21	70.00
Southern Counties	1877–79	70	37	52.86	35	9	25.71	105	46	43.81	73	44	60.27
Totals		8,316	4,051		2,613	764		10,929	4,815		4,768	2,640	
Mean or Average per cent				48.71			29.24			44.06			55.37
Aggregate of admissions 15,697; of recoveries 7,455													47.49

nation, can not well fail to throw light upon the question of curability as affected by duration, or by the fact of first or subsequent attack.

Nearly two years ago I collated the statistics of this table in a series of the annual reports of twenty-three of the British asylums, so far as relates to all cases of less duration than twelve months at the time of admission. For more than fifty years, all such cases have, in the United States, been called *recent*, in contradistinction to those of remoter origin, which have been called *chronic*; and my object in collecting the statistics was to ascertain the degree of curability to which those asylums had attained in the treatment of what we call recent cases.

Of each of twelve of the asylums these statistics, which are embodied in Table I, extend over a series of six consecutive years, the last of which was, in some instances, 1882, and in others, 1883. At three of the asylums they extend over five years; at one, over four years; and at seven, over three years. At each asylum the years are consecutive; and at no one is the last of the series later than 1878, the majority being either 1880, 1881, or 1882.

The results of these statistics may be briefly stated.

1st Class (First Attack, less than 3 months' duration) the admissions were 8,316; recoveries, 4,051; per cent of recoveries, 48.71.

2d Class (First Attack, 3 to 12 months' duration) admissions, 2,613; recoveries, 764; percent of recoveries, 29.24.

3d Class (Not first Attack, less than 12 months' dura-

tion) admissions, 4,768; recoveries, 2,640; percent of recoveries, 55.37.

By uniting the first two classes, we have all cases of first attack and of less duration than one year. Of these, the admissions were 10,929; the recoveries, 4,815; and the proportion of recoveries, 44.06 per cent.

Of the third class the admissions were 4,768; the recoveries, 2,640; and the proportion of recoveries, 55.37 per cent. Here we have another illustration of the fact that recovery takes place in a less proportion of cases of first attack than in cases subsequent to the first—a fact which was demonstrated in an article on curability in the report for 1880 of the Northampton Lunatic Hospital.

By a union of the three classes, all of which contain, exclusively, cases of less than twelve months in duration, and are consequently here known as recent cases, we obtain the subjoined results.

Admissions, 15,697; recoveries, 7,455; proportion of recoveries, 47.49 per cent.

Among this series of twenty-three asylums is the Retreat at York, the statistics of recoveries at which, from 1796 to 1819, have been quoted, ever since they were published, as one of the authorities for the eminent curability of mental disorders. It may not be uninstructive to bring into juxtaposition those statistics of three-fourths of a century ago, and those of the same institution for the five years from 1876 to 1880 inclusive. This is done in the following table [Table II].

The diminution of the proportion of recoveries on the

TABLE II. Per Cent of Recoveries at the York Retreat of Cases
of Less Duration Than Twelve Months

	Per Cent of 1st Class	Per Cent of 2d Class	Per Cent of 3d Class	Per cent of Total
1796–1819	85.10	55.55	61.76	68.25
1876–1880	50.00	42.86	36.11	43.30
Decrease of per cent	35.10	12.69	25.65	24.95

TABLE III. Recoveries of Cases of Less Duration Than One Year

Classes	Admissions	Recoveries	Per cent of Recoveries
Class I 1st attack; less than 3 months' duration	38,283	18,654	48.72
Class II 1st attack; 3 to 12 months' duration	12,126	3,421	28.21
Class III Not 1st attack; less than 12 months' duration	19,574	10,494	53.61
Total	69,983	32,569	46.52

admissions is, for the 1st class, 35.10 per cent on the admissions; for the second class, 12.69 per cent; for the third class, 25.65 per cent; and for the whole, 24.95 per cent, or, in round numbers, one-fourth of the admissions.

The proportion of diminution from the actual recoveries of the first period, is, for the first class, 41.17 per cent, or a fraction more than two-fifths; for the second class, 22.84 per cent, or a fraction more than one-fifth; for the third class, 41.53 per cent, or a fraction over two-fifths; and for the whole, 36.25 per cent. In other words, for each hundred of recoveries of what we call recent cases, three-fourths of a century ago, there are but sixty-four (63.75) recoveries now.

Some months after the collection of the foregoing statistics, but before any use had been made of them, Dr. T.A. Chapman, of the Hereford Asylum, England, published a similar but much larger collection, in *The Journal of Mental Science* for July, 1884. It contains the statistics of "46 English County and Borough Asylums, and the Edinburgh and Glasgow Royal Asylums, for (in most instances) 11 years, 1872 to 1882 inclusive." Here is a collocation of the remarkable number of 93,443 cases of insanity, all of them classified as in the foregoing table. The whole number of recoveries was 35,468, or 37.95 per cent of the admissions. But as the recoveries of *recent* cases are now, alone, under consideration, we will turn our attention especially to them. The subjoined table [Table III] shows the numbers, and the percentage, in each of the first three of Thurnam's classes.

Dr. Chapman's table includes, apparently, twenty-eight Asylums that are not in mine, and mine has five that are not in his. Of these five, two are in Scotland and three in England, the Retreat at York being one.

In regarding these two tables, so much alike and yet so different, almost the first impression received from them is the striking similarity of results. These are, indeed, so nearly identical as to justify one's faith in the sometime possibility of a close approximation to accuracy in this branch of vital statistics. The difference in the proportion of recoveries, as indicated by the two, are, for the first class of cases, only one-one-hundredth (.01) of one per cent; for the second class, one and three-hundredths (1.03) per cent; for the third class, one and seventy-six-hundredths (1.76) per cent; and for the total, ninety-seven hundredths (.97) of one per cent.

When Dr. Woodward, in 1833, took charge of the Worcester Hospital, he had before him, as exemplars, three well known pioneers in the field of high percentages of recoveries. Dr. Burrows, in 1820, had reported 91.32 per cent as the result of the treatment of 242 cases, of which 221

recovered. He also published the results, from 1797 to 1819, at the York Retreat, where, of 47 cases of less duration than three months, the recoveries were 40, or an equivalent of 85.10 per cent. [1] In 1827 Dr. Todd, at the Hartford Retreat, reported that, of 23 recent cases admitted 21 had recovered, a proportion of 91.3 per cent. In 1841, Dr. Woodward obtained his highest proportion of recoveries, 91.42 per cent, by the treatment of 70 cases, 64 of which recovered; and in 1842, Dr. Galt, at the Williamsburg, Virginia, Asylum, excelled all of his predecessors in the announcement that of thirteen recent cases under his care twelve had recovered, a percentage of 92.3.

Here we have five different, well-known medical authorities, each confirmatory and corroborative of the others, and all of which have, for an average of half a century, been regarded as a kind of oracular proclaimers of the possible achievement of recovery in about 90 per cent of recent cases. Yet, singularly enough, the whole of the five separate reputations were built, and the oracles established, upon the treatment of an aggregate of only 395 cases.

On the other hand we have before us, in Dr. Chapman's table, the results of treatment of a number of recent cases which lacks but seventeen to make it seventy thousand, and the recoveries are only 32,569, or 46.52 per cent. This ratio of curability is only 86 hundredths of one per cent more than half as large as that which was claimed by Dr. Burrows, and only 37 hundredths of one per cent less than one-half as large as that of Dr. Galt. Even in the cases of first attack and of only three months' duration, of which there were 38,283, the recoveries were but 18,654, or 48.72 per cent. In the light thrown upon the subject by this unparalleled collection of recent cases, what becomes of the once exceedingly fashionable assertion that "from seventy-five to ninety per cent can be cured?"

RECOVERIES AT THIRTY-NINE (15+24) AMERICAN INSTITUTIONS

Inasmuch as neither Thurnam's table nor its equivalent in any other form is used at the American institutions, it is impossible to group, or analyze the results at the latter on precisely the same basis, in all respects. Nevertheless, upon looking over the American reports, I find that a large

1 The fact should not be overlooked that, if the word *recent* be used in its American signification, applying to all cases of less duration than one year, the proportion of recoveries at the Retreat was only 68.25 per cent, the admissions being 126, and the recoveries 86.

TABLE IV. Whole Number of Recoveries, and Recoveries of Cases of Less Than Twelve Months' Duration, at Fifteen American Institutions

Asylums	Years	Admissions		Discharged Recoveries				
		Under 12 Months	Whole Number	Under 12 Months	Per cent of Recent cases	Whole Number	Per cent of Whole Number	Per cent of All Recoveries on Recent Admissions
Elgin	6	488	1,017	197	40.37	246	24.19	50.41
Concord	5	334	536	148	44.31	161	30.04	48.20
Worcester	5	593	1,254	191	32.21	254	20.26	42.83
Taunton	5	824	1,619	300	36.41	369	22.79	44.78
Utica	5	1,518	2,184	661	43.54	716	32.78	47.17
Harrisburg	5	395	716	117	29.62	133	18.58	33.67
Dixmont	5	646	1,117	238	36.84	288	25.78	44.58
Dayton	5	607	977	285	46.95	342	35.00	56.34
Ossawatomie	5	398	707	165	41.46	217	30.69	54.52
McLean	4	207	308	81	39.13	89	28.90	42.99
Northampton	4	224	511	75	33.48	104	20.35	46.43
Danvers	4	962	2,078	361	37.53	458	22.04	47.61
Columbia, S.C	4	408	702	110	26.96	161	22.93	39.46
Boston	3	174	275	66	37.93	80	29.09	45.98
Winnebago	3	285	561	117	41.05	162	28.88	56.84
Totals, and Mean per cent	68	8,063	14,562	3,112	38.59	3,780	25.96	46.88

amount of matter may be brought together, illustrative of the proportion of the reported recoveries of recent cases.

In the statistics of a majority of our hospitals, although, in reference to admissions, the duration of the insanity is given, and hence a distinction between recent and chronic cases rendered possible, yet no such discrimination is made in regard to patients discharged. The subjoined table [Table IV] contains the results, in regard to recovery, for a series of from two to six years, of fifteen American hospitals, in the reports of which the recoveries of cases of less than twelve months' duration are numerically given. The time during which each hospital furnished these statistical results was at Elgin, six years; at Concord, Worcester, Taunton, Utica, Harrisburg, Dixmont, Dayton, and Ossawatomie, five years each; at McLean, Northampton, Danvers, and Columbia, S.C., four years each; and at Boston, and Winnebago, three years each; the period ending, in most cases, in 1883.

The aggregate of the admissions of *all cases* is 14,562; the aggregate recoveries, 3,780; and the proportion of recoveries, 25.96 per cent. The largest proportion was 35 per cent, at Dayton; and the smallest, 18.58 per cent, at Harrisburg. At five others it was less than 23 per cent; and at still five others less than 30 per cent; while at three besides Dayton, it was over 30 per cent.

The aggregate of admissions of *recent* cases, is 8,063; that of recoveries of recent cases, 3,112; and the proportion of recoveries of recent cases, 38.59 per cent. The largest proportion of 46.95 per cent, at Dayton; and the smallest 26.96 per cent, at Columbia, S.C. Of the thirteen others, the proportion at one was less than 80 per cent; at two, between 30 and 35 percent; at five, between 35 and 40 per cent; and at five between 40 and 45 per cent.

Finding that, in despite of the traditional "75 to 90 per cent" of some of the fathers, not one of these hospitals discharged even 47 per cent of recoveries of recent cases, while the mean, or average of all of them was less than 39 per cent, I studied the relation between the *whole number of*

recoveries and the number of *admissions of recent cases*. The whole number of recoveries is larger by 668 than the recoveries of recent cases; and the number of admissions of recent cases is 6,499 smaller than the whole number of admissions. Yet, strange as it may appear, the total of recoveries is only 46.88 per cent of the admissions of recent cases! The largest proportion, 56.84 per cent, is at Winnebago; and the least, 33.67 per cent, at Harrisburg. Of the remaining thirteen hospitals, the proportion is less than 40 per cent at one; between 40 and 45 per cent, at four; between 45 and 50 per cent, at five; between 50 and 55 per cent, at two; and over 55 (56.34) per cent, at one. Thus, after aiding and assisting the recoveries of recent cases by a supplementary and a complimentary gift of the certainly not despicable number of 668 cases, we have been unable to swell them even to 50 per cent of the admissions of recent cases.

We now come to the hospitals which give the duration of the disease in the cases admitted, but give no such information in respect to the cases discharged. The following table [Table V] includes the statistics, for a term of from two to six years each, of twenty-four institutions of this class. Of six of them—Jacksonville, Ill., Mt. Pleasant, Iowa, Fulton, Mo., St. Joseph, Mo., Lincoln, Neb., and Jackson, La.,—the term was six years; of eleven—Hartford Retreat, Ct., Middletown, Ct., Middletown, N.Y., Trenton, N.J., Danville, Pa., Williamsburg, Va., Richmond, Va., U.S. Government Hospital, Washington, D.C., Jackson, Miss., Cleveland, Ohio, and Longview, Ohio,—five years; of six—Brattleboro, Vt., Staunton, Va., Weston, W.Va., Pontiac, Mich., Madison, Wis., and St. Peter, Minn.,—four years; and on one—Augusta, Me.,—three years.

The total of admissions is 18,756; the total of recoveries, 5,933; and the proportion of all recoveries on all admissions, 31.63 per cent. The largest percentage of recoveries 48.54, was at Fulton, Mo., and the smallest, 15.83, at Danville, Pa. Of the remaining 22 institutions, the proportion was less than 23 per cent, at four; from 25 to 30 per cent, at five; from 30 to 35 per cent, at five; from 35 to 40 per cent,

TABLE V. Recoveries at Twenty-Four American Institutions

Hospitals	Years	Admissions		Discharges		
		Under 12 Months' Duration	Total Admissions	Total Recoveries	Percent of Recoveries on All Admissions	Per cent of All Recoveries on Admissions of Less Than 12 Months' Duration
Jacksonville, Ill	6	1,000	1,605	440	27.41	44.00
Mt. Pleasant, Iowa	6	852	1,548	400	25.84	46.95
Fulton, Mo	6	675	1,162	564	48.54	83.56
St. Joseph, Mo	6	435	740	257	34.73	59.08
Lincoln, Neb	6	414	654	267	40.83	64.49
Jackson, La	6	83	231	63	27.27	75.90
Hartford Retreat	5	300	434	150	34.56	50.00
Middletown, Ct	5	492	1,168	241	20.63	48.98
Middletown, N.Y	5	503	775	300	38.71	59.64
Trenton, N.J	5	373	786	244	31.04	65.42
Danville, Pa	5	263	695	110	15.83	41.83
Williamsburg, Va	5	165	380	171	45.00	104.00
Richmond, Va	5	357	559	254	45.44	71.15
U.S. Gov't Hospital	5	549	1,099	357	32.48	65.03
Jackson, Miss	5	235	526	228	43.35	97.02
Cleveland, O	5	681	1,135	414	36.48	60.79
Longview, O	5	470	882	325	36.85	69.15
Brattleboro, Vt	4	199	344	88	25.58	44.22
Staunton, Va	4	207	467	201	43.04	97.10
Weston, W. Va	4	136	328	104	31.71	76.47
Pontiac, Mich	4	320	707	145	20.51	45.31
Madison, Wis	4	307	746	163	21.85	53.09
St. Peter, Minn	4	486	1,168	267	22.86	54.94
Augusta, Me	3	358	617	180	29.17	50.28
Totals	118	9,860	18,756	5,933	31.63	60.17

at three; from 40 to 45 per cent, at three; and from 45 to 46 per cent, at two.

The whole number of *recent cases* admitted was 9,860; the whole number of recoveries, as before stated, 5,933; and the percentage of *all recoveries* upon the number of *recent cases* admitted, 60.17. Here, then, by setting aside and disregarding the 8,896 cases of more than 12 months' duration, we have succeeded in raising the recoveries to a point above 50 per cent.

By the union into one group, so far as they are susceptible of such union, of the contents of these two tables, we obtain the following aggregate results.

In 39 American hospitals, during a period of from 3 to 6 years each, making an aggregate of 186 years of hospital work, the number of patients admitted was 33,318; the number of patients discharged recovered, 9,713; and the proportion of recoveries, as compared with admissions, 29.15 per cent. In the factors producing this result it will be observed that all the cases of duplicate, triplicate and manifold recoveries of one and the same person, are included, and yet the recoveries do not rise to 30 per cent.

The whole number of *recent* cases admitted was 17,923; the total recoveries of both recent and chronic cases, as already mentioned, 9,713; and the proportion of *all recoveries*, as compared with the admissions of *recent cases*, 54.19 per cent. But be it not forgotten that this result is obtained by the sacrifice, or annulment, of *fifteen thousand three hundred and ninety-five (15,395) admissions*, or, in other words, by calculating the proportion of recoveries upon a little more than one-half of the number of admissions.

RECOVERIES AT TWENTY AMERICAN HOSPITALS; THIRD TERM OF FIVE YEARS

It will, perhaps, be remembered that my monograph on the Curability of Insanity, which was prepared in 1876, contained a list of twenty institutions for the insane, so tabulated with their statistics as to show the proportion of recoveries at each of two quinquennial periods,—the first of those periods being the second quinquennium of the existence of those hospitals, respectively, and the last period being the quinquennium terminating in either 1876, or one of the two immediately preceding years. The longest time wholly intervening between those two quinquennia was 44 years, at the McLean Asylum, Mass; the shortest, 2 years, at the Mendota Hospital, Wisconsin; and the mean or average time, eighteen and one-half years. But the true mean time, as applied to the gathering of the statistics—that is, the time from the middle of the first quinquennium to the middle of the last—was five years longer, or twenty-three and one-half years.

The total of admissions in the first period was 14,516; the total recoveries, 6,689; and the proportion of recoveries on admissions, 46.08 per cent. The admissions of the second period were 24,383; the recoveries, 8,354; and the proportion of recoveries, 34.26 per cent, or a fall of 11.82 in that proportion. This diminution equalled one fourth, or, to be exact, 25.66 per cent, of the recoveries of the first period.

As eight years have elapsed since the close of the second period, it has appeared to me that some similar researches, at a still later date, might tend more fully to illustrate the

TABLE VI. Recoveries at Twenty American Hospitals; Third Term of Five Years

Institutions	First Five Years	Per cent of Recov's	Second Five Years	Per cent of Recov's	Decrease of Per cent of recov's	Third Five Years	Total Admitted	Total Recov'd	Per cent of Recov's	Per cent of Recoveries Compared With That of Second Five Years		Decrease of Per cent of Recover's From First Five Years
										Decrease	Increase	
Augusta, Me	1846–50	48.55	1871–75	36.62	11.93	1880–84	1,008	296	29.36	7.26		19.19
Concord, N.H	1848–52	46.92	1872–76	32.97	13.95	1880–84	623	158	25.36	7.61		21.56
Brattleboro, Vt	1841–46	43.50	1871–76	30.43	13.07	1878–83	551	124	22.50	7.93		21.00
McLean, Mass	1823–27	40.69	1871–75	21.66	19.03	1880–84	421	123	29.22		7.56	11.47
Worcester, Mass	1839–43	48.59	1871–75	29.75	18.84	1880–84	1,319	264	20.01	9.74		28.58
Taunton, Mass	1859–63	43.46	1871–75	23.11	20.35	1880–84	1,318	296	22.46	0.65		21.00
Butler Hospital	1854–58	39.78	1872–76	35.57	4.21	1880–84	635	191	30.55	5.02		9.23
Hartford Retreat	1829–33	57.40	1870–74	39.21	18.19	1880–84	453	162	35.76	3.45		21.64
Bloomingdale, N.Y	1826–30	47.55	1871–75	32.55	15.00	1880–84	626	200	31.95	0.60		15.60
Utica, N.Y	1848–52	43.17	1871–75	32.33	10.84	1880–84	2,020	610	30.20	2.13		12.97
Flatbush, N.Y	1861–65	41.88	1871–75	33.11	8.77	1880–84	2,071	336	16.22	16.89		25.66
Trenton, N.J	1853–57	42.79	1872–76	31.32	11.47	1880–84	836	251	30.02	1.30		12.77
Pennsylvania Hospital	1846–50	51.10	1871–75	42.30	8.80	1880–84	973	328	33.71	8.59		17.39
Dixmont, Pa	1861–65	37.78	1871–75	30.01	7.77	1880–84	968	216	22.31	7.70		15.47
Catonsville, Md	1838–43	51.59	1871–75	40.83	10.76	1880–84	656	209	31.86	8.97		19.73
Newburgh, O	1860–64	46.63	1871–75	30.03	16.60	1880–84	1,147	439	38.27		8.24	8.36
Dayton, O	1860–64	60.16	1870–74	45.25	14.91	1880–84	910	337	37.03	8.22		23.13
Indianapolis, Ind	1853–57	57.26	1871–76	52.48	4.78	1880–84	4,010	1,678	41.84	10.64		15.42
Jacksonville, Ill	1855–60	46.53	1869–74	31.96	14.57	1879–84	1,486	395	26.58	5.38		19.95
Mendota, Wis	1865–69	33.82	1871–75	25.86	7.96	1880–84	1,021	280	27.42		1.56	6.40
Totals, and Mean per cent		46.08		34.26	11.82		23,052	6,896	29.91	4.35		16.17

subject of curability, and perhaps secondarily, or indirectly, the general character of the disease. Accordingly, I have collected the statistics of admissions and recoveries at the same twenty institutions during a third period of five years, that period terminating, at nineteen of them, in or with 1884, and at one where the reports are biennial, in or with 1883. At two of the institutions, both of which issue biennial reports, the duration of the period is six years. Those statistics, together with the results in each of the first two periods, are contained in Table VI.

The aggregate admissions in the course of this third period is 23,052; the aggregate recoveries, 6,896; and the proportion of recoveries, 29.91 per cent of the admissions, a result which demonstrates that the reported recoveries have continued to diminish, during the last eight years, in very nearly the same annual ratio as they had diminished between the first and the second period.

The following is a summary of the results of the whole investigation—

Recoveries in the 1st period, 46.08 per cent of the admissions.

Recoveries in the 2d period, 34.26 percent of the admissions.

Recoveries in the 3d period, 29.91 percent of the admissions.

Decrease of recoveries from 1st to 2d period, 11.82 per cent of the admissions.

Decrease of recoveries from 2d to 3d period, 4.35 per cent of the admissions.

Total decrease of recoveries from 1st to 3d period, 16.17 per cent of the admissions.

The decrease of recoveries from 1st to 2d period, is 25.66 per cent of the recoveries of the first period.

The decrease of recoveries from 2d to 3d period, is 12.69 per cent of the recoveries of the second period.

The total decrease from the recoveries of the first period is equal to 35.09 per cent of the recoveries of the first period.

The numbers of the insane subjected to treatment being hypothetically the same at the three periods, then, for each hundred (100) that recovered in the first period only seventy-four (74.34) recovered in the second period, and only sixty-five (64.91) recover now.

The proportion of recoveries between the last two periods, from 1879 to 1884, did not diminish at all of the twenty institutions. At three of them it increased. At the McLean Asylum this increase was 7.56 per cent of the admissions; at the Newburg, Ohio, hospital, it was 8.24 per cent; and at the Mendota, Wisconsin, hospital, 1.56 per cent. But notwithstanding this augmentation, the actual decrease from the proportion recovered in the first period, at those three institutions, is still 11.47, 8.36, and 6.40 per cent, respectively.

The decrease from the second to the third period, and the total decrease from the first to the third period, at each of the seventeen other institutions, may be learned from the last two columns of the table. The decrease is more than one-half at the Worcester and the Flatbush hospitals; very nearly one-half at Brattleboro and Taunton; and more than one-third at Augusta, Concord, Hartford, Pennsylvania Hospital, Dixmont, Catonsville, Dayton and Jacksonville.

STATISTICS OF ONE YEAR,
AT FIFTY-EIGHT AMERICAN INSTITUTIONS

For the purpose of ascertaining the extent to which the results of one year of the current work at American insti-

TABLE VII. One Year at Fifty-Eight American Institutions

Institution	State	Year	Admitted	Recovered	Per cent of Recoveries	Died	Per cent of Deaths
Augusta	Me	1884	203	59	29.06	101	49.75
Concord	N.H	1884	141	18	12.77	24	17.02
Brattleboro	Vt	1884	82	23	28.05	29	35.36
McLean	Mass	1884	113	34	30.09	17	15.04
Worcester	Mass	1884	252	53	21.03	57	22.62
Northampton	Mass	1884	136	25	18.38	25	18.38
Taunton	Mass	1884	283	85	30.04	65	22.97
Danvers	Mass	1884	530	96	18.11	101	19.06
Boston, City	Mass	1884	121	34	28.10	32	26.45
Butler	R.I	1884	106	46	43.40	13	12.26
Hartford Retreat	Ct	1884	97	37	38.14	18	18.56
Middletown	Ct	1884	271	72	26.57	80	29.52
Bloomingdale	N.Y	1884	136	55	40.44	27	19.85
Flatbush	N.Y	1884	479	47	9.81	101	21.09
Utica	N.Y	1884	372[a]	89	23.92	56	15.05
Buffalo	N.Y	1884	275	80	29.09	43	15.63
Trenton	N.J	1884	175	52	29.71	64	36.57
Morristown	N.J	1884	210	37	17.62	57	27.14
Penna. Hos	Pa	1884	203	51	25.12	40	19.70
Harrisburg	Pa	1884	128	23	17.97	36	28.12
Dixmont	Pa	1884	189	28	14.81	69	36.50
Danville	Pa	1884	201	37	18.41	29	14.42
Norristown	Pa	1884	356	92	25.84	96	26.96
Warren	Pa	1884	203	36	17.73	46	22.66
Catonsville	Md	1884	95	29	30.53	30	31.57
Mount Hope	Md	1884	169	77	45.56	45	26.62
Washington	D.C	1884	347	79	22.77	67	19.30
Staunton	Va	1884	133	55	41.35	36	27.06
Richmond	Va	1884	119	97	81.51	61	51.26
Weston	W.Va	1884	176	74	42.05	39	22.15
Raleigh	N.C	1884	106	26	24.53	11	10.37
Goldsboro	N.C	1884	81	26	32.10	14	17.28
Morganton	N.C	1884	71	31	43.66	9	12.67
Columbia	S.C	1884	293	72	24.57	143	48.80
Austin	Texas	1884	254	66	25.98	41	16.14
Little Rock	Ark's	1884	82	42	51.22	21	25.61
Nashville	Tenn.[b]	1882–84	222	67	30.18	62	27.93
Columbus	Ohio	1884	282	164	58.16	59	20.92
Newburgh	Ohio	1884	220	87	39.55	37	16.81
Dayton	Ohio	1884	188	60	31.91	37	19.68
Athens	Ohio	1884	223	96	43.05	63	28.25
Longview	Ohio	1884	220	56	25.45	58	26.36
Indianapolis	Ind	1884	908	329	36.23	112	12.33
Pontiac	Mich	1884	192	62	32.29	29	15.10
Kalamazoo	Mich	1884	174	17	9.77	9	5.17
Jacksonville	Ill	1884	240	56	23.33	32	13.33
Elgin	Ill	1884	123	38	30.89	21	17.07
Anna	Ill	1884	220	67	30.45	33	15.00
Kankakee	Ill	1884	291	48	16.49	31	10.65
Mendota	Wis	1884	239	58	24.27	30	12.55
Oshkosh	Wis.[b]	1883–84	601	148	24.63	115	19.13
Mt. Pleasant	Iowa[b]	1882–83	534	120	22.47	98	18.35
Independence	Iowa	1883	233	38	16.31	34	14.59
St. Peter	Minn.[b]	1883–84	595	143	24.03	82	13.78
Rochester	Minn.[b]	1883–84	299	55	18.39	43	14.38
Fulton	Mo.[b]	1881–82	364	175	48.08	113	31.04
St. Joseph	Mo.[b]	1881–82	316	110	34.81	49	15.51
Napa	Cal	1884	500	130	26.00	90	18.00
Totals, and Mean per cent			14,372	4,007	27.88	2,980	20.74

[a]15 cases "found not insane" are deducted.   [b]Biennial.

tutions would enlighten us upon the subject of curability, I have collected and herewith present, in Table VII, the statistics of fifty-eight of them, taken, in fifty-one instances, from the reports for 1884. Of seven of the hospitals the reports are biennial, and consequently contain the results for two years each. In four instances the report from which these results were taken ended in 1884; in one instance in 1883, and in two in 1882.

I am well aware of the many influences, both favorable and unfavorable, which may, and often do, modify the number of recoveries, as well as of deaths, in public institutions, and which necessarily render the results of any one year unreliable as a test or measure of the work of a series of years, at any individual hospital. But at a large number of institutions on any given year, these influences would probably very nearly balance one another, and consequently the aggregate results would fairly represent the mean or average of the same group of institutions for a much greater length of time.

The aggregate of patients admitted at these fifty-eight institutions, in the course of the time specified, is 14,372; the aggregate of recoveries, 4,007; and the proportion of recoveries, calculated upon the admissions, 27.88 per cent, or a trifle more than one-fourth. The least relative number of recoveries, 9.77 per cent was at Kalamazoo; and the largest, 81.51 per cent at Richmond.

In the following schedule the hospitals are arranged in groups, according to the proportion of their recoveries, each group differing five per cent from the one above or below it.

Below 10 per cent, Flatbush and Kalamazoo.

From 10 to 15 per cent, Concord and Dixmont.

From 15 to 20 per cent, Northampton, Danvers, Morristown, Harrisburg, Danville, Warren, Kankakee, Independence and Rochester.

From 20 to 25 per cent, Worcester, Utica, U.S. Gov't Hospital, Raleigh, Columbia, S.C., Jacksonville, Mendota, Oshkosh, Mt. Pleasant and St. Peter.

From 25 to 30 per cent, Augusta, Brattleboro, Boston, Middletown, Ct., Buffalo, Trenton, Penna. Hospital, Norristown, Austin, Longview and Napa.

From 30 to 35 per cent, McLean, Taunton, Catonsville, Goldsboro, Nashville, Dayton, Pontiac, Elgin, Anna and St. Joseph.

From 35 to 40 per cent, Hartford Retreat, Newburg and Indianapolis.

From 40 to 45 per cent, Butler, Bloomingdale, Staunton, Weston, Morganton, and Athens.

From 45 to 50 per cent, Mount Hope and Fulton.

From 50 to 55 per cent, Little Rock.

From 55 to 60 per cent, Columbus.

Over 80 per cent, Richmond.

If there be no mistake in the record from the Virginia Central Asylum, at Richmond, that institution, so far as my knowledge extends, has exceeded every other of its kind, not in America alone but upon the whole surface of the earth, in the proportion of its recoveries. Forty years ago, it was doing well to report the recovery of eighty per cent of *recent* cases. At the present time, it is rare that even sixty per cent are so reported, and the average in the United States, as we have just seen, is below forty per cent. But here we are confronted with a proportion of 81.51 per cent of *recoveries of all the cases admitted!* The moral to be derived herefrom appears to be, that, if any person yet unborn be blessed with the pre-natal power of foreordination of his own physical organization, and desire to recover in case he be afflicted with insanity, he should elect to be born a negro. [2]

There is yet another useful moral to be derived from the case. At the Danvers Hospital, which, before it went into operation, had cost more than $3,500, for every patient for whom its accommodations were calculated, and more than $2,500, for each of the seven hundred patients who have been crowded into it, the per cent of recoveries was 18.11. At the Richmond Hospital, which apparently could not have cost over $100, and probably not more than $50, per patient, the recoveries were equal to 81.51 per cent. The moral is so conspicuously obvious, that it would be a work of supererogation to repeat it.

In Table VIII, the fifty-eight hospitals and their statistics are grouped according to the States in which they are respectively situated.

The proportion of recoveries was the smallest in New Hampshire, and that proportion increased in the other States in the following order, Pennsylvania, Iowa, New York, Michigan, Minnesota, District of Columbia, Massachusetts, New Jersey, Illinois, Wisconsin, South Carolina, Texas, California, Vermont, Maine, Connecticut, Tennessee, North Carolina, Indiana, Maryland, Ohio, Missouri, West Virginia, Rhode Island, Arkansas and Virginia.

If the statistics of recoveries be arranged in accordance with the groups popularly called the Eastern, the Middle, the Southern, and the Western States, the results are as follows;—and to them are appended the percentage of deaths, calculated, like the recoveries, upon the number of patients admitted.

In the Eastern States the total of admissions was 2,335; the total of recoveries, 582; and the proportion of recoveries, 24.92 per cent. The number of deaths was 562, and the proportion, 24.07 per cent. The number of recoveries exceeded that of deaths by only 20.

In the Middle States the number of admissions was 2,927; the number of recoveries, 627; and the proportion of recoveries, 21.42 per cent. There were 664 deaths, equal to a percentage of 22.69. The deaths have a majority of 37 over the recoveries; and the proportion of both recoveries and deaths is less than in the Eastern States. It has been suggested in one of the criticisms of a psychological periodical, that the small ratio of recoveries in Massachusetts is a consequence of the published writings of the superintendent of one of the hospitals in that State. As, according to these statistics, the proportion of recoveries is less in the Middle States than in Massachusetts, the proposition now is,— *Whose published writings were the cause of it?*

In the Southern States 1,844 patients were admitted; and 632, or 34.27 per cent, recovered. The total of deaths was 496, or 26.90 per cent. The proportion of recoveries is nearly ten per cent on the admissions in excess of those of the Eastern States; and that of deaths nearly three per cent. The proportion of recoveries is considerably increased by the statistics of the Richmond Asylum. If those statistics be set aside, and the computation made upon the returns from the other Southern institutions, the results are;—Admissions 1,725; recoveries 535; per cent of recov-

---

2 The Virginia Central Asylum is for colored persons.

TABLE VIII. State Groups, One Year

States	Number of Hospitals	Admissions	Recoveries	Per cent of Recoveries	Died	Per cent of Deaths
Maine	1	203	59	29.06	101	48.75
New Hampshire	1	141	18	12.77	24	17.02
Vermont	1	82	23	28.05	29	35.36
Massachusetts	6	1,435	327	22.79	297	20.69
Rhode Island	1	106	46	43.40	13	12.26
Connecticut	2	368	109	29.62	98	26.63
New York	4	1,262	271	21.47	227	17.99
New Jersey	2	385	89	23.12	121	31.15
Pennsylvania	6	1,280	267	20.80	316	24.69
Maryland	2	264	106	40.15	75	28.41
District of Columbia	1	347	79	22.77	67	19.31
Virginia	2	252	152	60.31	97	38.49
West Virginia	1	176	74	42.05	39	22.15
North Carolina	3	258	83	32.17	34	13.18
South Carolina	1	293	72	24.57	143	48.80
Texas	1	254	66	25.98	41	16.14
Arkansas	1	82	42	51.22	21	25.61
Ohio	5	1,133	463	40.86	254	22.41
Michigan	2	366	79	21.58	38	10.38
Indiana	1	908	329	36.23	112	12.33
Illinois	4	874	209	23.91	117	13.38
Wisconsin	2	840	206	24.52	145	17.26
Iowa	2	767	158	20.60	132	17.21
Minnesota	2	894	198	22.14	125	13.98
Missouri	2	680	285	41.91	162	23.82
California	1	500	130	26.00	90	18.00
Tennessee	1	222	67	30.18	62	27.93
Totals, and Mean per cent	58	14,372	4,007	27.88	2,980	20.74

eries, 31.21. Deaths 435; percentage of deaths on admissions, 25.21.

In the Western States the admissions were 7,266; the recoveries, 2,166; and the proportion of them 29.81 per cent. Of deaths there were 1,258, or a proportion of 17.31 per cent, which is more than five per cent of the admissions less than in either of the other sections.

Arranged in accordance with the *increasing* ratio of recoveries, that is, from lowest to highest, the sections stand as follows;—Middle, Eastern, Western, Southern;—and in accordance with the *decreasing* ratio, from highest to lowest, of deaths, as follows; Southern, Eastern, Middle, Western.

These results are derived from the work of but a single year, and hence are unreliable as an established formula. By the extension of the investigation over a sufficient series of years, something more reliable might be obtained. Then, and not now, will be the time to speculate upon the causes of the differences.

STATISTICS OF PENNSYLVANIA HOSPITALS

The table to which attention is now requested [Table IX] includes statistics of the seven hospitals in Pennsylvania, during a period of five years each, with the exception of that at Warren, which is of but four years. At all of them the period ended in, or with, the year 1884.

The whole number of cases admitted was 5,934; the total of recoveries 1,204; and the proportion of recoveries 20.29 per cent. But Norristown and Warren are both new hospi-

tals, and in their first years received many transfers from other institutions. Hence they are unfairly represented. We will therefore permit the statistics of only the last two years at these institutions to enter into the computation, retaining, for the others, the full period of five years. Those statistics are as follows: [Table IXa]

By a substitution of these figures for those contained in the next preceding table, it will be found that the whole number of admissions is 4,794; the number of recoveries, 1,102; and the proportion of recoveries, 22.98 per cent, or a gain of 2.69 per cent on the admissions, by the change.

At the four State Hospitals of Massachusetts, the proportion of recoveries in the three fiscal years ending in 1882, and the statistics of which form the basis of an article on curability in the Northampton, Mass. report for that year, was 22.25 per cent. This is seventy-three hundredths (.73) of one per cent less than that of the Pennsylvania hospitals, according to these statistics. But this difference is more than counterbalanced by the fact that the Massachusetts statistics relate to *persons* only, while those of Pennsylvania relate to *cases*. In the latter all duplicate, triplicate and multiplicate recoveries are included, while in the former they are all *rejected*.

By the first of the two tables [Table IX] the deaths were 1,158, and their proportion on the admissions, 19.51 per cent. By the last table [Table IXa] they were 1,054, and their proportion, 21.98 per cent, or an increase of 2.47 per cent. This increase is a natural result, as deaths are generally comparatively few in the first two or three years of a hospital's operations.

TABLE IX. Pennsylvania Hospitals

		Admitted	Recovered	Per cent of Recoveries	Died	Per cent of Deaths.
Frankford	1880–4	196	58	29.59	39	19.90
Penna. Hospital	"	973	328	33.74	147	15.11
Dixmont	"	968	216	22.31	277	28.61
Harrisburg	"	772	121	15.97	174	22.54
Danville	"	720	114	15.83	118	16.39
Norristown	"	1,458	275	18.86	290	19.89
Warren	1881–84	847	92	10.86	113	13.34
Totals, and Mean per cent		5,934	1,204	20.29	1,158	19.51

TABLE IXa

		Admitted	Recovered	Per cent of Recoveries	Died	Per cent of Deaths
Norristown	1883–1884	777	195	25.09	219	29.18
Warren	1883–1884	388	70	18.04	80	20.62
Totals, and Mean per cent		4,794	1,102	22.98	1,054	21.98

TESTIMONY OF THE DANVERS HOSPITAL

The experience at the newest State institution in Massachusetts is both instructive and disappointingly interesting, in the light which it throws upon the curable, or rather the incurable, condition of a great mass of the insane of the present epoch in that State.

The Danvers Hospital was opened for the reception of patients on the 18th of May, 1878. It is, emphatically, one of those establishments upon which a flood of money has been poured, for the purpose of creating a curative institution as nearly perfect as possible under the light of existing knowledge. If abundance of pecuniary means in construction, together with what was believed to be the highest embodied ideal of architectural arrangements, could cure insanity more rapidly than a less costly and more simple structure, that hospital, most assuredly, was prepared for a demonstration of the proposition. It was evident that great efforts were made to arrive at such a demonstration, and thus prove that the curative advantages of the institution were an adequate, or—since the value of reason restored is not to be measured by dollars and cents—more than adequate compensation for the excess of expenditure. The usual custom of a large transfer of chronic and incurable cases from older hospitals or asylums to the new one, was here omitted, and the supply of patients was derived chiefly from current commitments. By this means the proportion of recent cases was much higher than usual from the first; and as Boston and five other large centres of population—which usually furnish a larger ratio of recent cases than the rural districts—are within a comparatively short distance from it, that proportion was raised still higher.

The fiscal year of the State institutions terminated four and one-half months after the hospital was opened. During this period 305 patients were admitted; and 26, or 8.82 per cent, discharged recovered. In the course of the next—1878–79—fiscal year, 653 were admitted; and 115, or 17.61 per cent, discharged recovered. In 1879–80 the admissions were 581, and the discharge of recoveries 165, making the percentage of the latter 28.40. At this point the proportion of recoveries stopped upon its ascending scale, and took a retrograde direction. In 1880–81 the admissions were 497, the recoveries discharged, 124, and the percentage, 24.95; in 1881–82, admissions 512, discharged recoveries 89, percentage 17.38; in 1882–83, admissions 488, discharged recoveries 80, percentage 16.39; and in 1883–84, admissions 530, discharged recoveries 96, and the percentage of the latter 18.11.

The whole number of admissions, during the six years and four and one-half months, was 3,566; and that of discharged recoveries 695, or an equivalent of 19.49 per cent. In the first three full fiscal years, the admissions were 1,731, the discharged recoveries, 404, and the per cent of the latter 23.34; and in the last three fiscal years, admissions 1,530, discharged recoveries 265, per cent of recoveries 17.32. In the first period of three years, the deaths were 240, or 13.86 per cent of the admissions; and in the last period, 285, or 18.63 per cent of the admissions. In the first period the deaths were 240, a per cent of 59.4 on the recoveries; and in the last period, they exceeded the recoveries by 20, the deaths being to the recoveries as 57 to 53.

The new formulae for statistics in Massachusetts give the ability still further to illustrate the character of the recoveries,—an ability rendered by the reports of no other State in the Union. The new tables were adopted in 1879, and first used in the reports for 1879–80. In the course of the five fiscal years ending September 30, 1884, 554 patients, or cases, were discharged recovered from the Danvers Hospital; but 115 persons, who had been discharged recovered a total 121 times, had returned to it. Within the last three years,—which are included in the foregoing years—the discharged recoveries were 265; but, during the same time, 80 persons, representing 86 of those recoveries, were readmitted. So far as the community is concerned, these recoveries offset, or cancel, the same number of the discharged recoveries, and the added recoveries in the population, instead of being 265, is 265 minus 86, or 179, a diminution of about

TABLE X. Two Years at Massachusetts Hospitals

Hospitals	Admissions			Discharges
	Persons Admitted Who Had Previously Been Discharged Recovered	Number of Times They Had Recovered	Ratio of Recoveries to Persons	Persons Discharged Recovered
Worcester	43	118	2.73	109
Taunton	64	147	2.29	145
Northampton	21	39	1.85	53
Danvers	49	54	1.1	176
Totals	177	358	2.02	483

one-third, and only 11.70 per cent on the number of admissions during that period.

RE-ADMITTED RECOVERIES IN MASSACHUSETTS

The annual report for 1881–82 of the Northampton Lunatic Hospital, contains an article on the statistics of the State Hospitals of Massachusetts during the three years which had then elapsed since the adoption of the new series of tables. I desire to call attention to some points in the statistical history of recoveries, as illustrated by the same hospitals, during the two years since that article was published. For this purpose a table is here introduced [Table X] which shows, for the fiscal years 1882–83 and 1883–84:

1st. The number of persons admitted who had previously been discharged recovered;

2d. The number of times they had previously recovered;

3d. The ratio of recoveries to persons; and

4th. The number of persons discharged recovered during those two years, at each of the four hospitals aforesaid.

The number of persons admitted who had previously been discharged recovered, was 177; and they had been discharged recovered a total of 358 times. There were 181 more recoveries than persons. In other words, the number of recoveries was four more than twice as great as the number of persons. Each person had recovered, as a mean or average number, 2.02 times. Regarded, during the last two years, from a debt and credit point of view, those four institutions cancelled, by taking back from the general population, no less than 358 recoveries for which they had been credited. During the same time they discharged, recovered, 483 persons, which is only 125 more than the *recoveries*, (not persons) which they had taken back.

Summary. A brief résumé of the most important results of the foregoing studies, expressed in the percentages of recoveries, may be found convenient for reference.

1. Cases of first attack; duration less than three months.

a. Earle's 8,316 cases, at 23 British Asylums. Recoveries 48.71 per cent.

b. Chapman's 38,283 cases, at 46 British Asylums. Recoveries 48.72 per cent.

2. Cases of first attack; duration less than twelve months.

a. Earle's 10,929 cases, at 23 British Asylums. Recoveries 44.06 per cent.

b. Chapman's 50,409 cases, at 46 British Asylums. Recoveries 43.79 per cent.

3. Not first attack; duration less than twelve months.

a. Earle's 4,768 cases, at 23 British Asylums. Recoveries 55.37 per cent.

b. Chapman's 19,574 cases, at 46 British Asylums. Recoveries 53.61 per cent.

In neither of the three foregoing classes have we any American statistics, because our institutions, in the tabulation of their cases, make no discrimination which would render such a classification possible.

4. All cases of duration less than twelve months.

a. Earle's 15,697 cases, at 23 British Asylums. Recoveries 47.49 per cent.

b. Chapman's 69,983 cases, at 46 British Asylums. Recoveries 46.52 per cent.

c. Earle's 8,063 cases, at 15 American Institutions. Recoveries 38.59 per cent.

5. All recoveries, calculated on all admissions.

a. Chapman's 93,443 cases, at 46 British Asylums. Recoveries 37.95 per cent.

b. Earle's 33,318 cases, at 39 [15+24] American Institutions. Recoveries 29.15 per cent.

c. Earle's 23,052 cases; 3d period at 20 American Institutions. Recoveries 29.91 per cent.

d. Earle's 14,372 cases; in one year at 58 American Institutions. Recoveries 27.88 per cent.

It will be perceived that, so far as these statistics are an index, the recoveries in British Asylums, both of recent cases and of all cases admitted, exceed the recoveries in the American institutions by between 8 and 9 percent.

The most important general conclusions to be derived from the statistics included in this paper, are, first, that the old claim of curability in a very large majority of recent cases is not sustained, and that the failure to sustain it is more apparent and more striking than at any antecedent time; and, secondly, that the percentage of reported recoveries of all cases received at the hospitals in this country still continues to diminish.

It is believed that this diminution is, in part, to be attributed to the admission of a larger proportion of chronic cases, and of cases of greater degeneracy from their origin; in part, from the increasing though, as there is good reason to believe, still far from universal practice of not reporting, *as recoveries from insanity*, either mere restorations from a drunken debauch, or forced temporary suspensions from habitual intoxication; and, in part, perhaps, from the adoption of a higher degree of improvement as the standard or criterion of recovery. It may be that there is still another cause of that diminution. Drs. Bucknill and Tuke, in their treatise upon insanity, mention what they call "cooked" statistics. It is possible that, in the United States, this class of published results is decreasing, and that the reported statistics are more generally given to the public in the spirit of a conscientious loyalty to scientific truth.

In conclusion I would express the hope, that the time is not far distant at which the American Association of Superintendents will so perfect its statistical system as to make a distinction between persons and cases; and enable the reader to learn how many of the reported recoveries are first recoveries and how many subsequent to the first. This improvement was made in the Massachusetts statistical tables, as already mentioned, in 1879; and in those of the British Medico-Psychological Association in 1883. Surely our Association ought not to lag far behind in the matter.

PERSONALITY CHANGES AND UPHEAVALS ARISING OUT OF THE SENSE OF PERSONAL FAILURE

By A.T. Boisen

Chaplain, Worcester, Massachusetts, State Hospital, and
Research Associate, Social Ethics Department, Chicago Theological Seminary

The symptoms of a neurosis are not merely the result of past causes . . . . They are also attempts at a new synthesis of life . . . . I have seen more than one man who owed his entire usefulness and justification for existence to a neurosis which put an end to all the stupidities which were dominating his life and forced him into an existence which developed the truly valuable qualities which would have been choked out if the neurosis with its iron talons had not taken the fellow and plunked him down in the place where he belonged. There are men who have in their unconscious the true meaning of their lives and in the conscious that which is for them error and seduction. With others it is just the reverse. In the one case the neurosis means a thoroughgoing reduction or regression, in the other not at all.

These words of Jung[1] express admirably the outstanding conclusion which has resulted from a series of case studies in religious experience and functional mental disorder, the results of which are embodied in the accompanying chart. A neurosis or a psychosis is not necessarily an evil. It is at least in the acute forms an attempt at the reorganization of the personality which may and sometimes does result happily. As an attempt at reorganization it may result in many types of solution from the thoroughgoing unification and socialization of the religious conversion experience at its best, to the complete disintegration and stupor which may be seen on the back wards of our hospitals for the insane. This chart or diagram is an attempt to show some typical solutions and their relationship to the common modes of reaction which may be observed anywhere among ordinary people who are dealing with the problem of personal failure.

It should be distinctly understood that this scheme does not pretend to include all types of the personality. It does not deal with the self-sufficient, self-reliant, healthy-minded types. It is concerned only with the person who either consciously or unconsciously has been faced by the fact that, judged by his own standards, he is or is likely to become a failure and whose conduct is to be understood only in so far as we recognize it as an attempt to meet that situation. Even so it must of necessity do scant justice to the complexity of the problem.

The data upon which this chart is based include thirty-nine cases of mental disorder studied during the past three years at the Boston Psychopathic Hospital and at the Worcester State Hospital; thirty-six cases of religious experience obtained in a survey of the churches and missions of Roxbury, Mass.; the analysis of the experience of five men of outstanding religious genius for whom adequate autobiographical sources were available. Reference has also been made to case studies by other workers, particularly to the Judge Baker Foundation Case Studies and to one case reported by Kempf. Some important suggestions have been taken from the latter's "Mechanistic Classification of the Neuroses" and the central proposition embodied in this scheme finds striking support in a "preliminary communication" by Dr. Harry Stack Sullivan on "The Conservative and Malignant Features of Schizophrenia" in *The American Journal of Psychiatry* for July, 1924, which appeared after the chart had been worked out.

The chart has been prepared to read down and also across. The first four columns represent pre-psychotic modes of behavior, observable in the individuals under consideration as well as in multitudes of "normal" persons. The last three columns represent types of solution which are likely to result from the different reaction modes and the means of solution operative therein. The reaction mode of "shifting responsibility" and of "bluffing" are thus likely to result in systematized ideas of grandeur and of persecution which serve to maintain the individual's self-respect and which when accompanied by the attitude of suspicion and hatred will make him a menace to society. The two central columns divide the pre-psychotic reactions from those representing the solutions and are intended to show that the original reaction modes do not always go on developing into the typical end-products for that reaction, as is the case in most of those psychoses whose onset is gradual and insidious; but that the individual may become aware of the situation and his entire personality may be aroused to meet it and the psychosis may serve to bring the difficulty from the realm of evasion and concealment out into the open.

The cases used in this study are for the most part a selected lot. Most of the records of religious experiences come from groups which cultivate abnormal manifestations, while most of the cases of mental disorder have been chosen

---

1 Psychologie der Unbewussten Prozesse, p. 71.

Personality Changes and Upheavals Arising Out of the Sense of Personal Failure

Primary evil	Controlling desires	Degree of awareness	Reaction mode	Transition stage	
				Gradual	Abrupt
	Integrative. (a) The will-to-serve. (b) The will-to-power.	Clear.	Honest facing of the situation.	Steady and often imperceptible changes in the controlling desires, interests and attitudes without marked upheaval and without attempt at reconstruction, the symptoms to be explained as attempts to encyst the evil and to conceal the real situation.	Awareness of danger with resulting disturbance or panic, and attempts to open up and eliminate the evil and to effect reconstruction. The disturbance may be characterized by: (1) Narrowing of attention, sleeplessness, loss of appetite with resulting systemic toxaemia. (2) Mood changes, anxiety, despair, depression, elation (affective psychoses). (3) Dissociation, regression to lower levels of consciousness, symbolism, animism, ideas of death and world destruction, confusion and unsystematized distortion of belief and conduct, with extreme disturbance or stupor (catatonic schizophrenia).
Personal failure as judged by the personal standards.	Conflicting.	Vague to unconscious.	Concealment. 1. Compromise. 2. Bluffing. 3. Shifting responsibility. (a) Upon other persons or objects. (b) Upon an organic scape-goat. Emotional explosion.		
		Oblivion.	Withdrawal.		
	Segmental and regressive.		Surrender.		

because of their interest from the religious point of view. They are not therefore representative of the general run of religious people nor of the mentally disordered. Their value is therefore chiefly suggestive and the conclusions drawn from these cases must be accepted with caution.

THE PRIMARY EVIL

Three closely associated evils are to be observed in these cases: a sense of personal failure as judged by the personal standards, a sense of isolation, and an experience which compels a reorganization of the individual's world and of his modes of thought and judgment.[2] With the exception of nine cases of religious experience which seem to be cases of the "once-born" type without radical changes and upheavals and without much of the abnormal beyond in three of the cases a profound belief in inspirations and

promptings, this third factor, which is of course that which is not necessarily an evil, is probably common to all the cases. Eighteen cases of religious experience were thus characterized by an abnormal experience accepted by the individual as a manifestation of the Holy Spirit and as such serving as a basis for the reorganization of his life. In three of these cases that experience was a life decision made through the automatic processes; in three others an answer to prayer; in the remainder it was an eruption of the unconscious induced largely through social suggestion and taking the form of speaking with tongues, jumping, falling on the floor, etc. Twelve of these cases were individuals whose previous lives had been distinctly unsatisfactory but who through this experience seem to have succeeded in reorganizing their lives without going through any marked period of conflict or of consciousness of sin. In five cases of mental disorder such an experience is perhaps primary. In all other cases it appears coincident with the sense of per-

---

2 Janet in his "Medications Psychologiques" (vol. 2, p. 268 ff.) has an interesting discussion of "l'évènement non assimilé" which bears upon this problem. He explains the "psychic trauma" of the psycho-analyst as an obstacle which the individual in his development has not succeeded in clearing, a difficult situation which has not been "liquidated." The "stadium of triumph" is achieved when the personality is reorganized and the troublesome experience is put in its proper place.

	Solution	
Attitude	Means of solution	End result
Reverence. Faith.	Association with the universal community. Confession and forgiveness. Reinforcement of motives. Re-integration of the personality.	Progressive socialization and unification of the personality (valid religious types).
Confidence and self- reliance.	The finding of a task worth while. Participation in contemporary society.	The "normal" man.
Flippancy.	Release of tension through jokes. Making light of accepted standards.	
Carelessness.	Association with group of easy standards and lowering the conscience threshold.	The rounder. The criminal gangster.
Cynicism. Fault-finding.	Maintenance of self-respect through depreciation of others.	The misanthrope.
Usually intolerance.	Making a virtue of mere repression. Substitution of a minor for major virtue or loyalty. Substitution of a minor for a major offense.	The ascetic. The prude. The legalist. The super-patriot. The pathological thief.
Self-importance. Braggadocio.	Maintenance of self-respect through delusional misinterpretation.	Paranoic types. The braggart or crank. The religiously eccentric. The paranoiac. The paranoid schizophrenic.
Suspicion. Jealousy.		
Anxiety. Self-pity.	Escape from responsibility and bid for sympathy and attention through simulated or actual illnesses and other bodily symptoms.	Psychoneurotic types, hysterical, neurasthenic, etc.
Irritability. Self-pity.	Release of tension through outbursts of anger or of weeping.	Psychopathic personality.
Listlessness. Seclusiveness. Day-dreaming.	Loss of hope. Taking refuge in phantasy.	Schizophrenic types. (a) Simple.
Apathy. Silliness.	Regression to lower and irresponsible levels.	(b) Hebephrenic, progressive deterioration and disintegration, probably accompanied by structural changes.
Open eroticism.	Loss of self-respect. Dominance of segmental cravings.	

sonal failure and isolation as at least an important factor in the disturbance.

The term "personal failure" may be used in an inclusive sense. It may denote the loss of all that makes life worth living. It would thus in a very real sense be the experience of death. Freud suggests that such an experience lies at the basis of the schizophrenic and paranoic psychoses.[3] This at least is true, actual ideas of death and of imminent world catastrophe, which, according to Freud, stand for the going to pieces of the individual's inner world appear in more than half of the acutely disturbed patients included in this study. Probably however for the purposes of this study it may be better to limit the term to the sense of inner disharmony and isolation marked usually by a sense of sin or guilt, or attempts to escape the sense of sin or guilt. It is important to notice that in many cases where the primary factor is apparently an overwhelming catastrophe, the disturbance is characterized by a sense of guilt. In one of our cases a woman of high standards and good character, following the fatal illness of a beloved daughter, developed the idea that she had committed the unpardonable sin. She did just the opposite of Job. Instead of "maintaining her integrity" in the face of disaster, she sought the explanation in some possible sin of her own. In another case of depression the precipitating factor was the loss of the patient's savings, and in one case of religious conversion experience it was the death of the subject's two daughters. But in no other cases are there any manifest crushing experiences. The sense of inner disharmony and dissatisfaction seems very generally to be primary, although in eleven of the cases of mental disorder it has clearly been accentuated by long-continued social or economic inadequacy; so also in seven of our cases of religious experience. In twenty-two cases the symptoms are apparently traceable to attempts to evade the sense of responsibility or guilt. Limiting thus the conception of personal failure to the sense of inner disharmony, the difference between the law of the members and the law which we have accepted as our own, we may follow MacCurdy in looking upon the death experience as one of the ways of seeking reorganization or renewal.[4]

3 Freud: Psychoanalytische Bemerkungen über einen autobiographisch beschriebnen Fall von Paranoia. Neurosenlahre, Dritte Folge, p. 258 ff.
4 Psychology of Emotion, p. 126.

The sense of isolation is probably characteristic of the mentally disordered as a group. They are for the most part those who have been regarded as "queer" or different from their fellows. The individual who succeeds in becoming an integral part of some group even though that group be small and peculiar does not as a rule find his way into our hospitals. The "prophet" who obtains a following is usually left in peace and as he succeeds in getting social support, his pathological symptoms, if he has them, tend to disappear. The inferior person who finds a group which accepts him and whose standards he also can accept may become a criminal or a delinquent, but he seldom develops a psychosis so long as he maintains his relationship to the group.

A study might well be worked out from the standpoint of the sense of isolation. For the present study however the sense of personal failure has been taken as the primary evil because it has seemed that in the cases under consideration the particular modes of behavior which are observable can best be explained with reference to the "sense of personal failure as judged by the personal standards."

The addition of the latter clause is necessary in order to guard against the assumption that mental disorder implies actual failure or inferiority. The individual's judgment of himself may be very different from the general social judgment, even though it may be a social judgment in the sense that it represents his interpretation of what those whom he loves and honors would think of him, and his psychosis may be due very largely to the fact that he clings to his ideals and refuses to compromise or lower his conscience threshold.

CONTROLLING DESIRES

Three sets of desires are manifest in our cases:

1. Those which find their best expression in the task which gives a man outlet for his creative impulses and wins for him a recognized place among his fellows. These desires have been included under the term "*will-to-power*."

2. Those which find characteristic expression in a devotion to his family which enables him to slave for long hours at monotonous drudgery in order that those whom he loves may live and be happy; and which find their highest expression in the devotion to that which is conceived of as universal and abiding which enables a man to find life worth living even when all other satisfactions have run dry. These desires have been grouped under the heading "*will-to-serve*."

Both the "will-to-power" and the "will-to-serve" are grouped under the term "*integrative desires*" because they contribute to the individual's purpose in life as he conceives that purpose. An equally good term would be "desire for self-realization."

3. Those desires consisting chiefly of physical cravings or appetites which by their partial character tend to interfere with a man's purpose in life as he conceives that purpose. For the most part these will be sex cravings of a perverse nature, though a weakness for drink or drugs might come

under that category. To these the name "*segmental desires*" as been given.[5]

Between the "integrative" and the "segmental" desires there is a wide range of "*conflicting desires*."

According to Freud and his followers all mental disorders are due to sex maladjustments.[6] Janet takes exception to this but is ready to grant that sex maladjustments occur in 75 per cent of his cases.[7] An inspection of the forty cases of mental disorder and of the sixteen cases of religious experience which were marked by conflict indicates that sex maladjustments are clear in all but five.

Vocational failure is clearly a factor in ten of these cases. In four of the cases there was some degree of vocational success.

This preponderance of sex maladjustments over vocational maladjustments is not to be wondered at if we bear in mind that in them a man is concerned not merely with his own destiny but with the destiny of unborn generations. The importance of the sex problem is probably to be measured in terms of *function* rather than of craving. It is not the satisfaction of the cravings which matters, but the faithful discharge of the obligations to the race. The truth which there is in the concept of *sublimation* might just as well be expressed by saying that a man can dispense with the sex function whenever he is able to see his relationship to society at its best, which is what a religious man means when he says God, in terms of some altruistic task.

DEGREE OF AWARENESS

This is the factor upon which Kempf lays greatest stress in his "Mechanistic Classification of the Neuroses." His major division into the "benign" and the "pernicious" groups is made upon the basis of the degree of consciousness of the nature and effect of the ungratifiable cravings which he assumes to be the chief causative factor in mental disorders. In the benign neuroses he finds a tendency to accept the personal source of these cravings, in the pernicious neuroses a tendency to oppose or refuse to accept a personal source of such craving and to blame them upon external causes.

An examination of our cases seems to bear out some such distinction. The entire group of cases of religious experience, especially those coming from the rescue missions, is characterized by frankness and openness in regard to past sins and failures. These constitute the dark background against which the present "saved" condition is viewed. And not infrequently the testimonies include the confession of some recent misstep which some brother desires to put behind him. Among the cases of mental disorder, the four which were characterized by a sense of failure and guilt assumed by the patient have at least in three of the cases and probably in the fourth also made good recoveries.

Our cases do not indicate however that the presence of hallucinations or even extreme dissociation and regression is necessarily due to an attempt to evade personal responsi-

---

5 This term is borrowed from Kempf.
6 Freud "Einführung," Lectures 20 to 22. Kempf in his Psychopathology takes an extreme position.
7 Médications Psychologiques, vol. II, p. 236.

bility. In many cases, as will be shown later, the acute disturbance is rather to be regarded as an attempt to open up and eliminate an evil, the disordered condition serving to bring things out into the light. The psychosis often serves as a judgment day, the patient blurting out what before, for the life of him, he would not have dared to say.

By *oblivion* in contrast with the term *unconscious*, as used in this chart, is meant forgetfulness not of the "craving" or other difficulty which has been causing the distress, but of the ideals or standards which the individual has accepted as his own.

REACTION MODES

Adolf Meyer, August Hoch and others of the American School of Psychiatry have taught that the functional psychoses are to be looked upon, not as disease processes, but as reactions to life situations. The situation with which we are here concerned is a sense of inner disharmony which amounts to a consciousness of personal failure and involves a sense of guilt or attempts to evade the sense of guilt. The attempt is here made to bring together the common methods of meeting such a situation.

By the *honest facing of the situation* is meant the degree of honesty and frankness and rationality in dealing with the situation which is necessary to mental health and to normal human relationships and which constitutes the first step in any successful reorganization of the personality. The different solutions or types of reorganization which may result from meeting the situation in this manner will be considered after we have discussed the "abrupt transition stages" or acute conditions. For the other reaction modes it has seemed best to consider at the same time their logical end-products and their characteristic attitudes and means of solution.

Many cases of religious experience would furnish examples of the reaction mode of *compromise*. Here would belong the case of the minister with an unresolved sex conflict due to marital infidelity whose sermons were confined to such themes as keeping the Sabbath and of another minister with a similar conflict whose constant concern was correctness of ritual and loyalty to his denomination. These men by substituting a minor for a major virtue attempted to evade their sense of personal failure. Very commonly such attempts at compromise take the form of intense loyalty to some institution or cause or hobby. The individual attempts through his devotion to these things to find his purpose in life. This reaction mode of compromise through the substitution of a minor for a major virtue or loyalty is to be found in ritualism, legalism, pedantry, sectarianism, superpatriotism, etc., at least when these are characterized by the attitude of intolerance. A man may be very punctilious about the tithing of mint and anise and cummin precisely because he is deficient in the weightier matters of the law.

Under compromise we may also include that pacing of undue stress upon merely negative virtues which we see in *prudishness* or *asceticism*.

A very different form of compromise is to be found in *pathological stealing* such as is described in Case 5 of the Judge Baker Foundation Case Studies. Here the solution for a severe sex conflict was found in the substitution of what was in the boy's eyes a lesser offense associated with the sex interest.

The method of *bluffing* is to be found in many of our cases. The self-educated negro minister of a tiny church with his clerical coat, silk hat and pompous language interlarded with quotations from the Greek who was "to busy" to talk to the investigator is a good example. He was trying to compensate for a sense of inferiority which was both personal and racial. In cases of mental disorder this method of bluffing is the basis of many ideas of grandeur. It is commonly associated with the method of *shifting responsibility* or of "passing the buck" for one's own failures upon other persons or objects. In the psychotic cases this method of shifting responsibility is to be found in fifteen cases in the form of *delusions of persecution*. Among normal people this is a very common reaction mode as anyone can testify who has made a low mark on some examination or failed in some important test and has then found himself blaming the instructor or the chief. The end result of this method of dealing with this problem of personal failure when combined with the method of pulling the wool over one's own eyes is of course to be found in the various *paranoid* types, who *maintain some degree of self-respect by means of their systematized ideas of grandeur and of persecution*. Of our cases nine are of this type. Four of these are quite religious and their religion undoubtedly serves to keep them from going to pieces even though that religion is very eccentric.

The method of *shifting responsibility upon an organic scapegoat* is found in two of our cases. Of these the young man who took refuge from a sense of guilt due to auto-erotic indulgence by developing heart trouble and visiting physician after physician in the effort to find one who would support his alibi is the best example. This method represents an attempt to *escape responsibility* which is characteristic of *psycho-neuroses* of the *hysterical* and *neurasthenic* types and also of some of the war-neuroses.[8] The attitude is that of anxiety and self-pity. Its beginnings are to be found in the child who gets out of going to school by developing a headache or who escapes an unpleasant situation by fainting as was the case with one of our patients. Such methods are also very frequently bids for sympathy and attention.

The method of *emotional explosion* is of course genetically one of the earliest. It is represented by the bursts of anger and of weeping in the baby and the tantrums of the young child. Many persons never outgrow it. Two of our psychopathic cases are characterized by chronic irritability, while three, at least in their disturbed condition, show an attitude of tearfulness and self-pity.

Withdrawal is another early reaction mode. The child who fails in one thing may stop trying and turn to something else. If he keeps on failing he becomes listless and is regarded as lazy. Failure in one line of endeavor may of course lead to diversion into other and more profitable channels, but it is apt to take the form of sulking, brooding,

---

8 According to Georges Dumas (Troubles Mentaux et Nerveux de la Guerre p. 184) certain forms of shell-shock are to be explained in terms of confusion and suggestion and considerations of personal security and obscure desires have little to do with them.

day-dreaming and the loss of hope and ambition. The day-dreaming going to the point where the dream world becomes the real world, is apt to result in the development of bizarre wish-formations, and the sulking easily results in ideas of persecution.

When the failure is vocational and social, when there is no marked inner disharmony, we may find an attitude of resignation, of passive, perhaps stoical acceptance of the situation. One of our cases adjudged not psychotic is clearly of this type. Three others characterized by loss of hope and ambition are classed as schizophrenia of the simple type. These individuals are rated fairly well according to the intelligence test and were "good as gold" and religiously inclined, but without any purpose in life and becoming increasingly listless, inefficient, dependent and disorganized.

Where the erotic tendencies get the upper hand and the unfortunate loses not only hope but self-respect we have progressive deterioration and disintegration, silliness, apathy, and regression to an irresponsible and dependent stage. Such cases are generally labeled *hebephrenic*. Our hospitals are full of them. They offer little interest from the point of view of the psychology of religion except as examples of what takes place when the individual surrenders completely.

THE TRANSITION STAGE

Gradual Development.—We have already considered certain typical reaction modes to the experience of personal failure as judged by the personal standards and we have followed these through to their logical end-results. These end-results may be reached by *steady and often imperceptible changes in the controlling desires, interests and attitudes.* There may be a character change that is insidious and gradual until the point is reached where the individual becomes so queer or so dangerous or in some other way so socially impossible that he has to be segregated in an institution. When the onset is thus insidious and gradual, without upheaval and without determined effort at reconstruction, the prognosis is generally poor. Of the cases under consideration, seven show this type of onset. One of these has however since his commitment become greatly agitated and depressed with an attitude that is self-accusatory and ideas of death and world catastrophe. Of the seven cases the latter is the only one that has shown signs of recovery.

The Acute Condition.—Seven of our cases of mental disorder show a distinctly sudden onset, in some it comes as a veritable bolt from the blue. The patient may even have seemed strong and well and happy, when he becomes preoccupied and worried and all of a sudden greatly disturbed. It is such cases which furnish the "raving maniac" of the popular imagination. But the hospital experience shows that the chances of recovery are good, provided there is freedom from hatred and from erotic indulgence. In fact the more sudden the onset and the more disturbed the patient becomes, the better apparently are the chances of recovery, if only he can be protected from self-injury and from toxic infections such as pneumonia and mastoiditis to which two of our patients succumbed. Of these seven cases two died,

four made good recoveries and one developed a paranoid delusional system which has become firmly fixed.

The suggestion is here offered that the favorable outcome in this group of cases is due to the fact that there is here a sudden awareness of danger and an arousal of the entire personality to meet the situation. The cause of the inner distress or disharmony is brought from the realm of evasion and concealment into the open and there follows an attempt at reorganization. And this takes place before malignant personality changes haves reached an advanced stage. Apparently the profoundness of the disturbance and the depth of the regression do not determine the outcome. In all of these cases there was dissociation sufficiently marked to justify a diagnosis of schizophrenia and six were actually so classified at staff conferences. In one of these the regression was complete, the patient at the beginning of the disordered period talking about "being reborn" and apparently regarding himself as going through the various stages of development from the single cell up. And in this case the recovery has been excellent and has moreover been marked by favorable personality changes.

These conclusions are supported by those of Dr. Sullivan, which are worth summarizing here: Dr. Sullivan, taking account of a series of case studies extending over seven years, finds a group of cases diagnosed at staff conferences as "dementia praecox" which not only recovered but showed favorable personality changes. Individuals who before the psychosis had been emotionally unstable, excessively sensitive and extremely self-conscious, emerged from the psychosis relatively open and frank and with previous defects either mitigated or overcome. The rough clinical label on this group would be catatonic dementia praecox. They were all individuals who did not have recourse to a comprehensive projection of their own problems upon their colleagues, as in the paranoid group; who did not show the multiple form of splitting characteristic of one type of the hebephrenic group; who in sharp distinction from the pure hebephrenic did not effect adjustments through the loss of the ego-strivings and perverse pleasure taking. Because his problems are not solved in these socially destructive fashions, the severe conflict remains unabated and the schizophrenic dissociation becomes greater in the catatonic group than elsewhere. The regressive processes go deeper and it is in this type that we find the clearest demonstration of the intrauterine mind. Such states and early schizophrenia generally are to be viewed as attempts by regression to genetically older thought processes to reintegrate masses of life experience which had failed of structuralization into a functional unity. They are to be regarded as a series of major mental events, always attended by material changes in the personality, but in themselves implying nothing of deterioration or of dementia. The disorder is one in which the total experience of the individual is reorganized and a great eruption of the primitive thought processes takes place. The presence of illogical or bizarre persecutory delusions may be merely incidental to the psychical reorganization and indicate an unfavorable prognosis only when such beliefs become consistent logically.

According to the view here taken this group of cases would differ from the manic-depressive manic group chiefly in the type of personality which is involved. The one represents the acute excitement of the aggressive, confident, extraverted type which is alive to external stimuli and does not hesitate to think out loud. The other is the acute excitement of the shy, seclusive, introverted type whose behavior is determined chiefly by internal stimuli. There may also be a difference in depth of regression and profoundness of disturbance. Each type may be recurrent or periodic and each successive disturbance may be none the less an attempt at reorganization with each time a real though decreasing possibility of favorable outcome.

The question may be raised whether the disturbed or acute conditions, even though they may not have an abrupt onset, do not represent attempts at reorganization. Just as inflammation in the body represents the attempt at repair or elimination, so the emotional disturbance may represent the attempt to throw off the cause of the distress. The unfavorable outcome found in our three other cases of acute excitement would be explained by the fact that the hostile processes had gone so far that they could not be thrown off but took possession of the personality.

The stupor conditions may have a similar function. According to MacCurdy benign stupor is analogous to sleep. Just as a normal person seeks relief in his bed from physical and mental fatigue, so the abnormal person may seek relief from mental anguish in a stupor which shuts him off from the necessity of adaptation and enables the inner processes to work undisturbed. Of greatest significance is the fact that out of 36 cases of definite stupor he finds literal ideas of death in all but one.[9]

Of our cases of religious conversion experience there are ten which show changes of mood from depression and despair to joy and elation which were accepted as evidence of forgiveness. These cases are without clear hallucinatory phenomena. In the other thirteen cases the conflict and despair were more severe and the changes were accompanied by hallucinatory phenomena. Of these, at least four, including John Bunyan, George Fox and Henry Suso, were cases of undeniably valid religious experience which were also at certain stages characterized by equally undeniable mental disorder. It seems clear that here also we are dealing with attempts at reorganization, attempts which are made usually under group influence and positive suggestion, and attempts in which the better part of the personality to which Jung refers in the introductory quotation, actually takes possession.

In the genesis of the acute disorders there is one factor which is commonly overlooked by psychiatrists, *vis.*, the *narrowing of the attention* and its significance. Among students of the psychology of religion it is a well-known fact that mystical states marked by all sorts of automatic processes are induced by the narrowing of the attention. The Hindu holy man may fix his attention upon a bright object or upon a single idea until he passes over into an abnormal condition in which self-consciousness with its distinction

of "I" and "thou" lapses and God is all.[10] This narrowing of the attention is also one of the recognized methods of inducing the hypnotic condition. Another important shamanistic device is that of producing fatigue through dancing and other practices until an abnormal condition is brought on.[11] It is therefore to be observed that in practically all the cases characterized by sudden onset the narrowing of the attention seems to have been an important factor in the genesis of the abnormal condition. The individual becomes pre-occupied. He can think of nothing else but the one particular problem. He loses sleep and the first thing he knows he is across the line in the realm of the unconscious, the "Daemmerzustand" as the Germans call it. "Systemic toxaemia" due to sleeplessness and fatigue may have something to do with it, but it is probably none the less a form of auto-hypnosis characterized by a mood of worry and despair and bewilderment instead of that of confidence and trust found in ordinary hypnosis or in religious trance.

Attention has already been called to the fact that a primary factor in nearly all these cases is an experience which requires the reorganization of the individual's inner world and of his modes of thought and judgment. This experience may have been a bereavement or disappointment which deprives him of all that makes life worth living for him and turns his attention away from the external world to the internal world. The immediate factor however is probably an eruption of the unconscious processes. His attention becomes fixed upon the inner world. Everything is new and strange. Of one thing only he is sure. Things are not what they seem.[12] He looks for hidden meanings in each person or object which comes within his horizon and in each happening. His ideas are grotesque and absurd because he is constantly guessing, constantly changing. The paranoic condition with its poor prognosis sets in when he succeeds in working out some system which satisfies the requirements of logical consistency. When this happens he is sure he is right and it is as hard to change him as it is to change the ideas of a college professor who has written a book on philosophy or of a psychiatrist who has worked out a water-tight theory of the psychoses.

Among the ideas which are especially common in such conditions are the ideas of grandeur in which the patient identifies himself with God or with Christ or with some other important personage. These ideas are commonly interpreted as "wish-formations" or attempts at "compensation." It is perhaps not far-fetched to suggest that the acute psychosis is indeed in many cases almost literally the experience of death and that there occurs here an attempted shift of the individual consciousness to the higher entity with which in interests and aspirations it is most closely identified. It would be similar to the common experience in which a man feels himself no longer an individual but identifies himself with his college, his church or his country and it may be precisely the experience of the religious mystic. The idea of grandeur may then be associated with the re-

9 Psychology of Emotion, p. 115.
10 Coe, Psychology of Religion, p. 176 and 267.
11 Coe, Psychology of Religion, p. 176.
12 MacCurdy's description of the "perplexity state" describes admirably this condition. The view here taken is that this condition is to be found at the beginning of any acutely disturbed condition and that it is most marked in those cases in which there are no firmly fixed vicious reaction modes.

birth or renewal of life which is a cardinal doctrine with certain great religious teachers and the patient who thinks he is Christ may indeed in some partial fashion have shared the experience of the great religious genius who said "I have been crucified with Christ and it is no longer I that live but Christ liveth in me."

The occurrence of religious ideas seems to depend only in part upon the individual's previous interests and pursuits. Ten of our patients before their disturbance had not taken any very active interest in religion but with the disturbance religious ideas become prominent. This does not mean that religion caused the disturbance. It means only that they were making a somewhat belated attempt to organize their inner world from the standpoint of those things which they felt to be abiding and universal. It means that the better self is seeking to express itself or to make its stand against the forces of destruction.

A favorable outcome for such an attempt at reorganization, as judged on the basis of the present data, is most likely to occur under the following conditions:

1. When the attempt is made with group influence dominating. Positive suggestions then control and the eccentricities which appear tend to be those of the group. The greatest amount of deviation is found among the religious cases in those whose experience was solitary.

2. When the attempt is made on the individual's own initiative and volition before disaster comes crashing around his head and before hostile processes get possession of the field.

3. When the sufferer is able to open up and seek help from those who are competent to give it.

4. When the situation admits of satisfactory adjustment. The case is hopeless if the unfortunate hasn't it in him to be something of a success economically or socially or if according to Kempf his "autonomic cravings" are such that he cannot control them or own them.

THE FINAL SOLUTION

In the discussion of the various reaction modes, the end-products were also considered. It is not necessary to go over this ground again. We are concerned here only with the solutions which may be reached as a result of the attempt at reorganization which may follow the awareness of danger.

First of all there may be no particular change. The individual may come out of his disturbed condition and become normal again without solving his problem. He may stick his head into the sand and try to forget about it. He may go back to his former manner of life and to his customary reaction modes. He may continue to compromise or to pull the wool over his own eyes or to pass the buck and seek escape from responsibility. And the primary evil may still remain. Most of the patients discharged from our hospitals are probably of this type, and because the primary evil still remains and the sense of failure is aggravated by the discouragement and humiliation of the hospital experience, there is soon a recurrence and perhaps repeated recurrences. Five of our cases have thus made excellent recoveries, but that does not mean that their problems are necessarily solved.

In the second place the solution may be an unhappy one. The disturbance may result in permanent regression and dissociation. Such a solution is probably to be found in four of our cases of acute psychosis.

In the third place the problem may be to some extent solved and happily solved.

This is more easily effected when the primary difficulty is a social situation which it is possible to correct—an unhappy home situation or vocational maladjustment. The finding of a worth-while job is in many cases the key to the problem. Work well done enables a man to win a place in contemporary society and so to regain his self-respect. Staupitz, at the time Martin Luther was going through such severe conflicts over his sinfulness, sent him to teach at the University of Wittenberg. His new duties and interests and the success he won as a teacher probably contributed as much to the happy solution of his difficulty as the doctrine of justification by faith. Interesting work may at least help one to forget. At best it may serve as a "sublimination" of the sex instinct. It may give meaning to the past failures and synthesize a man's entire experience in some altruistic purpose. This is probably the secret of the success of some rescue mission work. They pick a man up out of the gutter and immediately they set him to work picking up others. He may thus feel that his very failures have become a source of power.

But where the difficulty is primarily the sense of isolation due to the consciousness of inner disharmony and guilt another method is in order.

One of the outstanding contributions of the psycho-analytic school is the discovery of the fact that the uncovering of the cause of the distress and talking it over with the physician is often in itself enough to effect a cure. Striking examples of this are to be found in Healy's "Mental Conflicts in Misconduct" and in his Case 5 of the Judge Baker Foundation Case Studies. In the latter a puzzling case of pathological stealing in a gifted boy of good family and comfortable circumstances was corrected without great difficulty as soon as it was discovered that the stealing was really due to a sex conflict. The Freudian literature describes many such cases. The means involved in such cures is not merely confession and subsequent release of tension. More important still is the influence of the physician. The Freudian doctrine of transference means simply this, that the patient must believe enough in the physician to accept him as a representative of society at its best. In other words he accepts the physician's standards. If then the physician does not condemn him and he learns to look at his problems through the physician's eyes an adjustment of his conflict becomes possible.

Many men solve the conflicts of their 'teens by a somewhat similar process. They talk over their personal problems with some friend or friends and discover perhaps that they are not alone in their difficulties. They thus put an end to the isolation which their sense of guilt has produced in them. And they accept the standards of their chums instead of those of their parents or of the Church. Kempf's Case AN 3 is an excellent illustration. A young man of fine ability and high standards solves a severe conflict over auto-erotic indulgence by opening up to his room-mate and accepting his room-mate's solution. He visits a house of prostitution. He thus socializes his difficulty. He is able to keep himself occupied with his scientific work and to find great satisfaction in the recognition which he wins in this field. The method of keeping one's self occupied with work or pleasure and of laughing and joking about those things of which there is a tendency to be ashamed solves or avoids many a conflict. The joke serves to let the cat out of the bag[13] and to relieve the individual of the sense of hypocrisy and isolation. But it may also represent a lowering of the standards. It then becomes *flippancy*. Still another method is that of *cynicism*. Here the individual retains his own self-respect by a depreciation of others. He escapes self-reproach by convincing himself that he is as good as anybody. The *criminal gang* is in many instances an attempt to socialize inferiority. An inferior person may escape a severe conflict by taking refuge in a group of easy standards where he can give himself frankly to tendencies which society as a whole could not countenance and the members of the inferior group may support each other in flippant, cynical, a-social attitudes.

Such methods may be regarded as happy solutions in so far as they work. The man who excused himself for his autoerotic tendencies by blaming them upon persecutors who were throwing electricity upon him and who at the same time maintained his self-respect through the belief that he had a mission to "bring light," is in a far better state than the man who has lost hope and self-respect altogether. The man who is able to help in carrying on the work of the world, even though it be at the expense of lowering his standards, is probably better off than he would be if the inner conflict had landed him as a permanent inmate in a hospital for the insane. But these are not the best solutions and they do not always work. The young scientist in Kempf's case gets along beautifully for awhile. But he finally meets the girl who reminds him of his mother, who stands for all that is best and holiest in his life. Then he runs away and later he goes to pieces. Kempf says the difficulty here was a "mother fixation." The real difficulty is probably that this man has been false to the standards by which he judges himself, the standards which in his case were determined for him by the mother whom he adored.

The only cases in this study which present solutions that seem to be happy and permanent are found among the religious group. John Bunyan in early manhood went through four years of very severe mental disturbance, which if he were living today would probably have landed him in an institution for the insane. But he emerges from that experience with his personality unified and he later spends twelve trying years in Bedford Jail showing throughout the greatest fortitude and all through his later life he shows himself even-tempered and self-possessed, capable of hard work and with great influence over men as leader, adviser and teacher. George Fox's disturbance was probably even more marked than John Bunyan's, but he also in his later years shows extraordinary powers of endurance in the face of fearful persecution and hardship and we are told that even the great and mighty would quail before his piercing eye. In such men we see solutions which result in the progressive unification and socialization of the personality, which are characterized by the attitude of reverence and trust and altruism, and which are produced and maintained in association with the group which has in it the elements of universality and permanence with is expressed by the word God and through confession and forgiveness without any lowering of the standards. We see such solutions no less truly in some of the humbler personalities included in this study.

It is perhaps clear now why it is that we find so many pathological manifestations in the experience of certain great religious geniuses as well as in the experience of persons who are religious without being geniuses. It may also be clear why it is that we find so many religious formulations in conditions of mental disorder. We are in all such experiences dealing with a common problem, that of personal failure and personal salvation. All religions are vitally concerned with that problem. The voices, the visions and other automatic phenomena may be merely incidental to the process of reorganization. And the experience may be none the less valid as a religious experience, even though the disturbance be so profound as to justify the diagnostic term of schizophrenia, provided only the result attained be characterized by those attributes and values which are termed religious.

---

13 Freud, Der Witz.

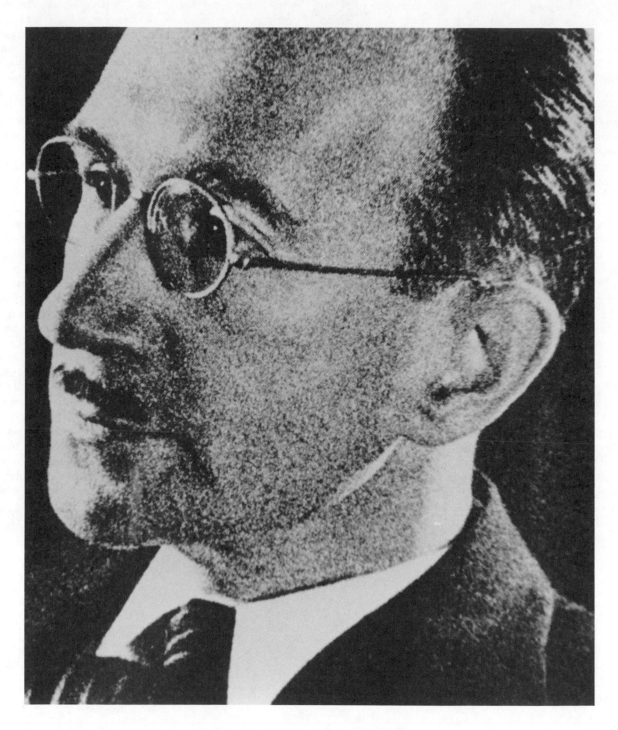

Harry Stack Sullivan, M.D., 1892–1949

The Onset of Schizophrenia

By Harry Stack Sullivan, M.D.

Psychiatrist, The Sheppard and Enoch Pratt Hospital, Baltimore, Maryland

Study of onset of disorder in male patients of this hospital seems to establish two factors preliminary to schizophrenic psychoses. Firstly, the appearance of the disorder is late in a long series of subjectively difficult efforts. Secondly, it seems never to occur in those who have achieved if only for a short time a definitely satisfying adjustment to a sex object. We have not been successful in our effort to identify exactly the factors which cause milder maladjustive efforts to pass over into schizophrenia. Neither do we believe we are justified by accumulated facts, to stress the sex factor as of exclusive importance. Much more data is needed to regard to the onset of the malady; at this stage, however, there seems little reason to doubt that cultural distortions provided by the home are of prime importance. We have not seen maladjustment which was without a foundation of erroneous attitudes which parents or their equivalent had thrust upon the child. We have found all sorts of maladjustments in the history of patients who suffered the grave psychosis, but regardless of vicious influences subsequently encountered, the sufferer had acquired the tendency to such an illness while in the home situation. Interpersonal factors seem to be the effective elements in the psychiatry of schizophrenia.

Objective manifestations of maladjustment are now divided among the three classes of psychoneurotic, psychopathic, and psychotic. The static implications of current teaching is unfortunate. The medical man in general envisages schizophrenia as a strange entity which befalls the predisposed. Teaching should emphasize the dynamic view of these situations.

The great number of our patients have shown for years before the break, clear signs of coming trouble. A number of them were brought to notice by the outcropping of behavior of a simple psychoneurotic sort. Unwitting attempts at hysterical incapacitations not only precede many psychoses, but actually make up much of the psychotic picture in some cases. Reactions by obsessive substitutions are seen in a small number to have preceded for years frank schizophrenic phenomena. Here, too, the maladjustive "psychoneurotic mechanism" is continued in the psychosis, and we may find with the autochthonous thoughts of schizophrenia, a mingling of doubts and scruples of a simple psychoneurotic nature. The gradations from neurasthenic picture into schizophrenia would be easy to observe, did we but attend more clearly to the mental state of quasi-normal adolescents. Anxiety conditions which deepen into schizophrenic panic occur in numbers.

The psychiatrist sees too many end states and deals professionally with too few of the pre-psychotic. To him, "ideas of reference" are apt to imply psychosis; to one who has comprehensive data on psychoneurotics, psychopathics, and eccentric "normals," such delusional content is recognized as wide spread and simply one of the signs of inefficient adjustment to the demands of life. The institutional physician, for that matter, cannot but realize that those who require supervision are but that portion of the psychotic who are so in the grip of their eccentricities as to be rendered conspicuous. He knows that many who leave as "social recoveries" have achieved nothing more remarkable than the ability to conform outwardly to certain standards—that they carry quite as extraordinary delusions as those of some others who cannot conform. With this in mind, it would seem as if we should lay great stress on the prompt investigation of failing adjustment, rather than, as is so often the case, wait and see what happens.

Most schizophrenics have shown evidences enough to excite even lay curiosity during more or less extended periods before mental disease was diagnosed. Not family physicians alone, but specialists in rhinology, laryngology, gastro-intestinal maladies, in urology and in gynecology, all these see the incipient schizophrenic and all too often "let things ride." I feel certain that many incipient cases might be arrested before the efficient contact with reality is completely suspended, and a long stay in institutions made necessary.

If there is anything at all in our present views of mind and its disorder, watchful expectancy is not the method of choice in the difficulties of youth, and the provision of useful experience is the only hope for insuring such patients against trouble.[1] If there is any good reason for a policy of

A part result of the study of schizophrenic motivation in progress in the clinical research service of the Sheppard and Enoch Pratt Hospital, Baltimore. Read in abstract before the joint meeting of The American Psychiatric Association and the American Psychopathological Association, New York, June 11, 1926.

[1] Experience as here used refers to anything lived, undergone or the like: to that which occurs *in* the organism, rather than directly to events in which the organism is involved. Experience is mental; *i.e.*, it is reflected to a greater or lesser extent in behavior and thinking. At the same time, experience often occurs without conscious awareness.

delay, it must reside in our lack of certainty as to what is to be done. In attempting to indicate promising lines, I shall review some of our notions of psycho-dynamics.

Ignoring that section of the population in the case of which serious physical factors exist,[2] we can distinguish three sorts of maladjustive processes which do not lead immediately to arrest of the individual's struggle.[3] They include *sublimatory resymbolizations* and *compensatory motivations*, neither of which interests us particularly here excepting in so far as they may antecede those processes more intimately related to schizophrenia. The *defense reactions*, infinitely diverse in their combinations, individual goals and explanatory rationalization, these are the maladjustive processes which can be seen to form a gradient from mere poses and trifling evasions of the obvious to the essential schizophrenia. They all show the characteristics that they are unwitting evasions and distortions of simple experience; means by which the organism interposes something artificial and relatively abstract in the complex of the individual and his environment, physical and cultural. From an objective viewpoint, the interposition seems "intended" to protect the creature from discomforts either internally conditioned as in conflict of deeper desires and ideals, or externally conditioned as in disconformity of supposed potentialities and environmental demands. Whether the individual struggles unwittingly to be other than he is, by poses and exaggerated reactions even amounting to psychotic excitements on the one hand, or substitute activities, rituals, etc; or seeks peace by transference of guilt and blame from himself to others or to social institutions; or, again, effects a modification of the stress by partial or total incapacitation as in the hysterical disabilities of the invalid reactions;[4] in all these cases we find the irrational, "unconscious" protection of the self a central theme. The *barrier* subvariety of defense reactions, more particularly, are of a piece with schizophrenia. Here we find a structure, so to speak, thrust between the creature's accepted self and everything else. Whether he has unwittingly adopted 1) an attitude of repulsion to those around him, or 2) a "physical" concealment by secretiveness or even seclusive behavior, or finally, 3) erected a complex relation which subtends all contact with personal and extrinsic reality (schizophrenia); all these processes reflect an increase in the complexity of life and a necessarily destructive influence upon personal efficiency.

It may be taken for granted that a clear appraisal of the factors entering into any difficult situation should precede efforts at its resolution. In our potential patients there is to be found a significant grouping of irrational factors. We find that the youth has developed many misapprehensions as to his real potentialities of achievement. He has come to exaggerate, misunderstand and conceal various requirements for his satisfaction; to believe that he needs certain end-situations which are superfluous; that he can dispense with certain others which are a part of the common biological heritage. Finally, we find him unwittingly elaborating a fabric of personal ideals which have but a complex order of relationship to possibility, and of notions concerning the estimation which others make of him that are simply fantastic. All these factors interlock in astonishing combinations, and his energy is dissipated in pseudo-problems and defensive processes. Feeling that an admission of his unhappiness—even to himself—is an indication of inadequacy or peculiarity, such an individual appreciates but vaguely that he is thwarted by an agency over which he has no control. That any increase in his correct insight would be helpful to him goes without saying.

Obvious though it should be, one must stress the factor of persons in all adolescent difficulties. The family physician seems often to accept the "physical" causation to which most patients refer their illness. Overwork, for example, enjoys great popularity as an excuse for mental disorder. Long hours, unsatisfactory working facilities, strain, even undernourishment—these masquerade as important much more frequently than not. The uncolored data from analytic investigation of patients quickly disabuses one of this "common sense" notion. Mental stress arises from societal relations, not from impersonal physical factors.[5] The question always to be answered is why the individual has proceeded into the state of physical depletion; what underlying societal factor has driven him to overwork, to deprivation of sleep, etc. When thus regarded, we find generally that the alleged causal factor is but a preliminary compensatory, sublimatory or defensive maneuver, to be regarded as the prodromal maladjustment which facilitated the more dramatic failure.

Of all the preliminary maneuvers by which youths seek unconsciously to safeguard themselves against the stress of conflict involving their societal relations, the use of alcoholic intoxication is probably the most impressive. This is to be regarded as a sub-variety of the defense reactions; it is seldom that one finds a case in which other defense processes are not also in evidence. Among alcoholic youths, one finds a continuous gradation of simple "comfortable" disso-

---

2 Roughly divisible among (1) the defective, whose equipment has low potential educability, so that he cannot undergo many varieties of experience, and so does not profit from many events; (2) the physically handicapped, *e.g.*, the hunchback; and (3) that group typified by the epileptics, in the case of which there appears to be a strong tendency to bizarre destructive reactions wholly injurious to the individual. Needless to say, "psychogenic" factors are important in every individual case in this group, as they are apt to be in the other two.

3 In contradistinction to (a) depression and (b) the anxiety processes, both of which are not only maladjustive but also methods which present no real attack upon the troublesome situation; as such, they may be regarded as a means of "standing still" before a problem.

4 Invalid reactions, in particular, may partake much of the nature of compensatory efforts. In these cases, all of which probably start as defense reactions, the acquisition of sympathy becomes a goal in itself, the kindly feelings of others making up for disappointments in more practical striving.

5 Fatigue as a phenomenon of the total organism has thus far escaped scientific measurement and study. That it includes an important psychic element cannot be gainsaid. Rest and recreation also belong largely in the category of mind, and physical quiescence—in so far as it can in fact be achieved under such circumstances—is unavailing in the presence of ineffective mental activity. *Vide*, in this connection, "Revery and Industrial Fatigue," Elton Mayo, Journal of Personnel Research, III, 1924, pp. 273–281.

Nothing herein is to be construed as denying to ill-health, toxaemia, loss of sleep, malnutrition, etc., an important place in the sequence culminating in many mental disorders. The point to be stressed is their entirely subordinate rôle. The data of our study do not minimize the importance of the *efficiency of the somatic apparatus* in the life situation. There may well be times when a cup of coffee would delay the outcropping of a mental disorder. We have onseted incipient depression and neurasthenic states follow unwitting denial of the accustomed caffeine dosage.

ciation bolstered by much drinking, to states of extreme discomfort with phobias, anxiety attacks, and hallucinatory phenomena.

It is never easy to say just when the schizophrenic patient has crossed the line into actual psychosis. In several cases we have found that there had occurred a brief phase of marked psychotic condition some considerable time before the final break. A patient, for example, when 17 underwent an operation firmly convinced that he would not survive the anaesthetic. He awoke minus his normal "grasp on reality." Things seemed for days to be quite entirely unreal— he "lived in a dream" in which all sorts of trifling and wholly unrelated occurrences seemed fraught with great personal import, to bear in some signal but incomprehensible way upon him: the operation had been the occasion for some strange mutilation: he was changed in some curious fashion. Then, one morning, all this was past; he "awoke his old self." He went on to the age of 25 years before the stress of heterosexual adaptation pushed him over into an exceptionally paranoid incipient schizophrenia. Another, receiving cocaine anaesthesia for a nasal operation, at 22, developed an extraordinary excitement like that seen in catatonia. This passed in some 30 hours, and nothing bizarre was shown for the next three months. As the date of his marriage approached, he passed swiftly into severe catatonic schizophrenia. Yet another, having accidentally discharged a gun in the direction of a beloved uncle, developed blocking and phenomena of stupor which lasted a few days. Eight months afterward, in circumstances when both his heterosexual efforts and his strivings for prestige among his fellows were baffled, he underwent a catatonic dissociation. In these few from a number of such cases, we observe fairly well demarcated psychoses following a major event.

Each one of this group of patients had come to a psychopathic type of adjustment quite early in life.[6] By this is meant a group of peculiarities in behavior and thinking which seem to be manifestations of, firstly, an unconsciously determined inability to profit from certain particular events. Unlike the defective, the psychopathic has no fundamental defect of educability; he has experience of unrestricted variety, but certain of it fails of elaboration and synthesis into a practical whole. This we mean when we refer to his "inability to profit by experience"—the impor-

tant point being that the experience from which he shows no practical learning lies in one or more circumscribed fields. These "resistant" areas are found to be the results of well known dynamics identical with those which we have identified in the psychoses and psychoneuroses. Secondly, psychopathic manifestations include characteristically a more or less distinct awareness of personal defect or abnormality, and this is accompanied by an exaggerated tendency to rationalize. Finally, there is a striking inability to advance considerations of the future into control over more immediate satisfactions. We know that the last mentioned characteristic applies to the immature, and, perhaps for this reason, we sometimes regard the psychopathic as instances of a selective arrest in mental development. Such a notion is permissible if it is understood as a general explanatory conception throughout psychopathology, rather than a specific conception of psychopathic states. By this, I refer to the identity of developmental sequences in this and all other groups. "Selective Arrest" then refers to distortion of customary development rather than to any stoppage in the accumulation and organization of experience. We have yet to determine what becomes of experiential material which is thus distorted; that problem is no less acute, however, than are many that we gloss over in our discussions of psychoneurosis.[7]

Psychopathic maladjustment is a product of the pre-adolescent phase of personality development. The adolescent upheaval in these individuals includes destructive phenomena of distinctive character. Schizophrenia is much more likely as an outcome than in those who have more coherently integrated the experience of infancy, childhood and the juvenile period. It is interesting, however, that the longer psychotic collapse is escaped, the less the chance of a grave disorder, and the less typical any illness which ensues. In other words a psychosis occurring in a psychopathic youth under, say, the age of 22, is in all likelihood frankly schizophrenic; but an initial psychosis occurring at, say, 30 will probably be a brief excitement—even if decidedly schizophrenic in type. This suggests that the psychopathic sort of maladjustment grows more effective as experience is accumulated, notwithstanding the fact that its interference with social efficiency may continue unchanged, or even increase.[8]

---

6 In "Regression, A Consideration of Reversive Mental Processes" (*State Hospital Quarterly*, XI, Nos. 1,2 and 3), we refer to this subject of the Psychopathic Personality, emphasizing the value of its study for the general theory of mental disorder. "Psychopaths" are not regarded as results of hereditary factors. It is true that germinal influences may prepare the soil for individual mental evolutions, for the maturation and growth by experience of the individual mind. There is nothing explanatory of the case before one, however, in this reference to hereditary defect or peculiarity. He is no product of pre-existing harmony or disharmony, but a product of growth, like anyone else. The analytic investigation of such individuals is most profitable research, even though its prosecution for therapeutic purposes may be discouraging.

It is regrettable that clinicians have not taken care to separate the group which they please to call "Psychopaths" into (a) those who show psychopathic type of maladjustment evolving from a basis of mental deficiency, and (b) the true psychopathic personalities, relatively stable maladjustments without mental deficiency in its accepted meaning. The former are problems of preventive medicine. The latter are an important field for study, and one almost entirely neglected.

7 To their credit be it said that the psychoanalysts are attacking the problem in their study of "Neurotic Dispositions." The outcome of investigations in this field has been somewhat concealed by the uniformity of "causal" factors that they uncover in all mental disorder. Analytically isolated factors have preoccupied them. We need to consider maladjustive syntheses as they occur in society, now that we have a grasp on abstract "mechanisms."

8 Brief excitements with schizophrenic "coloring"—which are sometimes indistinguishable from the gravest psychoses—are a profitable field for investigation. The fact of their occurring fairly late in the course of a relatively stable maladjustment, and their disappearance with as residuals an exaggeration of the pre-existing peculiarities, connects importantly with certain types of post-psychotic personality. We see after some cases of frank schizophrenia, "Social recoveries" amounting in fact to severe psychopathic states; *e.g.*, the paranoid personalities which arise from catatonic schizophrenics, in the case of many "spontaneous" recoveries. These post-psychotic states sometimes arise *de novo*—they are not foreshadowed materially in the pre-psychotic personality. In the one case, a decidedly peculiar person undergoes a brief schizophrenic dissociation and comes from the process with accentuated warp. In another, an imperfectly adjusted person (lacking marked psychopathic traits) undergoes a severe schizophrenia and achieves from it a relatively stable maladjustment. Something of the implication of this was outlined in "Schizophrenia, Its Conservative and Malignant Features" (*American Journal of Psychiatry*, IV, 1924, pp. 71–79). See for an interesting consideration not unharmonious with our views, Boisen "Personality Changes

Search for the phenomena actually constituting the onset of schizophrenia has brought several interesting facts to light. As already indicated in the case of delusions of reference, a great deal of the early phenomenology is an accentuation of what can be elicited from almost any mild case of mental disorder. A clear to vague content indicative of an unfriendly interest in him is general in psychopathological states. A great proportion of all maladjusted individuals believe that they suffer invidious discussion. The "neurotic tendency" to detract in a relatively unwitting effort to reduce others to a lower level than that adjudged to self, is evidenced not only in more direct behavior and thinking, but indirectly by projection as these persecutory trends. With any excuse, this progresses into notions that one is being slighted, annoyed, or definitely wronged. Were all those who entertained mild delusions of this sort to be assembled in institutions, the state would collapse immediately from depopulation. Phantastic meanings attached to the behavior of others, to one's own action, and even to events among inanimate objects—there too are non-specific. A remarkable number of those who are not regarded as psychotic entertain beliefs closely akin to delusions of mind-reading and of more or less mysterious control by another. Hypochondriacal notions form the rationalizations for innumerable maladjustive processes. Somewhat grandiose self-appraisals, on the one hand, and depressive depreciations and self-criticism, on the other, are easily uncovered in a great many patients. "Peculiar Thoughts" and even pseudo-spontaneity are not very uncommon: obsessions and preoccupations typify one large group of maladjusted.

In a study centering upon cognitive features,[9] I have demonstrated several points bearing particularly upon the evolution of schizophrenic panic, and somewhat upon the insidious forms. We have come to regard all initial manifestations of these illnesses as strikingly uniform. From the standpoint of content, there appear those processes and symbol elaborations customary in dreaming. Instead of turning "day-remnants" to the purpose, the schizophrenic cognitive operations deal with perceptions of reality, personal and impersonal. All these—like the figures of the dream—are distorted into use for representing the personal situation and for efforts at solving it. It is at this stage that the patient believes he is watched and followed; the observers personifying in some cases the ideals which cannot control his desires of lower cultural value by ordinary activity. In others, they are personifications of the "evil" desires which pursue him to assault or "rob" and degrade him. In the first situation, exteriorization takes the form of the "voice of God" and in the second, the hallucination of threats or foul epitaphs. This sort of content connects with a more or less terrible affective situation of a primitive sort—an "insane mood" which has pre-existed the clearcut cognitive phenomena. The motivation at work is in a general way conflicting groups of elaborated (and more or less successfully repressed) personal tendencies opposed by tendencies of the nature of ideals (cultural controls). The disturbance in reality-appraisal which has been slow in the predromal stages, is now very swift, progressing to a state in which everything is involved in the cognitive efforts. This stage in which nothing is without an incomprehensible meaning, and the ordinary exchange of intelligence is palsied, may continue in relatively simple elaboration. This is the catatonic type of schizophrenia. In it, the conflicts remain unresolved and the struggle expands into cosmic dramas and the psychic processes revert through the ontogenic repertory, perhaps down to the most primitive. At any time, however, this situation may pass into one of a few typical attempts at readjustment. There may be a massive resynthesis amounting to recovery with profit. There may be a fragile reorganization prone to relapse under fresh difficulties. Of grave portent, however, is the readjustment by paranoid processes. If it succeeds, we have a persistent paranoid state with more or less of schizophrenic residue (paraphrenias of Kraepelin). If it fails, we have an unhappy jumble of schizophrenic projections, any hopeful aspect of which is lost through the destructive hateful attitude of the patient ("paranoid precox," and many now classed as hebephrenic).

Finally, there is the practically irremediable hebephrenic type in which destruction of the conflict is achieved by disintegration of the acquired socially adopted tendencies, and along with this a dilapidation of the evolved structures influencing manifestations of simple native tendencies. The motivation of such patients then becomes juvenile, childish, or even infantile.

That which we have called the prodromal period of schizophrenia often includes characteristic features which should receive special attention. One sees many who were "depressed" for a long time before the outbreak of frank psychosis. The behavior and utterances of these individuals reflects much unhappiness, but is to be distinguished from the psychosis of depression. They do not slow up physically and mentally nor suffer preoccupation with a certain few grief-provoking notions to the exclusion of more practical thinking. Expressed loosely, they feel not that all is lost as a consequence of personal sins and errors, but that all is wrong for some more or less inscrutable reason, which may or may not pertain closely to some weakness or inadequacy or peculiarity of the individual—often alleged results of masturbation. The situation is always a maladjustment to assumed personal inadequacy, but this may elude the patient's awareness entirely. While the pure depression is preoccupied with thoughts of the enormity of the disaster, of punishment, hopelessness, and the like, the incipient schizophrenic is not the host of any simple content, but is burdened with pressing distresses and becomes more and more wrapped up in phantastic explanation and efforts at remedy. The distinction is one fundamentally dynamic: pure depression is practically a standstill of adjustment, the schizophrenic depression is a most unhappy struggle. Instead of literal or figurative sitting still, these people are striving to cut themselves off from painful stimuli, escape

---

and Upheavals Arising out of the Sense of Personal Failure" (*American Journal of Psychiatry*, V, 1926, pp. 531–552) [reprinted in this sesquicentennial anniversary supplement of the *Journal*].
9 "Peculiarity of Thought in Schizophrenia" (*American Journal of Psychiatry*, V, 1925, pp. 21–86. See in this particular pp. 56–63 and "Discussion," p.79, et seq.

the situation by mystic and more or less extraordinary efforts, and justify themselves by heroic measures. While the pure depression may end in suicide of a practical sort, the schizophrenic depression leads to fantastic methods of self-destruction often preceded by fear of being killed.

Perplexity also is an important phenomena of the incipient state. In this condition, extraconscious material influences perceptions of reality to such end that the patient becomes more and more entangled in contradictions, alternative notions, and illusions. Autochthonous thoughts appear and interfere unpleasantly with rational efforts. Insignificant characteristics of events persistently hold the attention and give rise to disturbing analogies.

Fear-states covering the gamut from phobia through terror, and from anxious feelings through apprehension, to the full-developed primitive panic,[10] are factors important in many incipient conditions. Whether or not rage—fighting fear—will make up part of the late picture depends in part on the character of the individual's former experience, in part on the particular explanatory delusions which he is entertaining.

All three of these phenomenon-groups combine in the evolution of most schizophrenic psychoses. [Case reports appended to the original article are not reprinted here because of space limitations. These can be found on pages 116–135 of the July 1927 issue of the *Journal*, vol. 84, no. 1.]

---

10 Affective experience related to fear can be divided into two major categories. Genetically it is evolved from the primordial experience including preliminaries to birth—the death-evil preconcept, as we have called it. See "Schizophrenia, Its Conservative and Malignant Features," *loc cit.*, and "The Oral Complex" (*Psychoanalytic Review*, XII, 1925, pp. 31–38). The differentiation proceeds along two lines, the basis lies in the external and internal character of reference. The former is through terror to fear. The latter is through apprehension to anxious states.

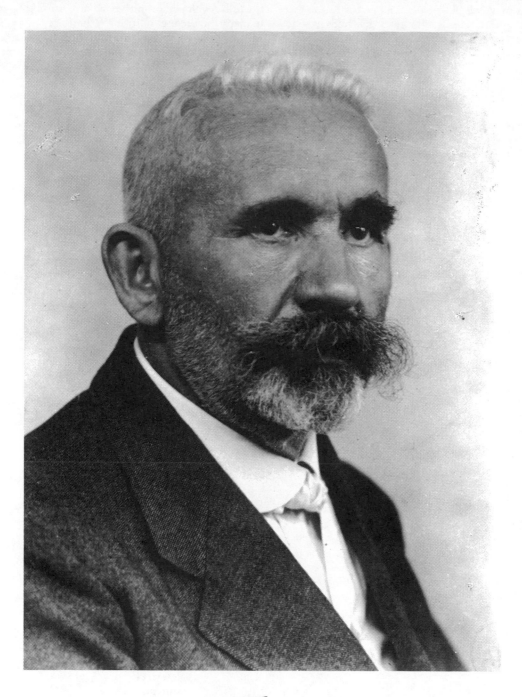

Dr. Emil Kraepelin, 1856–1926

In Memoriam: Emil Kraepelin

By Adolf Meyer, M.D.

Professor of Psychiatry, The Johns Hopkins University School of Medicine, Baltimore, Maryland

With Kraepelin psychiatry has lost its most widely known figure. During the last 25 years, no worker in psychiatry could have remained without at least a terminological impress from Kraepelin. Through him, diagnosis in psychiatry had become more than description. It committed the physician to certain implications, no doubt oversimplified in the minds of many, but definite and important implications of prognosis. Kraepelin himself demanded a definition of entities of definite cause, course and outcome, or at least groups of cases of a certain intrinsic unity, course and outcome. The psychiatric world in its broadest scope knew Kraepelin mainly for his distinction of manic-depressive psychoses and dementia praecox.

To a narrower group of workers in psychiatry Kraepelin meant more than a diagnostician. Indeed, just as diagnostician he was not generally considered to be the safest guide. His paresis diagnoses (before the serological definition of paresis) were too frequent; his zeal in the diagnosis of dementia praecox led him and his pupils far beyond the justified limits. But it was the unflinchingly psychiatric orientation of the man that impressed and attracted physicians and students.

Kraepelin is one of the few who entered psychiatry with unswerving determination and not by accident. Born in 1856, he entered upon the study of medicine in 1874, from the start with the goal of becoming a psychiatrist. The psychiatric courses of Rinecker in Würzburg attracted him even in his preclinical studies, and in his third medical year he already started work on the influence of acute diseases upon the origin of mental disorders—a topic which in 1887 produced his first and only strictly monographic piece of work, published in the Archiv für Psychiatrie. Wundt's fame attracted him to Leipzig for a summer course in psychology in 1877, and he returned to Würzburg as assistant in Rinecker's clinic while still a medical student.

When in 1879 Forel left the Munich Clinic to take the chair of psychiatry at Zurich, Kraepelin took his place as assistant to von Gudden, who was a remarkable personality, a distinguished investigator in experimental anatomy of the brain, and a level-headed and frank agnostic in psychiatric nosology, not ignorant and not indifferent but ready to say "I don't know" when the facts seemed to demand it. Forel in this respect always remained true to von Gudden's spirit; but Kraepelin was destined to aspire to a different course. In 1882, to be near Wundt, he went to Leipzig as first assistant of Flechsig, who, without any training in psychiatry, had been made director of a neuropsychiatric clinic because of his work on myelinization in Ludwig's laboratory. The psychiatrist and the anatomist clashed. Kraepelin resigned after a few months and turned whole-heartedly to Wundt and to his experimental work on the effects of drugs. He also wrote, in 1883, the first edition of his compend of psychiatry, destined to reach in the eighth edition the biggest scope of any treatment of psychiatry by any one writer. He returned to Munich, and in 1884 became first assistant in a non-academic institution at Leubus, in order to be enabled to get married, and in 1885 he was given the directorship of the psychiatric hospital at Dresden, only to be called to Dorpat in Russia in 1886, to the professorship of psychiatry, when he was 30 years old. Together with his wife, he organized the practical aspects of his new clinic, and with a group of co-workers he established his psychological laboratory and won a reputation which happily led to his call to Fürstner's place in Heidelberg in 1890, just before the Russification of Dorpat. When in 1888, I had my first instruction in psychiatry with Forel, we were told of Krafft-Ebing's book as clinically interesting, but of Kraepelin's third edition (written in Dorpat, 1887) as the psychologically best-founded introduction to the field. By the time I started work at Kankakee in 1893 I found stimulating help in the fourth edition published from the Heidelberg Clinic in 1891; and by 1895, when I was asked by Lindley (now Chancellor of the University of Kansas), one of my first hearers at Clark University and the Worcester Hospital clinics, where in Europe he had best continue his work in psychology, I had no hesitation in urging him to get work in Kraepelin's psychological laboratory in Heidelberg.

Kraepelin represented more than mere Wundtian psychology. He had worked out the method of "continued work," the utilization of the work-curve for the study of fatigue, of sleep, and of the effects of practice, of alcohol, of drugs. It is difficult to realize to-day what a relief it was to see a frankly functional principle stand before us in a field which had so far been either largely speculative or devoted to Weber's law and, we might say, to microscopic interests with ultra-accurate reaction-time methods. The method of continued additions, and the ergograph work, the technique utilized in Hoch and Kraepelin's study of the effect of tea, appeared like a big step towards reality, towards what occupied one in the observation of patients. I realized that the clinical aspects too were receiving a new impetus. Ziehen's Psychiatrie, published in 1894, was met by Kraepelin with a vigorous reaction and a promise to reply with a new book; and it was my good fortune, owing to the liberality of Dr. H. M. Quinby and the trustees of the then "Worcester Lunatic Hospital," to be in Heidelberg for six weeks at the time when that book appeared in the fifth edition of the Psychiatrie, no longer a Kompendium, but the greatest challenge that had ever come to psychiatry in the form of a text.

The Heidelberg Clinic at that time was the center of work on "processes." The psychological experiment and the clinic alike dealt with processes, i.e., specific modifications of structure and function, that might be underlying specific diseases. The static, purely descriptive period had come to an end. This is what attracted me. At the same time, the shape it took rather startled me. To find the thyroid disorders, paresis and the conditions terminating in "terminal dementia" all thrown together into a group of "metabolism disorders" was a pretty big dose to swallow, and to see the attack psychoses, mania and melancholia (apart from the involution depressions) dogmatically stamped as one group of periodic and circular disorders, non-deteriorating and rarely appearing but once in a lifetime, was another startling condensation. The favorable prognostic coloring of these attacks, even after continental psychiatry had become accustomed for a decade before Kraepelin to single out the less favorable confusions and delusional types now to be thrown together with dementia praecox, was not so clear either, to one coming from a large state hospital with the inevitable presence of some chronic circular cases. Furthermore, to find the constitutional background minimized if not wholly ignored, and even the "degenerative" character of the deteriorations, still upheld in the fourth (1891) edition, replaced by a "metabolism disorder" that anybody might get, never could convince me. With all my admiration and appreciation, I figured to some extent as a doubting Thomas when I left Heidelberg and published my review of the fifth edition in The American Journal of Insanity, Vol. 53, 1896–7, pp. 298–302. Nevertheless the Worcester State Hospital was probably the first hospital outside of Heidelberg to use the acceptable principles of Kraepelin's nosology in a mitigated form in its statistical accounts, from 1896 on.

What I always missed in the Heidelberg School was the publication of the casuistic material in monographic form. Kraepelin's chapters were monographs on his concepts, but not monographs on cases offered in toto. The monograph of Dreyfuss demolishing the melancholia picture (in the sense of involution melancholia) is one of the very few exceptions and even that a presentation leaving one in doubt as to whether the statement was altogether free of bias.

In the meantime Kraepelin's genius showed in another direction, viz., a determined fortifying of his position by attracting Nissl and Alzheimer to his group. What Kraepelin had done in the psychological laboratory, Nissl had pursued in the histological work: the experimental study of the effects of poisons with his cell-stain, unfortunately brought to a standstill (after the description of a number of cell changes found experimentally and others in the autopsies of the clinical material) because, on the one hand, of Nissl's

new fascination for the fibril-methods and his "diffuse gray," and the apparently fundamental harvest in his establishing histologically the "paresis process" together with Alzheimer. The observation of the characteristic, if not altogether specific, plasma cell infiltration and the spinal fluid studies and Alzheimer's remarkably clear pictures of the entire process reinforced Kraepelin's use of paresis as the very paradigma of a disease entity. Dementia praecox never was, however, morphologically defined to the same extent. It received just enough of a histological background in Sioli's work and some contributions of Alzheimer to Kraepelin's text to fortify that persistent but after all not probable claim of some kind of a nosological parallelism between general paresis and dementia praecox, and with it the demand for specific anatomical "processes."

Kraepelin's promotion to the directorship of the Munich Clinic led to the necessity of facing a new type of clinical material, viz., that brought in by a large city, the psychoneurotic material constituting the fourth volume of Kraepelin's eighth edition (1915). The chief attention on the part of the outside world was, however, absorbed by that further extension of Kraepelin's ideal in the direction of a large research institute, to which he was able to draw stars of the first magnitude—Alzheimer followed him; Nissl joined them again, although only to succumb to an early death; Brodmann, a pupil of Vogt, was attracted from Tübingen as the outstanding master of the cortex-map, but he also only to die, of septicaemia; Rüdin began his monumental collection of material for heredity study; Isserlin maintained the dignity of the psychological laboratory with his association studies; Plaut developed the serological work in syphilis; and Allers and later Wuth laid the foundations for the chemical studies. As his last big contribution Kraepelin aimed to add a valuable by-product of his love for travel, his comparative psychiatry. In all these developments, Kraepelin was fortunate to get the financial support of an American patient without whose assistance many steps of the great development would have been impossible. The broadening of Kraepelin's viewpoint shown in his "Erscheinungsformen des Irreseins" (Ztschr. f. d. ges. Neur. u. Psychiat., 62, 1, 1920) softened the extreme contrasts between nosological rigidity and the freedom of the reaction-type psychiatry without any great influence upon those who had once for all accepted the original simplification of diagnosis by classification.

The personality of Kraepelin appears more or less lost in this sketch of the career of the psychiatry connected with his name. His life and his work indeed were one. When he accepted the call to the new Munich Clinic nearly completed by Professor Bumm, he made it a condition that he be given an official residence attached to the clinic. In no other way could he have achieved the work he mastered.

A man of untiring energy, of very determined working habits and determined methods of self-protection; Kraepelin never allowed himself to be deflected from his sphere and goal by outside considerations. He rarely entered into polemic discussions with his contemporaries, nor did he give them much consideration in his writings unless they happened to furnish corroborative material. In this respect he treated them as he treated himself. Every edition of his work is to an unusual extent like the work of another man, with scant accounting for the changes. Things were just so in 1896, in 1899, in 1904 and in 1915 or 1920—new declarations without any concern for equally sure declarations made before.

Kraepelin was outside of the group that decided the choice of men for the academic vacancies and professorships of Germany or neighboring countries. Aschaffenburg in Köln is the one Kraepelinian placed as a Kraepelin pupil. Gaupp of Tübingen is fully as much a Wernicke pupil. Alzheimer was chosen for Breslau because he was Alzheimer. On his resignation from the directorship of the clinic, Kraepelin and his immediate associates in Munich were replaced by Bumke and his group, and it was natural that the continuity of the work of the Kraepelin group should have to come to depend on the continuity of the Forschungsanstalt which was fortunately saved through a donation from the Rockefeller Board. The wider influence of Kraepelin's doctrine was stronger than that of his personality. Even in his anti-alcoholic propaganda he worked rather single-handedly. In his political activity during and after the war he was an ardent nationalist.

His share in the medico-legal movements was that of outlining a very advanced program when still a very young man, in 1880, in a noteworthy plea for "the abolition of fixed terms of punishment." In Kraepelin's hand, the psychological laboratory never attained the vital connection with the clinic one had a right to expect at first; the intelligence-test wave and the "Thatbestand Diagnostik" outflanked him, and the lack of interest and capacity for a utilization of the "content" of the psychoses made him and his pupils miss a point of general interest in the association studies. A study of word-formations in dreams (Psychologische Arbeiten, Vol. V, 1, 1910) was completely overshadowed by the wave of dream-mythology with which Freud captured the world and to which Kraepelin devoted but a few condemnatory pages out of the 2372 pages of the last edition of his work. Kraepelin was too sincere to be unduly captivated by any endocrinological promises. The

strong impression left with the world was the dichotomy of psychiatric diagnosis according to the outcome. Even there it was not a utilization of a fundamental principle, that of studying complete developments, which might have suggested itself so strongly with dementia praecox as a disease entity. His steadfast Wundtian attitude and his temperament made him miss, and shrink from, the really dynamic aspect of the dementia praecox concept. His remarkable system of collecting the statistical essentials from the case records favored his being the last big creator of entities by classification.

Kraepelin was twice in this country, in 1908 in consultation with Dr. August Hoch and again two years ago on a trip devoted in part to a study of the Indians and negroes and their relation to paresis. It was a real pleasure to have him visit us in his most genial spirit and in an attitude of warm appreciation of what he saw, and with a capacity of work during his studies at the Government Hospital in Washington that would have done honor to a man 30 or 40 years younger. To hear Kraepelin and Dr. William H. Welch exchange reminiscences of their Leipzig days gave us a picture of a remarkable phase of medical history in the making. A little over a year later Kraepelin succumbed to a gastro-intestinal disorder which brought out an unsuspected myocardial insufficiency related to coronary arteriosclerosis, with a clear realization of the approach of the end. In plain sight of death, which occurred October 7, 1926, he sent a last appeal for support of his Forschungsanstalt to the Rockefeller Board and it must be a satisfaction to all Americans that his last wish was granted. Kraepelin had hoped to spend part of his seventy-first year in India in the pursuit of comparative psychiatry. May his staunch devotion to the cause be an ever impressive example to the many workers he stimulated.

On his seventieth birthday two large volumes of the two principal psychiatric journals of Germany came out as Festschrift, the biggest tribute ever paid to a psychiatrist. The Forschungsanstalt will be the lastingly active and productive monument. May it prosper!

THE ACUTE SCHIZOAFFECTIVE PSYCHOSES

By J. Kasanin, M.D.

Clinical Director, State Hospital for Mental Diseases, Howard, Rhode Island

When Kraepelin introduced his system of classification of mental diseases, it seemed that at last order had come into psychiatry, and that the first and most difficult task in the scientific approach to psychiatry had been solved. The classification which he offered was simple and empirically extremely useful, because it allowed the institutional physician to orient himself quickly in his case and even give a prognosis. On the other hand, its very rigidity, together with the underlying concept of an immutable disease process in dementia praecox was quite detrimental to the progress of psychiatry, as it discouraged any attempt at the understanding of the psychosis except in terms of chemical changes, hypothetical diseases of the endocrine organs, and cellular pathology. The famous observation (1) that the clinical picture of the various psychoses was the same in cultured Europeans as among the primitive Javans was used as an evidence that the same organic factors operated in the psychoses, in the same sense that tuberculosis was the same in the Negro as in the Eskimo. At the same time that the Kraepelinian classification found its ready acceptance in American psychiatry, a vigorous reaction was developed in the teachings of Meyer (2), who early in this century began to emphasize the study of the individual patient in terms of his total personality, rather than an investigation of the various faculties or separate systems. The emphasis on the study of the individual as a whole rather than the study of specialized functions was later incorporated into a philosophical system of psychobiology, a system on which most of us have been brought up. A parallel development took place in continental European thought where Kraepelinian classification was never adhered to as tenaciously as it was in America. Meyer injected a totally different, optimistic trend into psychiatry instead of the hopelessly fatalistic attitude of Kraepelin by stressing the necessity of utilizing and mobilizing all the patient's assets to bring him back into society, and also by pointing out how social conditions have to be modified to make them suitable for the patient. This social psychiatric point of view is what largely distinguishes the American psychiatry from the continental schools. It is by no means an accident that mental hygiene as a liaison of sociology and psychiatry originated in America. Finally, the psychoanalytical approach of psychiatry went even further into the study and therapy of the individual by attempting to reintegrate the various distorted elements of the patient's psyche.

A situation has developed in which a psychiatrist is taught to think in terms of what is fundamentally wrong with the patient and what can be done for him, rather than the application of a formal diagnostic label. On the other hand, the laws of scientific approach to any biological problem must be the same for psychiatry as for other biological sciences. Observations, in which psychiatry is very rich, must be classified if we expect to discover correlations and uniformities of sequence. True enough, the statistical method has thus far been inapplicable to psychiatry largely because psychiatric data are still in the descriptive stage and are not subject to measurement. It is the problem of the psychiatrist as a scientist to discover general laws which hold true of a large number of patients and a principle of classification must be found with establishment of definite differential criteria. The problem is extremely difficult. It took almost one hundred years to crystallize out the disease concept of general paresis and even then when the objective diagnostic criteria were established, it was found that mistakes in diagnosis reached as high as 50 per cent. In the so-called functional psychoses, the problem is still unsolved.

The development of general medicine brings out a large number of methods and techniques which are from time to time applied to psychiatric cases, but the research worker usually applies them to groups of cases which are diagnosed in terms of Kraepelinian classifications. These groups are so general and contain such a large number of heterogeneous cases with different clinical pictures that it is no wonder that the experimental results are quite worthless. I doubt very much if experimental research in psychiatry will ever yield any results unless we deal with fairly homogenous groups. This principle has to some extent been recognized by the younger research workers. Thus D'Elsaux, who is conducting extremely intensive metabolic studies in psychiatric cases, is studying stupors irrespective of diagnoses. In the attempt to bring out homogenous groups of cases Dr. Bowman and I were able to crystallize out a special group of the so-called "constitutional schizophrenics," which we are presenting elsewhere. Today, I wish to call your attention

Read at the eighty-eighth annual meeting of The American Psychiatric Association, Philadelphia, Pa., May 30–June 3, 1932.

Part of the work on this paper was done in connection with the special research on schizophrenia at the Boston Psychopathic Hospital under a grant from the Rockefeller Foundation. Due to limitation of space the detailed histories of Cases 2, 6, 7, and 9 are omitted from this report.

to a group of cases which are quite atypical. These are fairly young individuals, quite well integrated socially, who suddenly blow up in a dramatic psychosis and present a clinical picture which may be called either schizophrenic or affective, and in whom the differential diagnosis is extremely difficult. Of course, Bleuler (3) many years ago recognized such cases. He pointed out that at times it is extremely difficult to differentiate between the schizophrenic and the affective disorders. He stated that all manic-depressive symptoms may appear in schizophrenia but not reversely. Only prolonged observation will lead to a correct diagnosis with hallucinations and deterioration being the ultimate criteria. The clinical picture alone is not sufficient to make such a differentiation. While Bleuler pointed out that schizophrenic features never appear in the affective psychosis, Lange (4) in an extensive monograph gives a statistical review of frequency of the so-called catatonic phenomena in the manic-depressive psychoses. In some 700 cases he found thought disturbance in 53 cases, hallucinations in 46 cases, extremely odd and queer behavior such as stereotypy, catalepsy, passivity, impulsive and unmotivated conduct, extreme regression such as eating feces, etc, in 189 cases. Bowman (5) in his series of 1009 cases of manic-depressive psychoses found that about 20 per cent had delusions of persecution. Of course, his material may be questioned as to the diagnosis, as most of his cases were in the hospital less than ten days. Dunton, Jr., in 1910 described cyclic (6) forms and intermittent forms (7) of dementia praecox. The cyclic forms closely resembled manic attacks but instead of a flight of ideas there is usually stereotypy. Sometimes rigidity and cerea flexibilitas may be present. These patients have perfectly normal periods during which no dementia can be detected, but deterioration eventually takes place. By intermittent forms of dementia praecox the author described attacks beginning with excitements or depressions in which symptoms of deterioration gradually become apparent. Between attacks the patient may appear quite well but after each succeeding attack he usually shows more and more deterioration so that eventually hospital care is required. It is quite remarkable how this author with a very astute clinical sense is trying to fit his accurate observations into a formula which they do not always fit. On the other hand, Lewis (8) stresses the seriousness of the schizophrenic features in the affective psychosis. Claude (9, 10) in his several papers looks upon any deteriorating psychosis as dementia praecox. But this is usually a final stage. His cases go through successive stages of what he describes as schizomania, schizophrenia, and finally dementia. In schizomania, the most important thing is the extremely rich fantasy life of the patient in whom the creative imagination constructs the whole fabric of the delusions. In these cases there is a special schizoid personality make-up, early deprivation with unsatisfied wishes; and finally when the reality becomes too difficult, wish-fulfilling fantasy solves the impossible situation. Cases may be arrested at this stage or they may go further, become more serious with marked thought disturbance which he calls schizophrenia and which fit in fairly well with Bleuler's description of the disease, and finally the state of dementia in the Kraepelinian sense of complete deterioration. Claude (9, 10) points out that in

his cases of schizomania he finds the mechanism of ideo-affective compensation as a method of evasion of reality. There are many other workers who have discussed the same problem from different angles.

The group of cases which I describe can fit in any of the above mentioned groups except that the latter carry the implication of a definite disease process going on to deterioration and dementia which an unbiased study of cases of this type does not really justify.

My series included a small group of nine cases which I personally studied and which aroused my curiosity on account of the special clinical picture which they presented. They were all diagnosed dementia praecox. They were young men and young women in their twenties and thirties, in excellent physical health. The various biological tests of the urine, blood and cerebrospinal fluid were negative. They had average or superior intelligence, and they had no difficulty in coping with the work in which they were engaged. Preceding the attack there was, however, a difficult environmental situation which served as a precipitating factor. The environmental stress was chronic in some cases, and acute in others. It varied from the loss of a job, to a state of anxiety over a sudden promotion, a difficult love affair, alien environment or the usual case of hostile in-laws.

The personalities of our patients were not very much different from the general run of people in the community. They have been fairly well adjusted socially and were considered to be well integrated individuals who apparently got a good deal of satisfaction out of life. They are keen, ambitious, forward, some of them rather seclusive, others quite sociable. A subjective review of their own personalities reveals that they are very sensitive, critical of themselves, introspective, very unhappy and preoccupied with their own conflicts, problems, and sometimes with life in general. These conflicts and problems may go on for years before the patient breaks down, and they are not apparent to others. The interesting thing about the psychoses is that one is able to reconstruct them psychologically when one reviews the various symptoms and behavior with the patient after his recovery, and then they become fairly intelligible. The fact that there is comparatively little of the extremely bizarre, unusual and mysterious, is what perhaps gives these cases a fairly good chance of recovery. They do not exhibit any profound regression socially, although the thought processes show primitive and infantile modes of thought. There is very little passivity in these cases. Their reaction is one of a protest, or a fear, without the ready acceptance of the solution offered by the psychosis.

These psychoses occur in young men and women and tend to repeat themselves. In our series, there was usually a vague history of a previous breakdown with a complete recovery, and then a recovery again after the psychosis which we observed.

A review of the dynamic factors in the psychosis shows a severe conflict between the instinctive drives of the patient, usually sexual, and the barriers and repression imposed by the social group. Of course many of our patients are young people in whom one would naturally expect a great deal of pent up emotion and ideation about sex. But the unusual frequency with which the sexual conflicts stand out in the psychosis and the amount of emotion associated with it, suggests more than casual association between the sex maladjustment of the patient and the psychosis. There is also a marked feeling of inferiority, especially in the subjective notions of these patients that they are not able to adjust themselves socially. The psychosis is usually ushered in by a latent depression and a certain amount of rumination going on for some time until the more dramatic picture which we are describing here becomes apparent.

The clinical picture is best described by a review of some of the cases. A young girl of 19, Case 7, comes homes from work and suddenly becomes depressed and begins to carry on conversations with her dead father. Later on she expresses frank hostility toward her mother and sister, announces that she is pregnant with a rattlesnake, and brings up the fact that she is engaged to be married to all the Catholic boys in her neighborhood. After recovery, we find that there is a good deal of conflict over adjustment of a Protestant girl to a Catholic community in which she is living and working. The natural desire for companionship with boys of a different religion is suppressed. She shows hostility to one of her Catholic girl co-workers, and finally develops the feeling that all the Catholics are in a plot against her, including her own mother.

An ambitious, energetic, young mechanic, Case 3, becomes extremely upset over his promotion to a position of foreman in his plant and feels that he does not deserve it. This feeling of guilt is related to a large number of other conflicts and there is a profound interest in religion with several visits to the church of a very prominent evangelist, which brings to the patient the conviction that he was never really converted. God and the devil are constantly struggling over his soul. In a state of religious ecstasy, he runs to see the evangelical preacher, when his wife succeeds in taking him to the hospital. There the stage of ecstasy continued for some time with a feeling of electricity coming from the floor and that the food was poisoned. A subsequent review reveals a terrific conflict over his own instinctive drives, the attempt to repress it, the failure to do so, the feeling of guilt and inadequacy which become intensified when a promotion is given to him, and finally the attempt of solution by the religious conversion.

A young boy, Case 1, a happy-go-lucky musician, tests out the existence of God for over a year and finally when he begins to doubt it, the signs of impending death become so apparent that he runs in a panic and finally gets picked up by the police. After his recovery he was able to reconstruct the long period of interest in religion, his own emotional and instinctive conflicts, the solution of them by acquisition of religious beliefs, the environmental disappointments, the beginning of doubt, the premonition of punishment and death, and finally a panic.

The extremely primitive and archaic modes of thought can be seen in the reactions of the simple-minded boy, Case 2, who becomes over-stimulated by casual contact with a promiscuous woman and subsequent teasing by his co-workers. The sex drive comes to the surface, but the boy's super-ego tells him to sublimate it by worshipping St. Mary. His mother's name is also Mary and by laws of chain association, which is a residual from childhood, his mother becomes St. Mary. He wants to be a priest so that he can be nearer to his mother and he wants to be a bull so that he can have relations with all the girls in the world. He had intercourse only once and that was when he was born, by coming through his mother's sex organs. These utterances are not produced in a setting of an analytic treatment, but are the spontaneous productions of the patient.

Another young boy, Case 8, finally gets a date with a girl with whom he has been in love for a long time. A moderate amount of sex play after the movies arouses in him a sense of magnetism and results in a theory of a universe in which magnetism and spermatic fluids are curiously interwoven. The spermatic fluids travel all over his body producing a magnetic feeling in the various organs, the same as the sexual act. The fluid can be drawn from the various orifices of the body when touched. In a very crude and artless way the patient postulated a theory of pleasure closely akin to Freud's concepts of the polymorphous perverse.

The castration anxiety with the homosexual component in a paranoid setting is illustrated by a patient, Case 9, who showed, after the war, a strong suspiciousness that his cultured and superior brother-in-law was a German spy. Five years later, when the hopes of a love affair went to smash, and his brother-in-law spoke of Germans conducting the future warfare by emasculating all the males, the castration threat again arouses the hostility and suspiciousness to his brother-in-law and also his best friends, in a setting of a violent outburst.

It will be extremely interesting to analyze the reasons why our patients got well, whereas other patients with almost identical personalities and the same problems went on to ultimate deterioration. A deeper review of our cases shows that in all of them there was a pretty good grasp of life and a keen bite on its opportunities. These patients liked life, enjoyed it and wanted to have everything that life could afford. Together with this there is, however, marked sensitivity, a rich fantasy life, a facile return to more primitive modes of thought and behavior, but no complete withdrawal or passivity. Up to the very period of the breakdown these patients go on with their tasks, and we have no history of long years of rumination with the feelings of hopelessness, passivity and depersonalization, all of which differentiate them sharply from other less fortunate patients. The psychosis itself is a very dramatic affair with the attempt of a quick and intense compensation. It is an extremely severe emotional experience through which the patient goes without accepting it as an end in itself. Life has a good deal to offer to the patients, the capacity for reintegration is present. There isn't enough time for the thought processes to become disintegrated and thus the recovery is made easier. Perhaps the fact that the patient had mild attacks during adolescence confers a certain amount of immunity upon the patients in undergoing a more serious psychosis.

One sees these cases more frequently in private practice than in institutions, because often definite improvement takes place before hospitalization is seriously considered. In more serious cases, the change of environment and the treatment in a hospital are apparently beneficial, although the patient strongly objects to the residence in the hospital. It is quite curious to see how in a few days the patient begins to deny the existence of all sorts of queer and bizarre ideas which he expressed before. The return of the critical judgment is quick and definite, but a real psychological insight into one's own case is not usually present. It is fair to state that these cases have received more than the usual amount of psychotherapy which one finds in an active receiving hospital. These cases are so interesting and so unusual that they attract more than the passing attention of the ward physician. Whether this has anything to do with the recovery, I don't know. It does seem, however, that where the emotional conflicts are so obvious psychotherapy is strongly indicated, and probably a thorough analytical procedure would be in the best interest of the patient if one wishes to prevent the recurrence of such attacks.

CASE HISTORIES

CASE 1.—O.C., male, white, clerk, age 21, admitted to the hospital February 20, 1929; discharged to relatives, March 4, 1929. Diagnosis: *dementia praecox*.

Chief Complaint.—The patient suddenly decided that he was going to die and was found wandering in the New Jersey Flats, expecting his death. He was arrested by the police and sent to his relatives.

Family History.—The grandparents were fairly stable people although the maternal grandmother was quite emotional. The father is a musician, rather temperamental, but on the whole quite stable. The mother has extremely severe temper tantrums and at times she is difficult to manage. She also has a very limited intellectual endowment.

Personal History.—The patient is the oldest of four children. The birth history and the early developmental history are negative. He got along well in school, had a good many friends and graduated from high school at the age of 16. After graduation from high school the patient obtained a job as a clerk and took some courses at night in a local college. The whole family is quite temperamental but the members of the family got along well with each other, and made allowances for each other's peculiarities. The whole family was very musical and a great deal of time was spent in playing various instruments, with family interests revolving largely around musical topics. The patient began to write music quite early in life and cherished the ambition of becoming a great musician.

The patient was a lively child. He took part in athletics, was a good swimmer and skater. He played several instruments and earned extra money playing during the week ends. He had a good sense of humor and got along well with everybody, although very often he felt unusually sensitive about a deformed thumb of the left hand. He was not particularly aggressive although ambitious, and he intended to make his mark in the business world, if not in music. He was not prone to day-dreaming and had only fleeting interest in religion, attending the synagogue on the high holidays. The whole family worked very hard to maintain a decent standard of living, and the patient contributed to the family budget from his earnings.

Present Illness.—In September, 1928, the patient left for New York to obtain a position, and also to make some arrangements about publishing his songs. He apparently got along all right in New York until February 18, 1929, when the father got a telegram that the boy was psychotic and that he should come and take him home. When the father arrived in New York he found the patient in good condition. He gave a rambling story about a fear of an

operation which he was advised to undergo and also about a trip to New Jersey where the patient was picked up by police.

The father took the patient home. There he became extremely restless, began to argue with his parents and refused to stay in bed. He left the house and asked the police for protection. He was brought to the hospital February 28, 1929.

On admission the patient was found to be in good physical condition. There was an anomaly of the left thumb which consisted in the absence of the carpal bones. The examinations of the blood and urine were negative. At one time the patient showed a trace of sugar in the urine.

On the ward the patient was quiet, cooperative, talked freely and spontaneously. He tried very earnestly to go over his ideas, yet he smiled frequently when he discussed some of the more serious aspects of his illness. There was no evidence of any pronounced mood disturbance. On the whole, he appeared quite cheerful, but at times he seemed to be preoccupied. The patient said that he was worried over the fact that he was to have an amputation of his thumb. "On Sunday, the night before I was to get the operation for my thumb, I thought the Supreme Intelligence, or God, told me I was going to die soon, and I remembered this statement in the Bible or told me by a certain party: 'Resist not evil.' So I started getting thoughts about suicide but I got counter-suggestions also from my real self, which didn't believe in the Supreme Intelligence. One thought would say, 'At 12 you shall die,' then the other thought would say, 'Just for the hell of it see if that is a lie, and be sure to look at the clock.' I thought if I happened to touch a piece of metal I felt a slight electrical shock and I wondered if that was going to kill me.

"On Monday night, after I left the hospital, the suggestion came to me in two hours, while I was walking, that the blood-pressure test was to bind the artery and kill me, so my heart would fill up and burst.

"Losing my job was the thing that gave me a shock which sort of put me in a sort of trance, sort of dazed condition. I imagined God was speaking through me. It seemed to be an expression of what God was talking to me through my own voice. Just like a person mumbling or repeating someone else's advice. That's the explanation of the feeling or whatever you call it, hallucinations or whatever the technical word is."

The patient admitted that for the past year he had felt mystic contact with God and felt that he would be a success if he took God's advice if he did things in a perfect manner. He never had the actual sensory experience of hearing a voice or sound.

The intellectual functions were intact. The patient admitted auto-erotism, as well as serious conflict over it. Later he thought that a homosexual was a man who masturbated. He also admitted some mutual masturbation recently. Patient had several heterosexual experiences.

Within a few days the patient adjusted himself very well in the hospital life. He got along very well with the patients and the staff and there was nothing abnormal in his conduct. A psychological examination showed superior intelligence.

After the patient was in the hospital two weeks, although further treatment was recommended, the family refused permission for commitment and took him home against advice.

Since the patient left the hospital he rested for several weeks, then obtained a position where he has been very successful and which he likes very much. He seems to be perfectly adjusted at home and in the community. One of the patient's uncles is a psychiatrist who is in very close touch with him. He is quite satisfied with the patient's progress.

Sometime after the patient left the hospital he came to see me and during several interviews we were able to go over the whole situation.

Since early childhood he had worried about two things. He had a deformed left thumb, the boys in school teased him about it and he always tried to hide it. He wondered why he should not have been perfect, physically. The other thing which worried him was auto-erotism. He heard adults speak of masturbation as a cause of insanity and there was an occasional fear in him that if he didn't stop doing it something would happen to him.

The patient had formal religious Hebrew training but he was never especially interested in religion. In the summer and fall of 1928 he became interested in the question of fundamentalism versus modernism, which at that time occupied the attention of the Protestant religious circles, and which found its reflection in a good many of the popular magazines. He began to ask himself whether he believed in God or not. At times he felt that there was a God, at other times he felt there was no such thing. He decided that he would test God out. If God prescribed certain modes of conduct and he followed these modes, then success must crown his efforts. He did it several times and to his surprise he obtained good results. Thus, for several weeks, he behaved himself very well, did not go to movies, did not take out any girls, spoke only the truth, applied himself to his work and great energy, and all of a sudden he received a small increase in salary. On the other hand he could not accept wholeheartedly the idea of the existence of God, rejected many times the proofs of the existence of the Supreme Being, and scoffed at the whole idea. Finally the patient came to the conclusion that inasmuch as he did not know whether God existed or not, he would act as if God were existing, so that his efforts would be rewarded, providing that he acted in accordance with the ethical standards prescribed by the great religious teachers. Many times the patient had a vague feeling that in some way God was in touch with him, or at least supervised him and that he was destined for a great success. His friends liked his musical compositions, urged him to have them published, and jokingly called him the second Irving Berlin.

Early in the fall of 1928 he decided to go to New York to try his luck in getting a new job and also in publishing his songs. To his great surprise he found a very satisfactory job within a few days. The salary was small, but the prospects were excellent. The luck in finding this job so quickly was another proof to the patient that he was picked out for a big success in the financial world. However, things did not go well with the publishing of his songs and this was a disappointment. He was sent from publisher to publisher, and was finally told that there was no demand for songs on account of the advent of the talkies.

Through the winter of 1928 and January of 1929 the patient was quite preoccupied with the question of religious belief and his "heart was torn with doubt." Things began to look rather gloomy in his place of employment. Within a short time he was given a promotion without increase in salary and after three months he began to expect an increase in his salary. At the same time he conducted himself in a manner which he thought ought to bring reward from God, if He existed. The patient waited week after week but no increase in salary came. At the same time some of his co-workers became jealous of him, as he was generally liked by his superiors, and made things unpleasant for him. He began to neglect his work, paying less and less attention to it and finally on February 1, 1929, he was called in by his employer who told him that his work was unsatisfactory and that his services would not be required any longer.

The losing of his job was a tremendous shock to the patient. As he went home he began to feel a severe splitting headache. For several nights afterward he could not sleep. He was a complete failure. Ideas of suicide came to his mind. Then all of a sudden a "Biblical" saying flashed into his mind, "Those whom the gods destroy they first make mad." He knew he was mad or insane because he had the thoughts about suicide, which he knew were insane thoughts, and which he felt he could not control. And then he recalled the old fear that he would become insane on account of masturbation. Everything pointed to his death.

The patient was terrifically alarmed and went to see a physician who tried to quiet him and told him that the first thing he ought to do was to have his thumb amputated. He suggested that the patient should go to the Presbyterian Clinic in New York and have it done there. The night before the patient went to the clinic he could not sleep. He felt that God or the Supreme Being was in some way putting the thought into his head and that he was to commit suicide and that he was going to die. The thought of suicide was so alien to him as well as the thought of death, that he felt that in some way it was put into his head by an outside force. On the other hand "the scientific part of his personality" told him that it was all bunk, that nobody was putting thoughts into his head and as a proof of its strength suggested to him that he should go to the bathroom, open the medicine chest, look at a bottle of iodine, take it in his hands and then put it back. He did it. He knew that "the scientific part of his mind" had also some strength and that he was not altogether under the influence of the Supreme Being. In these thoughts, torn by his conflict and doubt, the patient spent the whole night. Toward morning the idea of death became stronger and stronger.

In the morning he went to the surgical clinic and told all his difficulties. A psychiatrist was called in, and suggested that he should walk to the Battery. This tremendously long walk was an additional proof that he was going to die. They wanted him to die and he knew he would die as the result of such a long walk. Blood was taken for a Wassermann test and it seemed to him that a tremendous amount of blood was withdrawn because the doctors wanted to give him the opportunity of a quick and painless death. He began his walk and on the way he stopped at his uncle's business establishment. The uncle suggested that instead of a walk he should go into a movie. The patient entered the vaudeville house and the first thing he saw on the stage was an actor producing a revolver and speaking about suicide. This of course convinced him that death was imminent.

Inasmuch as he knew he was going to die anyhow, he felt that there was no sense in walking himself to death and so he began to ride around in taxis. His headache was terrific and he felt that if he should leave the taxi, he would die on the street. The patient spent his two weeks salary riding in taxis. He told the taxi to drive him over to New Jersey and he got out in a quiet suburb near Paterson. It was a quiet and peaceful place and the patient thought that it would be a nice place to die and he began to walk slowly toward his destination—his death. A policeman approached him, asked him what he was going to do and when the patient told him he was going to die he took him to the police station and got in touch with his family. On the following morning his headache suddenly left him. He knew he was not dead, the whole threat and the thought of death suddenly left him, he felt differently, new, and in a way he was glad to be alive. Yet there was a tremendously dull feeling which did not leave him until he came to Boston. It was only after the patient left the psychopathic hospital that his head became clear and he knew what he wanted to do.

At the present time the patient is leading a very active life, he does not allow himself to indulge in rumination and introspection, realizing its hazards. He remembers very well the whole experience and feels that he is much more stable now than he has been for many years.

CASE 3.—A.C., male white, age 33, married, admitted to the hospital November 30, 1928; discharged December 10, 1928. Diagnosis: *dementia praecox.*

Chief Complaint.—On admission to hospital the patient complained of poor appetite for the past week, as well as unusual degree of anxiety and depression, worrying over the most trivial things.

Family History.—The parents were farmers in Canada, and the family history is negative for nervous and mental disease. Patient was brought up in a strict, puritanical atmosphere and he fitted in well (as a child) with his surroundings. He was a studious boy and applied himself to his studies.

Personal History.—Infancy and early childhood uneventful. Previous to his graduation from high school he was extremely nervous, and his parents feared a possibility of a breakdown.

Upon his graduation from high school, the patient tried teaching but did not like it, and worked for a while in a munition factory and afterwards was employed for seven years by a large industry, doing very well. A year ago he came East and did various odd jobs in Boston, and about nine months ago he got a job in a large factory nearby. He was an excellent workman and six months before admission he was appointed foreman in his department.

The patient has been married twice. His first wife, whom he loved a great deal, died very suddenly after a few years of married life. This was a great shock to the patient from which, as he states himself, he never recovered. Five years ago the patient remarried and his marriage was congenial.

The patient is described as a quiet, retiring, serious minded and studious individual. He has always been very considerate of others and overconscientious in discharging his duties. He was very sensitive and brooded for long periods over insignificant things. He was unceasing in his efforts to rectify mistakes despite his continual effort to better himself and forge ahead. He had a gross lack of self-confidence. He was adaptable, good natured and not the least impulsive. He liked to have people come and visit him. He enjoyed the company of others, but did not particularly seek it. He cared little for recreation, he preferred to study nights, after work, in the hope of bettering himself. He got the most recreation out of his violin which he played by ear. He loved music. He has already been of a religious nature, having been brought up in a strict Scotch Presbyterian household, where family worship was in vogue. Patient used to go to church Sunday mornings, but was never fanatical. For the past three years the patient has been taking up shorthand and typewriting as well as some other studies at night.

Present Illness.—Although the patient had for some time, as was his nature, fretted over his impoverished financial status, about a week before admission his worrying became much augmented. He seemed to be markedly preoccupied with his troubles; he had much less to say than usual and he was particularly glum. His appetite became poor and he slept badly at night. He expressed certain ideas about not doing his job as foreman properly. He felt he was not liked by his factory associates. They seemed not to respect his authority as a foreman. He felt that he was grossly inadequate. Then suddenly on Thanksgiving day he became very talkative on religious matters. Despite the fact that his family was over to spend the day, he seemed strangely out of harmony with the feasting and revelry of the others. He announced that he was an "awful sinner," his soul was unclean. He was worried over his conversion. Although when quite young he had been converted to the Christian faith and joined the Presbyterian Church, he felt now that his conversion was not genuine. He could not see how just joining the church and signing his name to the registry could make him a veritable convert. He had not experienced a change of heart thereby. He was extremely puzzled and bothered over his conversion. He felt that God and the devil were having a great struggle with regard to his conversion. He felt he must seek the spiritual advice of a certain Dr. Swift, the pastor of the temple, whom he had gone to hear on Sunday morning two or three times. He talked continually about the Bible. He stated that he thought family worship should be established in his household even as it had been in the home of his parents when he was a boy. Several times during the day he got down on his knees and prayed and stated that a spirit had come over him. He was restless and slept little during the night. Early the next morning his thoughts were still on religion and on his sinful ways. He expressed the notion that his wife and mother were working against him trying to thwart him in the struggle for salvation of his soul. He put on his hat and coat and started out to find Dr. Swift to acquire some spiritual advice. His wife and mother attempted to stay him but he would not listen to their pleadings. He merely remarked to them, "Get thee behind me Satan," and bolted through the door. His wife realizing that he was altogether too ill to set out for the Tremont Temple chased after him and called some nearby police who assisted her in getting him to this hospital.

On admission here he was in fair physical condition, although somewhat undernourished. The various chemical tests were negative. Neurological examination was negative. He was very quiet and uncommunicative. To most of the questions he replied that he couldn't tell the answer because it was for his Father in Heaven to decide. At times he would say, "God will tell you that I cannot tell." At one time he became quite talkative, and spoke about his "conversion." He also said that he felt that everybody should take more interest in spiritual things, stating that he himself had great difficulty in going through a spiritual rebirth and that he felt that everybody was interfering with him in his desire to do so.

"I am convinced more and more that men should have more spiritual things. I had the idea that my wife and mother were trying to stop me from getting converted and that all the powers of earth and hell were trying to trap me. To tell the truth about it, it was all imagination I guess. I felt that the men were trying to put the 'skids' under me at work. I began to feel this way about two or three weeks ago.

"One of the main reasons why I quit the job as foreman was because I was guilty of having stolen a cake of soap. I brought it home without paying for it. I felt that I might take more if the opportunity came; that if I were to be so dishonest as to steal soap, that if I were to take a more responsible position I might take something even greater. That is why I resigned the responsibility of foreman. When they allowed me to stay and granted my request, accepting my resignation, I felt that I was wrong in my belief that they were against me. I began to have a change of heart and I took a different viewpoint. I realized that they were working for my good, helping in my conversion. I felt moved by a power to a state of contentment when I realized this."

He said that he had a great many things on his conscience, especially in connection with his instinctive life. "Well, I've been too lustful. Here I've only been married five years and I have three children. I'm too highly sexed."

The intellectual functions were intact and there was good insight into his own condition. Within ten days the patient improved a good deal and was able to discuss his condition quite objectively. He went over his experience with me and stated that he always had been an unduly sensitive individual, too much preoccupied with fine ethical questions and trying to carry in his work the high principles which were the foundations of his mode of life. When he was promoted as foreman in his shop, he questioned himself for a long time whether he was the logical man for the job, and if someone else should have been given the promotion. He wondered whether it was the right thing for him to rise above his fellow workers and receive a higher compensation. He felt that his sex life was muddled up. He brooded over the love for his first wife, and yet his second wife was pregnant with the third child. The power of flesh was stronger than the spirit. He felt finally that he must completely change his life if he were to save his soul from eternal damnation, and he finally exhibited the conduct which led to his admission to the hospital.

When the case was presented at staff conference he was quite dramatic and said that the whole thing was a case of nerves. When he was asked if he ever heard any voices he said, "There never has been a man that hasn't heard the voice of God. Flowers in the field have heard the voice of God."

On December 10, 1928, the patient was transferred to a state hospital. He was calm and quiet on admission there and said that when he was in the other hospital he thought that the food was poisoned. It tasted peculiarly and he thought it must be poisoned. One day his sister brought to him a box of candy. He said it tasted peculiarly and he decided it must be poisoned. When he was in the hospital, he felt everybody was trying to poison him. He distrusted even his own people. At one time in the hospital he thought that electricity was coming up from the floor because he could feel it in his feet.

Inasmuch as the patient's conduct in the hospital was perfectly normal and only at times did he show signs of a mild depression, the diagnosis of the state hospital was manic-depressive—depressed. Patient's mood became quite stable after a few weeks, and on May 8, 1928, he was discharged to his family.

Inasmuch as the patient was a British subject, his deportation was requested by the United States immigration authorities. He went back to Canada on September 1, 1929. He obtained a satisfactory position in a large industrial plant in Canada, is doing very well, and has made a very satisfactory adjustment.

CASE 4.—F.P.A., male, white, age 42, business man, admitted to the hospital January 18, 1926; discharged April 3, 1926. Diagnosis: *dementia praecox.*

Chief Complaint.—A week before admission the patient suddenly began to talk about religion, said that God appeared to him, became very excited and on the day of his admission showed the family a razor, which greatly upset them.

Family History.—The mother was "nervous," not always adjusted; the father was intelligent. He took alcohol at times (probably rather excessively on occasions). One paternal uncle committed suicide and a second cousin on the mother's side is "subject to depression," and was a patient in a state hospital. The patient was the youngest of three children. Nothing is known about the grandparents. Paternal grandfather of a "nervous" temperament.

Personal History.—The patient was a premature baby. The birth and early developmental history, normal. He had the usual children's diseases with good recovery. As a small child he played a good deal by himself but when he entered school he made a few friends. He was a good athlete in school, but cared very little for girls. At home he was very distant to his sisters and brothers but was extremely fond of his mother. He depended a good deal on his mother and she on him. He was rather a cranky and fussy child at home but his behavior was excellent in school.

The patient has always kept away from girls and has practiced auto-erotism since childhood. In 1910 he fell in love with a girl and went out with her a good deal. They were unsuited to each other as she was too vivacious and flighty, and finally she threw him over.

The patient never took any drugs or alcohol; he was a "rigid teetotaller." His industrial career began at 15 and he was quite successful in the various positions he held. At 32 he established a business for himself and has done well since. He was extremely devoted to business and had it on his mind all the time.

The patient was always a rather serious person. He seemed to be always shy, quiet, never talked in the presence of strangers, capricious and fretful. He was a man of marked likes and dislikes, and he expressed his feelings to the family very freely. He was described as a disagreeable, dogmatic, dyspeptic old bachelor. His only amusement seemed to be to talk about business. About once a month he went out to see a physician, who was the only friend he had. With this friend he also spent his vacations. The patient always lived with his parents until recently when he has moved

across the street from his sister. His mother was staying with his sister since the death of patient's father one year before. Patient and father had never agreed.

Present Illness.—In 1919 the patient had a mild depression from which he recovered after several months.

On January 12, 1926, the patient suddenly began to talk about religion. This was very odd because he never cared for religion before. He said that God appeared to him and had chosen him to do certain things. He kept his coat on all day long and said he would not take it off until God told him to do so. He refused his cereal at breakfast saying that God told him not to eat it. The patient said that he was going to reform everybody and insisted that the whole family should go to church on Sunday mornings. The patient also spoke about his infatuation for his stenographer and the conflict he had in connection with her, as she belonged to a different religion. He lay awake nights thinking of what God told him to do. Finally on January 18 he became very excited and when his sister tried to quiet him he suddenly appeared with a razor in his hands. A physician was called in and sent the patient to the hospital.

Physical Examination.—The physical examination on admission showed an undernourished, middle-aged man in fair physical condition. The temperature was 100.2 but on the following day it became normal. The white blood count was 11,800. The examination of urine, blood and spinal fluid was negative.

Mental Status.—The patient's behavior underwent a definite change during the first week. For two days he was very irritable, suspicious, preoccupied and underactive; later more talkative, increasingly cooperative, alert but not overactive. He spoke quite freely about his difficulties after the first few days. The mood changed from an initial elation to a mild depression, not incompatible with his situation. The patient said that for a whole week he has been hearing God's voice which told him to do certain things. This was the reason why he woke up his family at 6:30 a.m. Sunday morning and told them to go to church. He said that the whole world was going to be changed and that his secretary should change her religion. The patient refused to go into details of his experiences when questioned further. The intellectual functions were intact. He had a fair insight in that he realized that he was depressed and worried lately but he felt that the whole situation should also be gone over with other people; *i.e.*, his landlady and his stenographer.

Clinical Course.—After a few days the patient related how shortly before his admission he went out with his stenographer. They had lunch together, and after this the patient felt that he was drugged. He felt that in some way she wanted to break his will. It was interesting that the name of his stenographer was the same as that of the girl with whom he was in love 15 years ago. The patient also spoke of his tremendous attachment to his mother and of his difficulty in breaking away from her. Several months ago, when he wanted to move elsewhere, she began to cry so he remained in the same neighborhood seeing his mother every day. The patient spoke quite freely about his sex life and admitted that the only sex experience he had was in early childhood. Since then he has practiced auto-erotism. He had no special conflict over auto-erotism. With reference to his religious experiences the patient said that he never thought about religion, that his interests were purely material, although his family was fairly religious. Lately he has felt quite worried about religious matters as this seemed to be the obstacle to his marriage to his secretary who was a Catholic.

On the night of January 13, 1926, the patient suddenly woke up in the middle of the night and was told there was a God. It was in the form of a very "strong thought." Another thought came to him that he was a strong Protestant. "A thought came to me that there was a God and other thoughts that I was a strong Protestant.

I loved my mother; I felt that some influence had changed me. I felt God making a direct communication to me . . . . The thought came to me that the stocks in the Elevated Company were going up and I would get par value. I ate breakfast and dinner in my overcoat and hat, I do not know why, it seemed to me that it should be left on. One night since I came here I felt the thoughts coming from under the bed."

The case was seen several times during the staff conferences and it was formulated as a condition arising in a setting of emotional turmoil. The patient's emotional life was blocked due to the fact that the girl with whom he was in love did not reciprocate his feelings.

There was marked tension of the sex instinct, then a formal decision by the girl prevented the expression of the instinct from being carried out.

The patient got along very well while in the hospital and gradually developed a healthier point of view of his problems. Cooperative, and had good insight finally.

He was discharged on April 3, 1926, to his family and after a short vacation was able to resume work. His stenographer resigned but she introduced him to a rather mature and intelligent young woman in whom the patient became very much interested. He married this young woman in 1927, and since that time made a very satisfactory adjustment.

CASE 5.—S.R., female, white, married, age 25, admitted to the hospital February 25, 1927; discharged March 3, 1927. Diagnosis: *dementia praecox.*

Chief Complaint.—The patient was sent to a psychiatric hospital from the city hospital where she was restless, excited and showed a "schizophrenic reaction type."

Family History.—The grandparents are dead and nothing is known about them. The patient's parents came to America from one of the Scandinavian countries and are average people. The patient's father is an eccentric and a very suspicious individual.

Personal History.—The patient is the seventh of nine children. The early developmental history is quite negative. She was always in good health and had the usual children's diseases with good recovery.

As a child she was quite a tomboy, liked to play outdoor games and was a leader in games. The patient graduated from the public school at the age of 13, took a year and a half in high school and then took a business course until she qualified as a stenographer. Her work in school was very good.

The patient was always an active, energetic, industrious person. She was ambitious, full of life, was very much interested in her house and held several positions after marriage. She was extremely affectionate, demonstrative and romantic. She liked to go out a good deal, danced, and was a very good mixer. Although she felt things very keenly she rarely annoyed her husband with her difficulties, realizing that he was under a good deal of stress.

The patient went out with boys as a young girl. When she was 18, she met her husband and married him six months afterward. The patient has one child, a boy of 6 years, to whom she was extremely devoted. There was quite a difficult situation at home on account of the mother-in-law disliking the patient. The patient's husband was petted and babied by his wife. At the same time his mother tried to prejudice him against the patient.

Present Illness.—The patient's husband was a policeman whose work involved a good many dangers and responsibilities. He liked to tell his wife about his work, getting a great deal of sympathy and support from her. In the fall of 1927, when the little boy began to attend school the patient felt that she ought to escort him to school. Her husband ridiculed her anxiety about the boy. She became upset and told the husband that if anything ever happened to the boy she would be through with him. Early in February, 1927,

a policeman in their neighborhood committed suicide. The husband came home, told his wife about the incident and said that such work would drive anybody to suicide. This seemed to have affected the patient and she became depressed afterward. When the husband asked the patient about the cause of her depression she told him that somebody was coming between them and complained about the interference of his parents. She dwelt upon the fact that they were of different religions and said that she would be glad to embrace his faith. The patient cried a good deal and on February 13 she said that her heart was bad and that she was going to die. In the middle of February, 1927, she became very upset, said something was going to hurt her and had a feeling that the chimney was going to fall down and kill her. She said that her house was a house of ill omen. Several times the husband was called away from his work on account of the patient's condition. The family physician advised the husband that he should take his wife to the country for a few days for a rest. About the 20th of February the patient suddenly got up in the middle of the night, dressed, packed her suitcase and said that she was going to her parents. The husband helped his wife to do it. Immediately on her arrival at her father's home the patient commenced to accuse her father and mother of being in league to influence her husband against her. She stayed there that day and the next night the sleeplessness was repeated. She got up and went into her brother's room. She accused him of intending to poison her husband and that he was trying to come between them. Suddenly she left the house, called up the police and asked them to come to her parents' house and rescue her, as something dreadful was going to happen. The husband succeeded in preventing the police from coming, and took her over to the city hospital.

When the husband came to see the patient at the city hospital she accused him of trying to wean the boy away from her and complained of all kinds of peculiar noises in the hospital. She felt that the other patients in the ward were discussing her affairs, swore at her, said that her husband was unfaithful to her and that he was going to steal the boy away from her. The other patients also said that her husband was "four in one," intimating that he was of mixed blood and part Negro. She thought that these voices were "rayed" from someone who was in a trance in one of the other rooms. When her husband visited her at the Boston City Hospital he appeared "funny"—his eyes were glassy and had a peculiar staring expression in them.

A psychiatrist who examined the patient at the city hospital felt that she was psychotic and he recommended her transfer to a psychiatric hospital.

On admission there the physical and neurological examinations were essentially negative. The temperature was 99.2 rectally, but rose to 102 five days afterward for no apparent reason. The blood count on admission was 15,200. Examination of urine and blood was negative.

The patient was very quiet most of the time, talked very little to other patients and brightened up when her husband came to visit her. She looked rather sad and discouraged. She said that she felt sad, unhappy and depressed. The intellectual functions were intact. She expressed a large number of ideas, revolving around her relationship to her husband. She complained that there was a good deal of interference in their home life. She also felt that she was going to be harmed, thought that her husband was going to shoot her rather than shoot himself. She also deplored the fact that she did not adopt her husband's religion. She said that when she was at the city hospital she heard her name being called out over the loud speaker. She denied any hallucinations in the psychiatric hospital. She also said that while at the city hospital she smelled many and various odors. The patient had fair insight in that she realized the difficulties which brought on her illness.

On March 3, 1927, she was transferred to a state hospital. There she was sullen, morose and made very little attempt to get interested in the ward. She was mildly depressed and was quite embarrassed when asked about her illness. She spoke freely about her illness and said that while she was in the psychopathic hospital she saw "studies" of her husband from childhood to manhood. She saw him as a boy, a sailor, and a police officer. She said that she had had many somatic sensations before she came to the hospital and had "funny impressions which seem to spell danger." She could not help but feel that something dreadful was going to happen to her child, and that her husband would blame her if anything happened to him. She had the suspicion that her husband was unfaithful to her, and that he had begun to take "dope," as he seemed very dull and stupid. She intimated that her gastric symptoms may have been due to poison.

Within a few weeks the patient changed a great deal. She began to laugh, appeared happy, talked very freely and spoke a great deal about "radio hypnotism," to which she attributed all her troubles.

The patient's relatives felt that she had improved and insisted upon taking her home. On April 17, 1927, she was discharged on a trial visit. At the state hospital the case was diagnosed as dementia praecox.

After the patient left the hospital she went to visit her relatives in the middle west. There she was entertained a great deal and came back to the city in the fall of 1927. She appeared perfectly well, resumed her care of the house and got a job in a department store during the Christmas rush. In the winter of 1928 she stopped working and devoted herself to the care of her family.

I saw the patient on January 10, 1929, when she came to see me. She was a well-developed, well-nourished, attractive woman, quite cheerful, happy, spoke very freely and frankly about her illness. She, herself, analyzed the whole situation and described the conditions which led to her breakdown. Following Thanksgiving of 1926, the patient moved into a new house which she bought with her own savings. She had a great deal of work to do, putting the house in order, as it was an old house. She wanted to get things done and she did not spare herself. At the same time she was troubled by the fact that the furnace was not working properly and she could smell some gas in the house. She lost her appetite, could not sleep and felt very badly. She vomited on several occasions and became cross, cranky and irritable. Things did not go very well with her personal life. Her husband loved and adored her, but he was under the influence of his mother who disliked the patient. She began to think a great deal about the difference in religion. She was a young woman, full of life and ambition, loved dances, music and people. Her husband, on the other hand, was a man 11 years older than she, and perfectly content to come home in the evening and read the newspaper. She was very ambitious for him and wanted him to take various examinations leading to a higher position on the police force, but he was slow and satisfied with his meager income.

Things began to assume a different aspect. She would occasionally become blue and the coarseness of her husband began to annoy her more than usually. The husband never was much of a ladies' man. She began to feel that he was excessive in his sex demands and that she should be left alone. She thought that he loved the boy a little bit too much, and only cared for her as the mother of his son. She exaggerated the difficulty between her and her husband. The husband's family was doing everything possible to estrange the two.

One night while she was in bed she saw three bright stars from her window. She could not fall asleep. The stars were bright red in color. She did close her eyes, but when she opened them again the stars would still be there. She felt that something terrible was going to happen. This was a bad sign and it meant that the husband should take her to his family, which he did.

The patient stressed the prominence of various physical factors in her psychosis.

A review of the family situation brought out the fact that there was a real foundation for some of the patient's beliefs. Both her family and her husband's family were doing everything possible to estrange the patient and her husband. The patient's father felt that she married a very inferior person, below her station in life. On the other hand, the husband's mother felt that the patient was inferior to her son. With reference to the voices the patient said that she heard the doctor's name called out over the radio at the city hospital, which was so. She denied other hallucinatory experiences.

The patient stated that she was facing essentially the same situation that she faced before, even worse, as the mother-in-law was in the house and constantly picking flaws in the patient. She was not afraid of her, however, because she knew how to manage the family and felt that she had the upper hand. She explained to us at the end of the interview that the whole marriage started out rather unfortunately. During the period of courtship he had attacked her and forced her to have relations with him. He was quite crude in their sex life and tried various perversions. She felt keenly the disgrace of a forced marriage, and would have preferred to marry her husband of her own free will. Her family hated and despised the husband. She was under constant pressure of getting along with her husband whom she really liked, of pleasing her mother-in-law, and of trying to reconciliate her own family with her husband. The patient said that the psychosis was a good thing as somehow it has helped to straighten out the various tangles in her life, and gave her courage, confidence in herself. The patient is doing very well now and handles unusually well the affairs which are just as complicated as they were before.

CASE 8.—E.F., male, age 20, single, laborer, white, admitted to the hospital March 15, 1929; discharged against advice to family, March 24, 1929. Diagnosis: *dementia praecox*.

Chief Complaint.—The patient was sent to the hospital by his family because about two weeks before admission he became overactive, exhibited queer behavior and spoke a great deal about his theories of life. Finally he became so excited that he was taken to the out-patient department from which he was referred to the house.

Family History.—Nothing is known about the patient's grandparents with the exception that they have lived to an old age. The parents were born in one of the southern European countries and settled in the 90's in southern Massachusetts. The father was a fisherman by occupation, was a kind and genial man, but at times drank excessively. He was drowned when the patient was a small child. The mother is an even-tempered woman with a great deal of patience, and is extremely devoted to her children. She has a very poor command of English. The patient is the fourth of seven children. His older sister developed an acute psychosis following the birth of her second child and was in a state hospital for a month. The diagnosis was an affective disorder. She was taken home but later it was necessary to commit her to a state hospital where she is at the present time. One of the patient's older brothers was psychotic in 1920 and was in a mental hospital for 10 days. The diagnosis was dementia praecox—hebephrenic. However, he made a good recovery. In 1926 this brother was arrested, the charge was a sexual offense, and he served a term in jail. He is doing quite well at the present time. It seems that both the psychosis and the sexual assault followed an alcoholic debauch.

The other siblings are fairly well-balanced individuals. There is a very fine family spirit, the children get along well with each other and are devoted to the mother. The family has few outside contacts and seems to have a close home life.

Personal History.—The patient was born in southern Massachusetts on February 21, 1909. The mother had been well throughout the pregnancy, the delivery was uneventful, the patient weighed 12 pounds. The early developmental history was normal. He was a well baby, had only the common children's diseases and exhibited no neurotic traits. At five and a half years patient entered school. He did well, according to mother, but left at the age of 15, after finishing his first year in high school, in order to go to work. The patient liked school, played on the baseball team and was well liked.

The patient did well in the various positions in which he was employed. Two years ago he obtained a job in a large rubber plant and worked up from $16.00 a week to $27.00 a week. He was a model employee, but very quiet and shy. For some time he complained to the factory physician that the work was too hard, but he was able to keep up with it.

As far as his personality is concerned he was quite an average young man. He was the mother's favorite and was much attached to her. He was rather quiet and shy in company, and did not care to go out. His outside interests were mostly athletic. He took part in several sports and played baseball with amateur groups. Baseball was his outstanding interest. He carefully followed the papers and often spoke about his ambition of becoming a professional baseball player. He tried to join one of the national baseball associations but he was rejected because he was too light. He was not much of a day-dreamer; on the contrary, he seemed like an active and energetic boy. He discussed his personal affairs with his family quite freely and was not especially sensitive. He worried often about his mother and took to heart other peoples' troubles. He had a good sense of humor and was not jealous. Like the rest of his family the patient was a devout Catholic. He took religion seriously.

Very little is known about the patient's sex life. He was extremely shy in the presence of girls and did not go out with them. Several months ago he fell in love with a girl who worked in the same factory where he worked and told his family about it. He wanted to bring the girl to the house but the mother told him he was too young to go out with girls. Although the patient spoke about having dates with the girl, she told her foreman that their acquaintance was very casual.

The patient drank some light wines in moderate amounts, as was customary in his family. He was never drunk, and smoked moderately. His reading was mostly confined to the sporting pages of the newspapers and adventure stories.

Present Illness.—Two weeks before admission the co-workers in the factory noticed that the patient began to talk a great deal and that he began to sing very loudly. Quite suddenly he declared that he was going to the stage or else would join a professional baseball team. The same behavior was observed at home. He sent a telegram to a Boston baseball team which was at that time playing in the South, asking the manager for a position. He told his family that he was going to make a great deal of money and they should finance him for the trip. He slept very poorly and was very restless at night. A week before admission he went to one of the Harvard physicians and offered him his body for scientific purposes. The latter referred him to the hospital. He was quite excited for several days and spoke a great deal about scientific experiments on his brain and the cure of insanity. Finally he was brought to the out-patient clinic.

On admission the patient was found to be in good physical condition. There was a slight leucocytosis of 13,800. Examinations of blood and urine were negative.

For several days the patient was quite active and restless, but responded very well to continuous baths. He was very cooperative and talked freely to the physician. He took a fair amount of interest in the ward routine and was friendly with other patients. His speech was relevant but at times incoherent and he spoke about a great many things. The patient spoke a great deal about his phi-

losophy of life giving several variants of his theory of personal magnetism. The main points of his theory were as follows. For some time the patient has had a conflict over auto-erotism which he has practiced since childhood. He also had six relations with a nine-year-old girl when he was of the same age and it disturbed him. The conflict was intensified by the fact that he was quite religious. He met a girl a year ago and fell in love with her, but it took him a long time before he was introduced to her. Finally he asked her for a date, about four months ago. She refused. He felt badly but he asked again three months ago, and she told him she was going to the beach with her parents. He finally got a date about a week prior to his admission to the hospital, they went to her house after the movies, and they "got to loving on the sofa." He felt magnetism go over him when he kissed her, and when he passed his hand over her hair he "felt the flow of magnetism just like in a wet dream."

This was the first time he had the sensation. After this experience all his thoughts were concentrated on her image and it made him desperate. He began to experiment in trying to recall her presence, or trying to imagine he was with her. He would imagine the pillow was her face and then he got the same flow of magnetism on passing his hand over the pillow. He began speculating about causes of this and thought he had made a new discovery.

The patient said that he was able to solve all his conflicts by this discovery. He found that the brain controlled the fluid which traveled throughout the whole body and could be drawn from mouth, teeth, roof of the mouth, lips and nose, if touched. This fluid would travel throughout the whole body producing a magnetic feeling passing over him, the same as a sexual act. When sound hits the ear drum it sets the fluid or brain in vibration and he harmonizes with it, and this pleasurable magnetic feeling passes over him. Similarly when he touches anything gently, this fluid, which is all over the body, is set in motion in waves which similarly give the pleasant feeling. Thus if he goes out with women he gets satisfaction by touch and sound, and he stated that if he leaves his wife for a few days (after he marries) he can go out with women and have no responsibility. Not only did he get this magnetic feeling when he touched an animate object but an inanimate object as well. When in church he felt that the holy images might be alive and that God was in communication with him. He stated that when he expectorated, the saliva was equivalent to spermatic fluid.

He went to Harvard Thursday, March 14, 1929, to tell of his discovery "for the benefit of science" and also because he felt his brain was developing, and for them to take an X-ray of his brain and if it was of any benefit to publish it and teach about it. He was willing to be experimented on if they thought it necessary. He was referred to the out-patient clinic. Friday early in the morning he awoke trembling and took to drawing a diagram of his brain letting his hand take its course.

He came the same morning to out-patient department for the purpose of showing his discovery. His brain was vibrating to all sounds and touch, and it was pleasurable. He felt mixed up in his head, it seemed queer to him the way sound affected him, but he enjoyed it.

"It is a magnetic force from above that is present on earth and is called magnetism and gravity. As the world spins round anything on the earth, if touched by humans, will receive this sensation. The sensation is the same as the sexual act. Misunderstanding in the past has brought shame, suffering, death, illness before death, if a person or any human it matters not what sex, will feel the effect of this sensation from above. The sensation comes from God to man and from man it travels through his body from finger tips to toenails, and if any object is held gently by a human the force of this effect will travel through said object into human, it matters not what sex. This power came to me from God. I'm in communication with God, it seems. It has been only recently that I have made the discovery by experimenting on brain and it has traveled throughout the human body."

The patient said that he could see God if he closed his eyes. He could see God moving about, saw Him moving His fingers and saw His features. He saw God sitting on the throne pointing His fingers and controlling the movement of the world. God never talked to him. At one time he saw God mold clay and blow the breath of life into it.

The patient's intellectual functions were intact. He was well oriented in all fields and his memory was good.

Clinical Course.—Within a few days the patient became quiet, cooperative but still insisted on elaborating his ideas. Commitment to a state institution was recommended but nine days after the patient entered the hospital he was taken home by his family. Within a few weeks he joined one of the branches of the governmental service and has been doing very well in his field of service.

SUMMARY

1. A group of 9 cases is presented in which there is a blending of schizophrenic and affective symptoms.

2. The psychosis is characterized by a very sudden onset in a setting of marked emotional turmoil with a distortion of the outside world and presence of false sensory impressions in some cases. The psychosis lasts a few weeks to a few months and is followed by a recovery.

3. Our patients are young people, in the twenties or thirties, in excellent physical health, in whom there is usually a history of a previous attack in late adolescence.

4. The prepsychotic personalities of our patients show the usual variation found in any group of people.

5. A good social and industrial adjustment, the presence of a definite and specific environmental stress, the interest in life and its opportunities, and the absence of any passivity or withdrawal are some of the factors favoring recovery.

REFERENCES

1. Kraepelin, Emil: Dementia Praecox and Paraphrenias, Edinburgh, 1919.
2. Meyer, Adolf: A Fundamental Conception of Dementia Praecox, British Medical Journal, 2:757, 1906.
3. Bleuler, E.: Lehrbuch der Psychiatric, 3 Auflage, Berlin, Julius Springer, 1920.
4. Lange, J.: Katatonische Erscheinungen in Rahmen Manischer Erkrankungen, Berlin, Julius Springer, 1922.
5. Bowman, Karl M., and Raymond, Alice F.: A Statistical Study of Delusions in the Manic-Depressive Psychoses, Proceedings of the Association for Research in Nervous and Mental Diseases, Vol. XI, Williams and Wilkins Co., 1931.
6. Dunton, W.R., Jr.: The Cyclic Forms of Dementia Praecox, American Journal of Insanity, 66:465, 1910.
7. Dunton, W.R., Jr.: The Intermittent Forms of Dementia Praecox, Proceedings of the American Medico-Psychological Association, 17: 239, 1910.
8. Lewis, Nolan D.C., and Hubbard, Lois D.: The Mechanisms and Prognostic Aspects of the Manic-Depressive Schizophrenic Combinations, Proceedings of the Association for Research in Nervous and Mental Diseases, Vol. XI, Williams and Wilkins Co., 1931.
9. Claude, Henri, Borel, S., et Robin, Gilbert: Démence Précoce, Schizomanie et Schizophrenie, L'Encephale, 19:145, 1924.
10. Claude, Henri: Schizomanie à Forme Imaginative, L'Encephale, 25: 10, 1930.

Symptomatology and Management of Acute Grief

By Erich Lindemann, M.D.

Instructor of Psychiatry, Harvard Medical School, Boston, Massachusetts

Introduction

At first glance, acute grief would not seem to be a medical or psychiatric disorder in the strict sense of the word but rather a normal reaction to a distressing situation. However, the understanding of reactions to traumatic experiences whether or not they represent clear-cut neuroses has become of ever-increasing importance to the psychiatrist. Bereavement or the sudden cessation of social interaction seems to be of special interest because it is often cited among the alleged psychogenic factors in psychosomatic disorders. The enormous increase in grief reactions due to war casualties, furthermore, demands an evaluation of their probable effect on the mental and physical health of our population.

The points to be made in this paper are as follows:

1. Acute grief is a definite syndrome with psychological and somatic symptomatology.

2. This syndrome may appear immediately after a crisis; it may be delayed; it may be exaggerated or apparently absent.

3. In place of the typical syndrome there may appear distorted pictures, each of which represents one special aspect of the grief syndrome.

4. By appropriate techniques these distorted pictures can be successfully transformed into a normal grief reaction with resolution.

Our observations comprise 101 patients. Included are 1) psychoneurotic patients who lost a relative during the course of treatment, 2) relatives of patients who died in the hospital, 3) bereaved disaster victims (Cocoanut Grove Fire) and their close relatives, 4) relatives of members of the armed forces.

The investigation consisted of a series of psychiatric interviews. Both the timing and the content of the discussions were recorded. These records were subsequently analysed in terms of the symptoms reported and of the changes in mental status observed progressively through a series of interviews. The psychiatrist avoided all suggestions and interpretations until the picture of symptomatology and spontaneous reaction tendencies of the patients had become clear from the records. The somatic complaints offered important leads for objective study. Careful laboratory work on spirograms, g.-i. functions, and metabolic studies are in progress and will be reported separately. At present we wish to present only our psychological observations.

Symptomatology of Normal Grief

The picture shown by persons in acute grief is remarkably uniform. Common to all is the following syndrome: sensations of somatic distress occurring in waves lasting from twenty minutes to an hour at a time, a feeling of tightness in the throat, choking with shortness of breath, need for sighing, and an empty feeling in the abdomen, lack of muscular power, and an intense subjective distress described as tension or mental pain. The patient soon learns that these waves of discomfort can be precipitated by visits, by mentioning the deceased, and by receiving sympathy. There is a tendency to avoid the syndrome at any cost, to refuse visits lest they should precipitate the reaction, and to keep deliberately from thought all references to the deceased.

The striking features are 1) the marked tendency to sighing respiration; this respiratory disturbance was most conspicuous when the patient was made to discuss his grief. 2) The complaint about lack of strength and exhaustion is universal and is described as follows: "It is almost impossible to climb up a stairway." "Everything I lift seems so heavy." "The slightest effort makes me feel exhausted." "I can't walk to the corner without feeling exhausted." 3) Digestive symptoms are described as follows: "The food tastes like sand." "I have no appetite at all." "I stuff the food down because I have to eat." "My saliva won't flow." "My abdomen feels hollow." "Everything seems slowed up in my stomach."

The sensorium is generally somewhat altered. There is commonly a slight sense of unreality, a feeling of increased emotional distance from other people (sometimes they appear shadowy or small), and there is intense preoccupation with the image of the deceased. A patient who lost his daughter in the Cocoanut Grove disaster visualized his girl in the telephone booth calling for him and was much troubled by the loudness with which his name was called by her and was so vividly preoccupied with the scene that he became oblivious of his surroundings. A young navy pilot lost a close friend; he remained a vivid part of his imagery, not in terms of a religious survival but in terms of an imaginary

Read at the Centenary Meeting of The American Psychiatric Association, Philadelphia, Pa., May 15–18, 1944. From the Department of Diseases of the Nervous System, Harvard Medical School and the Department of Psychiatry, Massachusetts General Hospital.

companion. He ate with him and talked over problems with him, for instance, discussing with him his plan of joining the Air Corps. Up to the time of the study, six months later, he denied the fact that the boy was no longer with him. Some patients are much concerned about this aspect of their grief reaction because they feel it indicates approaching insanity.

Another strong preoccupation is with feelings of guilt. The bereaved searches the time before the death for evidence of failure to do right by the lost one. He accuses himself of negligence and exaggerates minor omissions. After the fire disaster the central topic of discussion for a young married woman was the fact that her husband died after he left her following a quarrel, and of a young man whose wife died that he fainted too soon to save her.

In addition, there is often disconcerting loss of warmth in relationship to other people, a tendency to respond with irritability and anger, a wish not to be bothered by others at a time when friends and relatives make a special effort to keep up friendly relationships.

These feelings of hostility, surprising and quite inexplicable to the patients, disturbed them and again were often taken as signs of approaching insanity. Great efforts are made to handle them, and the result is often a formalized, stiff manner of social interaction.

The activity throughout the day of the severely bereaved person shows remarkable changes. There is no retardation of action and speech; quite to the contrary, there is a push of speech, especially when talking about the deceased. There is restlessness, inability to sit still, moving about in an aimless fashion, continually searching for something to do. There is, however, at the same time, a painful lack of capacity to initiate and maintain organized patterns of activity. What is done is done with lack of zest, as though one were going through the motions. The bereaved clings to the daily routine of prescribed activities; but these activities do not proceed in the automatic, self-sustaining fashion which characterizes normal work but have to be carried on with effort, as though each fragment of the activity became a special task. The bereaved is surprised to find how large a part of his customary activity was done in some meaningful relationship to the deceased and has now lost its significance. Especially the habits of social interaction—meeting friends, making conversation, sharing enterprises with others—seem to have been lost. This loss leads to a strong dependency on anyone who will stimulate the bereaved to activity and serve as the initiating agent.

These five points—1) somatic distress, 2) preoccupation with the image of the deceased, 3) guilt, 4) hostile reactions, and 5) loss of patterns of conduct—seem to be pathognomonic for grief. There may be added a sixth characteristic, shown by patients who border on pathological reactions, which is not so conspicuous as the others but nevertheless often striking enough to color the whole picture. This is the appearance of traits of the deceased in the behavior of the bereaved, especially symptoms shown during the last illness, or behavior which may have been shown at the time of the tragedy. A bereaved person is observed or finds himself walking in the manner of his deceased father. He looks in the mirror and believes that his face appears just like that of the deceased. He may show a change of interests in the direction of the former activities of the deceased and may start enterprises entirely different from his former pursuits. A wife who lost her husband, an insurance agent, found herself writing to many insurance companies offering her services with somewhat exaggerated schemes. It seemed a regular observation in these patients that the painful preoccupation with the image of the deceased described above was transformed into preoccupation with symptoms or personality traits of the lost person, but now displaced to their own bodies and activities by identification.

COURSE OF NORMAL GRIEF REACTIONS

The duration of a grief reaction seems to depend upon the success with which a person does the *grief work*, namely, emancipation from the bondage to the deceased, readjustment to the environment in which the deceased is missing, and the formation of new relationships. One of the big obstacles to this work seems to be the fact that many patients try to avoid the intense distress connected with the grief experience and to avoid the expression of emotion necessary for it. The men victims after the Cocoanut Grove fire appeared in the early psychiatric interviews to be in a state of tension with tightened facial musculature, unable to relax for fear they might "break down." It required considerable persuasion to yield to the grief process before they were willing to accept the discomfort of bereavement. One assumed a hostile attitude toward the psychiatrist, refusing to allow any references to the deceased and rather rudely asking him to leave. This attitude remained throughout his stay on the ward, and the prognosis for his condition is not good in the light of other observations. Hostility of this sort was encountered on only occasional visits with the other patients. They became willing to accept the grief process and to embark on a program of dealing in memory with the deceased person. As soon as this became possible there seemed to be a rapid relief of tension and the subsequent interviews were rather animated conversations in which the deceased was idealized and in which misgivings about the future adjustment were worked through.

Examples of the psychiatrist's rôle in assisting patients in their readjustment after bereavement are contained in the following case histories. The first shows a very successful readjustment.

A woman, aged 40, lost her husband in the fire. She had a history of good adjustment previously. One child, ten years old. When she heard about her husband's death she was extremely depressed, cried bitterly, did not want to live, and for three days showed a state of utter dejection.

When seen by the psychiatrist, she was glad to have assistance and described her painful preoccupation with memories of her husband and her fear that she might lose her mind. She had a vivid visual image of his presence, picturing him as going to work in the morning and herself as wondering whether he would return in the evening, whether she could stand his not returning, then, describing to herself how he does return, plays with the dog, receives his child, and gradually tried to accept the fact that he is not there any more. It was only after ten days that she succeeded in accepting his loss and then only after having described in detail the remarkable qualities of her husband, the tragedy of his having to stop his activities at the pinnacle of his success, and his deep devotion to her.

In the subsequent interviews she explained with some distress that she had become very much attached to the examiner and that she waited for the hour of his coming. This reaction she considered disloyal to her husband but at the same time she could accept the fact that it was a hopeful sign of her ability to fill the gap he had left in her life. She then showed a marked drive for activity, making plans for supporting herself and her little girl, mapping out the preliminary steps for resuming her old profession as secretary, and making efforts to secure help from the occupational therapy department in reviewing her knowledge of French.

Her convalescence, both emotional and somatic, progressed smoothly, and she made a good adjustment immediately on her return home.

A man of 52, successful in business, lost his wife, with whom he had lived in happy marriage. The information given him about his wife's death confirmed his suspicions of several days. He responded with a severe grief reaction, with which he was unable to cope. He did not want to see visitors, was ashamed of breaking down, and asked to be permitted to stay in the hospital on the psychiatric service, when his physical condition would have permitted his discharge, because he wanted further assistance. Any mention of his wife produced a severe wave of depressive reaction, but with psychiatric assistance he gradually become willing to go through this painful process, and after three days on the psychiatric service he seemed well enough to go home.

He showed a high rate of verbal activity, was restless, needed to be occupied continually, and felt that the experience had whipped him into a state of restless overactivity.

As soon as he returned home he took an active part in his business, assuming a post in which he had a great many telephone calls. He also took over the rôle of amateur psychiatrist to another bereaved person, spending time with him and comforting him for his loss. In his eagerness to start anew, he developed a plan to sell all his former holdings, including his house, his furniture, and giving away anything which could remind him of his wife. Only after considerable discussion was he able to see that this would mean avoiding immediate grief at the price of an act of poor judgment. Again he had to be encouraged to deal with his grief reactions in a more direct manner. He has made a good adjustment.

With eight to ten interviews in which the psychiatrist shares the grief work, and with a period of from four to six weeks, it was ordinarily possible to settle an uncomplicated and undistorted grief reaction. This was the case in all but one of the 13 Cocoanut Grove fire victims.

MORBID GRIEF REACTIONS

Morbid grief reactions represent distortions of normal grief. The conditions mentioned here were transformed into "normal reactions" and then found their resolution.

a. *Delay of Reaction*—The most striking and most frequent reaction of this sort is *delay* or *postponement*. If the bereavement occurs at a time when the patient is confronted with important tasks and when there is necessity for maintaining the morale of others, he may show little or no reaction for weeks or even much longer. A brief delay is described in the following example.

A girl of 17 lost both parents and her boy friend in the fire and was herself burned severely, with marked involvement of the lungs. Throughout her stay in the hospital her attitude was that of cheerful acceptance without any sign of adequate distress. When she was discharged at the end of the three weeks she appeared cheerful, talked rapidly, with a considerable flow of ideas, seemed eager to return home and assume the rôle of parent for her two younger siblings. Except for slight feelings of "lonesomeness" she complained of no distress.

This period of griefless acceptance continued for the next two months, even when the household was dispersed and her younger siblings were placed in other homes. Not until the end of the tenth week did she begin to show a true state of grief with marked feelings of depression, intestinal emptiness, tightness in her throat, frequent crying, and vivid preoccupation with her deceased parents.

That this delay may involve years became obvious first by the fact that patients in acute bereavement about a recent death may soon upon exploration be found preoccupied with grief about a person who died many years ago. In this manner a woman of 38, whose mother had died recently and who had responded to the mother's death with a surprisingly severe reaction, was found to be but mildly concerned with her mother's death but deeply engrossed with unhappy and perplexing fantasies concerning the death of her brother, who died twenty years ago under dramatic circumstances from metastasizing carcinoma after amputation of his arm had been postponed too long. The discovery that a former unresolved grief reaction may be precipitated in the course of the discussion of another recent event was soon demonstrated in psychiatric interviews by patients who showed all the traits of a true grief reaction when the topic of a former loss arose.

The precipitating factor for the delayed reaction may be a deliberate recall of circumstances surrounding the death or may be a spontaneous occurrence in the patient's life. A peculiar form of this is the circumstance that a patient develops the grief reaction at the time when he himself is as old as the person who died. For instance, a railroad worker, aged 42, appeared in the psychiatric clinic with a picture which was undoubtedly a grief reaction for which he had no explanation. It turned out that when he was 22, his mother, then 42, had committed suicide.

b. *Distorted Reactions*—The delayed reactions may occur after an interval which was not marked by any abnormal behavior or distress, but in which there developed an *alteration* in the patient's *conduct* perhaps not conspicuous or serious enough to lead him to a psychiatrist. These alterations may be considered as the surface manifestations of an unresolved grief reaction, which may respond to fairly simple and quick psychiatric management if recognized. They may be classified as follows: 1) *overactivity without a sense of loss*, rather with a sense of wellbeing and zest, the activities being of an expansive and adventurous nature and bearing semblance to the activities formerly carried out by the deceased, as described above; 2) *the acquisition of symptoms belonging to the last illness of the deceased*. This type of patient appears in medical clinics and is often labelled hypochondriasis or hysteria. To what extent actual alterations of physiological functions occur under these circumstances will have to be a field of further careful inquiry. I owe to Dr.

Chester Jones a report about a patient whose electrocardiogram showed a definite change during a period of three weeks, which started two weeks after the time her father died of heart disease.

While this sort of symptom formation "by identification" may still be considered as conversion symptoms such as we know from hysteria, there is another type of disorder doubtlessly presenting 3) a recognized *medical disease*, namely, a group of psychosomatic conditions, predominately ulcerative colitis, rheumatoid arthritis, and asthma. Extensive studies in ulcerative colitis have produced evidence that 33 out of 41 patients with ulcerative colitis developed their disease in close time relationship to the loss of an important person. Indeed, it was this observation which first gave the impetus for the present detailed study of grief. Two of the patients developed bloody diarrhea at funerals. In the others it developed within a few weeks after the loss. The course of the ulcerative colitis was strikingly benefited when this grief reaction was resolved by psychiatric technique.

At the level of social adjustment there often occurs a conspicuous 4) *alteration in relationship to friends and relatives* The patient feels irritable, does not want to be bothered, avoids former social activities, and is afraid he might antagonize his friends by his lack of interest and his critical attitudes. Progressive social isolation follows, and the patient needs considerable encouragement in re-establishing his social relationships.

While overflowing hostility appears to be spread out over all relationships, it may also occur as 5) *furious hostility against specific persons*; the doctor or the surgeon are accused bitterly for neglect of duty and the patient may assume that foul play has led to the death. It is characteristic that while patients talk a good deal about their suspicions and their bitter feelings, they are not likely to take any action against the accused, as a truly paranoid person might do.

6) Many bereaved persons struggled with much effort against these feelings of hostility, which to them seem absurd, representing a vicious change in their characters and to be hidden as much as possible. Some patients succeed in hiding their hostility but become wooden and formal, with affectivity and conduct *resembling schizophrenic pictures*. A typical report is this, "I go through all the motions of living. I look after my children. I do my errands. I go to social functions, but it is like being in a play; it doesn't really concern me. I can't have any warm feelings. If I were to have any feelings at all I would be angry with everybody." This patient's reaction to therapy was characterized by growing hostility against the therapist, and it required considerable skill to make her continue interviews in spite of the disconcerting hostility which she had been fighting so much. The absence of emotional display in this patient's face and actions was quite striking. Her face had a mask-like appearance, her movements were formal, stilted, robot-like, without the fine play of emotional expression.

7) Closely related to this picture is a *lasting loss of patterns of social interaction*. The patient cannot initiate any activity, is full of eagerness to be active—restless, can't sleep—but throughout the day he will not start any activity unless "primed" by somebody else. He will be grateful at sharing activities with others but will not be able to make up his mind to do anything alone. The picture is one of lack of decision and initiative. Organized activities along social lines occur only if a friend takes the patient along and shares the activity with him. Nothing seems to promise reward; only the ordinary activities of the day are carried on, and these in a routine manner, falling apart into small steps, each of which has to be carried out with much effort and without zest.

8) There is, in addition, a picture in which a patient is active but in which most of his activities attain a coloring which is *detrimental to his own social and economic existence*. Such patients with uncalled for generosity, give away their belongings, are easily lured into foolish economic dealings, lose their friends and professional standing by a series of "stupid acts," and find themselves finally without family, friends, social status or money. This protracted self-punitive behavior seems to take place without any awareness of excessive feelings of guilt. It is a particularly distressing grief picture because it is likely to hurt other members of the family and drag down friends and business associates.

9) This leads finally to the picture in which the grief reaction takes the form of a straight *agitated depression* with tension, agitation, insomnia, feelings of worthlessness, bitter self-accusation, and obvious need for punishment. Such patients may be dangerously suicidal.

A young man aged 32 had received only minor burns and left the hospital apparently well on the road to recovery just before the psychiatric survey of the disaster victims took place. On the fifth day he had learned that his wife had died. He seemed somewhat relieved of his worry about her fate; impressed the surgeon as being unusually well-controlled during the following short period of his stay in the hospital.

On January 1st he was returned to the hospital by his family. Shortly after his return home he had become restless, did not want to stay at home, had taken a trip to relatives trying to find rest, had not succeeded, and had returned home in a state of marked agitation, appearing preoccupied, frightened, and unable to concentrate on any organized activity. The mental status presented a somewhat unusual picture. He was restless, could not sit still or participate in any activity on the ward. He would try to read, drop it after a few minutes, or try to play pingpong, give it up after a short time. He would try to start conversations, break them off abruptly, and then fall into repeated murmured utterances: "Nobody can help me. When is it going to happen? I am doomed, am I not?" With great effort it was possible to establish enough rapport to carry on interviews. He complained about his feeling of extreme tension, inability to breathe, generalized weakness and exhaustion, and his frantic fear that something terrible was going to happen. "I'm destined to live in insanity or I must die. I know that it is God's will. I have this awful feeling of guilt." With intense morbid guilt feelings, he reviewed incessantly the events of the fire. His wife had stayed behind. When he tried to pull her out, he had fainted and was shoved out by the crowd. She was burned while he was saved. "I should have saved her or I should have died too." He complained about being filled with an incredible violence and did not know what to do about it. The rapport established with him lasted for only brief periods of time. He then would fall back into his state of intense agitation and muttering. He slept poorly even with large sedation. In the course of four days he became somewhat more composed, had longer periods of contact with the psychiatrist, and seemed to feel that he was being understood and might be able to cope with his morbid feelings of guilt and violent impulses. On the sixth day of his hospital stay, however, after skillfully distracting the attention of his special nurse, he jumped through a closed window to a violent death.

If the patient is not conspicuously suicidal, it may nevertheless be true that he has a strong desire for painful experiences, and such patients are likely to desire shock treatment of some sort, which they picture as a cruel experience, such as electrocution might be.

A 28-year-old woman, whose 20 months-old son was accidentally smothered developed a state of severe agitated depression with self-accusation, inability to enjoy anything, hopelessness about the future, overflow of hostility against the husband and his parents, also with excessive hostility against the psychiatrist. She insisted upon electric-shock treatment and was finally referred to another physician who treated her. She responded to the shock treatments very well and felt relieved of her sense of guilt.

It is remarkable that agitated depressions of this sort represent only a small fraction of the pictures of grief in our series.

PROGNOSTIC EVALUATION

Our observations indicate that to a certain extent the type and severity of the grief reaction can be predicted. Patients with obsessive personality make-up and with a history of former depressions are likely to develop an agitated depression. Severe reactions seem to occur in mothers who have lost young children. The intensity of interaction with the deceased before his death seems to be significant. It is important to realize that such interaction does not have to be of the affectionate type; on the contrary, the death of a person who invited much hostility, especially hostility which could not well be expressed because of his status and claim to loyalty, may be followed by a severe grief reaction in which hostile impulses are the most conspicuous feature. Not infrequently the person who passed away represented a key person in a social system, his death being followed by disintegration of this social system and by a profound alteration of the living and social conditions for the bereaved. In such cases readjustment presents a severe task quite apart from the reaction to the loss incurred. All these factors seem to be more important than a tendency to react with neurotic symptoms in previous life. In this way the most conspicuous forms of morbid identification were found in persons who had no former history of a tendency to psychoneurotic reactions.

MANAGEMENT

Proper psychiatric management of grief reactions may prevent prolonged and serious alterations in the patient's social adjustment, as well as potential medical disease. The essential task facing the psychiatrist is that of sharing the patient's grief work, namely, his efforts at extricating himself from the bondage to the deceased and at finding new patterns of rewarding interaction. It is of the greatest importance to notice that not only over-reaction but under-reaction of the bereaved must be given attention, because delayed responses may occur at unpredictable moments and the dangerous distortions of the grief reaction, not conspicuous at first, be quite destructive later and these may be prevented.

Religious agencies have led in dealing with the bereaved. They have provided comfort by giving the backing of dogma to the patient's wish for continued interaction with the deceased, have developed rituals which maintain the patient's interaction with others, and have counteracted the morbid guilt feelings of the patient by Divine Grace and by promising an opportunity for "making up" to the deceased at the time of a later reunion. While these measures have helped countless mourners, comfort alone does not provide adequate assistance in the patient's grief work. He has to accept the pain of the bereavement. He has to review his relationships with the deceased, and has to become acquainted with the alterations in his own modes of emotional reaction. His fear of insanity, his fear of accepting the surprising changes in his feelings, especially the overflow of hostility, have to be worked through. He will have to express his sorrow and sense of loss. He will have to find an acceptable formulation of his future relationship to the deceased. He will have to verbalize his feelings of guilt, and he will have to find persons around him whom he can use as "primers" for the acquisition of new patterns of conduct. All this can be done in eight to ten interviews.

Special techniques are needed if hostility is the most marked feature of the grief reaction. The hostility may be directed against the psychiatrist, and the patient will have such guilt over his hostility that he will avoid further interviews. The help of a social worker or a minister, or if these are not available, a member of the family, to urge the patient to continue coming to see the psychiatrist may be indispensable. If the tension and the depressive features are too great, a combination of benzedrine sulphate, 5–10 mgm. b.i.d., and sodium amytal, 3 gr. before retiring, may be useful in first reducing emotional distress to a tolerable degree. Severe agitated depressive reactions may defy all efforts of psychotherapy and may respond well to shock treatment.

Since it is obvious that not all bereaved persons, especially those suffering because of war casualties, can have the benefit of expert psychiatric help, much of this knowledge will have to be passed on to auxiliary workers. Social workers and ministers will have to be on the look-out for the more ominous pictures, referring these to the psychiatrist while assisting the more normal reactions themselves.

ANTICIPATORY GRIEF REACTIONS

While our studies were at first limited to reactions to actual death, it must be understood that grief reactions are just one form of separation reactions. Separation by death is characterized by its irreversibility and finality. Separation may, of course, occur for other reasons. We were at first surprised to find genuine grief reactions in patients who had not experienced a bereavement but who had experienced separation, for instance with the departure of a member of the family into the armed forces. Separation in this case is not due to death but is under the threat of death. A common picture hitherto not appreciated is a syndrome which we have designated *anticipatory grief*. The patient is so concerned with her adjustment after the potential death of father or son that she goes through all the phases of grief—depression, heightened preoccupation with the departed, a review of all the forms of death which might befall him, and anticipation of the modes of readjustment which might be necessitated by it. While this reaction may well form a safeguard against the impact of a sudden death notice, it can turn out to be of a disadvantage at the occasion of reunion. Several instances of this sort came to our attention when a soldier just returned from the battlefront complained that his wife did not love him anymore and demanded immediate divorce. In such situations apparently the grief work had been done so effectively that the patient has emancipated herself and the readjustment must now be directed towards new interaction. It is important to know this because many family disasters of this sort may be avoided through prophylactic measures.

BIBLIOGRAPHY

Many of the observations are, of course, not entirely new. Delayed reactions were described by Helene Deutsch (1). Shock treatment in agitated depressions due to bereavement has recently been advocated by Myerson (2). Morbid identification has been stressed at many points in the psychoanalytic literature and recently by H.A. Murray (3). The relation of mourning and depressive psychoses has been discussed by Freud (4), Melanie Klein (5), and Abraham (6). Bereavement reactions in war time were discussed by Wilson (7). The reactions after the Cocoanut Grove fire were described in some detail in a chapter of the monograph on this civilian disaster (8). The effect of wartime separations was reported by Rosenbaum (9). The incidence of grief reactions among the psychogenic factors in asthma and rheumatoid arthritis has been mentioned by Cobb, *et al* (10, 11).

1. Deutsch, Helene. Absence of grief. Psychoanalyt Quart., 6:12, 1937.
2. Myerson, Abraham. The use of shock therapy in prolonged grief reactions. New England J. Med., 230:9, Mar. 2, 1944.
3. Murray, H.A. Visual manifestations of personality. Jr. Abn. & Social Psychol., 32:161–184, 1937.
4. Freud, Sigmund. Mourning and melancholia. Collected Papers IV, 288–317; 152–170.
5. Klein, Melanie. Mourning and its relation to manic-depressive states. Internat. J. Psychoan., 21:125–153, 1940.
6. Abraham, C. Notes on the psycho-analytical investigation and treatment of the libido, viewed in the light of mental disorder. Selected Papers.
7. Wilson, A.T.M. Reactive emotional disorders. Practitioner, 146:254–258.
8. Cobb, S., & Lindemann, E. Neuropsychiatric observations after the Cocoanut Grove fire. Ann. Surg., June 1943.
9. Rosenbaum, Milton. Emotional aspects of wartime separations. Family, 24:337–341, 1944.
10. Cobb, S., Bauer, W., and Whitney, I. Environmental factors in rheumatoid arthritis. J.A.M.A., 113:668–670, 1939.
11. McDermott, N., and Cobb, S. Psychogenic factors in asthma. Psychosom. Med., 1:204–341, 1939.
12. Lindemann, Erich. Psychiatric factors in the treatment of ulcerative colitis. In press.

IRRELEVANT AND METAPHORICAL LANGUAGE IN EARLY INFANTILE AUTISM

By Leo Kanner, M.D.

Associate Professor of Psychiatry and Pediatrics,
The Johns Hopkins University School of Medicine, Baltimore, Maryland

During the past few years, I have had occasion to observe 23 children whose extreme withdrawal and disability to form the usual relations to people were noticed from the beginning of life. I have designated this condition as "early infantile autism." Phenomenologically, excessive aloneness and an anxiously obsessive desire for the preservation of sameness are the outstanding characteristics. Memory is often astounding. Cognitive endowment, masked frequently by limited responsiveness, is at least average. Most patients stem from psychometrically superior, though literal-minded and obsessive, families.

This condition offers fascinating problems and opportunities for study from the points of view of genetics, of the psychodynamics of earliest parent-infant relationship, and of its resemblances to the schizophrenias. Among numerous other features, the peculiarities of language present an important and promising basis for investigation. I should like to mention briefly the "mutism" of 8 of the 23 children, which is on rare occasions interrupted by the utterance of a whole sentence in emergency situations; the use of simple verbal negation as magic protection against unpleasant occurrences; the literalness which cannot accept synonyms or different connotations of the same preposition; the self-absorbed inaccessibility which has caused most of the parents to suspect deafness; the echolalia-type repetition of whole phrases; and the typical, almost pathognomonic, pronominal reversals which consist of the child's reference to himself as "you" and to the person spoken to as "I."

Frequently these children say things which seem to have no meaningful connection with the situation in which they are voiced. The utterances impress the audience as "nonsensical," "silly," "incoherent," and "irrelevant." These are the terms used by the reporting parents, physicians and nursery school teachers.

We were fortunate in having opportunities to trace some of these "irrelevant" phrases to earlier sources and to learn that, whenever such tracing was possible, the utterances, though still peculiar and out of place in ordinary conversation, assume definite meaning. I should like to illustrate this with a few characteristic examples:

Paul G., while observed at our clinic at five years of age, was heard saying: "Don't throw the dog off the balcony." There was neither a dog nor a balcony around. The remark therefore sounded irrelevant. It was learned that three years previously he had thrown a toy dog down from the balcony of a London hotel at which the family was staying. His mother, tired of retrieving the toy, had said to him with some irritation: "Don't throw the dog off the balcony." Since that day, Paul, whenever tempted to throw anything, used these words to admonish and check himself.

"Peter eater" was another of Paul's "nonsensical," "irrelevant" expressions. It seemed to have no association with his experiences of the moment. His mother related that, when Paul was two years old, she once recited to him the nursery rhyme about "Peter, Peter, pumpkin eater," while she was busy in the kitchen; just then she dropped a saucepan. Ever since that day Paul chanted the words "Peter eater" whenever he saw anything resembling a saucepan. There was, indeed, in the playroom a toy stove on which sat a miniature pan. It was noted then that Paul, while saying these words, glanced in the direction of the stove and finally picked up the pan, running wildly around with it and chanting "Peter eater" over and over again.

John F., at five years of age, saw Webster's Unabridged Dictionary in the office. He turned to his father and said: "That's where you left the money." In this instance the connection was established by the fact that John's father was in the habit of leaving money for his wife in the dictionary which they had at home. Upon being shown a penny, John said: "That's where play ten pins," as a sort of definition of penny. His father was able to supply the clue. He and John played ten pins at home with a children's set. Every time that John knocked over one of the ten pins, his father gave him a penny.

Elaine C. had been surrounded in her infancy with toy animals of which she was very fond. When she cried, her mother used to point out to her that the toy dog or toy rabbit did not cry. When Elaine was seen at seven years of age, she still kept saying when she was fearful and on the verge of tears: "Rabbits don't cry." "Dogs don't cry." She added a large number of other animals. She went about, when in distress, reiterating the seemingly irrelevant words: "Seals don't cry." "Dinosaurs don't cry." "Crayfishes don't

---

Read at the 102d annual meeting of The American Psychiatric Association, Chicago, Ill., May 27–30, 1946.

cry." She came to use the names of these and other animals in a great variety of connections.

Jay S., not quite four years old, referred to himself as "Blum" whenever his veracity was questioned by his parents. The mystery of this "irrelevance" was explained when Jay, who could read fluently, once pointed to the advertisement of a furniture firm in the newspapers, which said in large letters: "Blum tells the truth." Since Jay had told the truth, he *was* Blum. This analogy between himself as a teller of the truth and Blum does not differ essentially from the designation of a liar as Ananias, a lover as Romeo, or an attractive lad as Adonis. But while these designations are used with the expectation that the listener is familiar with the analogy, the autistic child has his own private, original, individualized references, the semantics of which are transferable only to the extent to which any listener can, through his own efforts, trace the source of the analogy.

The cited examples represent in the main metaphorical expressions which, instead of relying on accepted or acceptable substitutions as encountered in poetry and conversational phraseology, are rooted in *concrete, specific, personal* experiences of the child who uses them. So long as the listener has no access to the original source, the meaning of the metaphor must remain obscure to him, and the child's remark is not "relevant" to any sort of verbal or other situational interchange. Lack of access to the source shuts out any comprehension, and the baffled listener, to whom the remark means nothing, may too readily assume that it has no meaning at all. If the metaphorical reference to Ananias, Romeo or Adonis is not understood, dictionaries, encyclopedias or informed persons can supply the understanding. But the personal metaphors of the autistic children can convey "sense" only through acquaintance with the singular, unduplicated meaning which they have to the children themselves. The only clue can be supplied by the direct observation and recall of the episode which started off the use of each particular metaphorical expression.

Occasionally, though not very often, a chance gesture or remark of the child himself may lead to the understanding of a metaphor. This was the case when Jay S. happened to point to the Blum advertisement. This was also the case when five-year-old Anthony F. solved the puzzle of his frequently expressed fondness for "55." On one occasion, he spoke of his two grandmothers. We knew that one of them had shown little interest in him, while the other had reared him with much patience and affection. Anthony said: "One is 64 [years old], and one is 55. I like 55 best." The seemingly irrelevant preoccupation with a seemingly arbitrary number can now be recognized as being heavily endowed with meaning. It is Anthony's private way of expressing affection for his grandmother.

This phenomenon of metaphorical substitution is very common among our autistic children. Donald T., at seven years of age, was asked the Binet question: "If I were to buy 4 cents worth of candy and give the storekeeper 10 cents, how much money would I get back?" He obviously knew the answer. His reply, however, was not "6 cents" but: "I'll draw a hexagon." Two years previously, at 5 years of age, Donald had been scribbling with crayons; all the while he kept saying seriously and with conviction: "Annette and Cecile make purple." It was learned that Donald had at home five bottles of paint. He named each after one of the Dionne quintuplets. Blue became "Annette," and red became "Cecile." After that, Annette became his word for blue, and Cecile for red. Purple, not being one of the five colors, remained "purple."

It is mainly the private, original frame of reference which makes these substitutions seem peculiar. We witness similar processes in the introduction of trade names for perfumes, wines, cigarettes, cigars, paints and many other items. Etymology abounds with similar derivations. Common usage makes it unnecessary to know the original source in order to get the meaning. An ulster is a certain type of top coat whether or not you connect it with the county in Ireland from which it has its name. You need not know that a serpent is a "creeper" or that a dromedary is a "runner." It does not matter whether or not you know that filibuster is a corrupted form of "freebooter."

The autistic child does not depend upon such prearranged semantic transfers. He makes up his own as he goes along. In fact, he can keep transferring and retransferring to his heart's desire. Gary T., at five years, designated a bread basket as "home bakery." He did not stop there. After this, *every* basket to him became a "home bakery." This was his term for coal basket, waste basket or sewing basket. This procedure, too, has its etymological counterparts. The original meaning of "caput" is transferred from anatomy to anything which, literally or figuratively, is at the top or at the "head," whether this be "captain," the head of a group of people, "capitol," the top of a pillar, or "chapter," the inscription over a section of a book. The transfer does not even stop there for a "chapter" then becomes not only the "heading" of the section but the whole section itself.

From these observations we may safely draw a number of significant conclusions:

1. The seemingly irrelevant and nonsensical utterances of our autistic children are metaphorical expressions in the sense that they represent "figures of speech by means of which one thing is put for another which it only resembles." The Greek word metapherein means "to transfer."

2. The transfer of meaning is accomplished in a variety of ways:

a. Through substitutive analogy: Bread basket becomes "home bakery"; Annette and Cecile become "red" and "blue"; penny becomes "that's where play ten pin."

b. Through generalization: *Totum pro parte.* "Home bakery" becomes the term for *every* basket; "Don't throw the dog off the balcony" assumes the meaning of self-admonition in *every* instance when the child feels the need for admonishing himself.

c. Through restriction: *Pars pro toto.* The 55-year-old grandmother becomes "55"; a teller of the truth becomes "Blum"; the number 6 is referred to as "hexagon."

3. The linguistic processes through which the transfers are achieved do not as such differ essentially from poetical and ordinary phraseological metaphors. Etymologically, much of our language is made up of similar transfers of meaning through substitutions, generalizations and restrictions.

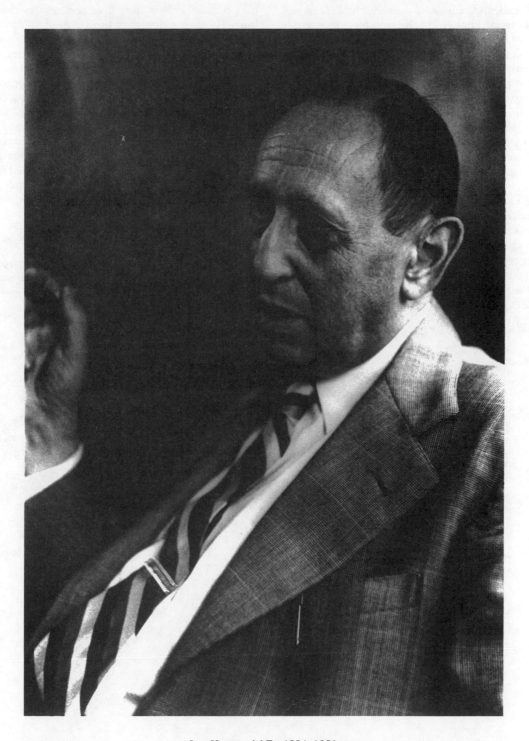
Leo Kanner, M.D., 1894–1981

4. The basic difference consists of the autistic privacy and original uniqueness of the transfers, derived from the children's situational and emotional experiences. Once the connection between experience and metaphorical utterance is established, and only then, does the child's language become meaningful. The goal of the transfer is intelligible only in terms of its source.

5. In contrast to poetry and etymology, the metaphorical language in early infantile autism is not directly communicable. It is not primarily intended as a means of inviting other people to understand and to share the child's symbols. Though it is undoubtedly creative, the creation is in the main self-sufficient and self-contained.

"The abnormality of the autistic person," say Whitehorn and Zipf, "lies only in ignoring the other fellow: that is, it lies in his disregard of the social obligation to make only those changes which are socially acceptable in the sense that they are both understandable and serviceable in the group. Naturally, once the autistic person pursues his own linguistic and semantic paths of least effort, the result may well appear to his perplexed auditor as a disorder of meanings, or even as a disorder of association. Yet the autistic speaker, in making his own language, without the nuisance of satisfying the auditor's needs, may employ the same prin-ciples of linguistic and semantic change as does the normal person, though not with the same care to insure community acceptance."

The above observations and conclusions gain additional importance because they give concrete evidence to the long-felt assumption that similar mechanisms prevail in the "irrelevant," "incoherent," and metaphorical language of adult schizophrenics. in the case of the latter, the earlier and earliest connections and pertinences have often been lost irretrievably, as they have been even for some of the expressions of our children at so early an age. But the examples cited (and the study by Whitehorn and Zipf) justify the conviction that schizophrenic "irrelevance" is not irrelevant to the patient himself and could become relevant to the audience to the extent to which it were possible to find the clues to his private and self-contained metaphorical transfers.

BIBLIOGRAPHY

Kanner, L. Autistic disturbances of affective contact. The Nervous Child, 2:217–250, 1943.

Kanner, L. Early infantile autism. J. Pediat., 25:211–217, 1944.

Whitehorn, J.C., and Zipf, G.K. Schizophrenic language. Arch. Neur. Psychiatr., 49:831–851, 1943.

III. Research: Methods, Mechanisms, and Causes

INTRODUCTION

The articles in this section of the sesquicentennial issue of *The American Journal of Psychiatry*, spanning a century, represent the foundation of the development of methods for the investigation of psychiatric disorders in modern times. Topics covered are of substantive historical interest, and theories, both explicit and implicit, are at once intriguing and embarrassing to the modern psychiatrist. Yet a reflective reading of these articles from the perspective of advances in investigative methods to explore that most challenging scientific frontier, the human mind, will be especially rewarding. First, the methods employed by these psychiatric pioneers derive from the investigations of the great women and men through the history of medicine, emphasizing the rightful place of psychiatry as a full partner among the medical specialties in both its public health importance and its scientific rigor. Second, these methods form the basis of modern explorations. For example, the twin method employed by Kallman in his classic 1946 article on the genetic theory of schizophrenia had its basis in the nineteenth century work of Galton (1). His work has since spawned the sophisticated modern twin studies of investigators such as Kendler (2), Cloninger (3), and Weissman (4).

The methods employed and the methodologic challenges encountered in these historical articles fall into six categories: reflective observation; the importance of accuracy in observation and measurement; the systematic review of data to provide insight into human illness; the analysis of the association of diseases and hypothesized risk factors; the application of unique design and statistical methods to the exploration of complex relationships between nature and nurture in the etiology of disease; and the use of experimental techniques to unlock the secrets of the brain, both in its normal and in pathological states. Each of these categories has precedent in physical medicine and progeny in modern psychiatric investigation.

Reflective observation is as old as recorded medicine. In the fifth century B.C., Hippocrates suggested that the maladies of humans may be associated with both the external as well as the personal environment (5). He encouraged the physician, on entering a city, "to consider the seasons of the year, and what effects each of the seasons produces. Then the winds, the hot and the cold, especially such as are common to all countries, and then such as are peculiar to each locality . . . and the mode in which the inhabitants live, and what are their pursuits, whether they are fond of drinking and eating to excess, and given to indolence, or are fond of exercise and labor." Sigmund Freud encouraged the application of reflective observation to the thoughts and behavior of persons, the substance of psychiatric formulation and diagnosis. Although psychoanalysis as a therapy has fallen on difficult times in an era of "cost effective" medicine, the techniques of observation initiated by Freud have served scholarship not only in psychiatry, but in anthropology, linguistics, and theology as well.

John Whitehorn, in the 1947 volume of the journal, extended the observational method in order to distinguish meaning and cause in the psychodynamics of the patient's mental life. He suggested that "much of one's supervisory assistance to trainees consists in helping them search and sift their facts and sharpen their observations about a patient to gain a well-justified formulation of the meaningfulness of a situation for a patient and the relevance of his reaction thereto . . . . The perception of an issue in a patient's life, which could clarify the meaningfulness of his reaction, is not infrequently misconstrued as if it were the discovery of *the cause* of the patient's illness." He went further to warn that the emphasis by supervisors on etiologic formulations that are too simplistic may lead to the development of "a crop of probe-pushers, clever in case presentations but not very competent in actual management and therapy of real patients." If we substitute DSM-IV diagnosis for case presentations, the warning is as applicable today as a half century ago. Central to all psychiatric method is careful, nonbiased, and nonconstrained observation.

Observation must not only be careful and thorough, it must be accurate and precise in the measurement of phenomena. Perhaps Darwin is our best example of taking care in observation not to overlook even the most minute variation and to record data accurately. Darwin's genius derived not from his theory of natural selection (the theory was not unique to Darwin); instead, it derived from his careful, logical, and perhaps overdetermined recording of data to support his theories. In the *Origin of Species* he described, in perhaps boring detail, his detailed and precise observations of domestic pigeons. "I have kept every breed which I could purchase or obtain . . . In the skeletons of several breeds, the development of the bones of the face in length and breadth and curvature differs enormously" (6). From these and multiple other observations, recorded with great precision, he substantiated his theory and revolutionized biological science.

Two articles in this section emphasize the importance of precise and accurate measurement to psychiatric investigations. N.S. Davis, in 1845, responded to the difficulties that psychiatrists might encounter in medicolegal settings. "Perhaps there is no one thing which tends more strongly to degrade the medical profession, in the estimation of enlightened men, than the various, uncertain, and often grossly contradictory testimony given by different medical men, on the same case in our courts of justice . . . . Doubtless by far the most prevalent cause, is the great carelessness and want of proper and minute investigation, on the part of the great body of physicians." He proceeded to describe the lack of precision in post-mortem analysis of specimens of brain and the propensity to "infer *a priori*, that disease in these respective portions of the brain, would be accompanied by derangement of the corresponding functions." He concluded with a warning that is as relevant today as it was a century ago. "It is proverbial that medical science abounds in false *theories*; but we believe even a slight examination will show that *false facts* are far more numerous than theories."

Adolf Meyer, in 1896, continued this theme. To dismiss this treatise on the basis of a now defunct theory—phrenology—is to miss the point of its inclusion in this section. No psychiatrist was more concerned with correct theory and the empirical testing of theories of psychopathology than Meyer. If the myriad of theories about body type, facial expression, and anthropomorphic characteristics of body parts were to be proven or dismissed, then a precise description of the physical structures must be developed. Meyer recognized that "the practical value of our *present* knowledge of the signs of degeneration is perhaps overrated by those who believe they have found a scientific phrenology. Probably for a long time to come the study of the mental capacity and potentiality will be best carried out by studying the psychical manifestations rather than the physical forms of a person." Yet he knew that if phrenology was to be systematically investigated, agreement in methods and instrumentation was essential. "In order not to rely only on our own observation, and in order to sum up our work, we must agree on definite methods . . . ." Later in the article he emphasized the importance of standardized instrumentation. "It is evident that one of the first conditions of work is excellence of the tools, of the measuring and recording instruments." Modern psychiatric investigators have available to them multiple and complex techniques for probing the structure and function of the brain. If these techniques are to advance our knowledge of psychiatric disorders, the instruments from various laboratories must be comparable and the measurement procedures standardized.

The application of statistics to the understanding of human illness was implemented by a haberdasher in London during the seventeenth century, John Graunt. He published *The Nature and Political Observations Made Upon the Bills of Mortality* in 1662, in which he analyzed the reports provided weekly of births and deaths in the city. This compendium permitted him to quantify the patterns of disease in the population through time (7, 8). As a result, he recognized the excess of both births and deaths in men compared to women. He also documented the ebbs and flows of the plague that devastated London during the seventeenth century.

Amariah Brigham, editor of *The American Journal of Insanity* in 1849, recognized the importance of collecting such descriptive statistics. For an intelligent readership, "we cannot believe that any harm whatever has resulted even from the occasionally defective tabular statements that have been published in reports upon insanity. On the contrary we cannot doubt in the least, that great, very great good has resulted from the publications of the statistics of institutions for the insane, and we have no hesitation in expressing our firm conviction that but for the statistical facts thus made known to the public, several of the best establishments for the insane in this country would not now be in existence." Brigham believed that clinicians could review the data presented, draw conclusions, and recognize potential bias, the elements of modern clinical epidemiology. His list of baseline data is virtually as relevant today as it was during the earliest days of the journal: "1. Time of admission. 2. Name. 3. Sex. 4. Married or single. 5. Occupation. 6. Place of residence. 7. By whom sent . . . . 14. Duration of present attack. 15. Number of previous attacks. 16. Age on first attack . . . . 20. How discharged; Recovered; Relieved; not improved; Died."

William Farr was among the first physicians to analyze public health data in order to determine if an association could be found between putative risk factors and disease (8, 9). Among the relationships identified by Farr was that between mortality and exposure to toxins related to the occupations of workers in Britain, such as metal mines and the earthenware industry. In the process of establishing these associations, Farr was forced to confront many of the methodological problems, such as the need for large numbers of population and biological inferences. "When the number of cases is considerable the relative mortality is most correctly expressed and . . . slight differences deserve little attention" (9, 10).

Karl Menninger, in his 1926 study of the relationship between influenza and a schizophrenic-like syndrome, employed the methods of Farr to establish that the apparent postinfluenza "dementia precox" following the influenza epidemic of 1918 was actually a separate syndrome. The construct of dementia precox, as delineated by Kraepelin, had not been formulated before previous influenza epidemics, and therefore Menninger had the opportunity to observe the relationship between the syndrome and influenza in a large sample for the first time. Unlike schizophrenia, the postinfluenza syndrome was followed by complete recovery in two-thirds of the subjects who could be traced. The association between the environmental agent and the disease was clear, and the unique clinical course of the syndrome substantiated separating these "toxic-infectious" psychoses from dementia precox.

The geographer, explorer, inventor, and statistician Francis Galton introduced the twin method to explore the relationship between nature and nurture in both normal behavior and disease (1, 12). Galton's basic question was whether twins who were alike at birth became more dissimilar in their anthropomorphic characteristics as a consequence of any dissimilarities in their nurture. He recognized the two types of twins, monozygotic and dizygotic. Among 35 monozygotic pairs (although he did not label them as such) reared under highly similar conditions, the similarities persisted into adulthood and after the twins had gone their separate ways. Among the 25 dizygotic pairs, they began to diverge from birth in characteristics. Galton concluded that nature prevails enormously over nurture.

Franz Kallman applied this same method, although with considerable more methodological rigor, in 1946, to the study of the nature-nurture controversy regarding schizophrenia. He included in his analysis family history, although he recognized the deficits in using pedigrees alone. "If the mating of two psychotic parents is found . . . to be capable of giving rise to seven definite cases of schizophrenia among the offspring . . . it would seem inadequate to disregard the possible significance of the biological factor prerequisite for inheritance . . . . On the basis of this single observation, however, the genetic hypothesis would be no more conclusive than either the assumption of *folie à neuf* due to 'psychic contagion' . . . ." He therefore encouraged the use of the twin family method, which remains the basis of population twin studies even today. Kallman recognized the importance of allowing for a combination of hereditary and environmental in the etiologic hypothesis. Modern statistical procedures have enabled us to quantify these relative contributions.

Claude Bernard, by most accounts, was the father of experimental medicine. He set down many of his observations in his *Introduction to the Study of Experimental Medicine* in 1865 (12). In contrast to Farr and Graunt, he believed the most useful path for advancing our understanding of physiology and medicine was to seek to discover new facts instead of trying to reduce to equations the facts that science already possessed. Subsequently he "discovered" the vasomotor nerves, the nature of curare on muscle function, the functions of the pancreatic juice in digestion, and the elucidation of the glycogenic function of the liver. Central to all of his discoveries was an enhanced understanding of the organ systems of the body in both their normal and abnormal function.

Seymour Kety and his colleagues followed in the tradition of Bernard. First they developed a procedure—the nitrous oxide technique—for exploring the normal physiological function of the brain through the window of cerebral blood flow. The noninvasive technique developed by these scientists has continued, virtually unaltered, as a tool of the neuropsychiatrist to this day. In their 1948 article in the journal, they applied this technique to understanding the pathophysiology of schizophrenia. Although their findings were negative, they recognized the future applicability of their procedure: "Our experience with this technique leads us to believe that it is worthy of extensive application in the study of the metabolic derangements in the brain associated with mental disease. It makes possible a new approach to psychiatric disorders, and gives the means of quantitatively determining the utilization or production of any substance capable of accurate analysis in the arterial and internal jugular venous blood."

Finally, Lawrence C. Kolb, in 1949, reminds us that some things never change, such as the lack of resources to fund quality research in psychiatry. The National Institute of Mental Health (NIMH) was established in 1948 under the auspices of the National Mental Health Act. Originally a part of the National Institutes of Health (NIH), NIMH left NIH in 1966, only to return recently. Concurrent with the formation of NIMH, Congress established the Mental Health Council and the Mental Health Research Study Section. Kolb noted that "Sufficient funds have never been available to support the total number of projects considered meritorious by the Advisory Council. At the present time 31 approved projects amounting to a total request of $377,272 remain uninitiated for this reason." Kolb also provides some insight into the workings of the multidisciplinary group. How could they decide which science is most worthy?

Some might state that the failure of the committee to agree that one or another area of investigation should have priority expresses a lack of decisiveness in regard to investigative opportunities in the field of psychiatry. However, it is doubtful that the way of a developing science has ever been along fixed and clearly predetermined paths. The committee has always supported the philosophy that any project should be considered solely on its merit; the merit to be determined on the competence of the investigator, the facilities available to him for carrying out the proposed plan, the delineation of the hypothesis to be tested, and the precision of the methodology outlined.

Let us hope and trust this will never change!

REFERENCES

1. Galton F: Hereditary Genius: An Inquiry Into Its Laws and Consequences. London, Macmillan, 1876
2. Kendler KS, Gruenberg AM, Tsuang MT: A family study of the subtypes of schizophrenia. Am J Psychiatry 1988; 145:57–62
3. Cloninger CR Bohman M Sigvardsson S: Inheritance of alcohol abuse: cross-fostering analysis of adopted men. Arch Gen Psychiatry 1981; 38:861–869
4. Weissman MM, Kidd KK, Prusoff BP: Variability in rates of affective disorders in relatives of depressed and normal probands. Arch Gen Psychiatry 1987; 39:1397–1403
5. Hippocrates: On airs, waters, and places, in Medical Classics, vol 3. Edited by Kelly EC. Baltimore, William Wood & Co, 1938, p 19
6. Darwin C: On the Origin of Species by Means of Natural Selection, or the Preservation of Favored Races in the Struggle for Life (1859). New York, Modern Library, 1967
7. Graunt J: Natural and Political Observations Made Upon Bills of Mortality (1662). Baltimore, Johns Hopkins Press, 1939
8. Hennekens CH, Buring JE: Epidemiology in Medicine. Boston, Little, Brown, 1987
9. Humphries NA (ed): Vital Statistics: A Memorial Volume of Selections From the Reports and Writings of William Farr, 1807–1883. London, Sanitary Institute of Great Britain, 1885
10. Lilienfeld DE, Lilienfeld AM: Epidemiology: a retrospective study. Am J Epidemiol 1977; 106:445–459
11. Plomin R, DeFries JC, McClearn GE: Behavioral Genetics: A Primer, 2nd ed. New York, WH Freeman, 1990
12. Bernard C: An Introduction to the Study of Experimental Medicine (1865). Translated by Green HC. New York, Dover Publications, 1957

DAN G. BLAZER, M.D., PH.D.

The Importance of a Correct Physiology of the Brain, as Applied to the Elucidation of Medico-Legal Questions; and the Necessity of Greater Accuracy and Minuteness in Reporting Post Mortem Examinations

By N.S. Davis, M.D.

Binghamton, New York

That some of the principles of Phrenology, if true, are not only of great practical importance in enabling us to determine from certain symptoms, more definitely, the nature and extent of many affections of the brain; but by affording a more definite idea of the natural functions of each individual part of the cerebral structure, greatly assists also in drawing rational conclusions from morbid appearances after death, can not be doubted. Perhaps there is no one thing which tends more strongly to degrade the medical profession, in the estimation of enlightened men, than the various, uncertain, and often grossly contradictory testimony given by different medical men, on the same case in our courts of justice. A great variety of cases are continually occurring, in which the testimony of physicians is required; and what other inference can be drawn from their conflicting statements and conclusions, made up ostensibly from the same facts, than that the whole is a mere system of "guessing" —"a pretended science without a singly permanent and well-established principle for its foundation." For instance, in testing the validity of a will, the attending physician is called, testifies that testator while making the will, was laboring under inflammation of the brain sufficient to confine him to bed, and to render active and direct depletion necessary—and further, that individuals under such circumstances, *would* be *likely* to retain *full possession* of their *mental* faculties.

Another of equal celebrity is called, and testifies with much apparent certainty, that a patient under such circumstances would *not* be likely to have possession of his mental faculties. A third equally entitled to confidence, comes forward and maintains that the brain is composed of a number of distinct organs, performing different functions; and that all would, therefore, depend on the particular organ or organs affected. If we suppose, as we are bound to do, that each of the witnesses is equally entitled to credit; is it not evident that no conclusion whatever can be legitimately drawn from their testimony. And yet, more contradictions than in the case supposed, are almost daily occurring before our various legal tribunals—to what then are they owing? To carelessness of observation, and want of candid investigation; or is it some radical defect or uncertainty in the science itself?

Doubtless by far the most prevalent cause, is the great carelessness and want of proper and minute investigation, on the part of the great body of physicians. Being often taught as a part of their primary education, the mental or metaphysical philosophy of the schools; and thus habituated to contemplate the mind unconnected with its physical organ, the brain; they too often enter upon, and even become eminent in the practice of their profession, without even investigating closely the connection between the mind and brain, and much less arriving at any clear and rational conclusions concerning it. But if it is true that the cortical or gray substance of the brain, is the seat of the mental operations, and the white or fibrous portion, like the nerves only transmitting in its functions; then we should infer *a priori*, that disease in these respective portions of the brain, would be accompanied by derangement of the corresponding functions. And further, if this cortical portion is again made up of as many distinct organs as there are separate mental faculties, then we should equally expect to find disease in any one of these organs always accompanied by derangement of the corresponding faculty. And hence, we not only arrive at definite conclusions concerning the functions of different portions of the brain, but we are prepared on the appearance of certain symptoms, or the derangement of certain mental faculties, to predict the location and extent of the disease; or on the appearance of certain morbid changes after death, to determine with some degree of accuracy, the symptoms and mental disorders which must have preceded. The direct practical bearing, and the importance of these views can not be doubted. The only question then, is, whether the fundamental propositions on which they are based are in fact true? If we appeal to morbid anatomy, the two following questions meet us for a candid examination:

1st. Is there a case on record, in which morbid appearances were observed in corresponding portions of the cortical substance of the brain, in both hemispheres, when the patient had not previously manifested corresponding mental derangement?

2d. Is there a case on record in which the morbid appearances were confined exclusively to the medullary substance, in which mental derangement had been present to any considerable extent?

Having carefully examined every thing within our reach, touching the subject, we must thus far answer the first question in the negative. It must be remembered that the question is not whether lesions of greater or less extent have been found in *one* hemisphere, without mental disturbance; neither is it whether organic lesions are perceptible in the brain, in every case where death takes place during the existence of insanity. As well might we suppose that plucking out the right eye would invariably destroy vision in the left also; or that organic lesions in the lungs would be found in every case of death, during difficult or disturbed respiration.

Destroying one eye might indeed lessen the field of vision, and so might destruction or disease of a portion, or the whole of one hemisphere of the brain, greatly lessen the strength and vigor of the mind. But has corresponding portions of the cortical substance of both hemispheres been found diseased, without derangement or destruction of some faculty of the mind? As we have already stated, we have yet been unable to find any such instance.

But it must be confessed that the subject is attended with some difficulty, on account of the ambiguity and indefiniteness, which characterize many reports of cerebral disease. Witness the following for example, taken from the Lancet, for Aug. 8, 1840. "A female aged sixty, had been declining in health for three or four years; and suffered occasional attacks of rheumatism. Of late her symptoms resembled those of subacute inflammation of the mucous membrane of the stomach. She vomited the blandest articles, and accompanying this, was a constant and severe headache over the right eyebrow. The headache, however, was always relieved for a time by the vomiting. But she continued to fail; and one day on being carried up stairs, her head struck with violence against the staircase. It produced no change in the symptoms—there was nothing to indicate an injury or disease of the brain, but she finally sunk, fourteen days after the blow. On dissection, the stomach was found contracted, its mucous membrane vascular, and there was a tumor adhering to the pylorus and duodenum. The membranes of the brain appeared healthy, and the left hemisphere was of its natural appearance, but on opening into the right, several ounces of coagulated blood were discovered. The walls of the cavity containing it, were of the consistency of cream. The blood had merely separated into serum and crassamentum." This case is reported as having an important bearing on Medico-Legal investigations; but what inference can be drawn from it, beyond the simple fact that a quantity of blood was found in the right hemisphere of the brain, around which the cerebral substance was altered in structure? But the questions, whether the disease implicated those parts connected with voluntary motion, as the optic thalami, the corpora striata, &c., or those parts connected directly with the mental faculties, as the cortical or cineritious substance forming the convolutions; or whether it was confined solely to that portion of the medullary substance, which only serves as a medium of communication between a portion of the cortical substance on the surface, and the cerebro-spinal centre in the medulla-oblongata, we are left entirely in the dark.

And hence we have no data, from which to draw a single inference of value. Whether the effusion of blood was produced by the blow against the staircase, without previous disease of the cerebral structure; or came on gradually only a short time before death, in a portion of the brain, already in a state of ramollissement from previous disease, is perhaps also difficult to determine. Though the circumscribed pain in the head, the softening of the brain around the blood, together with the simple seperation of that fluid into serum and crassamentum, would incline us to believe the latter was the case. The same want of precision exists in the detail of many cases related by Abercrombie, in his work on diseases of the brain.[1] And indeed, if we examine carefully, we shall find almost half of the cases reported in the various medical journals of the day, equally indefinite, and consequently equally valueless to the physiological inquirer. They may prove what every pathologist already knows, viz. that certain parts of the brain may be diseased, or totally destroyed, without producing mental derangement or disturbance. Or they may even prove what Prof. Sewall and other opponents of phrenological principles have asserted with so much apparent triumph, viz. that *every* part of the brain has been destroyed by disease and injury, without producing mental alienation. A fact of just as much physiological importance, as would be the assertion that ten men could be found in whom taken collectively, all the organs of external sense were destroyed, and yet, every individual of the ten, could feel, see, hear, taste, and smell.

It is true that facts form the foundation of all true science; but that foundation will only be useful and permanent, when the facts on which it rests are carefully observed, minutely recorded, and rightly arranged.—Hence, in studying the pathology of the brain, it is not enough that we ascertain, that half a pound of water has been effused; or that "there is an abscess in the right hemisphere;" or a "coagulum of blood in the left;" but we must first, if possible, rightly understand the symptoms during life, ascertaining not only that the intellect is sane, but that all the moral faculties and propensities are equally normal. And after death, we must bestow the necessary labor, to ascertain with minuteness, the precise seat and extent of the disease. If this was done by every observer, we are sure that Pathology would not long remain either barren or unfruitful in its contributions, to a correct physiology of the whole nervous tissue.

And if these remarks shall serve in any degree, to induce more care, and greater precision on the part of those who report cases of disease, the object for which they are written will be fully realized. Of the great importance, if not absolute necessity of greater accuracy and minuteness, in the detail of cases, every one will be convinced, who commences on examination of those already recorded, with the intention of drawing therefrom, any general conclusions. In the present state of our knowledge, we believe there is no case on record, contradicting the general rule, that disease in the cortical substance of the cerebral convolutions, in corresponding parts of both hemispheres is invariably at-

---

1 See pages 105, 108, 112, &c., of Abercrombie.

tended with derangement of some faculty or propensity of the mind. The cases which seem to militate most strongly against this rule, are those of superficial ulceration of the brain, related by Abercrombie, and others. But in those cases the ulcers were confined to one hemisphere, or affected different parts of both, and were evidently of a strictly chronic and local character. And the more recent investigations of pathologists would induce us to believe that in every case where death results from Insanity, there is well marked disease of the cortical substance of the brain. Thus Mr. Davidson, house-surgeon to the Lancaster county Lunatic Asylum, "has examined with much care, the bodies of more than two hundred patients who have died in the hospital since his appointment; and the result is, that he has scarcely met with a single instance, in which traces of disease in the brain, or its membranes, was not evident.[2] Again, M. Foville, Calmet, Falret, and Bayle, agree in asserting that "in mental alienation, the brain invariably presents lesions which can be distinctly recognized."[3] And Sir Wm. C. Ellis, resident medical Superintendent of the Pauper Lunatic Asylum, at Hanwell, [Eng.] states, "that of 154 male patients, examined after death, 145 had disease very strongly marked, either in the brain or its membranes. Of the nine remaining, two were idiots from birth; one died of dysentery, another of epilepsy; the other five had not been insane more than a few months, and died of other diseases. Of the females, 67 were examined, and 62 found with disease in the brain or its membranes. Two of the other five were idiots from birth, and with one exception, the others were recent cases.[4] The present list of cases on record, would lead us to the equally important conclusion, that disease affecting the central parts of the brain, as the corpora striata, the optic thalami, and the upper portion of the medulla oblongata, invariably deranges the powers of voluntary motion and sensation. For many cases illustrating this conclusion see American Journal of Medical Sciences, No. 32, August 1835; and Abercrombie on the Brain.

In these cases, the disease is generally insidious in its approach, and often fatal without any other marked symptom of cerebral disease, than paralysis of some one of the extremities, and sometimes convulsions. A third conclusion of no less practical importance than the preceding, is, that disease in a part of the medullary substance, which forms the comissures, or connecting fibres between the convolutions and the central parts mentioned above, when confined to one hemisphere, is seldom, if ever characterized by either mental derangement, or disturbance of the powers of sensation or volition. And hence its existence is often unsuspected, until revealed by a post mortem examination. These cases usually, (though not always) commence with paroxysms of severe pain, generally of limited extent in some part of the head, and not unfrequently vomiting; the skin is hot and dry, the pulse either slower than natural, or small and frequent; and though there is no real mental derangement, yet the patient almost always feels an unpleasant sensation in the head, either more marked or different from what is usual in attacks of ordinary fever. Of this description, are many cases of chronic asbcess, related in Abercrombie's work on the Brain. And we should place in the same class, the second case related by Prof. McNaughton in the American Journal of Medical Sciences, for July, 1842. Many of these cases resemble in the prominent symptoms, mild attacks of fever; and it must be confessed that we yet possess no certain means of diagnosis. But may we not hope that a more careful observation of symptoms, will yet enable us to detect disease in this part of the cerebral substance, as well as on its surface, or in the medulla oblongata. Practitioners have been too much in the habit of considering the brain normal, so long as the intellect remained sufficiently sane to answer questions correctly, and there was neither paralysis nor convulsions; and hence those hitherto less intelligible sensations, as pain, heaviness, dullness, vertigo, and other feelings in the head, have been too little attended to. The foregoing observations were originally suggested by an attendance on a legal process, for proving the validity of a will. And they are now published solely for the purpose of calling the attention of the profession to the important fact that reported cases of disease, are only valuable when all the circumstances are accurately and minutely detailed; and to report accurately, cases of cerebral disease, we must first study minutely, and correctly, cerebral anatomy. It is proverbial that medical science abounds in false *theories*; but we believe even a slight examination will show that *false facts* are far more numerous than theories.

---

2 See Combe on Mental Derangement, page 251.
3 See Ibid.
4 See American Journal Medical Sciences, page 157, for May, 1840.

STATISTICS OF INSANITY

By Amariah Brigham

Superintendent, New York State Lunatic Asylum, Utica, New York

S tatistical science is comparatively of modern date. The term itself was unknown until about the middle of the last century when a Professor in the University of Gottingen, first used it in describing the physical and moral and political condition of states. It is now generally used to designate a collection of facts respecting the state of society, the condition of the people in a nation or country, their health, longevity, domestic economy, arts, property and political strength, the state of the country, &c.

It has of late, attracted much attention, and now ranks among the most interesting and useful studies, though it has been cultivated much more assiduously and profitably in some countries than in others. In Germany the most so, which now possesses in her statistical works, an embodiment of the most valuable information respecting itself and other states. In England it is at present receiving much attention. Many individuals of great learning are devoting themselves to its improvement and perfection, and several statistical societies have been established. That of London, organized, we believe, in 1834, has already published eleven volumes of its Journal, which abound with most useful and interesting statistical information on a great variety of subjects. It is also doing much towards making known the true nature and objects of statistical inquiries and the correct method of pursuing them. The latter is much needed, as owing to incorrect data, defective registration, gross carelessness and other causes, many of the tabular statements and statistical details that have been published are erroneous. But that heretofore mistakes have occurred, and consequently erroneous conclusions sometimes drawn, is no reason why we should altogether relinquish the study, for in this as in other objects of human investigation, with perseverance and care, we may reasonably indulge the hope of improvement.

As respects the application of this science to the study and elucidation of insanity, which is more particularly the object of this article, it is supposed peculiar obstacles have to be encountered, and by some these have been deemed so insurmountable that they seem disposed to advise the total abandonment of the numerical method in the study of insanity.

Most persons, who have attended to the study of mental diseases, and especially those who have had the charge of institutions for the insane have perceived these difficulties, and many in the published reports of the institutions under their care, have so stated and cautioned their readers upon the subject, and given such explanations of the tabular statements, as to prevent their being misled. Thus as respects the causes of insanity, those who have published their opinions in a tabular form on this difficult subject, have usually been careful to state, that they gave not the certain or absolute cause, but merely the supposed or alledged cause.

Explanations of a like character, when the reader would be in danger of being misled by numerical statements have often been given, so that we cannot believe that any harm whatever has resulted even from the occasionally defective tabular statements that have been published in reports upon insanity. On the contrary we cannot doubt in the least, that great, very great good has resulted from the publications of the statistics of institutions for the insane, and we have no hesitation in expressing our firm conviction that but for the statistical facts thus made known to the public, several of the best establishments for the insane in this country would not now be in existence. The great curability of this disease when properly treated in its early stage, a fact, of which the public became fully convinced, from the tabular statements published in the annual reports of institutions established for the insane, led to the erection of others. This great truth, or argument, in favor of such institutions, has ever been the principal one relied upon by individuals and committees, whenever they wished to influence Legislators or other bodies of men to aid in providing new establishments; and we believe, in no way could this great fact have been brought convincingly before them but by the statistics of institutions already in operation. Admitting then, their partial imperfection, yet we must also admit they have accomplished much good.

But though many have seen the difficulty of giving, in a tabular form, certain facts relating to the insane entirely free from error, yet so far as we are informed, but few have thought of abandoning all attempts to impart information in this way. On the contrary, of late years increased efforts have very generally been made by those who have the care of institutions for the insane, to embody in a statistical form, numerous observations relating to those they have in charge. This is most particularly true in Germany, France and England; countries to which with good reason we are accustomed to look for proper examples in the investigation of truth and science. So essential is the embodiment in a tabular form of observations relating to the insane deemed in England, that by the late "Act of Parliament, for the Provision and Regulation of Lunatic Asylums," it is made an offence punishable by fine of the officers of an institution for the insane, for not keeping a register of the following particulars relating to the admission, treatment, discharge and death of patients. They are also required to transmit the same to the Commissioners of Lunacy. 1. Time of admission. 2. Name. 3. Sex. 4. Married or single. 5. Occupation. 6. Place of residence. 7. By whom sent. 8. Date of medical certificate. 9. By whom signed. 10. Form of mental disorder. 11. Supposed cause of insanity. 12. Bodily condition and name of disease if any. 13. Epileptic or idiotic. 14. Duration of present attack. 15. Number of previous attacks. 16. Age on first attack. 17. Names of patients under restraint and what kind. 18. Names of patients under medical treatment. 19. Date of discharge. 20. How discharged; Recovered; Relieved; not improved; Died. 21. Assigned cause of death. 22. Age at death. This act requiring the officers of institutions for the insane thus to Register their observations is a recent one, and was drawn up by men of ability and experience, after mature deliberation, with a full knowledge of all the objections to statistics, and with an entire survey of the whole subject of insanity and of the various methods of studying it.

Again, at the Annual Meeting of the Association of Medical Officers of Hospitals for the Insane, held at Lancaster, England, in June 1842, a form of Register was agreed to, that in *addition* to the particulars required by the act just mentioned, proposes that a record be made of the following particulars. 1. Degree of education of each patient. 2. Of what profession of religion. 3. Habits of life. 4. Temperament. 5. Original disposition and intellect. 6. Particular propensities and hallucinations. 7. Changes in the form of disorder before discharge. 8. Cause of death as ascertained by post-mortem examination. Thus it will be seen that we have the very highest testimony in favor of this method of studying insanity, and embodying particular observations relating to the insane, for the benefit of the public.

Still error should not be persevered in, even if supported by the most illustrious names. We therefore propose to examine a little farther, some of the objections that have been urged to the statistics of insanity; and see if there is any good reason for the abandonment of this method of studying the subject.

[The press being in the house, the printing of this article was commenced before the writer had completed it, and his illness is the cause of its appearing in an unfinished state.]

A Review of the Signs of Degeneration
and of Methods of Registration

By Adolf Meyer, M.D.

*Pathologist at the Worcester Lunatic Hospital
and Docent at Clark University, Worcester, Massachusetts*

Grown up in the Darwinian movement, we can hardly realize the primitive meaning of the general expression degeneration, as used by the writers who first introduced it. Morel speaks of the existence of a primitive perfect type of the human race; he calls it the master work and sum of the creation; as such, "it has received the threefold sanction of revelation, of philosophy, and of natural history." Degeneration is for him a pathological deviation from the biblical primitive type, a degradation of the progeny. While the physiological deviations are due to the influence of the climate, the nourishment, and the habits of life, the pathological deviation or degeneration is due to exaggerations and abnormalities of these influences: Intoxications, bad social surroundings and unhygienic conditions, diseases, moral defects, congenital or early acquired influences, heredity. Morel's studies on the very pronounced forms of degeneration in idiots, in cretins, etc., were subsequently extended more minutely to the insane, the criminals, and, since the importance of heredity in nervous affections has been more noted, to the "neuropathic family." At first the term merely comprehended the most obvious types of defectiveness. Lombroso, with his numerous followers in criminal and pathological anthropology, Benedikt, in his studies on the brain of criminals, and numerous writers on allied subjects, gradually extended the scope of their investigation and accumulated a great amount of interesting material. One of the chief features of this progress lies in the change of the philosophical position prevailing in our epoch. The originally perfect man has been swept away by the doctrine of evolution. Comparative anatomy, morphology, and ethnology have opened a great field for speculation in a new direction. The perfect man of the new school is he who is as free as possible from the characteristic features of phylogenetically less mature types. Everything that reminded strongly of possible ancestors of a lower degree was stamped with the term atavism. The ar-

dent search revealed indeed a great number of such features in the so-called defective elements of the human race, and the creation of the types of degeneration—the criminal, the neurotic, the imbecile, the insane, etc.—has, perhaps, been based too much on the "atavistic" features. The good influence of the general principles of evolution is quite evident; but just as in much of the evolutional literature, we find often that the existence of similarity with less mature types satisfied the minds that the features were "degenerative," and an investigation of the physiological reasons for the existence of the forms was dispensed with.

This movement could not help calling forth strong protest, and we may say that we stand at present in a wave of reaction. Quite a number of sober naturalists and anthropologists assume a non-committal position and approach the problem from a point of view similar to this: The so-called normal type is an arbitrary assumption and embraces a great number of physiological variations. It remains to be seen whether certain variations of form or function by themselves or in groups constitute actual signs of degeneration; *i.e.*, whether they are signs of constitutional inferiority, with a tendency to become more marked in the offspring. That there are such signs of degeneration, nobody would deny to-day; but their relative importance and the laws of their formation require a broader investigation. The number of observations is relatively so small that it is hardly ripe for general conclusions.

The practical value of our *present* knowledge of the signs of degeneration is perhaps overrated by those who believe they have found a scientific phrenology. Probably for a long time to come the study of the mental capacity and potentiality will be best carried out by studying the psychical manifestations rather than the physical forms of a person. The objection is raised that the study of the so-called signs of degeneration is not even of practical importance for the alienist. This is only true to some extent. Criminologists make use of the signs of degeneration in court. The physician must form an opinion of his own on the question if he will do justice as an expert. Or shall he simply repeat the conclusions drawn by others, on a very limited material? Why not unite for a broad, uniform investigation? Another problem is bound to become more and more important: the question of marriage in those afflicted with signs of degen-

---

The following notes were originally prepared for, and read as, the opening of a discussion of the "Study of Degeneration," at the meeting of the Association of Assistant Physicians of Hospitals for the Insane. As the desirability of studies in this line appealed to a majority of the association, the methods were taken as a starting basis for coöperative work, to be modified in subsequent meetings.

eration. The questions will arise: How far are the stigmata constitutional? How far do these localized brand-marks of the sins—unconscious or conscious—of the parents affect the entire personality? Which are the chief provoking agencies in their formation? Why do we find families with stigmata of degeneration going from bad to worse, and others grow up again and develop healthy and prospering children?

Let us admit that these questions touch problems which, to-day, are purely theoretical. Why? Because we do not know enough yet of the facts that underlie the acknowledged influence of heredity and the laws of growth and development.

That the alienist, who is every day confronted with the enigma of hereditary degeneration, will feel as deep an interest in the matter as any one, is evident. But he is also the one who, next to the criminologist, needs the most warning against premature conclusions.

For statistical purposes, for the mere study of frequency, our hospitals offer unique chances. But the great mixture of nationalities, with their strongly varying "normal" types, the great variety of diseases, the difficulty in ascertaining the history of the family and of the patient, make a great number of precautions necessary. The ideal method of procedure would be to examine whole families of one nationality, of the same locality, and the same conditions of life; to compare them with branches of the families which live in different climates and conditions; to study the results of inter-marriage, etc. Even if the chances for such work could be obtained it would be difficult enough to elucidate the causes of variations.

Our chances are not as favorable, but none the less worth our attention. If we make it a rule to look over our new patients at the physical examinations, and to use systematic methods of registration of whatever we find time to examine closely; if we further try to see the relatives; if we watch whether a person with signs of degeneration develops features of insanity different from those who have no stigmata in themselves or in their family; if we are able to gather a vast array of carefully, conscientiously collected data even on a limited number of factors only—if we have done all this, we have done ourselves and the patients and those after us our best service. We must not try to do too much at once, but be sure that we can carry out our plan within the domain that each of us may choose.

In order not to rely only on our own observation, and in order to sum up our work, we must agree on definite methods, and for this purpose the following notes are offered as a suggestion. A test by many will soon sift the unpracticable ones, and experience of a whole body of workers will establish a mutual ground.

Before entering upon the methods, we shall shortly review the classes of disorders to which the authors have drawn our attention:

A. *Morphological deviations from the normal.*
   I. Deviations of the general proportions of the body. The hands and arms, the feet and the legs, the trunk, the neck, the head (as a whole) and its various parts (skull, face, jaws, mouth, nose, etc.) may be too small or too large in proportion to the rest of the body.
   II. Asymmetries of skull, face, and rest of the body.
   III. Peculiar forms of special parts—skull (especially forehead and occiput), face (jaws, teeth, palate, lips, nose, ears, eyes), teratological peculiarities generally.
B. *Functional deviations from the normal.*
   I. Abnormal innervation of one side, or of special muscles, or of vasomotor nerves.
   II. Developmental irregularities—in dentition, learning to walk and to speak; enuresis nocturna, inclination to epileptic and other nervous attacks, etc. Lack of congruity between age and appearance.
C. *Purely psychical stigmata.*
   Abnormality of sensory perceptions (especially the pain sense); abnormalities of habits, of ideation, of action (sexual life, emotional attitude, egotism, disequilibration, imperative ideas, mental "tics," associated movements, explosive activity, periodicity, etc.).

For the latter group the book of Dr. J.L.A. Koch on "Die psychopathischen Minderwertigkeiten," and the one of Cullerre on the "Borderland of Insanity," offer a great number of instances.

In a general way, the examination of each case should extend over the principal features which determine the general anthropometric make-up of the individual, even if only a part is examined completely (for instance, the ear). An ear may be large in a small woman, small in a large man, etc. The following data should be given in every case:

No._____; name,_____; relation of No.,_____; sex,_____; age,_____; place of birth,_____; nationality,_____; religion,_____; occupation, ; weight,_____; height,_____; color of hair,_____; of iris,_____.

For the general relations of the body the following measurements were primarily chosen for use in the autopsies at the Kankakee Hospital:

Weight.
Height of vortex.
Height of vertebra prominens.
Height of perineum.
Height of spina ossis ilei—right; left.
Height of knee—right; left.
Height of tip of middle finger—right; left.
Height of acromion—right; left.
Length of acromion—elbow—right; left.
Length of acromion—tip of middle finger—right; left.
Girth of neck.
Girth of chest.
Girth of waist.
Girth of hips.
Girth of wrist—right; left.
Girth of arm—right; left.
Girth of forearm—right; left.
Girth of thigh—right; left.
Girth of knee—right; left.
Girth of calf—right; left.
Girth of ankle—right; left.
Length of foot—right; left.
Breadth of shoulders.
Breadth of hips.

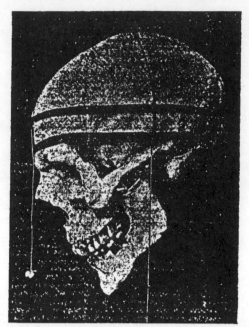

Fig. 1.

To these measurements should be added in the living:

Circumference of chest at deepest inspiration.
Circumference of chest at deepest expiration.
Capacity of lung (spirometer).
Strength of squeeze—right; left.

The points from which the measurements are taken are those described by Dr. E. Schmidt.[1]

For the elbow-joint we take the point between the humerus and the capitulum radii, for the knee-joint, the articulation is easily felt just outside of the patella or inside of it. The girth of the chest is taken over the middle of the sternum, just under the axilla; the girth of the waist in the middle between margin of ribs and crista ossis ilei; the girth of the hips below the crista. The girth of the wrists and of the ankles is taken as a means of comparison between size of the skeleton and of the soft parts, as given by the measurements of the arm and calf; it is therefore taken at the thinnest points, not around the epiphyses of the bones, but a little above them. The girth of the thigh is taken just below the gluteal fold.

Completer anthropometric blanks are used in many prisons and reformatories (see the report of the Elmira Reformatory). The above list of measurements appeals to me because it reveals asymmetries, atrophies, etc., sufficiently without being too long.

For the measurements of the head, Peterson[2] gives eleven measurements, with a full description of the method. In the autopsies at Kankakee I chose nine, one of which, the bi-temporal diameter, should be replaced by the binauricular diameter. The list is now:

Diameter naso-occipitalis.
Diameter biparietalis.

Diameter binauricularis.
Diameter mento-occipitalis.
Diameter zygomaticus.
Diameter of lower jaw (gonia).
Facial length.
Circumference of head.
Sagittal line.

On the whole, the points from which the measurements were taken coincided with those that form the starting point of Rieger's system of craniography. The facial length is taken from a point which lies in the connecting line of the two upper orbital margins to the chin. The upper end of this line is about five mm. above the actual root of the nose, which is sometimes a rather indistinct point.

For the study of facial asymmetries the following oblique measures should be taken:

Distance from the external angle of the eye to the angle of mouth—right; left.
Distance from tragus to chin—right; left.
Distance from tragus to root of nose—right; left.
Distance from tragus to tip of nose—right; left.
Distance from tragus to external angle of eye—right; left.

These measures, supplemented by a photograph profile view and one front view, will answer all the purposes, with the exception of the study of asymmetry of the skull, for which Peterson also recommends taking curves, either with a lead strip or lead wire, or with the instrument of Luys.

A great improvement on the separate measurement of the diameters and the circumferences is the method of craniography of Rieger.

The principal feature of Rieger's craniography is the registration of curves, of outlines instead of mere distances; further, the use of the so-called millimeter paper, which allows one to dispense altogether with the endless series of numbers. The plane of the fundamental curve corresponds approximately to the basis of the hemispheres and is easily ascertained; all the other transverse and longitudinal curves of the convexity are erected on it.

Rieger proceeds as follows: Two threads are tied together so as to form a cross. The ends are made heavy by attaching small weights of lead. The node of the cross is put on the vertex, in the median line; the anterior line goes along the dorsum of the nose, the posterior one through the middle of the nuchal groove; the lateral lines are conveniently put so that they pass over the anterior wall of the external auditory meatus. The fundamental circular curve, indicated by a rubber ring, is fixed by an anterior and a posterior point. The anterior point is chosen where a prolongation of the dorsum of the nose would cut the connecting line between the two upper orbital margins. The posterior point is given by the external occipital protuberance, or where it is not felt by the median point of the upper margin of the nuchal muscles. The rubber ring is so adjusted as to form a perfectly even horizontal plane. (Fig. 1.)

A square piece of millimeter paper is prepared, of about thirty cm. side. It is conveniently numbered, as Rieger's Fig.

1 Anthropoligische Methoden, von Dr. Emil Schmidt. Leipzig, 1888: Veit & Co.
2 "Craniometry and Cephalometry in Relation to Idiocy and Imbecility," by Frederick Peterson, M.D., American Journal of Insanity, Vol. 52, pp. 73-89.

15 shows, not from the real center, but from a point about two fields to the right of, and below, the center of the chart. This point forms the zero point of the graphic system of the two axes.

In order to obtain the fixed points of the rubber ring, the transverse diameter between the two lateral points is first measured. The distance is registered on the transverse axis of the paper, one-half of the distance to the left, the other half to the right, of the zero point.

The anterior point is obtained with a compass or caliper, one arm of which is armed with a pencil. We measure first the distance from the left lateral point and register it on the paper as a circle; then we take the distance from the right lateral point, put it also down as a circle, and the point of intersection of the two circles gives the exact location (Fig. 2). The posterior point is obtained in the same way. The distance between the occipital and frontal point obtained in this indirect way must, of course, be the same as when measured directly. This test will show the degree of accuracy of the measurements taken. If the points do not lie in the middle line, we are dealing with an asymmetrical skull.

The circular curve connecting the four points is next taken. Lead wire, pliable but absolutely unelastic, is the best material; it is pressed strongly against the head, only one quadrant being taken at a time. The line is, for the sake of accuracy, first marked with an ordinary pencil, and afterward repassed by a red pencil or with red ink. It is evident that the line obtained is somewhat vitiated by the temporal muscle. For this and other reasons it may be advisable to take one or more horizontal curves above the insertion of the temporal muscle. These planes must be perfectly parallel with the fundamental curve. A second rubber ring is applied; the measurements and curves are registered in identically the same manner as those of the first plane. Rieger marks this upper curve in blue color. If this blue curve is not larger than the red one, the head is more or less microcephalic.

The next curve is that of the median sagittal line. It would be too large to be obtained accurately at one time. It is therefore conveniently taken in two pieces, divided by the node of the cross. This node is ascertained by taking its distance from the four fundamental points with the compass or caliper (Fig. 3). The curve is drawn (in red) to the left from the median line, and does not interfere with the other lines of the drawing. If a depression should be taken, one or more parallel curves may be ascertained after the same plan. The chief condition is that the fixed points be first accurately registered, and that the lead wire be accurately applied and the curve tested before it is drawn with the pencil.

The transverse curves are to be taken in planes which are exactly perpendicular on the fundamental plane. If this rule is not observed caricatures may be the result, and artificial asymmetries will occur. The cross of thread may be, but usually is not, in this perpendicular plane. Fig. 3 shows that the point of intersection k is a certain distance in front of the transverse line, which goes through the zero

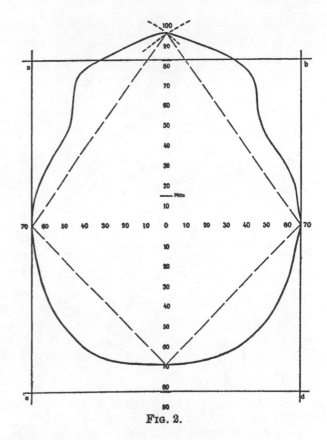

FIG. 2.

point and the two lateral fixed points of the cross; our curve must therefore be taken through that point of the sagittal line which lies just that distance behind the point of intersection. For planes anterior or posterior to the cross of threads the corresponding point of the sagittal line is also found with the help of the drawing (x' l' h' and x" l" h"). But, even if we know the correct point of the sagittal line, we must be careful to take the lateral halves of the curves exactly in the vertical plane, and not to choose the shortest way simply. In order to be quite sure, I should suggest a little brass instrument of T shape; the sagittal line is put on the median line; the cross branches must be of sufficiently firm material to keep the right angle when bent; i.e., it must not be readily twisted. Rieger enters the curves in green color, and forward.

To the comfort of the reader, I may say that the execution of the craniographic method is much easier than the study of a condensed description, and that it requires little practice to read from the drawing a mental reconstruction of the skull, with all its curves. At the same time all the measurements are registered without the burdensome array of figures, and any number of measurements can be read from the sketch, while the examination after the old method is unsatisfactory and inaccurate for the study of asymmetries, and, if the patient is gone, does not allow of any additional investigation.

This abstract of part of Rieger's paper[3] can not replace the original, which is herewith highly recommended as a very suggestive guide, and an argument in favor of accuracy. Even

---

3 Eine exacte Methode der Craniographie von Dr. C. Rieger, Würzburg. Jena, Gustav Fischer, 1885; $1.15.

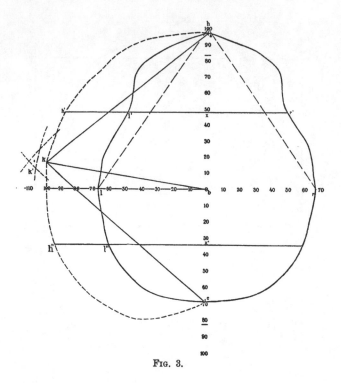

FIG. 3.

those who have not the time to take all the measurements do well to register the few they take after Rieger's plan.

A few words may be said here with regard to the deformities which may be met:

Virchow has given a very complete classification of the malformations of the skull, based largely on the observation that premature synostosis of suture produces shortness of the diameter perpendicular on the direction of the obliterated suture; the bone stops growing prematurely where the synostosis has occurred, whereas the not affected borders continue growing. Virchow's classification is as follows:

1. Simple macrocephalus:
   A. Hydrocephalus.
   B. Kephalones (without hydrocephalus).
2. Simple microcephalus (nannocephalus).
3. Dolichocephalus:
   A. Upper middle synostosis:
     Simple dolichocephalus (synostosis of sagittal suture)
     Sphenocephalus (synostosis of sagittal suture and compensatory growth in the region of the large fontanel)
   B. Inferior lateral synostosis:
     Leptocephalus (synostosis of frontal and sphenoid bones).
     Klinocephalus (synostosis of the parietal or sphenoid bones).
4. Brachycephalus:
   A. Posterior synostosis:
     Pachycephalus (synostosis of parietal bones with the occipital bone).
     Oxycephalus (synostosis of parietal bones with the occipital and temporal bones, with compensatory growth of the region of the anterior fontanel)—acrocephalus.
   B. Upper anterior and lateral synostosis:
     Platycephalus or chaemocephalus (extensive synostosis of frontal and parietal bones).

     Trochocephalus (partial synostosis of frontal and parietal bones in the middle of the half of the coronal suture).
     Plagiocephalus (unilateral synostosis of frontal and parietal bones).
   C. Inferior median synostosis:
     Simple brachycephalus (early synostosis of the basal and sphenoid bones).

Drawings of several of these extreme and well characterized types can be found in the paper of Dr. Peterson and in the "Reference Hand-Book for the Medical Sciences" (Frank Baker, the "Joints of the Skull," Vol. VI, p. 462). Dr. Peterson also mentions the scaphocephalus and trigonocephalus.

The following general features have been especially mentioned in connection with the insane:

1. Crania progenaea (L. Meyer), defective development of the posterior parts of the skull, breadth of the parietal and temporal bones, and projection of the maxilla.

2. Plagiocephalus.

3. Flat occiput (often due to rickets).

4. Low, sloping forehead.

Attention has also been drawn to deformities of the thorax (see the paper of Dr. Neff). Whereas the emphysematous, the paralytic, and the rachitic thorax has largely clinical interest, the skoliotic and kyphoscoliotic thorax may depend on a congenital weakness of the muscles of one side or on an acquired weakness, as in syringomyelia, etc. A peculiar retraction of the lower end of the sternum, called trichterbrust (funnel-breast), has been described as a sign of degeneration; the pectus carinatum, or pigeon-breast, might be called the reverse, and is also mentioned.

A very excellent system of dynamometric measurements for most muscles has been invented by Dr. Kellogg. As it belongs more into the field of clinical work and treatment than into that of the study of degeneration, we simply mention it here. It is of great practical value, and will help to introduce rational gymnastics.[4]

The Face.—While the facial angle is not so frequently mentioned in recent literature, various parts of the face have been the subject of much investigation regarding the signs of degeneration. The face and its expression are indeed the chief guides in daily life in judging people by their appearance.

General asymmetries of the face are already included in the measurements given above. There remains the study of the special parts. The eyes have not, so far, been much subjected to the study of degeneration. Whether any one of the five types of Metschnikow is prevailing can not be said. We find mentioned:

1. Congenital coloboma of the iris, which is so rare that it belongs among the monstrosities, and is of little importance among the insane.

2. Ptosis, congenital.

3. Asymmetrical coloration of the iris, in toto or in part.

4. Oval or eccentric pupil.

As functional stigmata nystagmus and strabismus are mentioned.

On the *nose* we have not been able to find any data. The

---

4 Kellogg, J. H., "A New Dynamometer for Use in Anthropometry," and various other papers. Battle Creek, Mich., 1893.

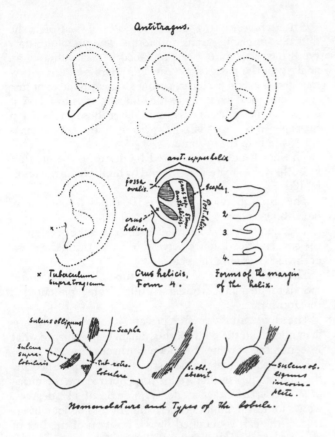

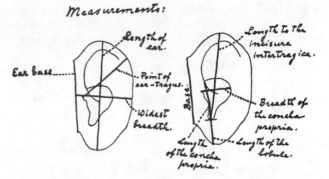

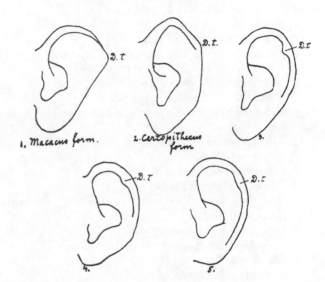

types of noses given by Topinard (Anthropologie) might form a basis for a study.

The *jaws* have attracted far more interest. Since Dr. Boody gives an excellent review of work done on this subject, I can limit myself to very short remarks. Most attention, so far, has been devoted to the upper jaw and palate; little has been done on the lower jaw, and even on irregularities of dentition. Dr. Channing, who has a collection of over 1,000 casts of palates of idiots, had the casts made in a systematic way and measured the casts, a plan which deserves imitation. If possible, a cast of both the upper and lower jaw should be made, and the relation in the position of the two must be ascertained. The dentists of the institutions will be able to demonstrate the methods; the measurements can be made later.

The typical stigmata are:

1. Prognathia, a projection of the mandibula. This point played an important rôle in the Prendergast trial, where the prosecuting attorney was pleased to formulate his question to the witnesses as follows: "Do you believe in the jaw-theory of insanity?"

2. Irregularity in dentition; persistence of milk-teeth (especially of an eye-tooth).

Irregularities of the position of the teeth.

Irregularities of the shape of the teeth.

3. The abnormal configuration of the palate.

a. The margin (alveolar circle) may be too wide, too narrow, pointed (V-shaped), saddle-shaped, asymmetrical.

b. The vault of the palate may be abnormally high, asymmetrical, etc.

c. There may be a longitudinal torus or ridge in the median line.

d. Cleft palate, hare-lip, etc.

Further, we find data on the thickness of the lips; especially thickness of the lower lip, is to this day called a sign of sensuality.

The ear has furnished the greatest number of types of degeneration, as the notes of Morel and the papers of Binder,[5] Gradenigo,[6] Váli,[7] Frigerio,[8] and Petrona Eyle[9] will show. G. Schwalbe,[10] the anatomist of Strassburg, has given the

5 Binder, Das Morel'sche Ohr, Arch. f. Psych., Vol. XX, 1889, p. 514 ff.
6 Gradenigo, Zur Morphologie der Ohrmuschel bei gesunden und geisteskranken Menschen und Delinquenten. Archiv für Ohrenheilkunde, XXX, 1890.
 —, Über die Formanomalien der Ohrmuschel. Ibid. Vol. XXXII and XXXIII, 1891.
 —, Centralblatt für d. medic. Wissenschaften, 1888.
7 Váli, Allg. Wiener Medic. Zeitung, Nov. 11, 1891.
8 L'oreille externe, Archives de l'anthropologie criminelle, 1888.
9 Petrona Eyle, Über Bildungsanomalien der Ohrmuschel. Zürich, 1891.
10 Schwalbe, Das Darwin'sche Spitzohr beim menschlichen Embryo. Anat. Anz., 1889.
 —, In wie fern ist die Ohrmuschel ein rudimentäres Organ? Archiv. f. Anat. und Phys. Anat. Anz., 1889. Supplement.
 —, Beiträge zur Anthropologie des Ohres. Internationale Beiträge zur wissenschaftlichen Medicin; Festschrift für R. Virchow. Bd. I, 1891.
 —, Zur Methodik statistischer Untersuchungen über die Ohrformen von Geisteskranken und Verbrechern. Arch. f. Psych., Vol. XXVII, p. 633.

subject the broadest study, and it will certainly be advisable in future study to follow his outline, which is based on the principles of Bertillon's Identification Anthropométrique (Melun, 1893).

Binder gives in his monograph the following analysis of Morel's ear (the ear of the degenerate):

1. Anomalies in the configuration of the ear as a whole:
    a. The variations in size.
    b. The implantation.
    c. Abnormalities in the general configuration.
    d. Inequality of the two ears.

2. Anomalies in the architecture and form of the parts composing the ear:
    a. The lobule may be excessively long or adherent, or absent. Coloboma, lobuli. Hypertrichosis.
    b. Anomalies of the helix.
    c. Anomalies of the anthelix.
    d. Anomalies of the crura furcata and fossa ovalis.
    e. Anomalies of the tragus and anti-tragus.
    f. Anomalies of the concha and fossa cymbae.
    g. Anomalies of the fossa scaphoidea.

From the analysis of these points he arrives at the following types of ears:

1. The defectively implanted ears.
2. Excessively large ears.
3. Excessively small ears.
4. The excessively folded ear.
5. The irregularly shaped ear (especially the ear with abnormally small upper portion).
6. Ears varying in breadth.
7. *Blainville's* ears (asymmetry of the two ears).
8. Ear without lobule.
9. Ear with adherent lobule.
10. *Stahl's* ear (1). The helix is very broad in the transverse portion and partly covering the fossa ovalis. The lower part of the helix is absent.
11. *Darwin's* ear (with marked tubercle at the beginning of the descending part of the helix).
12. *Wildermuth's* ear; anthelix prominent.
13. The ear without anthelix and crura furcata.
14. *Stahl's* ear (2). Wide bifurcation of crura; multiple bifurcation, especially of the upper crus.
15. *Wildermuth's* Aztek's ear. Lobule absent. The upper crus of the anthelix goes over the flat helix without any demarkation; the lower crus is very deep and apparently absent, the upper crus thus forming the margin of the concha.
16. *Stahl's* ear (3). Only the crus anterius present; the crus superius merely a node of cartilage. The concha apparently divided by an additional process starting from the anti-tragus.
17. The ear with double helix, the crus superius not even indicated; rare.
18. Concha too large or too small.
19. The ear with a scaphoid fossa extending into the lobule.
20. *Morel's* ear; flat and broad in the upper parts. Crus superius, broad, flat; scapha, broad, shallow.
21. Malformations of cartilage excluding the one caused by othaematoma.
22. Atypical malformations, coloboma, etc.

An attempt at using this tabulation shows at once the difficulty in placing transition forms. The use of arbitrary types has, therefore, been replaced by Schwalbe by an analysis of the parts of the ear. His chart contains thirty-four questions on each ear, perhaps a great number at first sight, but not over-accurate for him who tries to follow it for some time. The drawings made after those published in his paper in the *Archiv. für Psychiatre*, and a few explanations, will help the beginner.

The head-index is obtained by dividing the greatest breadth by the greatest length and by multiplying the result by 100.

The physiognomic ear-index is 100 times the quotient of breadth by length.

The morphological ear-index is 100 times the quotient of the base and the distance between the tragus and the point of the ear (Darwin's tubercle).

The various types of Darwin's tubercle, which corresponds to the point of the ear in animals, are represented in the drawings.

The satyrpoint is not often present; it forms what the layman might call the point of the human ear, similar to what is seen in the drawing of the cercopithecus form.

For the position of the ear to the skull, or more especially the mastoid process, Schwalbe does not require the measurement of the exact angle. The angle of 112 degrees, which forms the limit between straight and oblique insertion of the ear, is obtained by the position of the line of greatest length of the ear, and a line which passes through the lower orbital margin and the upper margin of the external meatus.

Next we have to consider the whole group of malformations:

Naevi and pigment-spots of the skin, abnormal growth of hair, vitiligo, patches of gray hair, club-foot, polydactyly, defective extension of the end-phalanges of the little finger, congenital luxations, narrow pelvis, tail-position of coccyx, gynaecomastia (development of breasts in the male); further, the whole array of malformations of the sexual organs—phimosis, epispadias, hypospadias, cryptorchism, abnormal smallness of testicles, azoöspermia aspermia, infantile uterus, atresia of vagina, partial or total redoublication of the vaginal and uterine canal, etc.

Little may be said on the functional deviations (strabismus, nystagmus, unequal innervation of the two sides of the face, tics, etc.) For the developmental irregularities the books of Emminghaus ("Psychosen des Kindesalters") and of Moreau ("La folie chez les enfants"), and also a few publications in the Transactions of the Illinois Child Study Association (published by the Werner Company in Chicago), will form a first guide. As to the psychical deviations, we should strongly advise the perusal of the books of Koch and Cullerre mentioned above.

It is evident that one of the first conditions of work is excellence of the tools, of the measuring and recording instruments. Those used by myself were contained in the anthropometric set of Virchow, made by Thamm, in Berlin. They can easily be imported by Eimer & Amend, in New York, or obtained directly from the maker. For other instruments the paper of Dr. Boody will give instructions, and

CHART FOR RECORDING DATA AS TO EAR, ETC.

No......	Name.				Disease.		Nationality.	Birthplace.	Heredity.	Other signs of degeneration.
Sex.	Religion.	Occupation	Age.	Height.	Color of Hair.	Color of Iris.	Length-breadth Index of Head.	Physiognomic Ear-Index.		Morphological Ear-Index.

							R.	L.		R.	L.
Greatest length of head............				Ant. upper helix near Darwin's tubercle (flat, 1; turned laterad, 2; reverted, 3)............					**LOBULUS AURICULÆ.** Attachment (prolonged on the cheek, 1; simply adherent, 2; partly separated, 3; free, 4)......		
Greatest breadth of head.........	R.	L.		Post. helix (flat, 1; turned laterad, 2, reverted, 3; reverted and adherent, 4)...................					Sulcus supralobularis (absent, 1; medium, 2; marked, 3; connected with scapha, 4)............		
Greatest length of entire ear......									Sulcus obliquus (absent, 1; only in antitragus region, 2; complete, 3).		
Greatest breadth of entire ear.....				Crus descendens (present, 1; absent, 0)					Tuberculum retrolobulare (absent, 1; medium, 2; marked, 3)............		
Length of ear base...........				**TRAGUS.**					Sulcus lobuli verticalis (absent, 1; medium, 2; marked, 3).........		
Length of concha propria.........				Tub. supratragicum (visible, 1; not visible, 0)................					Direction of lobule (bent inward, 1; straight, 2; bent outward, 3).....		
Breadth of concha propria........				**ANTHELIX.**							
Distance of upper end (Darwin's tubercle) to upper margin of tragus				Stem of the anthelix (retracted, 1; in the level of the ear, 2; prominent, 3).					Lobule split (split, 1; not split, 0)...		
Length to incisura intertragica				Crus anthelicis superius (absent, 1; indicated, 2; medium, 3; strongly developed, 4)............					Position of ear (closely attached, 1; medium, 2; almost at right-angle, 3)		
Length of lobule..............				Crus anthelicis tertium (present, 1; absent, 0)					General form of the ear...........		
HELIX.				Other accessory crura anthelicis (describe, if present; absent, 0)..					Insertion of ear (straight, angle less than 112°, 1; oblique, angle more than 112°, 2)...............		
Darwin's tubercle (Macacus, 1; cercopithecus, 2; reverted pointed, 3; reverted rounded, 4; indicated, 5; absent, 6)................				**ANTITRAGUS.**							
				Direction of upper margin (horizontal, 1; medium, 2; oblique, 3)....					Auricular appendices.............		
Satyr point (present, 1; absent, 2)..				Inclination outward (absent, 1; medium, 2; pronounced, 3).......					Fistula auris congenita...........		
Crus helicis (weak, 1; medium, 2; marked, 3; connected with anthelix [see figure] 4)...............				Form (straight, 1; slightly arched, 2; with marked prominence, 3)....					Anomalies of teeth...............		

those used in the military departments of this country are described in the article of Albert L. Gihon, on "Physical Measurements," in the "Reference Hand-Book of the Medical Sciences," Vol. V., pp. 667-673. The best guides will further be the little work of Schmidt, quoted above, the anthropology of Topinard and of Ranke.

For American literature, and also on account of several valuable papers on the principles in working out the results, a reprint of "Papers on Anthropometry" will be of use, from the publications of the American Statistical Association, by the American Statistical Association, Boston. (Price, 50 cents.) It contains a very useful list of literature. We also refer to the article "Head," in Hack Tuke's Dictionary of Psychological Medicine.

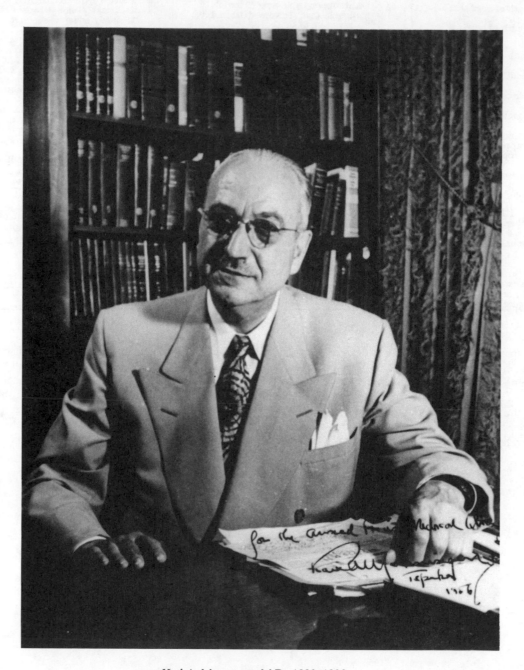

Karl A. Menninger, M.D., 1893–1990

April 1926

Influenza and Schizophrenia

An Analysis of Post-Influenzal "Dementia Precox," as of 1918, and Five Years Later

Further Studies of the Psychiatric Aspects of Influenza

By Karl A. Menninger, M.D.

Psychiatrist, Menninger Clinic, Topeka, Kansas

Of the psychoses appearing in close conjunction with influenza, as observed during the 1918 epidemic, the schizophrenic syndrome was by far the most frequent. The previous epidemics of influenza occurred prior to Kraepelin's formulation of "dementia precox," hence 1918 was the first opportunity afforded for the determination of the relationship of these two widespread afflictions as presently conceived. Because of the almost unequalled neurotoxicity of influenza, it should prove to be a critical test of the pathological basis of schizophrenia.

The facts are that of about two hundred acute post-influenzal psychoses at the Boston Psychopathic Hospital, one-third looked like and were labeled "dementia precox"; and follow-up inquiries made one to five years later reveal that of about fifty of these that could be traced, two-thirds had apparently completely recovered, and certainly only ten living cases showed no improvement.

This would seem to indicate the need of new diagnostic criteria or new prognostic conceptions (in re reversibility) for the acute schizophrenic syndrome.

We have previously presented various studies of the psychoses associated with influenza as observed at the Boston Psychopathic Hospital in the epidemic of 1918-19 (1, 8). Apparently all forms of mental disease are evoked by influenza in various ways and to various degrees. Neurosyphilis, (2) hypophrenia, (3) epilepsy, (4) manic-depressive syndromes, (5) and deliria, (6) have been dealt with in special articles. The present presentation concerns the association of the dementia precox syndrome with influenza.

Schizophrenia occurred during and following acute attacks of influenza in precisely the same ways as did the other psychoses. In some instances it was apparently a bolt from the blue, without any evidence of predisposition in the patient so far as we could learn. In other cases, influenza seemed to precipitate a psychosis which was perhaps imminent, or at least predetermined by temperamental and characterological twists known to have existed in the individual before the attack of influenza. Illustrations of both occurrences were recited in detail in the reports made soon after the epidemic, and cited above. A more comprehensive study of the problem of the association of schizophrenia and influenza is now possible because of the accumulated material and the perspective of time.

Quantitative

The first consideration might well be the relative frequency of schizophrenia as a post-influenzal psychosis. In a study made at the height of the epidemic, when about 80 cases all in the acute stage had been observed, dementia precox was the diagnosis in 25 of these 80; this to be compared with 16 cases of delirium and 23 cases of other psychoses, and 16 unclassified. We then thought that eight of these cases of dementia precox were latent processes activated by the influenza and that 17 of them were psychoses newly instigated.

Subsequent to this report there was the usual flood of literature relating to the effects of influenza on the nervous system, some of which warmly supported our data to the effect that schizophrenia was a very frequent, if not the most frequent, psychosis observed and others insisting that it was seen rarely, and even not at all.

Influenza is the only acute febrile disease which occurs with sufficient ubiquity and morbidity to make possible any considerable statistical study of its psychic effects. Dementia precox had not been born at the time of the last previous influenza epidemic (1890-1892). The rather bulky literature dealing with the psychoses associated with the influenza of that epidemic is a little difficult to interpret in present-day psychiatric categories. Occasionally, however, it is likely that the author refers to what would now be called dementia precox, as, for example, Sir William Gowers, (9)

Read in abstract at the eighty-first annual meeting of The American Psychiatric Association, Richmond, Va., May 12, 13, 14, 15, 1925.

who wrote in 1893: "Just as the depression develops into melancholia, so the delirium which occasionally attends the acute affections may have for its special sequel chronic delusional insanity (read dementia precox) and, very rarely, acute mania." Again, without entering into a discussion of the proper distribution of the entities composing the heterogeneous, ill-defined and fortunately obsolescent syndrome "amentia," it will be recalled that Kraepelin pointed out that many cases so diagnosticated proved to be dementia precox, and that Regis (10) regarded a prolongation of "confusion mentale" (essentially the same concept as amentia) as practically identical with one of his two forms of dementia precox (constitutional and incidental). And as "amentia" and "mental confusion," etc., are frequently mentioned as sequelae of influenza in the older literature (including Regis' textbook), one may presume that the occurrence of dementia precox after influenza, although frequent, by a confusion of nomenclature escaped signalization.

The few authors who mention it specifically do so in an apologetic manner, generally ascribing its occurrence to a coincidence. Kirn, (11) Bonhoeffer (12) and others mentioned above have referred to it, but generally add reassurance that definite stigmata of psychotic tendencies were previously manifest, or were apparent in the family history. Paton (13) remarks the occasional precipitation of schizophrenia by influenza, but ascribes to it only a minor rôle. Gosline (14) reported a series of necropsies with histologic brain findings, and pointed out the similarity of findings in a case of influenza with delirium, and cases of dementia precox, drawing the obvious inference, "that . . . . certain cases of dementia precox are due to infectious or toxic processes."

Fell (15) in the study of 20 post-influenzal psychoses at the Walter Reed Hospital in 1919, reports dementia precox as the diagnosis in 5, i.e., 25 per cent; he also comments that "the occurrence of dementia precox symptoms is not a sure indication of permanency, but such cases run a longer course and recovery is less likely." He also comments on the fact that schizophrenic symptoms combined with confusion and similar falsifications on the basis of emotional depression constitute the characteristic picture. He concludes that predisposition as shown by the family or personal history was marked only in the manic-depressive group.

The same author in another study (16) again emphasizes the mixture of delirium with schizophrenic symptoms for which he thinks the designation suggested by the present writer is particularly apt, namely, delirium-schizophrenoides.

Sandy, (17) in the study of the neuropsychiatric cases reported to that department of the office of the surgeon-general in the army, reports that from among over 70,000 neuropsychiatric cases only 73 could be ascribed to influenza, but of these 73, 7 were cases of dementia precox (as compared with 32, of the infective-exhaustive type, and 4, manic-depressives). Sandy is impressed by the fact that service in this country and in France and one or more previous neuropsychiatric examinations probably eliminated soldiers having mental abnormalities prior to influenza, and feels that the occurrence of these 7 cases confirms our findings of a schizophrenic psychosis occurring out of a clear sky following influenza.

Jelliffe (22) in a general study, discusses the mechanisms of the production of schizophrenic symptoms in post-influenzal lines in some detail, giving no statistics.

Harris (18) studied 18 cases of post-influenzal psychosis admitted to the Worcester State Hospital, of which 8 were diagnosticated dementia precox. In 4 of these 8 there was apparently no predisposition.

Schlesinger, (19) in a study of the delirium accompanying influenza, describes the varieties of delirium observed by him in Geneva mentioning catatonic states, peculiar automatisms and stereotypies such as singing or whistling one tune indefinitely. He says it is impossible to tell in some of these cases whether or not

dementia precox is beginning but that in general the prognosis is good. He divides the deliria into: (1) The acute; (2) the sub-acute of the mental confusion of a schizophrenic type; and (3) the alcoholic (delirium tremens).

Riese (25) describes 5 cases in detail, one called "amentia," two probably schizophrenia. Although holding to the usefulness of the amentia concept, he concedes that many cases so called, subsequent to influenza must to-day be classed as dementia precox or manic-depressive psychosis, and he adds that the fact that hebephrenic and paranoid processes may develop for the first time under the influence of influenza is so apparent that it scarcely needs emphasis.

Waterman and Folsom (26) studied 51 cases of psychosis associated with influenza at the Manhattan State Hospital in 1918-1919. Of the 23 male cases, 17 were diagnosticated at the first staff presentation as belonging to one or another of the well defined clinical groups, 4 of these were dementia precox, all of them predisposed. Of 28 female cases, 3 were regarded as definitely dementia precox, and 5 others strongly suggestive of dementia precox, all of whom seemed to have recovered.

In sharp contrast with these findings are such studies as that of Harris and Corcoran (20) of the Brooklyn State Hospital, who found no cases of dementia precox in 50 consecutive admissions in which influenza or influenza with pneumonia precipitated a psychosis. In a printed discussion of the work of Waterman and Folsom mentioned above, Kirby (27) stated that it seemed improbable in the light of their observations that dementia precox is precipitated abruptly by influenza, although conceding that peculiar catatonic-like symptoms are frequently observed and also conceding that "as soon as we get away from the ordinary febrile deliria we come immediately into a very obscure field and most recognize that mixed types occur . . . in very puzzling combinations." Similarly, in an elaborate study of 160 pages, Walthauer (21) of the University of Berne, describes 60 cases of post-influenzal psychoses from the canton of Berne, without anywhere in the book mentioning the words schizophrenia or dementia precox. The author makes much of the old concept of amentia which he divides into four types, comprising 16 cases. He seems to have been cut off entirely from American and English literature.

Bleuler (24) is exceedingly ambiguous in reference to this subject. In one place (page 442) in discussing the causes of schizophrenia, having just dispensed with "onanism" and overwork, he says curtly, "Neither the grippe nor the war have added to the existence of schizophrenia." Elsewhere, (page 363) he says, "Like Kraepelin, I saw several influenza deliria . . . . in which parasthenias were interpreted illusionally. At all events (whatever that may mean here!) in grippe psychoses it is mostly a question of a schizophrenic sort of dissociation of the mental stream, which appears all the more similar (sic!) to the schizophrenic (what?) because irritations of the nervous system readily give occasion to a kind of physical hallucination; the affectivity invariably, however, continues to fluctuate . . . . Fever deliria without a schizoid character, ... also occur . . . . In my experience all grippe psychoses which do not look from the first like schizophrenia are curable, that is to say, if the schizophrenia does not *just happen to appear* (italics, our's) at the same time as the infections."

Our final figures are that in approximately 175 cases in which the diagnoses were definitely determined, 67 were regarded by us at the time as dementia precox. Retrospectively we have changed the diagnosis and culled out a few of these, but even so amended, our figures make it appear that one-third of all the psychoses associated with influenza presented in the acute phase a schizophrenic syndrome.

CONFIRMATORY DIAGNOSES

Of course the question immediately arises as to the correctness of our diagnoses. Other psychiatrists seeing the patients at the same time might have had a different opinion; we, ourselves, seeing the patient some months later, might have had a different opinion. Concerning the first contingency there is nothing to say except that our diagnosis represents the final conclusion of the staff of the Boston Psychopathic Hospital after at least ten days study of cases which were not singled out by them in any way (i.e., the staff had no statistical predilections about the probabilities of post-influenzal cases being schizophrenic). To err is human, and there is no doubt but that some of our diagnoses would not have been concurred in by another group of psychiatrists. It is reasonable to suppose, however, that this percentage of error is relatively small and Lowrey has presented several studies (7) to show that the diagnostic acumen of the staff of the Boston Psychopathic Hospital was relatively high as judged by the confirmations of diagnoses by other state hospital staffs.

The second contingency, namely, that seeing the case later in the disease might have led us to change our diagnosis, is an exceedingly important although somewhat treacherous assumption. Of course it is true that some psychiatric cases cannot be adequately studied in a week, and the conception of dementia precox as an established, progressive splitting of the mind with dementia, can be no more than inferred from a picture observed during a week's time. Nevertheless if there are cross-sectional psychopathological criteria of the schizophrenic syndrome, they should be just as detectable in a week as in a year. Of course it is possible for the psychiatric picture to change such that a syndrome distinctly schizophrenic may within a month or two become distinctly hypomanic and in such a case the subsequent students of the case are of course justified in making a diagnosis to fit the picture which seems to last the longer or to terminate the case.

That such psychopathological criteria for the diagnosis of the schizophrenic syndrome exist is tacitly admitted or assumed by most psychiatrists. The Kraepelinian conception was to the effect that such syndromes characterized what was almost always a progressive dementing psychosis, and made the diagnosis of "dementia precox" depend upon the schizophrenic syndrome in cross section plus this dementing course in longitudinal section. Orthodox adherents of the early Kraepelinian tenets still tend to take the position that if a picture regarded as schizophrenic resolves itself into a fairly definitely normal readaptation, i.e., "gets well," the original observations or conclusions with reference to its schizophrenic qualities were at fault. In other words, they hold in most cases that since schizophrenia is a dementing process, cases that do not dement but go on to recovery are not schizophrenic, and the symptoms so regarded were misinterpreted.

This sort of diagnosis-by-outcome is the logical result of the psychiatric fundamentalism that accompanied the introduction of Kraepelin's useful but acknowledgedly premature groupings to a practical and suggestible American profession. It has required nearly two decades for the French attitude of pluralism to make perceptible alterations in the diagnostic attitudes of American psychiatrists, in spite of the persistence of such leaders as Adolf Meyer with his designation of "reaction types" and (with specific regard to dementia precox) Bleuler and Ernest Southard with their insistence upon the word (and concept) schizophrenia.

This schizophrenic syndrome, in the opinion of the writer, can be recognized in cross section without the necessity for a prolonged period of observation. For this reason we have no unusual compunctions about the diagnoses of schizophrenia made by the Boston Psychopathic Hospital staff in these cases. Nor are we in the least disconcerted by the (roughly) 40 per cent[1] of these cases in which the diagnosis of schizophrenia was not concurred in by a state hospital staff observing the cases subsequently, knowing as we do that the diagnosis-by-outcome habit is or has been deeply ingrained in state hospital staffs.

A discussion of the precise criteria upon which the recognition of the schizophrenic syndrome depends is scarcely within the scope of this paper, being a nosological and theoretical rather than a practical problem. From a pragmatic standpoint we all know the general outlines of intrapsychic ataxia, of ideational-emotional-volitional incongruities with the queer alterations of behavior in bizarre directions, with delusions of reference, persecution and influence, and hallucinations, particularly of vague, senseless sorts; in brief a projection of autistic or dereistic dejecta in varying degrees of organization and with varying degrees and kinds of accompanying emotional disharmonies. (23)

It was such pictures that we observed in these sixty odd cases of acute mental illness subsequent to influence, and we called them "dementia precox" because at that time (and still) this is the accepted statistical nosological designation for the idiopathic schizophrenic syndrome. As we knew it then, these cases looked like, i.e., were, dementia precox in the acute (hence not yet "demented") stage.

These cases lend themselves to a variety of analyses. They might be studied from the standpoint of the time relations of the influenzal precipitation, the types of onset, the developmental patterns. Considerations of heredity, temperament and predisposition might justify much sifting of the data. Detailed symptom analysis might well be in order in view of the diagnostic disputes. The principles of dereistic mentation as increasingly laid bare by psychoanalysis and dynamic interpretative psychology might be applied to the symptom manifestations with scientific profit.

So comprehensive an analysis would take on the nature of a monograph. Nothing of the sort has been essayed here. The present study is an effort to present merely the outstanding features of the influenza-schizophrenia relationships.

Of such outstanding features there are three: 1) The high relative frequency of schizophrenia among the post-influenzal psychoses; 2) the fact that it occurred with and without evidences of hereditary taint or predisposition; and 3) the unexpectedly high recovery rate.

Of these, the statistics of relative frequency have already

---

1 Statistics appear below.

been cited. The questions of predisposition and hereditary taint have been previously reported. (8) It remains to present the facts of a follow-up investigation indicating the outcome of 50 of these cases.

Follow-up inquiries were sent at intervals during the five years subsequent to the observations made on these patients in Boston in 1918. Letters from the state hospitals, from relatives and friends, and in some instances from the patients themselves, were collected and correlated with the case histories, some of which are to be presented in detail below. [Case reports not reprinted here because of space limitations. These can be found on pages 479–527 of the July 1927 issue of the journal, vol. 82, no. 4.]

The statistics of the follow-up findings are as follows:

Of 50 cases which we have followed from one to five years, upon which a diagnosis of dementia precox was made at the Boston Psychopathic Hospital during the acute psychosis precipitated by influenza, 21 had this diagnosis confirmed by other state hospitals in which they had a subsequent and longer residence, and 14, who went home directly from the psychopathic hospital, did not have the diagnosis confirmed or contradicted because of this fact, while in 16 other cases the diagnosis of dementia precox was contradicted by a subsequent state hospital. The revised diagnoses in these 16 were as follows: Manic depressive, 9; toxic infectious, 4; psychosis with mental deficiency, 1; undiagnosticated, 2.

Of the entire 50 cases, 35 were apparently completely recovered within the five-year period. In addition to this, 5 were apparently improved. Five were apparently unchanged and 5 apparently worse.

STATISTICAL SUMMARY

Total number of post-influenzal psychoses	175
Total number of diagnosticated schizophrenia	60
Total number schizophrenics traced in follow-up	50

Statistical Analysis of 50 Traced Cases

Recovered		35
Diagnosis confirmed	9	
Diagnosis unconfirmed	12	
Diagnosis contradicted	14	
Improved		5
Diagnosis confirmed	3	
Diagnosis unconfirmed	1	
Diagnosis contradicted	1	
Unimproved		5
Diagnosis confirmed	5	
Diagnosis unconfirmed	0	
Diagnosis contradicted	5	
Worse (dementing)		5
Diagnosis confirmed	4	
Diagnosis unconfirmed	0	
Diagnosis contradicted	1	

THEORETICAL IMPLICATIONS

The astonishing indication of these data is that the vast majority of cases regarded as "dementia precox" did not de-

ment, but actually recovered. That 70 per cent of supposed cases of dementia precox should get entirely well and an additional 10 per cent be "improved" within five years of the onset of the psychosis is incredible to anyone who preserves the older idea of the nature of dementia precox.

Such findings indicate either that our diagnoses were wrong or that our older conceptions of dementia precox were wrong, or that influenza produces a curious atypical type of dementia precox which tends to recover.

We can partially eliminate the first possibility by considering only those cases in which the diagnosis of one staff was, after a longer or shorter period of subsequent observation, confirmed by a second staff of psychiatrists in modernly conducted and equipped state hospitals. Even thus, however, we have 12 cases improved or recovered as compared to 9 unchanged or worse, and this again is not the usual history of dementia precox.

Concerning the possibility that influenza evokes a picture of a specific type of psychosis, schizophrenic or whatever, we have already dealt in previous discussions. (1) This was a thesis strongly advocated by Kraepelin and vigorously combated by Bonhoeffer and the French psychiatrists. Influenza precipitated and created too great a variety of psychotic pictures to be regarded as possessed of a specific psychiatric syndrome. Frequent as was the schizophrenic picture, it would not be justifiable to regard it as influenzal until we have carefully considered the comparable results of other infectious diseases. The presumption is that a schizophrenic picture appeared as the result of the neurotoxic effects of the influenzal infection, but it is definitely known that other infections, such as typhus fever, typhoid fever, etc., can similarly produce schizophrenic pictures. (29) Accordingly there may be an acute, reversible, post-influenzal schizophrenia, but there is no justification for regarding it as specifically influenzal at the present time and it is much more productive to consider it merely as a generic problem, viz., the schizophrenic syndrome produced by acute infectious somatic illness.

The cases under discussion differ from those ordinarily regarded as "toxic-infectious" psychoses chiefly in the duration of the symptoms and in the multiplicity of psychopathology. There was once a diagnosis in vogue which would probably have included many of the cases, at least in the acute phase, namely, amentia (Meynert). Amentia was given up because it was indistinguishable by many psychiatrists from dementia precox, while others regarded it as merely a severe chronic delirium.

After all, a diagnosis of "toxic-infectious psychosis" is merely to say that the given patient has a psychosis for which there is believed to be a more or less obviously somatic cause. It requires no long citation of histories, which however, could be done page on page, to point out that from a descriptive standpoint there is little fundamental difference between delirium and dementia precox. Both embrace the same elements, and if the perceptual obnubilation and incoherence (often ambiguously labeled "clouding of consciousness") are apparently greater in what we call delirium, and if bizarre behavior is a little more marked in most cases of what we regard as "dementia precox," some explanation might be sought in questions of duration, intensity and cell layer. This seems more plausible now that epidemic encephalitis has appeared in such definitely symptomatically schizophrenic as well as "delirious" forms. In both there are the same emotional disharmonies, and other evidences of fragmented dissociation. It is the author's thesis that between the mildest attack of so-called simple delirium and the most profound dementia of late schizophrenia there is an essential unity, and also progressive gradation, not (necessarily) in the intensity of symptoms but in the degree of reversibility. Theoretical implications are deferred for presentation elsewhere. (29)

CONCLUSIONS

1. There are three outstanding features in the analysis made of the data pertaining to post-influenzal psychoses of the schizophrenic type:

(a) Schizophrenia was relatively the most frequent psychiatric syndrome; (b) it occurred with and without evidences of hereditary taint or predisposition; (c) most of the cases so diagnosticated made more or less complete recoveries.

2. If we retain the Kraepelinian conceptions of dementia precox, we must think that influenza precipitated many cases which seemed in the acute phase to be dementia precox, but of which relatively few ultimately verified this early diagnosis, and were somatic psychoses or cyclothymic psychoses of strongly schizophrenoid coloring.

3. For those, including the author, who reject Kraepelin's conception of dementia precox in favor of the conception of a schizophrenic syndrome, representing certain kinds or phases of psychic disintegration arising upon varied bases and following varied courses (i.e., showing varied degrees of reversibility), the conclusions from the influenza series would be that many such schizophrenic syndromes occurred immediately subsequent to influenza, but of the entire series the great majority ultimately recovered, some promptly, some only after a year or more; a few progressed to various degrees of dementia. This would indicate a relative benigninity of this process.

4. This schizophrenic picture has been reported under a variety of names by most of the writers on post-influenzal psychoses. All agree that the syndrome occurs in both predisposed (schizoid) and unpredisposed (syntonic) individuals. There is some disagreement as to the relative frequency of the schizophrenic syndrome, but the general agreement as to the good prognosis.

5. The small incidence of all the major psychoses subsequent to influenza relative to the enormous morbidity of influenza would indicate that while the influenza-schizophrenia relationships offer much subtle material for elucidating the inner structure of mental mechanisms, they do not offer many direct problems of management or treatment.

BIBLIOGRAPHY

1. Menninger, Karl A.: Psychoses Associated with Influenza. J.A.M.A., 72:235 (January, 1925), 1919.
2. Menninger, Karl A.: Influenza and Neurosyphilis. Arch. of Internal Med., July, 1919, Vol. XXIV, pp. 98–115.
3. Menninger, Karl A.: Influenza and Hypophrenia. J.A.M.A., October 16, 1920, Vol. 75, pp. 1044–1051.
4. Menninger, Karl A.: Influenza and Epilepsy. Am. Jour. of Med. Sciences, June, 1921, No. 6, Vol. CIXI, p. 784.
5. Menninger, Karl A.: Melancholy and Melancholia. Jour. Kansas Med. Society, February, 1921.
6. Menninger, Karl A.: Reversible Schizophrenia. Am. Jour. of Psychiatry, Vol. 1, No. 4, April, 1922.
7. Lowrey, Lawson G.: Medicine and Surgery, March, 1918; also Bulletin Mass. Com. on Mental Disease, Vol. II, No. 3; Am. Jour. Insanity, Vol. 75, 1919; Boston Med. and Surg. Journal, Vol. 183, September, 1920; also Bull. Mass. Com. on Mental Disease, Vol. III, No. 3. Am. Jour. Insan., January, 1921.
8. Menninger, Karl A.: Psychoses Associated with Influenza. Archives Neurol. and Psychiatry, September, 1919, II, 291–337.
9. Gowers, W.R.: The Nervous Sequelae of Influenza. Lancet 2:1 and 73, 1893.
10. Regis: Psychiatrie, Paris, and Delire de la convalescence. Ann. med.-psych., Paris, 1883, p. 393.
11. Kirn: Ueber Influenza Psychosen. München. med. Wchnschr. 37: 299–301, 1890. Die nervoesen und psychischen Stoerungen der Influenza. Samml. klin. Vortr., n. F. 23: Leipzig, 1891; Die Psychosen der Influenza, Allg. Ztschr. f. Psychiat. 48:1–15, 1891–1892.
12. Bonhoeffer: In Aschaffenburg's Handbuch (Leipzig and Vienna), 1912.
13. Paton, S.: Psychiatry, Philadelphia. J.B. Lippincott Co., 1905.
14. Gosline, H.I.: Newer Conceptions of Dementia Precox. J. Lab. & Clin. Med. 2:691 (July), 1917.
15. Fell, Egbart W.: Postinfluenzal Psychoses. J.A.M.A. 72:1658 (June 7), 1919.
16. Fell, Egbert W.: Psychoses Accompanying Influenza. Boston Med. and Surg. Jour. CLXXII, No. 5, pp. 113–116, January 29, 1920.
17. Sandy, Wm. C.: The Association of Neuropsychiatric Conditions with Influenza in the Epidemic of 1918. Arch. Neuro. and Psych., August, 1920, IV, pp. 171–181.
18. Harris, A.F.: Influenza as a Factor in Precipitating Latent Psychoses and Initiating Psychoses, with a Brief History of the Disease and Analysis of Cases. Boston M. and S. J. 180:610 (May 29), 1919.
19. Schlesinger, Alfred.: Des Delires infectieux au cours de la grippe. Revue med de la Suisse romande XXXIX, No. 4, April, 1919.
20. Harris, I.G., and Corcoran, David.: Psychoses Following Influenza. State Hospital Quarterly, August, 1919.
21. Walther, F.: Ueber Grippepsychosen. Bircher, Berne, 1923.
22. Jelliffe, S.E.: Nervous and Mental Disturbances of Influenza. N.Y. Med. Jour., October, 26, November 2, November 9, 1918.
23. Greenacre, P. The Content of the Schizophrenic Characteristics Occurring in Affective Disorders. Am. Jour. Insan. 75, 197.
24. Bleuler, Eugen.: Textbook of Psychiatry. Translated by Brill. Macmillan, 1924.
25. Riese, Walther.: Psychic Disturbances after Spanish Grippe. Neurol. Centralbl., Nov. 1, 1918, No. 21, Vol. XXXVII. Abstr. in Jour. N. and M. Dis., Vol. 56, No. 2, August, 1922, pp. 115–125.
26. Waterman, Chester, and Folsom, R.P.: Psychoses Associated with Influenza. State Hospital Quarterly, Vol. IV, No. 4, August, 1919.
27. Kirby, Geo. H.: Psychoses Associated with Influenza. State Hospital Quarterly, Vol. IV, No. 4, August, 1919.
28. Bleuler, E.: Dementia Precox. Aschaffenburg's Handbuch, Section 4, 1st half, p. 280.
29. Menninger, Karl A.: The Schizophrenic Syndrome as a product of Infectious Disease. Read at the annual meeting of the Association for Research in Nervous and Mental Diseases, New York, December 28, 1925.

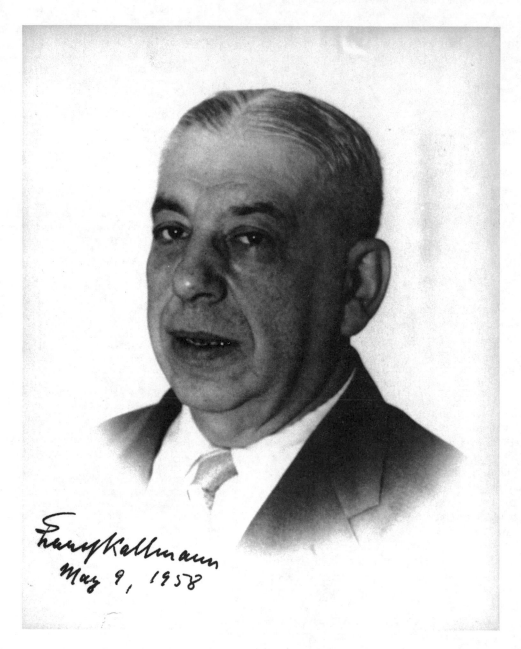

Franz J. Kallmann, M.D., 1897–1965

THE GENETIC THEORY OF SCHIZOPHRENIA
An Analysis of 691 Schizophrenic Twin Index Families

By Franz J. Kallmann, M.D.
New York, New York

Despite notable changes in the attitude of contemporary psychiatry toward the constitutional problems of psychosomatic medicine, there is still a tendency to perpetuate the genetic theory of schizophrenia as a controversial issue.

Some arguments thrive largely on dialectic grounds and, from a scientific standpoint, are more apparent than real. Others are based on preconceptions which are kept alive by an ambiguous terminology and the pardonable tendency either to oversimplify a complex causality or to mistake it for obscurity. A main source of misunderstanding is the erroneous belief that acceptance of causation by heredity would be incompatible with general psychological theories of a descriptive or analytical nature, or that it might lead to a depreciation of present educational and therapeutic standards. Evidently, there is no point in presenting evidence of the inheritance of schizophrenia, if in subsequent statements the etiology of schizophrenic psychoses is likely to be listed as unknown, or if reservations are made regarding a similar psychotic syndrome labeled dementia praecox, or if the given genetic mechanism is finally dismissed as unessential or non-Mendelian.

From a genetic point of view, the main question to be clarified is whether or not the capacity for developing a true schizophrenic psychosis is somehow controlled by inherited, predispositional elements. In order to settle this problem beyond any reasonable doubt, only three types of investigative procedure are available. They are:

1) The pedigree or family history method,
2) The contingency method of statistical prediction, and
3) The twin study method.

The investigation of individual *family histories* is the oldest, simplest, and most popular method of recording familial occurrence of an apparently hereditary trait. Such a pedigree is often impressive to behold and sometimes as suggestive of the operation of heredity as is true with respect to the family unit[1] presented in Fig. 1. If the mating of two psychotic parents is found, under certain circumstances, to be capable of giving rise to seven definite cases of schizophrenia among the offspring, that is, in all the children of this union who reached the age of maturity, it would seem inadequate to disregard the possible significance of the biological factor prerequisite for inheritance, namely, consanguinity. On the basis of this single observation, however, the genetic hypothesis would be no more conclusive than either the assumption of *folie à neuf* due to "psychic contagion" or the supposition that the psychosis of the father of this remarkable sibship was not "inherited" because his parents had apparently been ordinary first cousins without schizophrenia.

Obviously, the general usefulness of the pedigree method is limited to the study of relatively rare unit characters which are easily traced and fairly constant in their clinical appearance. In more common traits and especially in irregularly expressed anomalies such as schizophrenia, it is necessary to employ statistical methods which demonstrate more clearly the effect of blood relationship.

This objective is accomplished by the *contingency method*, which compares the morbidity rates for representative samples of consanguineous and non-consanguineous groups. The results of such a procedure will indicate whether or not a given anomaly occurs more frequently in blood relatives of unselected index cases than is to be expected in the light of the normal average distribution of the trait in the general population. The available morbidity figures for schizophrenia, obtained with the contingency method, are summarized in Fig. 2. The rates refer to different population and consanguinity groups and may have been compiled with different degrees of statistical accuracy. The samples differ in size as well as in uniformity, and many of them seem to have lived under socio-economic conditions which cannot be compared directly.

However, one essential point has been confirmed by all of these studies, namely, that the incidence of schizophrenia tends to be higher in blood relatives of schizophrenic index cases than it is in the general population. Concerning the offspring of schizophrenic index cases it has been shown that their morbidity rates range from 16.4 to 68.1 per cent, that is, from nineteen to about eighty times average expec-

Read at the 102d annual meeting of The American Psychiatric Association, Chicago, Ill., May 27–30, 1946. From the Department of Medical Genetics of the New York State Psychiatric Institute and Hospital, New York 32, N.Y.

[1] The investigation of this family was carried out in collaboration with Miss Jean Mickey. The psychiatric aspects of this study will be discussed in another publication. As all the other charts and tabulations, the pedigree was arranged by Mrs. Helen Kallmann.

FIGURE 1.—Pedigree of a Family Showing Unusual Accumulation of Schizophrenic Cases

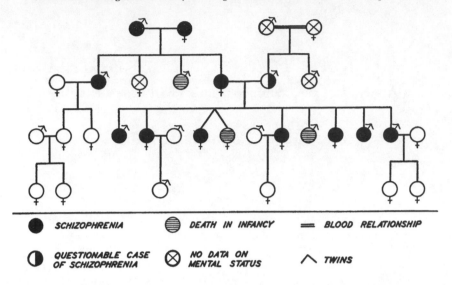

● SCHIZOPHRENIA   ⊕ DEATH IN INFANCY   ══ BLOOD RELATIONSHIP

◐ QUESTIONABLE CASE OF SCHIZOPHRENIA   ⊗ NO DATA ON MENTAL STATUS   ∧ TWINS

FIGURE 2.—Schizophrenia Rates Obtained With the Contingency Method of Statistical Prediction

	Incidence of Schizophrenia in Consanguineous Groups Related to:										
								Two Ordinary Index Cases		One Twin Index Case	
	Incidence of Schizophrenia in General Population	One Ordinary Index Case of Schizophrenia									
		Nephews and Nieces	First Cousins	Grand children	Half Siblings	Parents	Full Siblings	Children	Siblings	Children	Dizygotic Cotwins	Monozygotic Cotwins
Previous morbidity studies of Kallmann	0.85	3.9	—	4.3	7.6	10.3	11.5	16.4	20.5	68.1	12.5	81.7
Range of morbidity rates of other investigators	0.3–1.5	1.4–3.9	2.6	—	—	7.1–9.3	4.5–11.7	8.3–9.7	20.0	53.0	14.9	68.3

tancy, according to whether one or both of their parents are schizophrenic (Fig. 3). It is to be verified, therefore, that the chance of developing schizophrenia in comparable environments increases in direct proportion to the degree of blood relationship to a schizophrenic index case. If such evidence can be supplied, intransigent supporters of purely environmental theories should be expected to demonstrate with equally precise methods that a consistent increase in morbidity is found associated with particular environmental circumstances *in the absence* of consanguinity.

In order to establish the hereditary nature of a psychosis beyond the possibility of random contingency and in relation to the interaction of predispositional genetic elements and various precipitating or perpetuating influences acting from without, the best available procedure is the *twin study method* in conjunction with an ordinary sibling study. Such a combination method[2] has been adopted in our long-range studies of specific behavior disorders and has been called by us "Twin Family Method" (Fig. 4). This approach provides six distinct categories of sibship groups reared under comparable environmental conditions; namely, monozygotic twins, dizygotic twins of the same sex, dizygotic twins of opposite sex, full siblings, half-siblings, and step-siblings. If

the assumed genetic factor exists and the part played by the twinning factor is negligible, the statistical expectation will be that the morbidity rates for full siblings and dizygotic twin partners should be about the same, but they should clearly differ from the rates for the other sibship groups.

One-egg twins are expected to show the highest concordance rate for a genetically determined disorder, even if brought up in different environments. Two-egg twins may be either of the same or of opposite sex, but genetically they are no more alike than any other pair of brothers and sisters who are born at different times. Half-siblings with only one parent in common should be about midway between the full siblings and the non-consanguineous step-siblings, if the given morbidity depends on the closeness of blood relationship rather than on the similarity in environment.

In order to obtain statistically representative material for the application of this method, our survey was organized on a state-wide basis. The twin index cases (Fig. 5) were collected from the resident populations and new admissions of all mental hospitals under the supervision of the New York State Department of Mental Hygiene. The danger of bias on account of technical selective factors in the sampling of the material was avoided by referring the determination of

2 A more detailed description of the method can be found in a previous report of F.J. Kallmann and D. Reisner, "Twin Studies on Genetic Variations in Resistance to Tuberculosis," Journal of Heredity, Vol., 34, No. 9.

FIGURE 3.—Expectation of Schizophrenia and Schizoid Personality
in Descendants of Schizophrenics

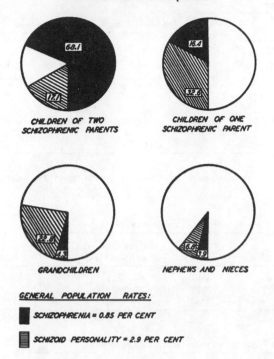

GENERAL POPULATION RATES:

█ SCHIZOPHRENIA = 0.85 PER CENT

▤ SCHIZOID PERSONALITY = 2.9 PER CENT

FIGURE 4.—Degree of Consanguinity in Twin Family Method

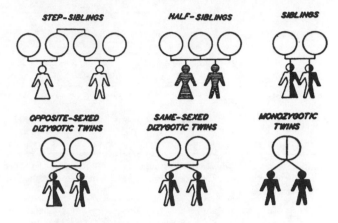

the twin index cases to the staffs of the hospitals cooperating in the survey. The only criteria for selection were that the reported cases be born by multiple birth and that they had been admitted with a diagnosis of mental disease.

The classifications of both schizophrenia and zygocity were made on the basis of personal investigation and extended observation. The twin diagnosis was based on findings obtained with the similarity method, since it is known now that monozygotic twins are not necessarily monochorial. The statistical analysis was limited to the families of 794 schizophrenic twin index cases whose cotwins were available for examination at the age of fifteen years. These index cases were reported within a period of nine years by twenty institutions, which in 1945 had a total resident population of 73,252 patients with 47,929 schizophrenics and 12,316 new admissions.

The random sampling of the 691 index pairs is indicated by the close correspondence between the statistically expected figure of 25.6 percent for the proportion of monozygotic twin pairs in an unselected American twin group, and the actual percentage of 25.2 as obtained with the Weinberg Differential Method for the present study. It is in accordance with expectation that the main deficit is on the part of dizygotic twins of opposite sex. Altogether, there are 174 monozygotic and 517 dizygotic index pairs with schizophrenia in at least one member or, more precisely, 691 pairs constituted by 1,382 twins, of whom 794 were legitimate index cases. Of the dizygotic sets, 296 are same-sexed and 221 are opposite-sexed.

The excess of female over male index cases is almost 20 percent. The ratio of white to non-white index cases is about 14:1. Approximately 70 percent of the index cases are unmarried. The proportion of nuclear cases, characterized by

hebephrenic or catatonic psychoses with the tendency to progression and deterioration, amounts to 68 percent.

The various groups of relatives included in the analysis of these 691 twin index families are identified in Fig. 6. There are 1,382 twins, 2,741 full siblings, 134 half-siblings, 74 step-siblings, 1,191 parents and 254 marriage partners of twin patients, making a total of 5,776 persons who have been uniformly classified according to their mental, social and genealogical conditions.

The collective schizophrenia rates for the different relation groups are compared in Fig. 7. The variations in age distribution have been corrected by the use of the "Abridged Weinberg Method." The resulting morbidity rates are average expectancy figures valid for persons above the chief manifestation period, which in this study was assumed to extend from the age of fifteen to forty-four.

Regardless of whether the uncorrected or corrected rates are taken into account, they are in definite accordance with genetic expectation regarding both schizophrenia and schizoid personality. The corrected schizophrenia rate for full siblings amounts to 14.3 percent, corresponding closely with the collective concordance rate for dizygotic twin pairs (14.7 percent), although it clearly exceeds the rate for half-siblings (7.0 percent). A comparison with our previous sibship figures reveals only minor variations which seem sufficiently explained by the different sampling procedures of sibship and descent studies. Our previous schizophrenia rates were 7.6 percent for half-siblings, 11.5 percent for full siblings, and 12.5 percent for dizygotic cotwins.

The newly obtained morbidity figures for step-siblings and marriage partners of schizophrenic index cases are 1.8 and 2.1 percent, respectively, showing a small excess over the general population rate of 0.85 percent. So far as this excess is statistically significant, it is referable to the effect of mate selection rather than an expression of socially induced insanity.

By contrast, the difference in concordance between two-egg and one-egg twin partners ranges from 14.7 to 85.8 percent. An almost equally striking difference remains, if the comparison is limited to the groups of same-sexed dizygotic and separated monozygotic twin pairs (Fig. 8). Their morbidity rates vary from 17.6 to 77.6 percent, and this differ-

FIGURE 5.—Racial and Diagnostic Distribution of the Twin Index Cases

| | All Schizophrenic Twin Index Cases Reported[a] | | | | | | | All Complete Index Pairs Studied[b] | | | | |
| | Marital Status | | Racial Distribution | | Diagnostic Distribution | | Total Number | Mono-zygotic | Dizygotic | | | Total Number |
	Single	Married	White	Non-white	Nuclear	Peripheral			Same Sex	Opposite Sex	
Male	292	70	337	25	253	109	362	75	132	$\frac{221}{2}$	317½
Female	266	166	405	27	290	142	432	99	164	$\frac{221}{2}$	373½
Total number	558	236	742	52	543	251	794	174	296	221	691

[a]Without index cases whose cotwins were unavailable at the age of 15 years.
[b]The difference between 794 index cases and 691 index pairs is explained by the fact that in 103 pairs both twin partners were reported as index cases and acceptable as such.

FIGURE 6.—Number and Relationship of the Persons Included in the Survey

	Twins	Full Siblings	Half-Siblings	Step-Siblings	Parents	Husbands and Wives of Index Cases	Total Number
Living	1198	1682	84	47	618	221	3850
Dead	184	1059	50	27	573	33	1926
Total number	1382	2741	134	74	1191	254	5776

FIGURE 7.—Incidence of Schizophrenia and Schizoid Personality in the Twin Index Families

| | Relationship to Schizophrenic Twin Index Cases | | | | | | |
	Parents	Husbands and Wives	Step-Siblings	Half-Siblings	Full Siblings	Dizygotic Cotwins	Monozygotic Cotwins
Statistically uncorrected rates							
Number of persons	1191	254	85	134	2741	517	174
Cases of schizophrenia	108	5	1	4	205	53	120
Incidence of schizophrenia[a]	9.1	2.0	1.4	4.5	10.2	10.3	69.0
Corrected morbidity rates							
Schizophrenia[b]	9.2	2.1	1.8	7.0	14.3	14.7	85.8
Schizoid personality	34.8	3.1	2.7	12.5	31.5	23.0	20.7

[a]Related to all cases of schizophrenia and to all persons over age 15.
[b]Related only to definite cases of schizophrenia and to half of the persons in the age group 15-44 (plus all persons over age 44).

ence is still so pronounced that explanations on non-genetic grounds are very difficult to uphold. The total morbidity distribution as summarized in Fig. 8 is a rather clear indication that the chance of developing schizophrenia increases in proportion to the degree of consanguinity to a schizophrenic index case. The only other syndrome showing a significant increase in the index families is that of schizoid personality changes, whose genetically heterogeneous nature has been discussed in previous reports.

Concerning the total morbidity rate of 85.8 percent for monozygotic cotwins it should be borne in mind that the figure expresses the chance of developing schizophrenia in a comparable environment for any person that has survived the age of forty-four and is genetically identical with a schizophrenic index case, but is not distinguished by the fact of having been selected as the child of such an index case. The last point needs particular emphasis, since it apparently explains the difference between the morbidity rates of 68.1 and 85.8 percent as found for the children of two schizophrenic parents and for the monozygotic cotwins of schizophrenic index cases, respectively. In fact, it

is only by a comparison of these two figures that a satisfactory estimate can be obtained of the extent of biased sampling in a morbidity study dealing with children of schizophrenic index cases. In order to provide such a sample, schizophrenics must have had a chance of getting married and producing offspring.

According to our previous fertility studies (Fig. 9), the total reproductive rate of schizophrenic index cases is not more than about half that of a comparable general population. However, the decrease in fertility is much more pronounced in the nuclear group of schizophrenia, comprising the deteriorating types of hebephrenia and catatonia, than it is in the paranoid and simple cases. The consequence is that milder schizophrenic cases have a better chance of reproducing a schizophrenic child than have the more severe cases. If the children of one schizophrenic parent will often be the offspring of patients with lessened severity of their symptoms, the children of two schizophrenic parents may be expected to represent an even greater selection of potential schizophrenics in the direction of a highly resistant constitution. Obviously, such a process of natural se-

FIGURE 8.—Expectancy of Schizophrenia and Schizoid Personality in Blood Relatives of Schizophrenic Twin Index Cases

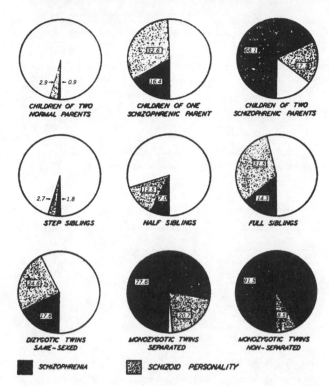

FIGURE 9.—Marriage and Birth Rates of Schizophrenic Hospital Patients

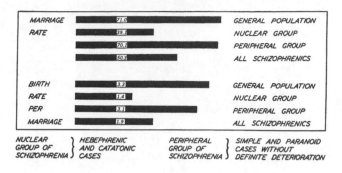

lings. In this evaluation of significant similarities and dissimilarities in the life conditions of various relationship groups in our index families, a credible explanation should be sought especially for a finding which is never accounted for by exponents of purely "cultural" theories of schizophrenia. This rather striking observation is that over 85 percent of our groups of siblings and dizygotic cotwins did *not* develop schizophrenia, although about 10 percent of them had a schizophrenic parent, all of them had a schizophrenic brother or sister, and a large proportion shared the same environment with these schizophrenics before and after birth.

For anatomical reasons, prematurity of birth, instrumental delivery and reversal in handedness are more common in twins than in single-born individuals. It is shown in Fig. 10, however, that no one of these factors has any bearing on the occurrence of schizophrenia in persons who happen to be twins. There is practically no difference between concordant and discordant twin pairs in the frequency of premature birth (14.3-15.4 percent) or of instrumental delivery (4.1-4.2 percent). In discordant index pairs, over 82 percent are alike in regard to handedness, the vast majority (81.8 percent) being right-handed. In the unlike pairs, left-handedness occurs about as often in the non-schizophrenic twin partners (9.1 percent) as in schizophrenic twin index cases (8.2 percent). It is in accordance with expectation that most of the concordant twin pairs showing dissimilarity as to left-handedness are monozygotic.

The collective morbidity rates for the cotwins are modified by a variety of secondary factors, genetic as well as nongenetic, but certainly not to an extent which would explain the marked difference between the two types of twins. Variation in relation to the sex factor cannot exist in monozygotic twin pairs and is of equally limited extent in the groups of siblings and dizygotic twins. The range of the former group is from 12.3 to 16.1 percent, and that of the latter group from 10.3 to 17.6 percent (Fig. 11). The difference in morbidity remains constant regardless of whether the siblings and cotwins are male or female. This sex variation is an indication that fraternals belonging to the same sex as a given index case have a greater chance of being alike in any particular circumstances which may favor the manifestation of the schizophrenic genotype. It is clear, however, that these sex variations are by no means extensive enough to permit a non-genetic explanation for the entire differ-

lection does not operate in persons who have only the distinction of being the monozygotic cotwins of schizophrenic twin index cases.

Clinically it is very important that neither the offspring of two schizophrenic parents nor the monozygotic cotwins of schizophrenic index cases have a morbidity rate of 100 percent as would be expected theoretically in regard to a strictly hereditary trait. This observation indicates a limited expressivity of the main genetic factor controlling schizophrenia, but it should not be misinterpreted in the sense that the extent of the deficit is an adequate measure of the part played by non-genetic agents in the production of a schizophrenic psychosis. From a biological standpoint, the finding classifies schizophrenia as both preventable and potentially curable. The implication is that the main schizophrenic genotype is not fully expressed either in the absence of any particular factor of a precipitating nature or in the presence of strong constitutional defense mechanisms which in turn are partially determined by heredity. The statistical difference between observed and expected morbidity rates for unquestionably homozygous carriers of the schizophrenic genotype does not mean, however, that heredity is effective in only 70 to 85 percent of schizophrenic cases, or that it is essential merely to the extent of 70 to 85 percent in any one case.

In order to exclude the possibility that the entire difference in morbidity between monozygotic and dizygotic cotwins might be sufficiently *explained by factors other than genetic*, it is necessary to analyze the morbidity rates for the various sibship groups in relation to any developmental or environmental circumstances peculiar to twins and sib-

FIGURE 10.—Handedness and Instrumental Delivery in the Twin Index Pairs

| | Similarity of Delivery and Handedness in Twin Partners | | | | | Dissimilarity of Instrumental Delivery and Handedness in Twin Partners | | | |
| | | | | | | Instrumental Delivery in | | Left-Handedness in | |
	Normal Delivery	Premature Birth	Instrumental Delivery	Right-Handedness	Left-Handedness	Schizophrenic Twin	Non-Schizophrenic Twin	Schizophrenic Twin	Non-Schizophrenic Twin
Both twin partners schizophrenic	79.6	14.3	4.1	72.1	2.5	2.0	—	25.5[a]	—
One twin partner schizophrenic	76.2	15.4	4.2	81.8	0.9	2.4	1.8	8.2	9.1
All twin index pairs	77.1	15.1	4.2	67.4	1.2	2.3	1.3	12.9	6.6

[a]Of 41 twin pairs in whom only one of the two schizophrenic twin partners was found to be left-handed, 33 pairs were monozygotic

FIGURE 11.—Variations in the Schizophrenia Rates of Siblings and Twin Partners
According to Sex and the Similarity or Dissimilarity in Environment

| | Siblings of Twin Index Cases | | | Dizygotic Cotwins | | | Monozygotic Cotwins | | |
	Male	Female	Total Number	Male	Female	Total Number	Separated	Non-Separated	Total Number
Same-sexed	15.9	16.3	16.1	17.4	17.7	17.6	77.6	91.5	85.8
Opposite-sexed	12.5	12.0	12.3	10.5	10.2	10.3	—	—	—
Total number	14.0	14.5	14.3	14.3	14.9	14.7	77.6	91.5	85.8

FIGURE 12.—Concordance as to Schizophrenia
in Separated and Non-Separated Pairs of Monozygotic Twins

	Separated[a] Pairs	Non-Separated Pairs	Total Number
Number of cotwins	59	115	174
Corrected morbidity rate of cotwins	77.6	91.5	85.8

[a]Separated for five years or more prior to the onset of schizophrenia in the index twin.

ence, or a major part of the difference, between the concordance rates of monozygotic and dizygotic twin pairs.

The main variations in the morbidity rate of monozygotic cotwins are apparently associated with age at disease onset, type of psychosis, and a variety of extrinsic factors causing significant changes in the physical development and general health status of one twin partner. Most of these modifications in susceptibility or resistance do not lend themselves to statistical analysis, and it is impossible here to enter into a discussion of individual twin histories. It is essential, however, to stress the great variability of such contingent influences, because it is this point which makes the etiology of schizophrenic processes so complex and a carefully adapted program of constructive therapeutic measures so important. Many of our twin histories indicate that incidental factors such as pregnancy, intercurrent disease, or a reducing diet which may have been responsible for the crucial difference between health and psychosis in one twin pair, will not have the same vital effect in others.

The morbidity rate for monozygotic cotwins varies from 77.6 to 91.5 percent for those twin partners who were or were not separated for over five years prior to disease onset in the index twin (Fig. 12). It has already been emphasized

that this statistical difference is no adequate expression of the relative effect of extraneous circumstances on the development of schizophrenia in genetically alike persons. Separation is no exact measure of dissimilarity in regard to environmental agents precipitating schizophrenia. There are numerous factors of potential etiological significance, which are practically universal. In fact, our group of separated one-egg pairs includes twins who developed schizophrenia at almost the same time, although their separation took place soon after birth and led to apparently very different life conditions.

Conversely, even with similar environment it cannot be expected that the time of onset of a schizophrenic psychosis in genetically identical persons will be exactly the same. It is shown in Fig. 13 that simultaneous occurrence of schizophrenia is found in only 17.6 percent of monozygotic twin pairs. In about one-half of the index pairs (52.9 percent) there is a difference of one month to four years, and in over one-quarter the difference may be from four to twelve years. Psychobiologically it is of interest to note that significant dissimilarities in symptomatology are observed only in twin partners who show a definite variation in age of onset.

The age discrepancies between twin partners remain about the same if the comparison is based on the dates of first admission. The average age at disease onset is 22.1 years for the index twins, and 25.6 years for the cotwins.

There are also certain differences in the period of time during which either the twin partners were under observation before they were classified as concordant or discordant as to schizophrenia, or during which the concordant pairs had been separated before the index twins developed their psychosis. A glance at Fig. 14 will reveal, however, that these differences are entirely insufficient to explain the variations in morbidity between one-egg and two-egg types

FIGURE 13.—Variations in the Average Age at Disease Onset and First Admission
of the Monozygotic Twin Index Pairs Concordant as to Schizophrenia

| | Average Age in Years | | | Percentage of Twin Pairs Showing Differences in Age at Onset of Schizophrenia | | | | | |
	First Twin	Second Twin	Difference Between Twin Partners	No Difference	0.1–4 Years	4.1–8 Years	8.1–12 Years	12.1–16 Years	16.1–20 Years
Onset of disease	22.1	25.6	3.5	17.6	52.9	18.6	10.8	—	—
First admission	26.0	30.3	4.3	26.5	38.2	21.6	7.8	3.9	2.0

FIGURE 14.—Distribution of Concordance and Discordance in Twin Index Pairs in Relation to Disease Onset and Environment

| | Number of Index Pairs | | Average Duration in Years | | Discordant Pairs in Per Cent | |
	Concordant	Discordant	Separation in Concordant Pairs	Discordance in Discordant Pairs	With Similar Environment	With Dissimilar Environment
Monozygotic	120	54	11.1	8.5	61.1	38.9
Dizygotic same-sexed	34	262	12.9	12.5	57.3	42.7
Dizygotic opposite-sexed	13	208	13.8	11.1	50.5	49.5
All twin index pairs	167	524	11.8	11.5	55.0	45.0

FIGURE 15.—Relationship Between Similarity or Dissimilarity in Environment and Concordance or Discordance
as to Schizophrenia in the Twin Index Pairs

| | Cotwins With Similar Environment | | | Cotwins With Dissimilar Environment | | | All Cotwins | | |
| | | Rate of Cotwins in Per Cent | | | Rate of Cotwins in Per Cent | | | Rate of Cotwins in Per Cent | |
	Number of Cotwins	Concordant	Discordant	Number of Cotwins	Concordant	Discordant	Total Number	Concordant With Dissimilar Environment	Discordant With Similar Environment
Monozygotic	114	71.1	28.9	60	65.0	35.0	174	22.4	19.0
Dizygotic	276	7.6	92.4	241	10.8	89.2	517	5.0	49.3
Total	390	26.2	73.8	301	21.6	78.4	691	9.4	41.7

of twins. The separated concordant twins had lived apart for an average of 11.8 years before disease onset in the first twin, and the discordant index pairs had reached a total average age of thirty-three years at the time of their examination for this survey. All categories of cotwins had at that time been discordant for over eight years since the development of schizophrenia in the index cases.

It is more significant that similarity and dissimilarity of environment are almost equally distributed among the discordant index pairs. The ratio for all discordant pairs is 5.5:4.5, and that for monozygotic pairs alone is 6:4.

Additional evidence against a simple correlation between closeness of blood relationship and increasing similarity in environment with correspondingly intensified pressure toward development of a psychosis is obtained by an investigation of the distribution of concordance and discordance in similar and dissimilar environments in both groups of index pairs (Fig. 15). This analysis indicates that 22.4 percent of all monozygotic pairs are concordant without similar environment, and that 49.3 percent of all dizygotic twin partners remain discordant although they have been exposed to the same environment as an index case.

It may be of some interest that the concordance rate of monozygotic pairs varies from 65.0 to 71.1 percent accord-ing to dissimilarity or similarity of environment, while there is no corresponding increase in the dizygotic group (10.8—7.6 percent). There can be no doubt, however, that any such variation in relation to environment does not suffice to explain a ratio of 1:6 or 14.7:85.8 percent, as has been obtained for the morbidity rates of dizygotic and monozygotic twin partners.

That heredity determines the individual capacity for development and control of a schizophrenic psychosis is demonstrated still more clearly, if the similarities in extent and outcome of the disease are taken as further criteria of comparison. This is the objective of the remaining tabulations (Figs. 16-18) which compare the cotwin groups with completely and incompletely similar or dissimilar behavior to schizophrenia, instead of comparing the twin groups with and without psychotic symptoms as was done by the use of morbidity rates.

Complete similarity has been assumed when both twins either recovered from a mild psychosis with little or no defect (Group II) or reached about the same degree of medium (Group III) or extreme deterioration (Group IV). On the basis of this classification, complete concordance is found in 67.5 percent of the concordant one-egg twin pairs, but only in 6.4 percent of the dizygotic pairs (Fig. 16).

FIGURE 16.—Distribution of Concordance in Relation to Similarity of Environment and Clinical Course of Schizophrenia

	Concordant Pairs in Percent				
	Not Separated	Separated— Similar Environment	Separated— Dissimilar Environment	Completely[a] Concordant	Incompletely[a] Concordant
Monozygotic	50.8	16.7	32.5	67.5	32.5
Dizygotic	42.5	2.1	55.3	6.4	66.0
All twin index pairs	48.5	12.6	38.9	50.3	49.7

[a]As related to the following four classifications: Group I: No schizophrenia despite similar environment. Group II: Schizophrenia with little or no deterioration (recovery). Group III: Schizophrenia with medium deterioration. Group IV: Schizophrenia with extreme deterioration.

FIGURE 17.—Variations in Resistance to Schizophrenia in the Twin Index Pairs

Degree of Resistance to Schizophrenia	Clinical Behavior to Schizophrenia in Twin Index Pairs				Number of Twin Pairs	
	First Twin		Second Twin			
	Subgroups	Clinical Classification	Subgroups	Clinical Classification	Monozygotic	Dizygotic
Complete dissimilarity	IV	Extremely deteriorating type of schizophrenia	I	No schizophrenia despite similar environment	0	91
	IV	Extremely deteriorating type of schizophrenia	Ia	No schizophrenia with dissimilar environment	0	62
Less complete dissimilarity	IV	Extremely deteriorating type of schizophrenia	II	Schizophrenia with little or no deterioration	9	21
	III	Schizophrenia with medium deterioration	I, Ia	No schizophrenia (regardless of environment)	0	197
Complete similarity	II	Schizophrenia with little or no deterioration (recovery)	II	Schizophrenia with little or no deterioration	19	2
	III	Schizophrenia with medium deterioration	III	Schizophrenia with medium deterioration	33	0
	IV	Schizophrenia with extreme deterioration	IV	Schizophrenia with extreme deterioration	29	1
Less complete similarity	II	Schizophrenia with little or no deterioration	I, Ia	No schizophrenia	54	120
	III	Schizophrenia with medium deterioration	II	Schizophrenia with little or no deterioration	20	14
	IV	Schizophrenia with extreme deterioration	III	Schizophrenia with medium deterioration	10	9
Total number of pairs		All dissimilar pairs			9	371
		All similar pairs			165	146
		Grand total			174	517
Ratio		No schizophrenia to extremely deteriorating schizophrenia			0:174	1:2.5
		Dissimilar resistance to similar resistance			3:55	3:1

Complete dissimilarity means that the cotwins developed no psychosis despite similar environment (Group I), while the index twins showed an extremely deteriorating type of psychosis. Such a difference does not occur in the group of monozygotic twins, but it ensues in about every sixth dizygotic pair under dissimilar environmental conditions (Fig. 17). This finding implies that the chance of a rapidly progressive psychosis (low resistance) is practically zero for a schizophrenic patient who is the monozygotic twin of, or genetically identical with, a person who remains free of schizophrenic manifestations under similar environmental circumstances. However, the chance of developing a very destructive type of psychosis is 1:3.5, if the person is merely the patient's sibling or dizygotic twin, which means that he is as likely to differ in the inherited elements for a satisfactory resistance as are two brothers or sisters.

In comparing the total groups with dissimilar and similar behavior to schizophrenia, incomplete similarity denotes a difference of only one step between two of the four sub-groups; and incomplete dissimilarity, a difference of two steps. This comparison yields a ratio of 3:55 for the monozygotic pairs, and a ratio of 3:1 for the dizygotic pairs. The difference in similarity of resistance between the two types of twins is expressed by a ratio of 1:55, which far exceeds the difference found in their original morbidity rates. In other words, similar behavior to schizophrenia is about eighteen times more frequent than dissimilar behavior in monozygotic twins, although dissimilarity predominates in dizygotic twin partners.

Fig. 18 expresses the same difference in resistance between one-egg and two-egg twins in rates rather than in ratios, identifying less complete and complete dissimilarity in behavior to schizophrenia with favorable and very favorable resistance, and similar behavior in the deteriorating subgroups with insufficient resistance. In the monozygotic group, five out of 100 cotwins of schizophrenic index cases show a tendency to favorable resistance and none shows very favorable resistance, if their twin partners are insufficiently resistant. In the dizygotic group, however, favorable resistance is seen in seventy-two out of 100 cotwins of insufficiently resistant index cases, and very favorable resistance in about 30.

This finding indicates that *constitutional resistance* to the main genotype of schizophrenia is determined by a genetic mechanism which is probably non-specific and certainly multifactorial. Taking into account the results of biometric investigations, there is reason to believe that this constitutional defense mechanism is a graded character and somehow correlated with the morphological development of mesodermal elements. For various reasons it does not seem likely, however, that the genetic mechanisms controlling susceptibility and lack of resistance to schizophrenia, that is, the ability to develop a schizophrenic psychosis and the inability to counteract the progression of the disease, are entirely identical with each other. If they are identifiable, it is possible without qualification to accept the recent suggestions of Penrose and Luxenburger that inheritance of schizophrenia may be "the result of many factors."

As far as the *specific predisposition* to schizophrenia is concerned, that is, the inherited capacity for responding to certain stimuli with a schizophrenic type of reaction, the findings of the present study are conclusively in favor of the genetic theory. Our conclusion is that this predisposition depends on the presence of a specific genetic factor which is believed by us to be recessive and autosomal.

The hypothesis of recessiveness is borne out by the taint distribution in the ancestry of our index cases and by an excess of consanguineous marriages among their parents. Of 211 twin index pairs without schizophrenia in their known ancestry, twelve sets (5.7 percent) originated from consanguineous parental matings. Of the remaining index pairs, 95 were found to have a schizophrenic parent; 283 had no schizophrenic parent, but schizophrenic cases in the collateral lines of ancestry; and in 102 pairs the available information about the ancestors was considered inadequate. This excess of consanguineous parental marriages in the present survey appears quite convincing, even if a part of it may be due to the fact that our index cases are twins.

Psychiatrically it should be evident that the *genetic theory of schizophrenia* as it may be formulated on the basis of experiment-like observations with the twin family method, does not confute any psychological concepts of a descriptive or analytical nature, if these concepts are adequately defined and applied. There is no genetic reason why the manifestations of a schizophrenic psychosis should be not be described in terms of narcissistic regression or of varying biological changes such as defective homeostasis or general immaturity in the metabolic responses to stimuli. Genetically it is also perfectly legitimate to interpret schizophrenic reactions as the expression either of faulty habit formations or of progressive maladaptation to disrupted family relations. The genetic theory explains only *why* these various phenomena occur in a particular member of a particular family at a particular time.

The general meaning of this genetic explanation is that a true schizophrenic psychosis is not developed under usual human life conditions unless a particular predisposition has been inherited by a person from both parents. Ge-

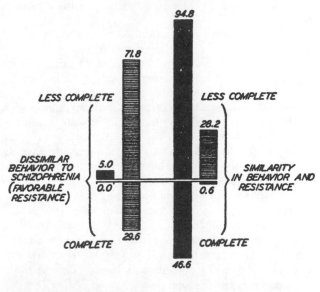

FIGURE 18.—Rates of Similar and Dissimilar Resistance to Schizophrenia

netically it is also implied that resistance to a progressive psychosis does not break down without certain inherited deficiencies in constitutional defense mechanisms, the final outcome of the disease being the result of intricate interactions of varying genetic and environmental influences. Another genetic implication is that a schizophrenic psychosis can be both prevented and cured. The prerequisite is that the psychosomatic elements, which may act as predispositional, precipitating or perpetuating agents in such a psychosis, are morphologically identified, and that the complex interplay of etiologic and compensatory mechanisms is fully understood. Pragmatic speculation will be no aid in reaching this goal.

SUMMARY

1. The methods available for genetic investigations in man are the pedigree or family history method, the contingency method of statistical prediction, and the twin study method.

2. A study of the relative effects of hereditary and environmental factors in the development and outcome of schizophrenia are undertaken by means of the "Twin Family Method." The study was organized with the cooperation of all mental hospitals under the supervision of the New York State Department of Mental Hygiene. The total number of schizophrenic twin index cases, whose cotwins were available for examination at the age of fifteen years, was 794.

3. In addition to 1,382 twins, the 691 twin index families used for statistical analysis include 2,741 full siblings, 134 half-siblings, 74 step-siblings, 1,191 parents, and 254 mar-

riage partners of twin patients. The random sampling of these twin index pairs is indicated by the distribution of 174 monozygotic and 517 dizygotic pairs, yielding a ratio of about 1:3.

4. The morbidity rates obtained with the "Abridged Weinberg Method" are in line with the genetic theory of schizophrenia. They amount to 1.8 percent for the step-siblings; 2.1 percent for the marriage partners; 7.0 percent for the half-siblings 9.2 percent for the parents; 14.3 percent for the full-siblings; 14.7 percent for the dizygotic cotwins; and 85.8 percent for the monozygotic cotwins. This morbidity distribution indicates that the chance of developing schizophrenia in comparable environments increases in proportion to the degree of blood relationship to a schizophrenic index case.

5. The differences in morbidity among the various sibship groups of the index families cannot be explained by a simple correlation between closeness of blood relationship and increasing similarity in environment. The morbidity rates for opposite-sexed and same-sexed two-egg twin partners vary only from 10.3 to 17.6 percent, and those for non-separated and separated one-egg twin partners from 77.6 to 91.5 percent. The difference in morbidity between dizygotic and monozygotic cotwins approximates the ratio of 1:6. An analysis of common environmental factors before and after birth excludes the possibility of explaining this difference on non-genetic grounds.

6. The difference between dizygotic and monozygotic cotwins increases to a ratio of 1:55, if the similarities in the course and outcome of schizophrenia are taken as additional criteria of comparison. This finding indicates that constitutional inability to resist the progression of a schizophrenic psychosis is determined by a genetic mechanism which seems to be non-specific and multifactorial.

7. The predisposition to schizophrenia, that is, the ability to respond to certain stimuli with a schizophrenic type of reaction, depends on the presence of a specific genetic factor which is probably recessive and autosomal.

8. The genetic theory of schizophrenia does not invalidate any psychological theories of a descriptive or analytical nature. It is equally compatible with the psychiatric concept that schizophrenia can be prevented as well as cured.

BIBLIOGRAPHY

1. Gralnik, A. The Carrington family. Psychiat Quart., 17:2, 1943.
2. Hoskins, R.G. The biology of schizophrenia. The Salmon Memorial Lectures, New York, 1945.
3. Kallmann, F.J. The genetics of schizophrenia. New York, 1938, J.J. Augustin.
4. Kallmann, F.J. The scientific goal in the prevention of hereditary mental disease. Proc. of Seventh International Genetical Congress, Edinburgh, 1939, Cambridge University Press.
5. Kallmann, F.J., and Barrera, S.E. The heredoconstitutional mechanisms of predisposition and resistance to schizophrenia. Am. J. Psychiat., 98:4, 1942.
6. Kallmann, F.J., and Reisner, D. Twin studies on the significance of genetic factors in tuberculosis. Am. Rev. Tuberc., 47:6, 1943.
7. Luxenburger, H. Erbpathologie der Schizophrenie. Part II, Vol. II of Guett's Handbuch der Erbkrankheiten. Leipzig, 1940, G. Thieme.
8. Myerson, A. Some trends of psychiatry Am. J. Psychiat., Cent. Anniv. Iss., 1944.
9. Penrose, L.S. Heredity. Part IV, Vol. I of Hunt's Handbook, Personality and the Behavior Disorders. New York, 1944, Ronald Press Co.
10. Pollock, H.M., Malzberg, B., and Fuller, R.G. Heredity and environmental factors in the causation of manic-depressive psychoses and dementia praecox. Utica, 1939, State Hospital Press.
11. Rosanoff, A.J., Handy, L.M., Rosanoff Plesset, I., and Brush, S. The etiology of so-called schizophrenic psychoses. Am. J. Psychiat., 91:247, 1934.
12. Rosenberg, R. Heredity in the functional psychoses. Am. J. Psychiat., 101:2, 1944.
13. Slater, E. Genetics in psychiatry. J. Ment. Sci., 90:3, 1944.
14. Strecker, E.A. Fundamentals of psychiatry. Philadelphia, 1945, J.B. Lippincott Co.
15. Weinberg, W. Zur Probandenmethode und zu ihrem Ersatz. Ztschr. Neurol., 123:809, 1930.

THE CONCEPTS OF "MEANING" AND "CAUSE" IN PSYCHODYNAMICS

By John C. Whitehorn, M.D.

Professor of Psychiatry, The Johns Hopkins University School of Medicine, Baltimore, Maryland

There is much that is irrational in the behavior of neurotic and psychotic patients which had been considered in the descriptive age of psychiatry as psychologically nonunderstandable and therefore insignificant, except as evidence of disease. In large part the apparently irrational has been found intelligible and personally meaningful as reaction pattern, in the modern, biologically oriented frame of reference of personality functions, particularly through the aid of the facts brought to light by psychoanalytic study of the unconscious. One may say that conceptual means have been found to "unscrew the inscrutable." We appreciate now that even irrational symptoms have personal meanings (for the patient although he may not tell us or even know it, as well as to the psychiatrist). Yet these forms of behavior presumably also have causes; and meanings and causes are not the same.

Some psychiatrists profess a belief in absolute psychic determinism as a scientific dogma, but this is an affirmation of metapsychological faith, not a statement of fact. The hypothesis of psychogenesis is not the only reason for the close scrutiny of a patient's attitudes and the searching of issues at stake in his reaction to his situation. For the strategy of psychotherapy there is much practical value in recognizing the *meaning* of reactions, even though causal explanation be lacking. In modern psychodynamic psychiatry, as distinguished from the preceding stage of descriptive psychiatry, one of the main principles is to conduct an individualized study of each patient adequate to point up the main recurrent theme or issue of dissatisfaction and conflict, to assess the individual's currently unused potentialities for dealing with this issue and to evoke a well-founded and self-assured mode of resolving the issue more satisfactorily.

Some persons show perspicacity in discerning the themes or issues which make understandable much psychopathology that is otherwise apparently irrational. Such perspicacity can be cultivated and made useful for psychotherapy. Much of one's supervisory assistance to trainees consists in helping them search and sift their facts and sharpen their observations about a patient to gain a well-justified formulation of the meaningfulness of a situation for a patient and the relevance of his reaction thereto. The catch-word "psychogenesis" has become something of an impediment in this task. The perception of an issue in a patient's life, which could clarify the meaningfulness of his reaction, is not infrequently misconstrued as if it were the discovery of the *cause* of the patient's illness. Some young doctors are made foolishly happy thereby, feeling that they have "explained the illness"; some others, more discerning, perceive that the explanation is not complete, and so, obsessed with the fancied necessity for getting a complete psychogenetic explanation as a preliminary to therapy, they frantically attack the patient again and again, picking him to shreds in the ingenious effort to ferret out the true "cause," while neglecting the large strategic possibilities of aid to the patient which might be rendered through the appreciation of "meanings" implied in current and past experience.

I wish to make clear that it is not my purpose in this discussion to deny the validity of the psychogenetic concept. I believe that, among the many facts whose combination determines the development of a neurotic or psychotic condition, psychological experiences are of critical importance. One could even say, *in some instances*, that *single traumatic events* are of crucial importance, as in some of the combat neuroses. In general, however, we have probably all come to the realization that *clinical study seldom reveals a single crucial traumatic event as the specific cause of a neurosis*. Most commonly one finds anamnestically, a wealth of symptomatic anecdotes, *expressive* of the pathological attitude, rather than *causative* of it. It is also commonly true, in an intensively studied and treated case, that many small items come to light indicative of a general pressure of many psychogenetic influences which have combined in shaping one's neurotic attitudes. It is possible, thus, in a fair proportion of thoroughly studied cases, to construct a fairly plausible but rather complex etiological hypothesis for the individual case.

The plausible etiological hypothesis, finally elaborated, may, however, be of considerably less strategic importance in therapy than the mutual understanding, reached much earlier, by which physician and patient both come to understand the meaning of some of the patient's neurotic behavior in terms of emotional need, rather than in terms of historical cause and effect. To arrive at a mutual understanding of the theme of a repetitive pattern may provide at once an opportunity for a "corrective emotional experi-

Read at the 103d annual meeting of The American Psychiatric Association, New York, N.Y., May 19-23, 1947.

ence" or an "attitudinal interaction," setting into motion powerful therapeutic impulses. Some physicians are disposed, however, by personality and by doctrine, to disregard such opportunities to deal with meaning, in an obsessive insistence upon a routine continuation of the search for *the cause*. In the long run, there is great scientific potentiality in this obsessive search for specific etiology. In individual instances, however, the particular patient does not always benefit. The patient may thereby suffer loss of time, loss of rapport, and loss of a helpful focus for his own efforts. It is important in treating the individual patient not to miss the opportunities for mutual understanding of a meaningful theme, out of a scientific zeal to get all the details pinned down rigidly for an etiological hypotheses. Particularly if the patient has schizoid tendencies, such obsessive insistence provides one of the quickest and surest ways of losing a therapeutic relationship.

Personal experiences color professional thinking. My own earlier psychotherapeutic experiments were with psychotic patients, who, in comparison with neurotic patients, usually require a more personal support and more mature appreciation from the therapist, as encouragement to their shattered egos. One has many opportunities to notice in the early phases of the psychotic patient's progress toward recovery that the patient does begin by making tentative and hesitating steps of his own. Without some spontaneity, the therapist is stymied. How to elicit and encourage spontaneity in a constructive direction is the most difficult technical problem, and in this task the therapist's grasp of the potential meaningfulness of the life-situation and the meaningfulness of the patient's reaction does give opportunity for helpfulness at a time before one has been able to get from the patient sufficient evidence to form a valid etiological hypothesis. The following incident may serve as an example:

A manic patient, Robert S., 50 years old, a business executive, upon being addressed by a certain doctor as "Mr. S.", repeatedly requested that he be called just "Bob." When the doctor inquired into the reason for his request the patient replied, "You are my superior—you are No. 1." The doctor then questioningly repeated the word "superior," while raising an eyebrow at the same time. This resulted in an outburst of seemingly incoherent talk, which included the sentence, "Well, okay, you are not my superior, so you may call me 'Mr. S.' " This little episode helped the doctor considerably to understand the patient's need in his relationship with him, and with other people as well. He was a proud, prestige-oriented person who resented being dependent and attempted to minimize his dependence on the doctor by caricaturing it in a way which is so typical of the manic patient.

A discerning comparison of the patient's attitudes in the current situation, with his attitudes during his periods of better previous functioning, grows naturally out of this interest in issues and attitudes (that is to say, meanings), whereas a physician obsessed with a thirst for discovering "the cause," tends to neglect the therapeutically helpful review of the patient's best period, and to focus exclusively on the traumatic and the pathological.

These matters mark out, however, differences of emphasis rather than completely different principles in the psychotherapy of the psychoses and of the neuroses. In both there is great importance in timing the steps of therapy to fit the need and the mood of the patient at a given time. In psychotherapeutic strategy, when one bears in mind the meaning or theme of the patient's pathological reaction, there are opportunities to evoke memories and attitudes constructively useful in relation to this meaning, but such strategic opportunities will be missed if the psychiatrist is continually obsessed with the necessity to pin down the cause as the preliminary to psychotherapy.

Experience in the psychotherapy of neurotic patients makes one very familiar with the patient who has cooperated nicely with a psychiatrist's efforts to explore early memories and emotional traumata, and who has arrived at a fairly neat psychogenetic formulation, but without benefit in the form of personality growth or even relief of symptoms. The intellectual insight, or pseudo-insight, of such patients is a dubious benefit. It is not infrequently a considerable handicap to more effective therapy. Such experiences demonstrate the fallacy of the glib phrase: "Find the psychogenetic cause and eliminate it." As Franz Alexander has expressed it, the essence of psychotherapy is the "corrective emotional experience." The therapist has a considerably greater chance of helping his patient to achieve a "corrective emotional experience" if he directs his attention to the indications of the "meanings" implied in the patient's experiences, current and past, rather than focussing merely on indications of potential "causes."

Since the psychoanalytic school of thought has particularly emphasized psychic determinism and the etiological focus of therapy, it would be only natural that one would expect to find among psychoanalysts more than among other psychiatrists those who are, in a doctrinaire way, obsessed with the necessity to discover the psychic etiology as preliminary to psychotherapy. It is my impression, however, that this doctrinaire attitude is more characteristic of the psychoanalyst of limited experience. There is still, however, a persisting attitude in psychoanalysis, carried over from the phase of overemphasis "on the intellectual understanding of the past that made psychoanalytic treatment almost synonymous with genetic research."[1]

For one, concerned as I am, for purposes of psychotherapeutic strategy, to place much emphasis upon the *meaningfulness* of neurotic or psychotic reactions, in terms of the themes or issues involved in those reactions, it would be somewhat ungracious to appear in any way to make unduly critical remarks about psychoanalysis, just because some analysts have given too exclusive an emphasis to doctrines of etiology. We owe to psychoanalysis, more than to any other method or school of psychiatric study, the appreciation of meaningful issues in neurotic reactions. Historically, this has also been accompanied by many valuable etiological studies. The principal purpose of my discussion today has been, not to deplore the interest in "cause," but rather to deplore, and to seek to correct, the haziness of thinking which tends to obscure the distinction between

---

1 P. 20. Alexander, Franz, French, T.M., et al. Psychoanalytic Therapy, The Roland Press, New York, 1946

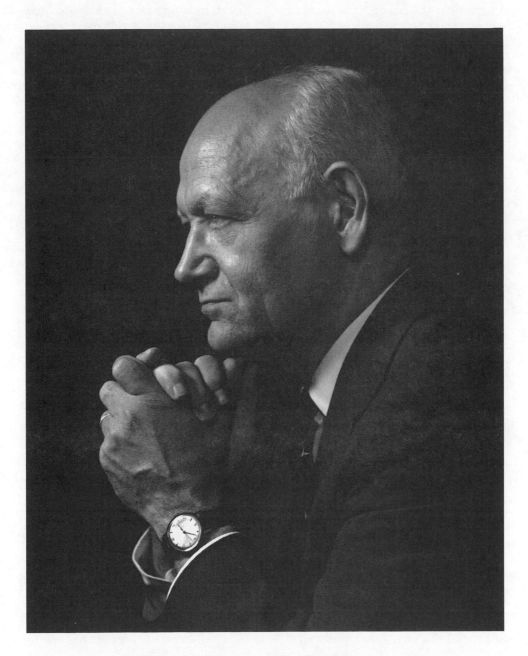

John C. Whitehorn, M.D., 1894–1973

"meaning" and "cause," so important for psychotherapeutic strategy.

Etiological research must of course continue, and it has better prospects of success through the increasing understanding of the meaningfulness of symptoms. Meaning and cause are not mutually contradictory; but neither are they synonymous. The understanding and practice of psychotherapy will be improved by the more general recognition of this distinction.

At the present time there are two special reasons for emphasizing the therapeutic implications of the distinction between meaning and cause.

One reason lies in public misunderstanding. Many persons have gotten from the movies, novels, and Sunday papers a mistakenly simplified notion that psychiatric salvation lies wholly in recapturing some specific forgotten memory and thereby finding and removing "the cause" of emotional ill health. The simplicity of this concept and the implications of painless magical therapy give it a special appeal to neurotic patients; and a special investment of time, effort, and tactful education is now often required to circumvent this romantic expectation. The psychotherapist needs to keep in his own mind a fairly clear-cut distinction between cause and meaning in order to avoid the pitfalls set by the patient's misled expectations. A clear distinction also helps to avoid aimless quibbling with the patient about this issue.

The other main reason for emphasizing at this time the distinction between "cause" and "meaning" of symptoms lies in the overcrowded condition in most of the good institutions training young psychiatrists. Increased numbers in training dilute the advisory supervision and favor a tendency toward didactic patterns. The bright young trainee discovers that, in seminar and staff conference, interest and approval are aroused by case presentations well padded with so-called "etiological" probings in the direction of early memories and traumatic episodes. The techniques of personality dissection are easier and more spectacular than those of plastic reconstruction. If we fail to keep the young psychiatrist clearly oriented to current issues and attitudes in the patient's life, we are likely to develop a crop of probe-pushers, clever in case presentations but not very competent in actual management and therapy of real patients.

The present situation has seemed to me, therefore, to require some clarification of concepts along the lines of the distinctions herein made between "meaning" and "cause."

CEREBRAL BLOOD FLOW AND METABOLISM IN SCHIZOPHRENIA
The Effects of Barbiturate Semi-Narcosis, Insulin Coma and Electroshock

By S.S. Kety, M.D., R.B. Woodford, M.D., M.H. Harmel, M.D., F.A. Freyman, M.D., K.E. Appel, M.D., and C.F. Schmidt, M.D.

Quantitative measurement of the blood flow and the metabolism of the living brain in psychotic states is a fundamental prerequisite to a better understanding of the possible metabolic derangements associated with these conditions. Unfortunately the lack of a suitable method has hitherto barred this approach. Determination of the cerebral arteriovenous oxygen difference is of little value in this problem since this measurement is determined by both blood flow and metabolism, neither of which can be assumed to be normal on the basis of a priori reasoning. The recent development by Kety and Schmidt (1) of a technique for the quantitative measurement of cerebral blood flow in unanesthetized man offers a method for determining whether a primary defect in total cerebral circulation or metabolism exists in the psychoses, and the effects of various therapeutic procedures upon these important functions.

Methods.—In all, 23 schizophrenic patients were studied. Cerebral blood flow was measured by the nitrous oxide technique (8). This necessitates the insertion of needles into the femoral artery and superior jugular bulb from which samples of blood are drawn over a 10-minute period while the patient breathes a mixture containing 21% oxygen, 64% nitrogen, and in addition 15% nitrous oxide, a concentration of nitrous oxide low enough to be without appreciable effect. From the shape of the arterial and internal jugular nitrous oxide blood curves cerebral blood flow can be calculated. Mean arterial blood pressure was recorded directly from the femoral artery by means of a mercury manometer. Blood samples were analyzed for oxygen and carbon dioxide contents by the Van Slyke-Neill technique (2), for pH potentiometrically by means of a glass electrode at 37° C.

Cerebral metabolism was estimated in terms of oxygen or glucose consumption as the product of the cerebral blood flow by the respective arteriovenous difference. In the case of pentothal seminarcosis, studies were done 20 minutes after an initial control blood flow was obtained. Control blood flow determinations for insulin coma and hypoglycemia were obtained on the previous day. The nitrous oxide technique measures cerebral blood flow as an integrated function over a 10-minute period and requires a fairly steady state. For this reason as well as the necessity that the patient breathe the gas mixture and keep needles in place it was not possible to make measurements during convulsions induced by electroshock. Rather, a control study was completed and the needles withdrawn; a convulsion was then produced and as soon thereafter as the patient relaxed the needles were reinserted and a second determination was performed. It was usually possible to begin this determination 10 minutes after the onset of convulsions.

RESULTS AND DISCUSSION

The results obtained in 30 control determinations on 22 patients are presented in Table 1 and compared with similar data obtained by Kety and Schmidt in 35 observations in normal young males (3). It is seen that the cerebral blood flow and cerebral oxygen consumption in the schizophrenics are identical with the normal, nor do any of the measurements made show a significant deviation from the normal. If the patients are divided into two groups showing respectively acute and chronic aberrations no significant difference between the groups appears. On the basis of these data a generalized change in circulation or oxygen utilization by the brain of schizophrenics may safely be ruled out although there remains the possibility that local disturbances confined to small but important regions may still occur since the method used yields only mean values for the entire brain. Furthermore although over-all oxygen utilization may be normal there may be qualitative aberrations in any of a vast array of metabolic processes which would remain undetected. However, with the means for measuring cerebral blood flow now available, it becomes possible to determine quantitatively the utilization or production by the brain of any substance capable of accurate analysis in arterial and internal jugular venous blood.

Read at the 103d annual meeting of The American Psychiatric Association, New York, N.Y., May 19-23, 1947. From the Departments of Pharmacology and Psychiatry, University of Pennsylvania School of Medicine, and the Delaware State Hospital.

This investigation was partly financed through the National Committee for Mental Hygiene from funds granted by the Committee on Research in Dementia Praecox founded by the Supreme Council, 33 Scottish Rite, Northern Masonic Jurisdiction, U.S.A.

We are indebted to Dr. F. D. W. Lukens of the University of Pennsylvania for the glucose determinations.

Dr. Harmel is a National Research Council Fellow in Anaesthesiology.

TABLE 1. Schizophrenia; Resting Values

Patient	Age	Sex	Arterial blood				Internal	
			CO_2 Content (vol. %)	CO_2 Tension (mm. Hg)	O_2 Content (vol. %)	pH	CO_2 Content (vol. %)	CO_2 Tension (mm. Hg)
J.McH	31	M	48.2	37	19.8	7.45	54.4	45
V.Z.	31	M	54.6	45	16.2	7.40	59.9	53
R.B.	40	M	50.5	41	19.0	7.43	56.4	50
R.B.	40	M	49.3	48	17.9	7.33	55.2	56
W.R.	30	M	52.8	44	20.0	7.42	57.9	50
W.R.	30	M	49.5	42	19.8	7.40	54.9	50
W.R.	30	M	48.6	44	19.8	7.38	53.6	49
J.Sk.	37	M	52.7	44	17.3	7.40	57.8	53
J.Sk.	37	M	53.3	41	16.8	7.44	58.4	47
G.A.	31	M	44.5	38	16.3	7.40	49.6	44
U.P.	21	M	42.5	31	19.5	7.47	49.7	41
U.P.	21	M	40.4	29	19.2	7.50	51.5	40
W.L.	34	M	49.0	43	18.0	7.39	55.1	52
W.L.	34	M	49.7	48	17.9	7.34	56.2	58
G.H.	29	M	47.1	37	17.9	7.44	53.5	44
E.F.	42	F	48.3	41	16.4	7.40	55.4	49
G.C.	33	M	51.4	43	17.4	7.41	57.5	51
C.A.	27	F	58.3	46	13.5	7.41	63.1	54
P.W.	33	M	54.3	46	18.5	7.41	60.0	54
E.McC.	56	F	49.3	38	13.0	7.42	54.9	45
C.O.	34	F	47.0	41	16.6	7.39	52.5	51
E.G.	54	F	50.4	43	15.2	7.39	56.4	54
E.B.	44	M	50.4	45	19.2	7.39	55.0	53
E.B.	44	M	51.8	47	18.7	7.38	58.2	55
R.C.	35	M	50.2	46	17.9	7.36	55.2	55
L.R.	25	F	50.6	45	16.9	7.38	58.2	58
S.S.	34	M	52.6	45	17.0	7.40	57.6	53
S.S.	34	M	50.2	39	16.3	7.43	56.9	48
M.T.	46	F	51.6	43	17.2	7.40	58.3	53
L.B.	19	M	50.3	52	17.8	7.30	55.8	62
Mean			50.0	42	17.6	7.40	56.0	51
Mean			49.5	43	17.3	7.39	55.8	52

TABLE 2. Effects of Pentothal Seminarcosis on Arterial and Cerebral Venous Blood Constituents, Cerebral Blood Flow, and Cerebral Oxygen Consumption

Patient Diagnosis	Age	Response to Pentothal	Arterial Blood								Internal	
			CO_2 Content (vol. %)		CO_2 Tension (mm. Hg)		O_2 Content (vol. %)		pH		CO_2 Content (vol. %)	
			Control	Pentothal or Amytal	Control	Pentothal or Amytal	Control	Pentothal or Amytal	Control	Pentothal or Amytal	Control	Pentothal or Amytal
J.McH. –Catatonic	31	Excellent	48.2	49.2	37	36	19.8	18.7	7.45	7.47	54.4	56.3
V.Z.–Catatonic	31	Good	54.6	53.7	45	43	16.2	15.7	7.40	7.41	59.9	60.0
R.B.–Catatonic	39	Fair	50.5	53.2	41	40	19.0	18.3	7.43	7.45	56.4	59.3
W.R.–Simple	30	Good	52.8	52.1	44	41	20.0	19.8	7.42	7.44	57.9	58.2
J.Sk.–Simple	37	Fair	52.7	53.4	44	47	17.3	16.9	7.40	7.38	57.8	58.4
G.A.–Paranoid	31	Good	44.5	48.1	38	41	16.3	16.0	7.40	7.38	49.6	53.3
U.P.–Simple	21	Good	42.5	47.5	31	40	19.5	18.6	7.47	7.41	49.7	53.6
W.L.–Paranoid	34	Excellent	49.0	49.5	43	44	18.0	17.7	7.39	7.38	55.1	56.1
Mean: Early schizophrenic			48.4	50.9	40	41	18.3	17.7	7.42	7.43	55.1	56.9

SEMINARCOSIS PRODUCED BY BARBITURATES

Table 2 illustrates the data obtained on 8 patients before and during the seminarcotic state produced by the intravenous administration of sodium pentothal or sodium amytal. Sufficient drug was administered intravenously to produce marked clinical change in the patients: marked increase in accessibility in the paranoid patients, and spontaneous verbalization in previously mute catatonics. It is to be noted that at no time did the patient lose consciousness. There was no significant change in cerebral blood flow, cerebral metabolism, nor in any of the other functions studied.

| Jugular Blood | | | Cerebral | | | Schizophrenia | |
O2 Content (vol. %)	pH	A-V O2 (vol. %)	Cerebral Respiratory Quotient	Cerebral Blood Flow (cc/100g/min.)	Cerebral Metabolic Rate (cc. O2/[100g/min.])	Type	Duration of Hospitalization (years)
12.8	7.41	7.0	0.87	48	3.4	Catatonic	10
10.7	7.36	5.5	0.96	50	2.8	Catatonic	3
12.3	7.38	6.7	0.88	57	3.8	Catatonic	16
11.6	7.30	6.3	0.94	61	3.8		
14.7	7.39	5.3	0.96	59	3.1	Simple	4
14.2	7.37	5.6	0.97	51	2.9		
12.6	7.36	7.2	0.70	47	3.4		
11.8	7.35	5.5	0.93	57	3.1	Paranoid	11
11.0	7.43	5.8	0.88	68	3.9		
11.2	7.36	5.1	1.00	62	3.2	Paranoid	4
11.2	7.41	8.3	0.87	36	3.0	Paranoid	5
11.1	7.45	8.1	1.37	52	4.2		
12.0	7.35	6.0	1.02	61	3.7	Paranoid	3
11.2	7.31	6.7	0.97	56	3.8		
10.1	7.41	7.8	0.82	44	3.4	Hebephrenic	5
9.1	7.36	7.3	0.98	45	3.3		
10.7	7.37	6.7	0.91	51	3.4	Catatonic	9
8.0	7.36	5.5	0.87	59	3.2	Catatonic	4
12.5	7.37	6.0	0.95	49	2.9	Catatonic	11
7.3	7.39	5.7	0.98	53	3.0	Hebephrenic	15
11.4	7.32	5.4	1.02	60	3.2	Catatonic	11
9.2	7.32	6.0	1.00	53	3.2	Catatonic	26
14.0	7.34	4.6	0.89	64	2.9	Simple	4
12.5	7.35	6.2	1.03	44	2.7		
13.4	7.32	4.5	1.11	64	2.9	Paranoid	6
10.2	7.32	6.7	1.13	47	3.1	Simple	8
10.7	7.35	6.3	0.79	58	3.7	Paranoid	8
10.8	7.39	5.5	1.22	64	3.5		
10.0	7.36	7.2	0.93	48	3.5	Catatonic	9
13.2	7.27	4.6	1.20	43	2.0	Paranoid	<1
11.4	7.36	6.2	0.97	54 σ7.63	3.3 σ±.43		
10.9	7.34	6.2	1.02	54 σ8.9	3.3 σ±.43	Normal males, 35 observations	

| Jugular Blood | | | | | | Cerebral | | | | | | | |
| CO2 Tension (mm. Hg) | | O2 Content (vol. %) | | pH | | A-V O2 (vol. %) | | Cerebral Respiratory Quotient | | Cerebral Blood Flow (cc/100g/min.) | | Cerebral Metabolic Rate (cc. O2/[100g/min.]) | |
Control	Pentothal or Amytal	Control	Pentothal or Amytal	Control	Pentothal or Amytal	Control	Pentothal or Amytal	Control	Pentothal or Amytal	Control	Pentothal or Amytal	Control	Pentothal or Amytal
45	46	12.8	11.9	7.41	7.0	6.8	0.87	1.04	48	42	3.4	2.9	
53	53	10.7	9.6	7.36	5.5	6.1	0.96	1	03	50	46	2.8	2.8
50	50	12.3	11.3	7.38	7.40	6.7	7.0	0.88	0.87	57	57	3.8	4.0
50	50	14.7	13.8	7.39	7.39	5.3	6.0	0.96	1.02	59	57	3.1	3.4
53	56	11.8	11.3	7.35	7.33	5.5	5.6	0.93	0.89	57	60	3.1	3.4
44	47	11.2	10.2	7.36	7.36	5.1	5.8	1.00	0.90	62	55	3.2	3.2
41	48	11.2	12.7	7.41	7.36	8.3	5.9	0.87	1.03	36	50	3.0	3.0
52	54	12.0	11.6	7.35	7.33	6.0	6.1	1.02	1.08	61	56	3.7	3.4
49	51	12.1	11.6	7.36	7.37	6.2	6.2	0.94	0.98	54	53	3.3	3.3

HYPOGLYCEMIA AND COMA INDUCED BY INSULIN

The results of our investigations in hypoglycemia and insulin coma in schizophrenic patients are given in Table 3. Our results corroborate the fall in oxygen and glucose arteriovenous differences observed by others (4, 5) but, in contrast to the suggestion of Loman and Myerson (6) that cerebral blood flow is diminished in hypoglycemia, we found that the cerebral blood flow is well maintained. The measurement of cerebral blood flow together with arteriovenous oxygen and glucose differences permit us to calculate both oxygen and glucose consumption. As the arterial blood

TABLE 3. Effects of Insulin Hypoglycemia and Coma on Arterial and Cerebral Venous Blood Constituents, Cerebral Blood Flow, and Cerebral Oxygen Consumption

I—Control.   II—Hypoglycemia.   III—Coma.

| | Arterial | | | | | | | | | | | | | | |
| | Blood Pressure | | | Glucose | | | O_2 | | | CO_2 | | | pH | | |
Patient	I	II	III	I	II	III	I	II	III	I	II	III	I	II	III
E.B.	95	79		73	23		19.2	18.8		50.4	48.2		7.39	7.33	
R.C.	78	84		64	20		17.9	18.3		50.2	50.7		7.36	7.29	
L.R.	88	89	79	56	16	6	16.9	16.7	13.3	50.6	53.0	56.3	7.38	7.41	7.39
S.S.	110		96	65		13	17.0		18.0	52.6		44.4	7.40		7.39
L.B.	100	90	115	113	18	9	16.1	17.8	17.3	56.6	50.3	56.5	7.49	7.30	7.39
C.R.			85			6			18.0			42.4			7.30
C.R.			90			6			16.6			54.5			7.42
Mean	94	85.5	93	74	19	8	17.4	17.9	16.6	52.1	50.6	50.8	7.40	7.33	7.38

[a]Not included in the mean.
[b]Indicates statistically significant changes.

TABLE 4. Effects of Electroshock Convulsions on Arterial and Cerebral Venous Blood Constituents, Cerebral Blood Flow, and Cerebral Oxygen Consumption[a]

| | | Mean Arterial Blood Pressure | | Arterial | | | | | | | | Internal | |
| | | | | CO_2 Content | | pCO_2 | | O_2 Content | | pH | | CO_2 Content | |
Patient	Minutes After Convulsions	I	II	I	II	I	II	I	II	I	II	I	II
J.Sk.	11	77	78	53.3	33.5	41	39	16.8	17.9	7.44	7.24	58.4	40.9
W.L.	12	75	83	49.7	23.8	48	39	17.9	19.1	7.34	7.08	56.2	31.9
R.B.	13	102	93	49.3	23.5	48	37	17.9	18.8	7.33	7.10	55.2	32.7
L.B.	31	100	97	56.6	43.6	52	38	16.1	15.7	7.49	7.38	62.0	50.0
S.Se.	10	109	114	50.2	29.3	39	35	16.3	17.6	7.43	7.23	56.9	37.2
U.P.	13	80	73	40.4	26.4	29	29	19.2	19.7	7.50	7.29	51.5	36.1
W.R.	10	93	91	49.5	26.9	42	39	19.8	20.4	7.40	7.15	54.9	34.0
Mean		91	90	49.9	29.6	43	36	17.7	18.5	7.42	7.21	56.4	37.5

I—Control. II—Postconvulsion.

sugar falls there is a progressive fall in cerebral glucose utilization and oxygen consumption. In deep insulin coma the glucose consumption has fallen 83% while oxygen utilization has decreased only 45%. The expected ratio of O_2 to glucose utilization if all the O_2 were being used to burn glucose would be 0.75. In the resting state this ratio is 0.77, additional evidence that glucose is the only foodstuff of the brain normally. As hypoglycemia develops this ratio increases, indicating either the utilization of some other foodstuff or consumption of the carbohydrate stores of the brain itself.

THE POSTCONVULSIVE STATE

In Table 4 are summarized the changes found in 7 patients during the period from 10-20 minutes after a generalized convulsion induced by electroshock. The changes consist of a severe acidosis characterized by a sharp drop in CO_2 content and pH, probably due to the severe muscular exercise plus anoxia which would augment the anaerobic production of lactic acid. There is a moderate fall in cerebral oxygen consumption and a marked decrease in cerebral

blood flow. The exact cause of the decrease in circulation is somewhat obscure although the constant blood pressure and the increased A.V. oxygen difference would indicate that it was neither extrinsic to the brain nor dependent on the decreased metabolism. Data from other studies (7) indicate that the response to changes in carbon dioxide tension of the magnitude encountered here would be about an 18% reduction in cerebral blood flow. The decreased pH would tend to counteract even this effect. The decrease in cerebral circulation can be explained only partially on the basis of the reduced carbon dioxide tension, for the circulatory reduction under these circumstances is 36%. The increased arteriovenous oxygen difference is probably related to the decrease in cerebral blood flow.

SUMMARY

Studies by the use of the nitrous oxide technique on 22 schizophrenic patients show no deviation from values obtained in normal young males for cerebral blood flow and oxygen consumption.

A clinically significant change in 8 patients given sodium

Cerebral																				
A-V O$_2$			A-V glucose			Cerebral Respiratory Quotient			Cerebral Blood Flow			Cerebral Metabolic Rate (cc. O$_2$/100g./min.)			Cerebral Metabolic Rate (mg. glucose/[100 g./min.])		
I	II	III	I	II	III	I	II	III	I	II	III	I	II	III	I	II	III
5.2	4.7		6	6		0.89	1.04		64	58		3.3	2.7		3.8	3.5	
4.5	3.8		5	5		1.11	0.95		64	68		2.9	2.6		3.2	3.4	
6.7	4.4	1.5	8	1.5	0.3	1.13	1.20	1.33	47	73	72	3.2	3.2	1.1	3.8	1.1	0.2
6.3		5.6	8		3.5	0.79		1.18	58		47	3.7		3.0	4.6		1.6
6.6	4.6	1.95	11	3.0	1.7	0.81	1.20	0.49	59	43	113[a]	3.9	2.0	2.2	6.5	1.3	1.9
		2.6			0.3			0.55			68			1.8			0.2
		2.5			0			1.04			63			1.6			0
5.9	4.4	2.8	8	3.9	1.2	0.95	1.10	0.92	58	61	62.5	3.4	2.6[b]	1.9[b]	4.4	2.3[b]	0.8[b]

Jugular						Cerebral							
pCO$_2$		O$_2$ Content		pH		A-V O$_2$		Cerebral Respiratory Quotient		Cerebral Blood Flow		Cerebral Metabolic Rate	
I	II	I	II	I	II	I	II	I	II	I	II	I	II
47	49	11.0	9.7	7.43	7.22	5.8	8.2	0.88	0.90	68	36	3.9	3.0
58	46	11.2	10.9	7.31	7.03	6.7	8.2	0.97	0.99	56	38	3.8	3.1
56	60	11.6	9.5	7.30	7.02	5.3	9.3	0.94	0.99	61	40	3.8	3.7
62	48	9.5	7.9	7.42	7.33	6.6	7.8	0.81	0.82	59	41	3.9	3.2
48	49	10.9	9.3	7.39	7.18	5.4	8.3	1.24	0.95	64	38	3.5	3.1
40	47	11.1	10.0	7.45	7.20	8.1	9.7	1.37	1.00	52	33	4.2	3.2
50	53	14.0	13.5	7.37	7.11	5.8	6.9	0.93	1.03	45	30	2.6	2.1
52	50	11.3	10.1	7.38	7.16	6.4	8.3	1.02	0.95	58	37	3.7	3.1

pentothal or amytal intravenously is not associated with a measurable change in cerebral blood flow or cerebral oxygen consumption.

Insulin hypoglycemia and coma is associated with a progressive decrease in cerebral utilization of oxygen and blood glucose, the cerebral circulation remaining unimpaired. The fall in blood glucose utilization is greater than that of oxygen.

Electroshock is followed by a moderate decrease in metabolism and a marked decrease in cerebral blood flow in the face of a severe acidosis.

Although there were no demonstrable deviations from the normal in this group of schizophrenic patients, our experience with this technique leads us to believe that it is worthy of extensive application in the study of the metabolic derangements in the brain associated with mental disease. It makes possible a new approach to psychiatric disorders, and gives the means of quantitatively determining the utilization or production of any substance capable of accurate analysis in the arterial and internal jugular venous blood.

BIBLIOGRAPHY

1. Kety, S.S., and Schmidt, C.F. Am. J. of Physiol., 143:54, Jan. 1945.
2. Van Slyke, D.D., and Neill, J.M.J. Biol. Chem., 61:523, Sept. 1924.
3. To be published.
4. Himwich, H.E., Bowman, K.M., Wortis, J., and Fazekas, J.F. J. Nerv. and Ment. Dis., 89:273, March 1939.
5. Dameskek, W., Myerson, A., and Stephenson, C. Archiv. Neurol. and Psychiat., 33: I, Jan. 1935.
6. Loman, J., and Myerson, A. Am. J. Psychiat, 92:791, Jan. 1936.
7. Kety, S.S., and Schmidt, C.F. J. Clin. Investigation, 27: July 1948 (in press).
8. Kety, S.S. Measurement of cerebral blood flow in man; in Methods in Medical Research, vol. I, Year Book Publishers, Chicago, 1948.

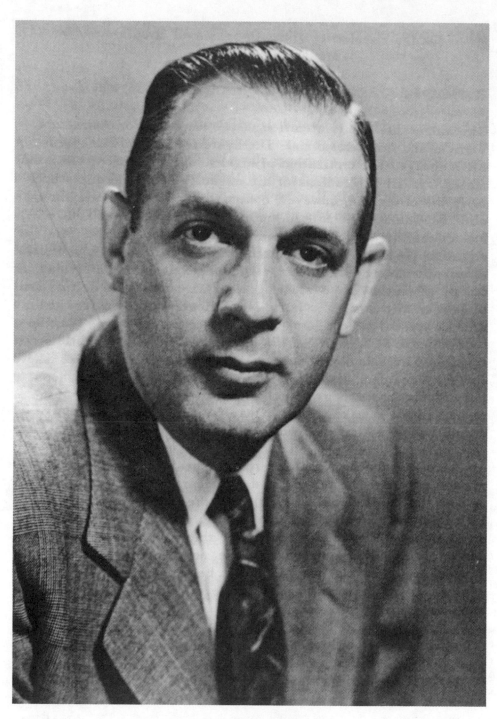

Seymour S. Kety, M.D., 1915–

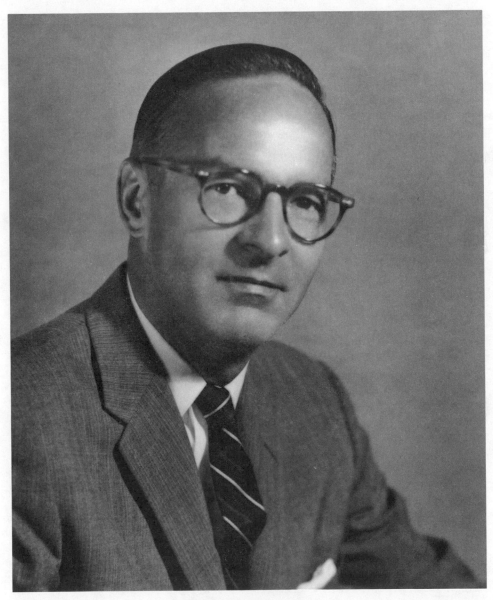

Lawrence C. Kolb, M.D., 1911–

Lawrence C. Kolb, M.D., 1911–

RESEARCH AND ITS SUPPORT
UNDER THE NATIONAL MENTAL HEALTH ACT

By Lawrence C. Kolb, M.D.

Research Projects Director, National Institute of Mental Health, U.S. Public Health Service, Bethesda, Maryland

I t is fitting that a symposium on the objectives and first achievements of the National Mental Health Act be presented at this time. My report and those of my associates represent, essentially, statements on the outcome of a decade of planning and action to provide the assistance of the Federal government in attacking the vast problem of mental illness. In his 1938 report the Surgeon General of the United States Public Health Service stated that mental diseases constituted the most important public health problem to the people of this country at that time. Immediately following publication of this report, plans were initiated which led eventually to the passage of the National Mental Health Act of 1946 and to its activation during the past 3 years.

The soundness of the early basic plans and recommendations concerning the course to be pursued by the U.S. Public Health Service in stimulating an attack upon the mental health problem of the country is apparent as one reviews the present operation of the National Mental Health Act. Yet it is also of interest to note the modifications that were introduced into the early plans concerning support of research and the changes in emphasis in regard to the disciplines which might contribute and the types of studies which might be pursued since the first advisory committees met.

In December, 1940, an advisory committee on nervous and mental diseases met with the Surgeon General and his associates. This Council recommended Federal support for investigations pertaining to mental diseases. The discussion emphasized not only the need for the establishment of a Federal institute for research but, also, the need for a grant-in-aid program to provide support to non-Federal institutions, hospitals, and physicians throughout the country to stimulate investigations relating to mental disease. It was pointed out that a Federal service alone would be in a position to conduct long-term studies, if necessary over several generations, which might shed light on the etiology, course, and treatment of chronic mental illnesses, that epidemiological studies were properly the function of the Federal government, and finally, that support from private funds for

this important field had proved inadequate. At that meeting interest was focused on the biological approach to the causation of mental diseases while considerably less weight was given to the possibilities of psychological investigation. Little mention was made concerning the contributions which social science investigations might make to understanding mental disease.

In May, 1940, the Council of The American Psychiatric Association endorsed the recommendation of the Surgeon General of the U. S. Public Health Service for the establishment in the Public Health Service of an institute for the study of mental and nervous diseases and urged the authorities to take appropriate action for the establishment of such an institute.

The immediate exigencies of the war led to the postponement of these early plans. However, after the cessation of World War II, a group of consultants met with the Surgeon General and the Chief of the Division of Mental Hygiene and again proposed a Federal program for supporting research on mental disease. After a lapse of 6 years, the contribution of the social sciences to psychiatric investigation was now stressed and the need defined for a more diversified attack on the sources of mental disease.

The research program developing under the provisions of the National Mental Health Act is proceeding along 3 broad avenues. First is the support of research projects initiated by individuals and institutions throughout the United States and presented for consideration to the National Advisory Mental Health Council and its technical sub-committee, the Mental Health Research Study Section. The Council, with the assistance of the Research Study Section, reviews research programs submitted to the Public Health Service and recommends to the Surgeon General support for projects that show promise of making valuable contributions to human knowledge with respect to psychiatric disorders. The Council is also authorized to collect information on studies being carried on in the field of mental health and to make such information available through appropriate publications to health and welfare agencies, physicians, or any other scientists, and the general public.

Secondly, a research fellowship program has been instituted to provide aid to young investigators in obtaining additional and specialized training.

Read at the 105th annual meeting of The American Psychiatric Association, Montreal, Quebec, May 23-27 1949.

TABLE 1

	Fiscal years					
	1947		1948		1949	
	Number	Sum	Number	Sum	Number	Sum
Projects						
Received	76	$1,101,361	94	$1,105,525	79	$1,059,389
Approved	28	271,639	27	314,870	25	330,494
Paid	0	0	0	363,791	14	186,150
Terminated	0	0	2	0	2	0

Thirdly, Federal participation in the research program is provided by authorization of the construction of the National Institute of Mental Health. Each of these aspects of the research program will be described.

Research Grants-in-Aid.—Those procedures and policies which have been developed to facilitate the review of the requests for grants-in-aid for research presented to the Public Health Service in relation to mental disease during the past 3 years deserve further comment. The Mental Health Research Study Section has as its function the review of applications for research grants-in-aid and the initiation of any research project deemed particularly worth while. This study section was organized in 1947 under the chairmanship of Dr. John Romano. In contrast to research study sections of other Advisory Councils of the Public Health Service, which are concerned with the research in other spheres of medicine, the Mental Health Research Study Section has a larger number of members (20) representing a wide variety of disciplines. It has representatives from the biological fields of chemistry, pathology, physiology; the clinical fields of psychiatry, neurology, medicine, surgery, and pediatrics; and the social science fields of anthropology, sociology, and psychology. Doubts were expressed by some when this committee was first formed as to whether a body representing so many diverse viewpoints of science and consisting of such a large number of members could function efficiently. The work performed by the Research Study Section in the initial 3-year period dispels these earlier questionings. The extent of the work done and the breadth of the research program developed and now being supported through the activities of this committee is presented in Table 1.

The large number of applications submitted in the brief span of 3 years demonstrates that no dearth of ideas exists in regard to psychiatric investigation. On the other hand, the fact that only a third of the applications submitted were considered meritorious enough to warrant recommendation for support by the National Advisory Mental Health Council does show weakness in terms of available and competent investigators, appropriate techniques, and facilities for undertaking the studies proposed.

Analysis by categories of the applications submitted makes evident the extensive coverage of subjects in which investigation related to psychiatric problems is being planned and pursued. The subjects range through anatomy, anthropology, biochemistry and metabolism, electroencephalography, genetics, preventive methods, pathology, personality development, physiology, psychosomatic medicine, psychology, sociology, and therapy.

The largest concentration of approved grants, 10 in number, falls in the field of psychology. Nine grants, respectively, have been made for psychophysiological and neurophysiological studies, 9 for various therapeutic investigations, and 8 each in the fields of personality development, psychosomatic disorders, and social psychology. The majority of the grants-in-aid have been made to teams working under the direction of a physician. Nine grants have been made to clinical psychologists and 2 to psychiatric social workers.

Sufficient funds have never been available to support the total number of projects considered meritorious by the Advisory Council. At the present time 31 approved projects amounting to a total request of $377,272 remain uninitiated for this reason.

From time to time the question has been asked as to whether the research committee has selected certain areas of study as being of the highest priority. Similar questions are asked in regard to the research program to be developed under the auspices of the National Institute of Mental Health. This problem was placed before the Research Study Section at its earliest meeting and has also been discussed in the National Advisory Mental Health Council meetings. In these discussions, no less than 20 different areas of investigation have been mentioned as meriting priority. Nevertheless, a number of the members expressed outright the opinion that a priority listing of investigative areas should not be considered at this time, and no semblance of consensus for consideration of priority of support could be reached.

Some might state that the failure of the committee to agree that one or another area of investigation should have priority expresses a lack of decisiveness in regard to investigative opportunities in the field of psychiatry. However, it is doubtful that the way of a developing science has ever been along fixed and clearly predetermined paths. The committee has always supported the philosophy that any project should be considered solely on its merit; the merit to be determined on the competence of the investigator, the facilities available to him for carrying out the proposed plan, the delineation of the hypothesis to be tested, and the precision of the methodology outlined.

In addition to its activities in reviewing research grants, the National Advisory Mental Health Council, through the study section, has also made a beginning in its second function of initiating projects and collecting information on studies being carried on in this field. Recommendations have been made for a survey of current active research re-

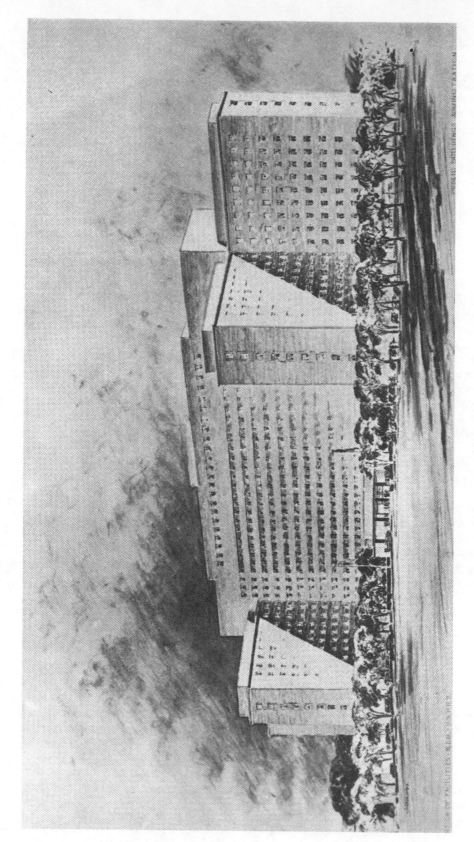

FIGURE 1.—Clinical Center of the National Institutes of Health

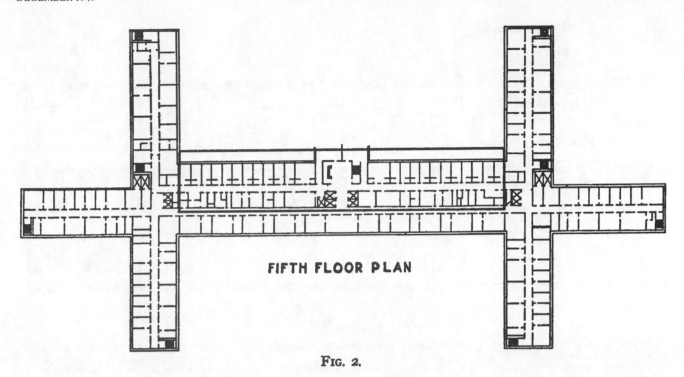

FIFTH FLOOR PLAN

FIG. 2.

lating to mental disease. The survey would cover not only projects strictly relating to psychiatry, but also projects in the socio-psychological and anthropological disciplines which contribute to our understanding of mental health or disease. Secondly, it has been recommended that a series of research conference groups be supported over a period of years. These conference groups would have as their purposes the free interchange of knowledge between various investigators and the encouragement of the pursuit of new leads. The initial series of conferences are to be concerned with psycho-surgery; the proceedings to be published under the auspices of the National Institute of Mental Health for distribution to interested workers.

Research Fellowships.—The research fellowship program appears to be less well known to the membership of The American Psychiatric Association than the research grant-in-aid and the training grant-in-aid programs. During the several years of operation of the fellowship program, 39 research fellowship appointments in this field have been made by the Surgeon General. Twenty-four are now active. Again, it is evident that the emphasis on investigations as applied to psychiatry is broad. Of the 24 active fellows, 4 are principally concerned with studies directly related to clinical psychiatry, 2 in neurology, 7 in psychology, 7 in neurophysiology, 1 in biophysics, and 3 in biochemistry.

The Research Study Section has recommended that special consideration in awarding of fellowships be given to individuals desiring further training in investigative techniques in disciplines other than those in which they were originally trained.

Research Branch of the National Institute of Mental Health.—The third avenue of the research program initiated with the passage of the National Mental Health Act is the development of the Research Branch of the National Institute of Mental Health. Planning for the construction

and staffing of this research activity has been pursued during the past 2 years. The original plan for the National Institute of Mental Health called for a separate structure. However, during 1948 Congress appropriated a sum of money to build a clinical center in relation to the National Cancer Institute, National Heart Institute, and other Institutes of the Public Health Service. It was decided that the clinical and laboratory facilities for the various Institutes should be congregated into a single clinical facility which will be known in the future under the title of the Clinical Center of the National Institutes of Health.

Construction of the Clinical Center of the National Institutes of Health commenced in August of 1948 on a plot of land in Bethesda, Maryland. This structure will have bed space for 500 patients and extensive laboratory space. One-hundred and fifty beds and 100,000 square feet of laboratory space will be devoted to the activities of the Research Branch of the National Institute of Mental Health.

Much assistance in the specialized planning for the Research Branch of the National Institute of Mental Health has been provided by members of this Association acting as consultants to the Public Health Service. Certain details concerning the architectural plans for this structure and its eventual staffing represent in themselves experimental approaches and, therefore, are of more than passing interest.

The Clinical Center is to be constructed in the form of a Lorraine cross, the central block to contain the clinical areas; and the six wings, the laboratory areas. The architect's sketch of the north exposure is shown in Fig. 1.

Of particular importance in the planning of the central block is the use of the double corridor plan (Fig. 2). This plan, which requires air-conditioning throughout the building, makes possible the use of the central section for nursing services, therapeutic rooms, various utility and housekeeping rooms. All rooms on the southern exposure

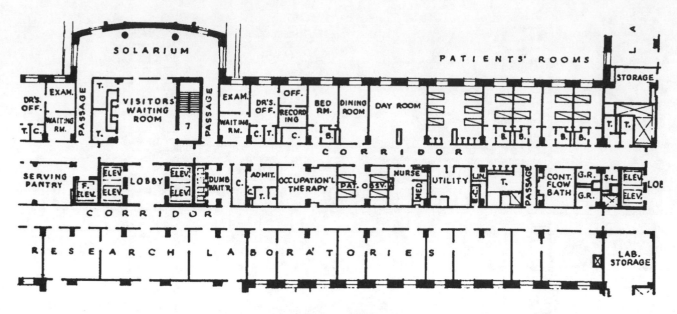

LEGEND

ADMIT.	= ADMITTING ROOM	F. ELEV.	= FOOD SERVICE ELEVATOR	MED.	= MEDICINE ROOM		
B.	= BATH ROOM	G.R.	= GEAR ROOM	OFF.	= OFFICE		
C.	= CLOSET	J.C.	= JANITOR'S CLOSET	PAT. ØBSV.	= PATIENTS OBSERVATION		
E.C.	= WIRE CLOSET	LIN.	= CLEAN LINEN	S.L.	= SOILED LINEN		
EXAM.	= EXAMINING ROOM	LKR.	= LOCKER ROOM	T.	= TOILET		

FIG. 3.

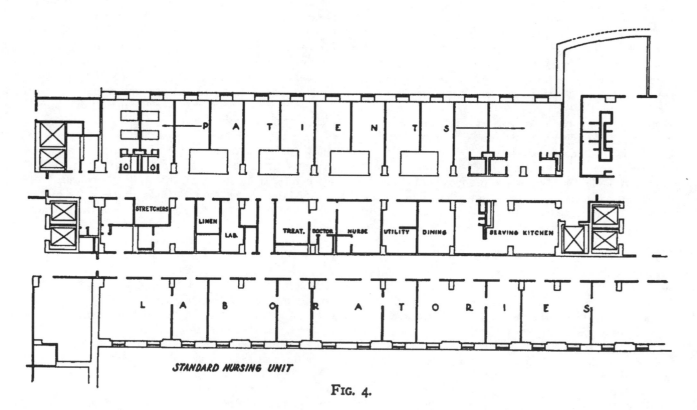

STANDARD NURSING UNIT

FIG. 4.

can then be used for patients, and those on the north for laboratory spaces. These laboratory spaces are thus immediately adjacent to patient areas and will prove highly useful for clinical-laboratory research. On the psychiatric floors

such spaces will allow the development of adequate interviewing rooms often so lacking in modern psychiatric hospital construction.

In the 13-floor central structure the second, third, and

fourth floors with bed capacity of 100 will have specialized arrangements for closed psychiatric nursing units. This arrangement is shown in Fig. 3. The fifth floor, with bed capacity of 50 patients, will be arranged in the standard 2-bed nursing unit (Fig. 4) being utilized in the other clinical areas for psychiatric and neurological patients who require only ordinary hospital facilities.

The ancillary therapeutic units of recreational, occupational, and physiotherapy (physical therapy) are to be located in the 5-story southwest wing immediately adjacent to the psychiatric clinical floor areas. The administrative unit and the outpatient area for the Institute will also be housed on the lower floors of this wing. The large outside area in the southwest angle of the Clinical Center is planned as a recreational section for restricted patients.

The clinical accommodations represent an attempt, on a moderately large scale, to house severely disturbed patients in a general hospital for long-term study and treatment. Visual segregation is to be afforded by the horizontal separation of floors and auditory segregation through the use of sound-proofing. If this type of construction proves successful, the future planning of psychiatric units may be materially modified.

There will be ample provisions for audio-visual recordings of human behavior. The development of excellent equipment of this type over the past 10 years now makes it possible to record in detail verbal and non-verbal action of and between individuals.

The laboratory spaces are to be constructed on the module principle with movable steel partitions, which have been used with success in laboratories constructed for industrial research. Thus, laboratory spaces may be expanded or contracted at any time as required for the particular experimental project in operation. The use of the movable steel partition will also be tried in certain partitions of the psychiatric nursing units.

The opening of the Clinical Center of the National Institute of Mental Health is not expected before 1952. A gradual development of the clinical and scientific staff is envisaged so that complete occupancy of this structure will not be attained in less than 5 or 6 years thereafter. Through this gradual growth, it is hoped to bring together a strong and talented staff. In accordance with the recommendations of the Public Health Service consultants, the research program in the National Institute of Mental Health will be multidisciplined. The fellowship, training grant, and in-service training programs developed in connection with the National Mental Health Act are expected to produce the younger men who will participate in the activities of the Institute in the future.

The National Mental Health Act has provided a strong impetus to investigations relating to mental disorder since its activation 3 years ago. The progress reported here gives high promise of meeting the expectations of the early progenitors of this Act, many of whom, it is a pleasure to observe, are in attendance at this symposium.

IV. Developments in Somatic Treatment

INTRODUCTION

P sychiatric diseases have somatic treatments that are, for the most part, empiric. The development and application of these treatments in American psychiatry over the last 150 years have been fascinating—reflecting a developing astuteness in clinical observation, diagnosis, assessment, pharmacology, and, most recently, neurobiology. All treatments have been empiric because no understanding yet exists of the biological basis of psychiatric illnesses. Where pathophysiology is known, treatment development can be focused on correcting a pathologic mechanism and outcome can be specifically measured. In psychiatry, strategies for new treatments have derived either from mimicking past successes, making small advances within a strategy, testing speculative new ideas, or serendipity. Serendipity, coupled with critical clinical observation, has already played a critical role in the development of successful treatments for psychiatric diseases. These successes are represented in this section by articles on electroconvulsive and tricyclic treatments for depression and neuroleptic treatment for schizophrenia. The clinician has played an important role in advancing these treatments, as directed by clinical need, current scientific ideas, and basic pharmacology. This section provides us with a one and a half century time line of the best psychiatric somatic treatments: how they were applied, how evaluated, and their hypothetical mechanisms.

The articles in this section demonstrate astute clinical observation, with growing sophistication, in a number of different psychiatric diseases practiced largely by psychiatrists who were both caregivers and scientists. Attention has been given to observation of pattern and type of symptoms, treatment rationale, response to medication, and overall outcome. The basic treatment strategy was description in Samuel Woodward's article "Medical Treatment of Insanity." Practical need drove the basic strategy in A.E. Bennett's article on curare, while Sakel, Moniz, and Barrera used the study and presentation of representative case vignettes. The lack of real knowledge about the physical and mental effects of malaria (Wagner-Jauregg), hypoglycemia (Sakel), and lobotomies (Moniz) made these particular treatment strategies ill-fated, not an inattention to symptom observation or practical need. Accurate and timely observation by clinician scientists, with creative formulation of data, has always been the basis for the advances in our field. Because of this, diagnosis and definition of symptoms and outcome assessment has been practiced in a more exacting fashion in psychiatry than in many other medical specialties. In these articles, despite the often inadequate formulations and premature conclusions, it is a joy to read the observations and vignettes that have arisen from the efforts of intelligent and thoughtful physicians trying to improve outcome for patients. The advantage for psychiatry in the twenty-first century will be the ability to organize our clinical observations on the basis of the growing biologic understanding of brain function.

In most of medicine the emphasis on differential diagnosis arises from the fact that differential treatments exist for different disease entities. Diagnosis assists in identifying the treatments that will produce optimal response of the illness. Diagnosis is most precise when the defining characteristics of the disease can be assessed biologically, as in anemia or diabetes. Even when this is not the case however, as in most psychiatric illness, diagnosis can be drawn from phenomenologic characteristics with reasonable precision. Diagnosis has clearly advanced in the last 150 years. Increasing emphasis has been given to defining categories of illness and differential diagnosis. At present, diagnoses are based on standard criteria, supported by information about symptoms and psychosocial function gathered in a standardized way, across the disease history. Specific diagnoses are associated with particular treatment regimens of recognized efficacy. But brain diseases have not always been clearly distinguished. While insanity as a diagnosis was subdivided into types in 1846, these categories no doubt included not only schizophrenia but also depression, dementia, vitamin deficiencies, communicable diseases (e.g., syphilis), and genetic conditions (e.g., Huntington's disease). Treatments for insanity, as detailed by Woodward, were understandably symptomatic and complex, without attention to selective symptom response. Some more delimited diagnostic categories such as "general paralysis" (Wagner-Jauregg) and "psychosis" (Sakel) were represented transitionally in our history, before the nearly modern diagnostic categories of alcoholism (Barbera), depression, and schizophrenia (Kinross-Wright). Today, diagnostic categories have assumed great importance for suggesting a typical treatment regimen and for the discovery of new, selective treatments.

Increasingly rigorous and controlled strategies for assessment in treatment trials have developed over the last 150 years in theory and in practice. Whereas assessment was global and imprecise in the nineteenth century, throughout the twentieth century assessment techniques have become progressively more specific and scientific. Assessment instruments have been developed that are sensitive and selective, and more attention has been given to their application. The ideas that 1) assessment is necessary not only in individuals but across populations (as in Sakel's article) and 2) that a control treatment is an important design element (as in Barbera's study) are pivotal to modern treatment evaluation. In modern psychiatric drug development, valid, reliable, sensitive, and precise clinical assessment has become a key to contemporary advances in somatic therapies. This ingredient for treatment testing has been increasingly recognized over the last 150 years, and its growth is represented in this section.

Gradually over this time line, sound principles of clinical pharmacology have also emerged. Whereas in 1846, Woodward advocated many treatments for insanity without clear attention to mechanism of drug action, drug dose, or kinetic considerations, subsequent articles demonstrate the application of these kinds of pharmacologic techniques. By the early twentieth century, scientists made hypotheses on the basis of critical observations (e.g., Wagner-Jauregg's observance that psychosis remitted following a febrile illness). Sakel articulates this directly: "The great advances in treatment made by modern medicine in recent years have taught us to expect that every successful treatment has to be based on sound biological principles." Bennett, in his article on curare, made a further step: he reviewed the pharmacologic characteristics of curare and found that these properties answered a pressing clinical need—muscle relaxation for electroshock. In testing his hypothesis, he first did drug dose finding and studied duration of drug action for muscle relaxation. This optimized his final treatment design. The more recent articles on chlorpromazine (Kinross-Wright), imipramine (Pollack), and lithium (Wharton and Fieve) paid increasing attention to rigorous pharmacologic principles of protocol design. These include establishing a selective diagnostic group, clarifying drug dose, including adequate control groups, performing an unbiased clinical assessment, fixing drug doses, specifying duration of treatment, and evaluating side effects. Sound principles of pharmacologic evaluation have grown throughout this century, and they continue to be developed, debated, and challenged today. At present, all adequate treatment trials include: a delimited target population, a treatment agent with known characteristics, a study hypothesis with clear outcome predictions, and appropriate rating scales for primary outcome symptoms. An adequate drug dose range with demonstration of CNS activity, an adequate placebo group or period, and structured side effect evaluation are all a regular part of evaluation and demonstration of drug treatment efficacy. The background for these current practices has been based on practices in our modern history.

An inadequate neuroscience database routinely misled these clinicians in their scientific speculations about psychiatric diseases. Neuroscience is a young field. It was not until the

1890s that Cajal (1852–1934) first proposed that brain tissue is composed of specialized cells, which he named neurons. At the turn of this century, a furious debate still raged over the mechanism of neurotransmission: was it electrical over neural networks, or was it chemical at synapses? The general acceptance of the process of chemically mediated neurotransmission laid the foundation for the whole field of modern psychopharmacology. Chemically mediated transmission is important, because it is at the "nodes" of neuronal information transmission, called the "synapse," where drugs have a pivotal influence on neuronal function. The first neurotransmitter (acetylcholine) was not discovered and described until the late 1930s; norepinephrine was not demonstrated to be active at sympathetic ganglia until the mid-1940s; dopamine and serotonin were accepted as transmitters in the 1950s. The most prevalent neurotransmitters in brain are amino acids, which include γ-aminobutyric acid, glutamate, glycine, histamine, and taurine. These were not described or demonstrated until the 1950s and 1960s. Thus, it has only been possible to describe the basic principles of transmitter-mediated neurotransmission in the latter part of this century. Earlier investigators did not have the basic theoretical tools to explain drug action. In general the authors of the articles in this section realized the lack of adequate knowledge to explain their treatments. They realized the power that biologic understanding would provide. Some tried to substitute reasoning for real knowledge; this demonstrated a proper intent but produced an ineffective outcome nonetheless (e.g., the malarial and hypoglycemic treatments). Therapeutic developments for the future will rest on increasingly sophisticated advances in basic neuroscience knowledge.

The treatment of mental illness over the centuries, especially before the time of modern medicine, has reflected the moral characteristics and societal assumptions of an age. Some premodern ages failed to identify psychiatric syndromes as diseases at all; other ages built mystical causes for mental aberrations. The Greeks identified the brain as the organ providing thought, judgment, and memory to the spirit but through a mystical mechanism. Later, Galen postulated that nerves were specialized ducts, conveying brain fluid along with information to the periphery of the body. During the Middle Ages, while the intellectuals identified the brain's cavities (cerebral ventricles) and its fluid (cerebrospinal fluid) as the "soul's power," political leaders were burning the insane at the stake as devils. Moral treatments were initiated in Europe and in America with the increasing social awareness of its citizens.

Treatments in psychiatry over the last 150 years have not been limited to somatic treatments. Ours has been perhaps the first field to recognize the often critical nature of psychosocial treatment and the contribution of psychodynamic considerations to overall recovery. These treatments are represented in other sections of this issue and not discussed here. This perhaps represents the focus in the journal of reports on therapeutics to somatic treatment. It has been only recently that studies have begun to evaluate the individual and combined benefit of drug and psychosocial treatments. Considerable opportunity exists for new work in this area.

What has our own field of American psychiatry done with the formulation and treatment of mental illness over the course of its recorded history in *The American Journal of Psychiatry*? Our early ideas for treatments were developed with little understanding of neurobiologic mechanisms. During the later nineteenth and in the early twentieth centuries, treatment concepts have been set within the medical model of a biologic disorder, responsive to pharmacologic treatment. Thus, physicians have assumed the existence of biologic explanations, even in their absence, and have always experimented with "scientific" explanations. We can see from the articles presented here that while the treatment directions of the past may have been based on naive and contextual ideas, they contain treatment pearls and pieces of wisdom relevant today.

One might wonder what lessons we can learn today from the record of our past successes and failures. What strengths were demonstrated in this history? First, most of these past successes were built on a history of observations and discoveries. Treatments in general did not come from entirely unanticipated directions. Rational treatment development brings progress. Moreover, strategies brought increasing success when they were based on hypotheses and tested scientifically. The more solidly the hypothesis was based on biologic data or on known facts of brain or body function, the more likely was the success of the treatment. And the more scientific the methodology, the clearer the answer. Strategies designed to answer a specific clinical need tended to bring progress. The more specific the question and the more focused the design, the more likely was a positive outcome. In sum, the gradual advances in clinical observations, diagnosis, assessment, pharmacology, and neurobiology over the last 150 years have contributed to the increasing success of our psychiatric treatments.

In the next 150 years, considerable opportunity for advances will belong to us and to our students. Sakel echoed a pertinent sentiment in 1937 when he counseled that "Psychiatrists need no longer have that paralyzing feeling of insufficiency toward their psychotic patients that they used to have." What are our opportunities? Which are the fruitful research directions in treatment? We are equipped with good clinical methods for treatment testing. We have delineated psychiatric diseases as entities requiring treatment. We continue to have the same strong desire for improved treatments as our predecessors, fueled by clinical need. But, perhaps different than the past, we are entering a time of great scientific advantage, because the mechanisms of brain function are now being elaborated. These discoveries will undoubtedly unfold over an extended period of time because of the complexity and inaccessibility of the brain. The brain speaks in electrical impulses to cells organized in embedded networks to guide the human body not only in movement, coordination, and verbalization but also in less tangible functions such as thought, attention, memory, and consciousness. It will be our challenge to apply the burgeoning neuroscience knowledge base to the treatment of psychiatric diseases in the twenty-first century. Moreover, tools for human brain research exist at present and are continuously being developed. Woodward, in 1846, already articulated a useful attitude: "Good influences are everywhere operating, and we may confidently hope that what is overlooked by the passing generation, which might have been beneficial to them, will be supplied by their successors."

CAROL A. TAMMINGA, M.D.

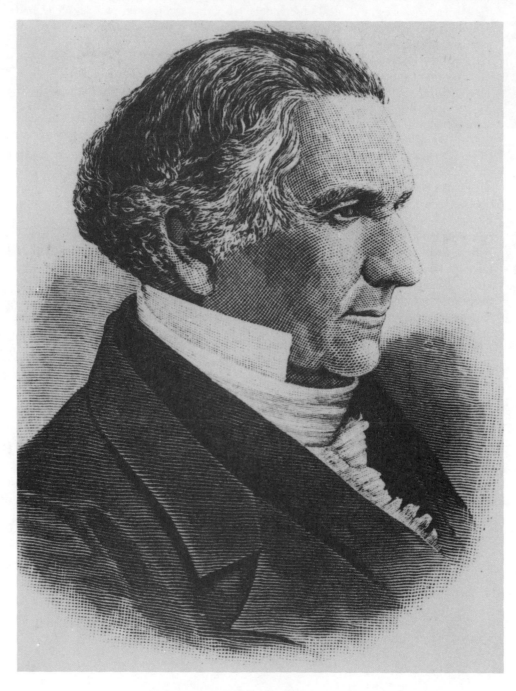

Samuel B. Woodward, M.D., 1787–1850
Co-Founder of APA and Its First President

OBSERVATIONS ON THE MEDICAL TREATMENT OF INSANITY

By Samuel B. Woodward, M.D.

Late Superintendent of the Massachusetts State Lunatic Hospital, Worcester, Massachusetts

The medical treatment of insanity includes, strictly, all the appliances available in any form of the disease.

Moral influence is nearly as important in the treatment of any physical disease as in insanity. The mind must be managed, hope inspired, and confidence secured, to insure success in the treatment of any important disease.

The ancients taught that insanity was a disease requiring the use of medical remedies, but while they prescribed hellebore, and other drugs to effect its cure, they recommended that the mind be diverted and the feelings soothed and assuaged. For this purpose they directed the insane to be taken to the temples of their gods, that they might participate in their religious rites, look upon the beauties of nature from these elevated situations, and, in the temples of Æsculapius, consult the records of experience engraven on the tablets of their walls.

All cases of insanity do not require a medical prescription. Many will recover spontaneously after a time, and many more by simple regulations of diet and such gentle means as will aid the powers of nature in effecting salutary changes. This is also true of many other diseases affecting the vital organs. The judgment must be exercised in all cases to decide where to withhold and when to use remedies.

Insanity has been divided into Mania, Melancholia and Dementia, and each of these into acute and chronic forms. Without inquiring whether these divisions embrace all the forms of disease included under the general term, insanity, it is sufficient for the present purpose to give some account of these diseases with some of their complications, and the remedies that have been found useful in their treatment.

Acute Mania is the most violent and apparently the most formidable and dangerous form of insanity. Its accession is generally sudden, often violent, and its symptoms unequivocal. It is usually attended with increased heat of the head, frequent pulse, warm and soft skin, with extremities inclined to coldness, furred tongue, constipated bowels, sleeplessness, disposition to loud talking, great volubility, dissociation of ideas, rapid changes of the feelings, impetuosity of manner, extravagance of expression, delusion, perversion of the moral powers, disorder of the senses, and inordinate muscular strength. When at rest the pulse is not often found to be hard or strong, neither is there much evidence of vascular excitement, but when the maniac puts forth his power in physical efforts, his strength is amazing, his power of endurance incredible, and an excitement is produced in the system which is a fallacious guide to the treatment. Those who are not extensively acquainted with insanity frequently prescribe for this group of symptoms as they would in phrenitis, though the diseases vary essentially.

In phrenitis the head is extremely painful. The arteries of the head and neck throb violently. They eyes are inflamed, and light is intolerable. The pulse is hard and strong when the patient is at rest. The skin is hot and dry, the appetite gone, the strength prostrated, and the mind is affected with muttering delirium instead of maniacal excitement. Inflammation of the most acute character attends this disease. Not so with acute mania. The symptoms are different. The head is rarely painful, the eyes are not inflamed, light is seldom distressing and sometimes there is great insensibility to it. The appetite is generally unimpaired, sometimes excessive, the pulse is full but not hard, the strength increased, not prostrated, and the reaction, if there is any, not general, not affecting the extremities and the skin as in acute inflammation.

The first requires free bleeding, active and saline cathartics, applications of ice to the head, exclusion of light, and a strict antiphlogistic regimen. The latter is more favorably treated by long continued warm baths, cold applications to the head with pediluvia and other stimulants to the feet, laxatives and narcotics, with all the soothing influences which can be adopted to calm the agitated state of the system and procure repose.

General bleeding has been almost universally prescribed in the treatment of acute mania before the patient is received into an hospital. The report of its effects in diminishing the violence of its symptoms is various. Occasionally it is said to give permanent relief, more generally it affords a temporary respite of the violent symptoms which soon after recur with increased severity. In a very large proportion of cases it is said to have done no good, in many, positive evil.

Copious bleeding is almost universally injurious. It diminishes the strength of the patient without lessening the excitement or removing the delusions of the disease, and brings on a train of symptoms often more difficult of cure than insanity itself. The old physicians used to speak of bleeding below a crisis in pneumonia, by which was under-

Read at a Meeting of the Association of Medical Superintendents of American Institutions for the Insane, May, 1846.

stood that the remedy had been carried so far as to interfere with a regular crisis, and induce irritations, and awaken susceptibilities which prolonged and rendered complicated a disease originally simple. Such is in some degree the effect of too copious bleeding in mania. Unless there are complications of disease indicating the use of the lancet, acute mania can be managed with more safety and success without it.

The effect of local bleeding is more favorable, and often decidedly beneficial. The great excitement of the brain tends to produce a congestion of the blood vessels which local bleeding will obviate with more certainty than general bleeding, leaving none of the evil effects. When the head is constantly hot, the temporal and carotid arteries throb when the patient is at rest, and the general strength will admit the loss of blood, leeches to the temples, and cupping to the back of the neck may afford present relief and prepare the system for more efficient remedies.

In a great majority of cases bleeding is unnecessary, giving little temporary relief and producing no permanent benefit. In some cases a considerable loss of blood changes the character of the disease from excitement to dementia, a change quite undesirable.

Next to bleeding, purging with active cathartics is a remedy in common use in the treatment of acute mania. Cathartics prescribed for the purpose of reducing excitement, are liable to the same objections as blood letting. It is rare that even temporary benefit arises from their use, and they frequently disturb the stomach, destroy the appetite, produce an irritable and irregular state of the bowels, difficult to manage, the tendency of which is evil, especially if the strength is considerably prostrated.

Laxatives are important remedies, and not as objectionable as active cathartics. It is common for the bowels to be constipated in mania, but gentle remedies are usually sufficient to produce all necessary evacuations. Mercurial purges are useful not only to produce desirable laxative effects, but they cause changes in the secretions which are often necessary to the restoration of health. In warm climates, and in those sections of the country where bilious diseases are common, calomel or blue pill becomes a very important remedy. Mercurial purges are also useful when the healthy functions of the uterus are suddenly suspended or when these functions are performed in an irregular manner.

In the early states of acute mania, when the tongue is coated, the secretions of the skin deficient or vitiated, the patient sleepless, and the bowels constipated, calomel combined with Dover's powder is a very valuable remedy. So also the blue pill in combination with some of the narcotics, especially with Conium and other deobstruents, in certain conditions of the digestive organs, is a useful auxiliary in the cure of insanity. Costiveness should not be suffered to continue long, and yet too much anxiety need not be had if the bowels do not move daily. Diarrhoea is more to be dreaded than costiveness; it is rarely useful and is more difficult to regulate and control. A regular, daily movement of the bowels is desirable. There is a condition of the bowels occasionally occurring in mania but more frequently in dementia, in which the patient has liquid or thin discharges when at the same time there is considerable accumulation of foecal matter in the rectum. Such a condition of the bowels is relieved at once by cathartics. The case is sometimes deceptive but experience soon designates the cases of this description from ordinary diarrhoea, and the remedy is always easy and effectual.

Emetics, as a remedy for insanity, have been variously estimated. Some practitioners have great confidence in them, others esteem them of little value. The late Mr. Haslam said that he had given them by thousands, but could not say they were beneficial. They are useful only as in other cases of disease. In cases of high excitement nauseating doses of emetics sometimes produce quiet and composure of the mind, and are useful auxiliaries in the treatment by narcotics. In those sections of the country where bilious diseases prevail they may be more frequently indicated. No great reliance, however, can be placed upon them. They rarely produce any permanent benefit and are sometimes injurious in their effects by causing too much determination of blood to the head while operating, and by deranging the stomach and bowels afterwards. Some remedies of this class alone or combined with opium and other narcotics, produce a favorable influence on the skin, and allay general irritation and excitement. Of these the preparations of antimony are most effectual but less safe than Ipecacuanha, Actoea Racemosa and Sanguinaria, the last two of which are both emetic and narcotic remedies.

As a means of exciting nausea, in violent cases of mania, the circular swing was recommended by the highest medical authority. Dr. Darwin speaks well of it and Dr. Cox relied upon it almost exclusively to remove maniacal excitement. It is a very effectual means of producing sickness, vertigo and vomiting, and usually prostrates the system remarkably. It is not always a safe remedy. It is extremely unpleasant to the patient, and always regarded as a punishment rather than a means of cure. It has been very properly discarded in modern practice.

The warm bath is a safe and useful remedy in this form of disease. In many cases it is more efficacious if cold be applied to the head at the same time or in the interval of its use. The temperature of the bath should be from 90 to 100 degrees, and the patient may be continued in it an hour or more at a time. This bath may be repeated at least every night till the violence of the excitement is removed. A combination of other remedies makes the bath more effectual than when prescribed alone. The cold shower bath has been recommended as a remedy. It may do good if agreeable to the feelings of the patient, but, like the circular swing, it is too frequently considered as a punishment, the patient dreads its application and is frightened when it is applied. In such cases it is injurious rather than beneficial. The simple application of cold water to the head is not usually unpleasant, and is a mode of procuring tranquility in cases of great excitement. When the head is hot there is an instinctive desire to apply cold water to the head an[d] many patients will seek it themselves whenever an opportunity presents. If the efficacy of cold applications to the head in removing paroxysms of excitement was generally understood, the resort to copious bleeding would be less frequent, and greater numbers of patients would recover from insanity, more speedily, and with less evil influences to be overcome by remedies, or to be endured in after life.

In this disease there is often a vitiated state of the skin, the secretions are unhealthy, of peculiar smell, and offensive. This state of the skin is more generally and effectually relieved by baths than any other remedies. Eruptions, existing or repelled, are often the supposed cause of insanity. Simple or medicated baths are useful in such cases. The general cold bath is an important remedy but not usually applicable to acute mania. Baths are everywhere useful in insanity, but in warm climates where the functions of the skin are of more importance to health than elsewhere, they are not only preventives of disease but efficient remedies in its cure.

Certain sedative medicines, principally narcotics, have been extensively used in this disease. Of these perhaps the Digitalis has had the longest and highest reputation. The effect of this remedy in controlling the action of the heart, and diminishing the frequency of the pulse, doubtless first led to its use in insanity, and in some cases it is decidedly tranquilizing.

Narcotics have little power in controlling maniacal excitement unless prescribed in large doses. This is true of Digitalis. The unpleasant and sometimes dangerous effects of this powerful medicine, when prescribed freely, should prove a caution as to its use, and has probably led to its very general disuse at this time in the simple form of this disease. This is not to be regretted, as there are many remedies of this class more efficacious in the removal of insanity, and far more safe and agreeable. Digitalis should not be wholly discarded in the treatment of mania. There may be cases and combinations of disease in which it may be useful. When prescribed its effects should be narrowly watched, and the medicine withdrawn when its specific action takes place, without apparent mitigation of the symptoms of the case.

Next on the list of narcotics, which has been relied upon in the treatment of acute mania is the Datura Stramonium. Twenty-five years ago this remedy was in general use in the treatment of insanity. It is no common encomium of its virtues that it was highly esteemed and frequently prescribed by the celebrated Dr. Todd, late Superintendent of the Retreat at Hartford, Conn., whose knowledge of insanity and its remedies, and whose thorough acquaintance with narcotics generally entitle his opinions to great weight.

The objections to the use of the Stramonium and Digitalis are similar. In large doses they destroy the appetite, produce dryness of the tongue, disturb the vision, and, in some cases, prostrate the strength to an alarming degree, without controlling the maniacal excitement. The Stramonium, in particular, produces illusions of sight which frequently coincide with the delusions of disease and increase the excitement. There are cases in which the effect of Stramonium is more favorable, controlling the symptoms and inducing sleep, when given in such doses as do not develop its hazardous influences.

The Hyoscyamus has a reputation equal to its merits in the treatment of insanity. It is extensively used both in this country and Europe, and its effects are spoken of as certain and efficacious. This is a remedy, of far less power than the Digitalis or Stramonium, but more agreeable in its effects, and is not attended by the danger which the others produce in full doses. In mild cases of nervous excitement the Hyoscyamus alone, or in combination with other narcotics of equally mild character, produces sleep, controls troublesome excitement, and makes the patient feel better. It is not a powerful medicine, and is far less efficacious than some others of the same class that are equally safe.

Camphor has had a good reputation in allaying maniacal excitement. It is a medicine of some power, and, in large doses, produces decided narcotic effects. The reputation which it once had is lost, and, with Hyoscyamus is used only to promote sleep and tranquilize the nervous system in a mild form of disease.

Lupuline is less of a narcotic than either of the above, but with an influence quite favorable on the nervous system, it possesses a tonic power that is beneficial in some forms of insanity.

The combination of Hyoscyamus, Camphor and Lupuline forms a valuable medicine to induce sleep, and is a remedy of no small power in controlling irregular nervous excitement.

Ether, Valerian, and the fetid gums have a reputation quite above their merits in the treatment of insanity. They are of little use and cannot be relied upon to effect any changes in a disease so formidable.

The Cannabis Indica, the Indian hemp of the East Indies, has recently been introduced into the English hospitals as a remedy for insanity. Doctor Conolly, in his lectures on insanity recently published in the London Lancet, bears testimony to the favorable influence of this remedy in controlling the symptoms of mania. This medicine has also been used in France with apparent success. In this country some trial has been made of it and the reports of its utility are anything but satisfactory. Some attribute to it considerable power, others esteem it of little efficacy. Doctors Nellegan and Mease consider it the same as the Apocynum Cannabinum of the United States Pharmacopoeia. This is doubtful. If it is the same the difference in climate may make a difference in medicinal power. However this may be it is probable that it will prove a remedy of secondary importance. Favorable trials of the foreign article and the extensive use of the native Indian hemp, have not at all sustained the high encomiums bestowed upon it by foreign writers. At one time it gained a reputation in dropsy as a stimulant diuretic. It is probably a stimulant narcotic as it has long been used in India and Persia to produce intoxication. It has but recently been introduced into the materia medica in India by the late Dr. O'Shaughnessy of Calcutta. The native article has long been used in this country as a popular remedy.

Of all the narcotic or sedative remedies useful in this form of mania the salts of Morphia, and other preparations of opium, are the most effectual and salutary. It is of little consequence what form of this remedy is selected for use. The sulphate and acetate of morphia are more generally approved, and perhaps the least exceptionable. Liquid preparations of opium are always preferable to solid, especially if the doses to be used are large, as the effect is less liable to accumulate, the influence is sooner felt, and the remedy more easily managed. The tincture of opium is, in many cases, the best preparation, and is equally safe when cautiously and judiciously prescribed. The Dover's powder is one of the best forms to commence this remedy, especially if there is any unnatural heat or dryness of the skin, or determination of blood to the head. The cases in which the preparations of opium are clearly indicated are those in which the excitement is more purely nervous, the surface moist and of no unusual heat, the pulse soft and full, the tongue moist, and the head not unusually hot. If, on the contrary, the head is hot, the eyes red, the skin hot and dry, the tongue red and dry, and especially if there is tenderness in the epigastric region, some preparation is necessary before the opium should be freely given.—When administered it should be combined with Calomel, Antimony, Ipecacuanha or the Actoea Racemosa. Calomel or the blue pill may be first given in such cases, blisters or the tincture of Iodine applied over the epigastrum and the warm bath used sometime before opium is commenced. The warm bath and cold applications to the head may also accompany the use of opium in many cases.

When the case is well selected and the system well prepared for the use of opium, or when the case first presents itself indicating its use, it is potent in relieving the excitement and in removing the symptoms of disease. It should be given in liberal doses once in six or eight hours, or if it disturbs the stomach, in smaller doses repeated more frequently. When one preparation disagrees, another may sometimes be substituted with benefit. To gain all the good effects of this remedy it is essential that the system be kept under its influence, and that the doses be repeated sufficiently often that the effect of one shall not be lost till another is administered. It is contrary to all true experience in mania to expect to gain much by the use of opium in single doses at night to promote sleep. Whatever good may occasionally arise in this or any other form of disease from this practice, it is far better that the system be kept under its influence till the excitement is subdued and the disease removed.

In acute mania the patient requires but little sleep. The condition of the brain is such that the replenishing of sleep is not needed as in health, and after sleep the excitement is often increased rather than allayed.

Costiveness if present, or if it supervene in the progress of treatment, should be obviated by the gentlest remedies. The bowels are not usually very torpid in this disease, and costiveness is attended with less evil than would be expected. A regular state of the bowels is most desirable.

In all cases of acute mania that do not recover spontaneously, or yield at first to other remedies, the preparations of opium should be prescribed unless symptoms exist which forbid their use. It is exceedingly rare that some favorable influence will not be produced, the violence of the symptoms be lessened and the period shortened by their use. Many cases of mania recover without narcotics or other active treatment, but when they are indicated more confidence can be placed in opiates than in any other remedies, and their effects, in removing disease, are often sudden. If when first administered, opiates do not produce the desired effect, or any unfavorable circumstance attends their use,

they may be suspended for a time, till further preparation is made for them, or till the indications for them are more clear, and they may then be resumed with advantage. It is impossible always to foresee the objections to this remedy, but if the symptoms be carefully watched the medicine can be varied or so combined with others as to obviate objections that may occasionally arise to its use. Less doses will be needed to control excitement in many cases when diaphoretic or nauseating remedies are combined with it.

Dr. Conolly remarks that "whatever sedative is given in mania, the dose should be large; less than a grain of acetate of morphia is productive of no good whatever, and laudanum requires to be given in doses of a drachm, or at least forty or fifty drops."

It is better, however, to give smaller doses at the first and repeat them every four or six hours, than to give such large doses at a longer interval. The symptoms of disease yield more readily and the system suffers less when the remedy is managed in this way. Many cases of acute mania require even larger doses than these mentioned by Dr. Conolly, and it is necessary to repeat them frequently before the disease will subside and a healthly condition take place.

Aged people, the intemperate, persons affected with dyspepsia, liver complaints, and general palsy, do not bear opium in large doses as well as the more healthy. The doses should not be less, but, in such cases, the medicine usually does best in combination with other remedies.

When opium has been used with benefit in full doses, and the patient becomes more quiet and rational, the medicine may be slowly withdrawn. At first it is better that the dose be diminished than that the number of doses be lessened. If no excitement occur there may be a gradual withdrawal of the medicine till it is wholly removed. When this medicine is taken off too rapidly neuralgia of the lower limbs, with restlessness and general pain over the whole body, or toothache will sometimes occur, coryza and other symptoms of a severe cold frequently follow, and a diarrhoea prevents the entire withdrawal of opium at once. It is desirable that the patient continue under care till the health of body and mind is fully established, and all remedies are abandoned.

Cases of mania following cases of acute disease which have exhausted the energies of the system, in delicate and highly susceptible nervous constitutions, and in those where excitement has been so severe as to waste the powers of the system rapidly, require that the strength be sustained by cordials, tonics, and generous diet.—Preparations of bark, vegetable bitters, aromatics, wine and porter are the remedies to be relied upon when the physical powers flag, and the danger is from exhaustion and debility. The combination of porter and lime water is one of the best cordials in dyspeptic cases with acidity and loss of appetite. The diet in this condition of the system, should be generous.

Convalescents from mania require substantial food in liberal quantities. The tendency of this great excitement is to exhaust the powers rapidly, and frequent and full replenishing is necessary. Moderate exercise in the open air is one of the best restoratives, tending to produce quiet sleep, good appetite, and physical and mental vigor. Insane persons usually sleep better after full suppers. Much of the noise and violence that was formerly found in institutions for the insane, arose from insufficient food, harsh treatment, and severe and painful restraints.

RECAPITULATION

The Medical Treatment of mania may generally be commenced by a long continued warm bath, especially on going to bed, cold applications to the head, if agreeable to the patient, and the bowels must be moved by a mercurial purge or other laxative. If it is then decided that opiates are appropriate remedies, the Dover's powder with small doses of calomel may be first used, and the solution of the sulphate of morphia, acetate of morphia, or the tincture of opium may be given, either alone or with small doses of Antimony, Ipecac, or Actoea Racemosa to determine to the surface. The operation of these remedies should be narrowly watched, and the dose increased or varied according to the effect. If the patient becomes more quiet the doses may be gradually lessened, but the medicine should not be suddenly withdrawn lest the excitement return. If the excitement continues, the remedy may be increased gradually or rapidly till it controls the symptoms, produces quiet, and the mind becomes rational. The warm bath may be renewed if the effect is favorable, and cold may be applied to the head if there is much heat, or if it is grateful to the patient. If the excitement is moderate, the case may be left for a time without medicine, or the milder narcotics may be tried. If, however, narcotics are indicated, no substitute can be found for these different preparations of opium. The strength must be supported by good nourishment, diffusible stimulants, and tonics if needed, and all the appliances moral and physical that can be useful should be added to medical treatment to insure a favorable restoration to health.

CHRONIC MANIA

The treatment of chronic mania differs considerably from that of the acute forms of the disease. Depletion, as such, either local or general, will rarely be indicated. The period of vascular excitement, if it has ever existed is past. When the patient is quiet, the head is not hot, neither is the pulse excited nor accelerated. If there is any increased heat about the head the extremities will be cold, and the action of the capillary vessels deficient. The functions of digestion are often well performed, the appetite is good, sometimes excessive. In many cases there is no apparent derangement of the physical system which indicates medical treatment except the insanity itself.

If the health is not good the first object should be to improve it. The condition of all the important organs of the body should be attentively examined before the case is abandoned as hopeless. The appetite, apparently good, may be morbid, the functions of the liver may be disturbed, the bowels may be constipated, the evacuations may be unhealthy or a tendency to diarrhoea may exist. The functions of the skin are often badly performed, the secretion is defi-

cient or unhealthy, and a peculiar fetor attends it. The functions of the uterus are frequently disturbed, and an unnatural irritation in that organ affects the general health and gives character to the symptoms of mental alienation.

The warm and cold bath, laxatives, alteratives, deobstruents, tonics, narcotics, a generous diet and active exercise are often indicated in different forms and stages of chronic mania. If the liver is diseased or inactive, the bile vitiated or deficient, and the bowels torpid, mercurials will be indicated for a time, and tonics and narcotics accompany or follow their use. The Conium with Iron is a useful combination to effect salutary changes in the secretions of the liver, to quiet the irritability and restlessness of the patient, and promote sleep. The doses must be large to produce any perceptible effect. In some cases other preparations of iron combined with narcotics and diffusible stimulants, answer the purpose equally well. Malt liquors, porter, ale, and strong beer are much used in some foreign institutions, and may be prescribed with advantage in many cases. Porter and lime water in equal quantities, form one of the best remedies to invigorate the system, to correct the stomach when dyspeptic, and promote sleep.

In chronic mania there is rarely continued excitement, some periodicity is apparent, and in the intervals neuralgia is frequently troublesome, affecting the face, teeth, and limbs, causing much suffering, and greatly increasing the irritability of the patient. When the excitement comes on, all these symptoms vanish, and a violent mania, equal in severity to a recent attack, continues for some days. In proportion to the length and severity of this excitement will be the corresponding depression and melancholy, and the case will continue in this way for many years. In this form of insanity the mind is less liable to become demented than when either melancholy or mania continues with little or no interruption, and the case is more hopeful of cure than most others found, of chronic mania. Whatever tends to lessen the excitement in one condition, or prevent or remove the melancholy in the other, will diminish the severity of the disease, and aid in accomplishing the cure. Many such cases are but little affected by medicine; some, however, yield favorably to its influence, and finally recover. The diet and regimen that will produce the most perfect bodily health, with tonics, stimulants, and narcotics, have a favorable tendency in this form of mania. In no case is the perseverance in the use of means attended by more encouraging results. In some cases full doses of opium are very effectual in diminishing the violence of the excitement and preventing the severity of the following depression. A continuance of this remedy for a long period has finally resulted in the removal of disease, and a complete restoration of health. Such favorable results cannot be anticipated in a majority of the cases.

The long continued use of Conium and Iron in large doses, occasionally effects favorable changes, and is worth a fair trial, especially if neuralgia intervenes between the paroxysms of excitement. This remedy is not at all calculated for acute mania, certainly not till the active symptoms have subsided, but in chronic mania its use is often indicated. These indications are torpor of the liver, neuralgia, unhealthy secretions of the intestinal and dermoid surfaces, amenorrhoea, dysmenorrhoea, glandular enlargements, general strumous habit, dyspepsia with gastrodynia and an irritable excited state of the nervous system often observable in insanity, producing irascibility, restlessness, indescribable peevishness, discontentment, and variableness of feeling. Sometimes this remedy will relieve the symptoms before its narcotic effect is distinctly perceived, sometimes slight narcosis takes place before relief is procured, but in general its full effect is not felt in relieving the disease for which it is prescribed till narcosis, more or less obvious is produced. These effects are slight vertigo, pain over the eyes, gastric sinking and faintness, and coldness of the extremities. It is safe to give the medicine in gradually increasing doses till these results are produced, and it may be continued with entire safety for months, the doses being occasionally increased to show that the nervous system is under its influence.

Nitrate of Silver in combination with narcotics, is often a valuable remedy in mania where there is an epileptic tendency, or where the actions of the heart are involved in disease. Sulphate of Zinc, Quinine, the arsenical solution, Nux Vomica, Guaiacum, aromatics, and all the list of diffusible stimulants are useful to fulfill certain indications and promote the general health.

If the mind has not become demented, no case of chronic mania should be abandoned till all the appliances, medical and moral, that the case may indicate, have had a fair trial, and even a failure under some circumstances should not discourage further attempts to make impressions upon a disease, the symptoms of which sometimes recur only in obedience to established habits, and not from any organic lesion of the brain.

ACUTE OR RECENT MELANCHOLY

The attack of melancholy is generally less sudden than that of mania; the symptoms come on gradually and progress slowly; the health is more generally and obviously impaired.

In melancholy, one subject, and frequently a single idea, occupies the mind. It may be property, reputation, the present or future well being of the person affected, that engrosses the thoughts and overwhelms the mind with agitation and alarm. With the melancholic there is no present enjoyment, no hope, no confidence, every thing wears a gloomy aspect, every contemplation is sad, and nature, with all its loveliness, is sombre, darkened and cheerless.

In cases of this description the health usually suffers some time before the mind exhibits impairment. The digestive organs are often involved in disease, the biliary secretions are deficient or unhealthy, the bowels are torpid, the evacuations dark, glutinous, and offensive, the appetite is often deficient or morbid, the tongue is furred, though sometimes clean, smooth and often red, the skin is unusually dry, frequently cold, and the capillary action sluggish.

In the treatment of melancholy the first object is to remove the obvious symptoms of disease, and improve the general health. The bowels should be moved by calomel or blue pill, which may be occasionally repeated, care being taken that salivation be avoided, as this effect of mercury is not desirable. After the first impression is made upon the secretions by mercurial remedies, other laxatives may be substituted which will keep the bowels regularly open, and least disturb the stomach or reduce the strength. Drastic purges are rarely if ever indicated, but sometimes active remedies are required to produce moderate effects when the bowels are quite torpid.

It was in this form of insanity that the ancients prescribed hellebore successfully, and considered it little less than specific. This medicine is nauseating and drastic, and finds little favor in modern practice.

The infusion of Senna, pills of Aloes, and Colocynth, extract of Butternut, and especially the Guaiacum in tincture or powder, answer well to obviate costiveness. The Guaiacum possesses other medical qualities besides its power as a laxative. It is a favorable stimulant, improving the appetite, invigorating the muscular fibre of the bowels, promoting the action of the capillary vessels of the skin, and, in amenorrhoea, acting favorably upon the uterus. It may be given in doses much larger than are usually prescribed if necessary to obtain its laxative effects. After it has been used some time costiveness does not frequently follow when it is omitted; it leaves a permanent good effect in habits of costiveness.

Next in value to those remedies that make favorable impressions upon the digestive organs, are those that act upon the skin. Baths, friction, and counter irritation are often useful. When the skin is dry, and the capillary action sluggish, warm and tepid baths followed by friction, are valuable remedies. The invigorating effects of the cold bath and shower bath, followed by friction, are often useful in this form of insanity. This will hardly fail to be true if reaction speedily follows their use. If, however, chilliness, coldness and paleness of the surface follow, and little or no reaction takes place after them, the warm or tepid bath will be found to do better. In many cases, pediluvium answers a better purpose than general bathing, especially if the extremities are inclined to be cold, and the blood is too much determined to the head. Medicated foot-baths are often valuable remedies. For this purpose, mustard, common salt, or the nitro-muriatic acid may be used with benefit.

In many cases of insanity blisters are of doubtful utility, they often produce, rather than allay, irritation, and promote, rather than control excitement, but in some cases of melancholy, especially if there is disease of the digestive organs, and tenderness of the epigastric region, blisters applied over the part are valuable remedies. The tincture of Iodine applied externally, instead of blisters, often answers a valuable purpose and produces less irritation. The antimonial ointment has also the same good effect, but is often more painful than blisters, and sometimes disturbs the stomach with nausea and vomiting.

Tonics and stimulants are valuable remedies in melancholy. Quinine, Iron bitters, aromatics, malt liquors, and other diffusible stimulants, answer a good purpose, in many cases, either alone or in combination with laxatives. The milder narcotics are often useful in allying irritation and promoting sleep. Conium, Hyoscyamus, Camphor, and Lupuline, may be prescribed for this purpose with advantage, but in many cases the preparations of opium are better than all other medicines for this object. Opium does not usually require to be given in such full doses in melancholy as in mania, and night doses do better in the former than in the latter disease.

The combination of Conium and Iron is better adapted to melancholy than mania; its deobstruent effects are often as necessary as its tonic influence, and the combination is a more efficient remedy than either of the articles alone. In neuralgia, attending melancholy, its effects are often very beneficial, also in cases attended by glandular enlargement, indicating scrofula.

The combination of the extract of Hyoscyamus, Camphor and Lupuline often promotes sleep when other remedies fail, but where decided narcotic influence is required the preparations of opium are decidedly the best, and are more to be relied upon than all others. In certain cases of melancholy the patient is made tranquil and comparatively happy by the use of this remedy, the sleep becomes more quiet, and under its influence the person is able to pursue labor and amusement, when without it his suffering and despondency would wholly prevent him from engaging in any employment. Opiates are particularly indicated in suicidal cases by relieving the extreme suffering which impels to that fatal and deplorable act.

Setons, issues and cupping may be beneficial to certain cases of melancholy, especially where there have been eruptions, permanent or repelled, and where habitual ulcers have ceased to discharge. In ordinary cases they avail little in improving the condition of the patient, but, by the irritation which they excite, sometimes do injury.

Riding and other exercise, amusements, labor, whatever diverts the mind or improves the health of the patient, is of importance in the treatment of melancholy. Confidence in the medical adviser, and encouragement constantly held forth to the sufferer, greatly aid the effect of remedies.— Perseverance with medicine often achieves good when a short trial is attended with little or no benefit.

CHRONIC, OR LONG CONTINUED MELANCHOLY

In all cases of insanity which have passed into a chronic stage, where the health is not good and medical treatment has been neglected, a trial of remedies should be made. If the disease is not cured, the condition of the patient may be improved, the health made better, the sufferings diminished, and the enjoyments increased. The symptoms should be examined with care and every circumstance of health be attended to. Costiveness, habitual and obstinate, often attends chronic melancholy, morbid appetite is also common, and the functions of the liver are performed imperfectly, or in an unhealthy manner. The state of the skin is frequently bad, and cleanliness has generally been neglected. To remedy this baths are indispensable. Exercise, a very important means of cure, is usually but little attended to, and the extremities become cold, peculiarly soft and livid. With these evidences of physical derangement the mind dwells intently on one subject, broods over it to the neglect of every other till its sphere of action becomes ex-

tremely limited. Under these circumstances the energies of physical power, no less than those of the mind, become greatly prostrated, general debility and listlessness follow, exertion is painful and difficult, and no ordinary effort of the individual can relieve this condition of apathy and prostration.

All the appliances of art should be held in requisition to arouse the dormant physical and mental energies. Tonics, alteratives, baths, friction, purgatives, external and internal stimulants, generous diet, exercise, and narcotics may, in different cases, or in succession in the same case, be found useful. Occasionally one individual may be cured, many may be made essentially better, while with some all remedies will fail, and the patient, by imperceptible changes, will grow worse, and finally become permanently demented.

CHRONIC AND ACUTE DEMENTIA

Dementia is a term usually applied to a state of disease in which the mind is so weakened as to afford little or no hope of improvement. It commonly follows long continued mania and melancholy, and, in most cases, is probably the result of organic disease of the brain. This disease is of course, rarely cured, and can hardly be said to be a subject for medical treatment, except so far as the general health is impaired. In many such cases the health is bad, and the habits of life are perverted. Both medical and moral treatment may here be beneficial. There is often derangement of the digestive organs, vitiated appetite, constipation of the bowels, and a bad condition of the skin, which may be remedied. Baths, laxatives, tonics, and perseverance in the efforts to correct impaired and irregular habits, will greatly improve the condition of the patient. In such cases the brain is not always irreparably injured; great debility, and extreme inaction produce the phenomena instead of organic lesion.

ACUTE DEMENTIA

There is a form of dementia of recent accession in which the symptoms assume the character of this disease quite early after the attack, which is hopeful, and in which medical treatment is very successful. The appearance of the patient does not differ essentially from the protracted and chronic form. The physiognomy of the case may not be quite so bad, but the indications of loss of mind are nearly as distinct. The length of time which the symptoms have existed being less, the encouragement for the trial of remedies is greater, and the success of them is often exceedingly favorable. The treatment is various, according to the symptoms of the case. Alterative and laxative remedies, baths, tonics, aromatics, stimulants, blisters and irritants are indicated in different forms and stages of the disease. Exercise, active and passive, friction and every means of arousing the mind from its torpor and invigorating the system, will be found useful auxiliaries in the treatment of this form of insanity.

PERIODICAL INSANITY

No form of insanity is more troublesome to manage, or difficult to cure, than this, especially if it assumes at periods the two extremes of violent mania, and deep melancholy.

Such cases have, at each occasion, all the symptoms of recent mania, and at their period of depression the discouragement, wretchedness, and suicidal tendency of the most marked recent melancholy. These transitions take place at different period, sometimes annually, semi-annually, and at shorter intervals. The violence of one form of the disease may generally be predicted by the severity of the other. The condition of the mind in the transition state differs considerably, and this is longer or shorter in different cases. In some cases the mind seems to be nearly rational for a long period; in others, the delusions remain though the excitement subsides, and the extremes of the case are at long intervals. Sometimes the transition is very sudden, and the patient is most of the time greatly excited or much depressed. Some cases recover after years of suffering, in others the paroxysms diminish in frequency and intensity, and the patient is greatly improved if not entirely cured.

The treatment of this form of insanity may be conducted upon the principles before mentioned as applicable to the acute forms of mania and melancholy, with the use of such remedies in the interval as will tend to break up the periodicity of the disease. If, by the use of remedies, the excitement can be lessened, the corresponding depression will probably be less; so if extreme melancholy can be prevented the succeeding excitement will be less severe.

In such cases it is of the greatest importance that all the causes which have a tendency to bring on a renewed attack of disease be cautiously avoided. The health should be preserved as perfect as possible, all excitement should be shunned, especially that intensity of application of mind or body that tends to disturb the nervous system and bring it within the range of disease. By these means confirmed habits of periodicity may, doubtless, be avoided, in many cases, and the recovery may be perfect. If the business or occupation of a person affected with insanity is suspected to act as a cause of disease, it should be abandoned, and such others chosen as will have no such tendency, but rather a counteracting influence. The sedentary should become active, the irregular should become systematic, and those who are fond of excitements should avoid them. In this manner many may escape a return of disease and periodicity be avoided. There are many discouragements in these cases but hope may be entertained while the mind retains its vigor and the physical energies continue. The best efforts will, however, sometimes prove abortive, and though remedies may be used, the disease will remain unchanged, and a long life be spent in the extremes of this form of insanity.

When the maniacal excitement subsides in periodical insanity, neuralgia of the limbs, joints, teeth or face, often follows, and severe bodily suffering attends the gloom and wretchedness of the mental depression. In this form of disease the health is not usually good; this is more manifest in the period of depression. The remedies usually prescribed in neuralgia succeed in relieving the suffering of the patient, and improve the health. Of these the preparations of opium, bark, Nux Vomica, Conium and Iron, the arsenical solution, and Veratrine, are the most effectual.

PUERPERAL INSANITY

Insanity occurring in the puerperal state is a dangerous complication, and requires some modification of the treatment usually pursued. The symptoms are generally severe, the mania furious, and the indications of physical disease considerable. The hot skin, frequent pulse, wild delirium, and coated tongue resemble inflammation so strongly that there is danger of mistaking the case, and adopting a course of treatment which these deceptive symptoms seem to indicate. General bleeding is rarely useful, but leeching may often afford present relief and prepare the system for other remedies. Cold applications to the head give much relief, and local warm bathing to the feet, at the same time, or a general warm bath may be frequently beneficial. Calomel alone or in combination with Dover's powder may then be given till it moves the bowels freely, and be repeated in small doses till the secretions are favorably affected, the skin becomes soft, and the tongue moist. If the insanity continues, the preparations of morphia may then be given in such doses as the patient will bear, cautiously watching its effects. If they are favorable, the symptoms usually subside rapidly, the case terminates favorably, and the recovery is soon complete. Tonics and stimulants often aid in the speedy restoration of health.

INSANITY COMPLICATED WITH PALSY

The complication of insanity with palsy is usually unfavorable, and is rarely entirely removed. With partial palsy the mind is subject to certain impairment which is relieved and occasionally is nearly restored. But even in the most favorable cases, a peculiar imbecility follows, attended by a propensity to shed tears from the slightest cause, especially if there is any allusion made to the condition of the individual.

General palsy complicated with insanity is always fatal. Remedies may be prescribed with some advantage to relieve particular symptoms and improve the general health, but the benefit is temporary: fatal symptoms, in the form of epilepsy or apoplexy, occur when least expected, and, if not at the first attack, it will, at some subsequent period, assuredly result fatally.

When apoplexy or repeated epileptic paroxysms occur under such circumstances, and the patient lies insensible for hours or days, a full dose of calomel, repeated every six or eight hours, will, when it operates, relieve the symptoms and restore the patient to his former condition. Stimulant injections are often beneficial in such cases, sinapisms and blisters may also do good.

In the treatment of apoplexy following general palsy, bleeding is injurious, and in the condition of general palsy opiates have almost always an unfavorable effect. Acrid stimulants are often beneficial, such as tincture of Lytta, Ammonia, Veratrine, Nux Vomica, and wine and malt liquors, with generous diet.

The brain of intemperate persons is in much the same condition as that of those affected with general palsy, and when they become insane, bleeding is always injurious, and opiates are frequently unfavorable in their effects. In some cases of delirium tremens opiates do well.

The relaxation of the sphincter of the bladder attending general palsy, which makes the condition of the patient uncomfortable, is often entirely relieved by the use of the Nux Vomica. This remedy is also useful in may cases of palsy to relieve the attendant neuralgic pain and restore the muscular system.

INSANITY COMPLICATED WITH EPILEPSY

This form of insanity is most difficult to manage and hardly admits the hope of cure. In many cases, the patient is so impulsive, and the fits of violence so sudden and dangerous, that he cannot be trusted to associate with others unless constantly under the eye of an attendant, or in some kind of restraint. Forlorn as is this form of insanity, it can be favorably influenced in a majority of cases, by medical treatment, not to the extent of effecting a cure, but to lessen the violence of the case, and diminish the number and severity of the paroxysms. In some cases, the insanity seems to be much relieved or cured when the epilepsy continues.

The use of the nitrate of silver, in this complication of insanity, often produces obvious effects. The doses should be liberal, and the medicine continued for some time. The extract of Stramonium, in such doses as slightly to impair the vision, is also a valuable remedy. The combination of these two articles is usually more effectual in epilepsy than either, alone. In a large proportion of cases a liberal use of them will be attended by obvious and favorable results, though they rarely cure the disease when complicated with insanity.

The next most favorable remedy in the treatment of epilepsy alone or complicated with insanity, is the arsenical solution of Fowler. This must also be given so as to produce its specific effects or little benefit is derived from its use. It is more effectual in controlling the paroxysms when combined with morphia in moderate quantities, and its unpleasant effects are thus obviated. It is a valuable remedy and may be continued for a long time as its effects are never accumulative.

In cases of epilepsy with constipation of the bowels, the Croton Oil alone, or in combination with other remedies has proved useful. Costiveness should be avoided in epilepsy, especially when it is combined with insanity. It should be cautiously obviated in all cases of insanity, but undesirable as it is in this class of diseases, a diarrhoea is much more to be dreaded. The Croton Oil can be managed so as to act as a drastic purge or a mild and safe laxative. In this respect it differs from most active cathartics.

Nux Vomica is often prescribed with benefit in epilepsy. In some cases it is useful in combination with nitrate of silver and stramonium.

INSANITY COMPLICATED WITH DYSPEPSIA

Dyspepsia is frequently found to be the cause of insanity, and is often complicated with it when not strictly the cause. Obstinate costiveness attends in many cases, and such a total loss of appetite and loathing of food that the patient will often suffer from starvation if not urged and persuaded to take nourishment. Patients frequently vomit their food and have great derangement of the secretions of the stomach, flatulency, acidity, and morbid bile. Diarrhoea with red and dry tongue is worse than costiveness, and is an unfavorable complication of disease. Costiveness is easily obviated and produces less ill effect than would be supposed, but diarrhoea is often difficult to control, and when it has been suppressed it will recur again from the slightest cause.

Tonics, laxatives, baths, gentle exercise, friction, and a proper regulation of diet constitute the treatment of insanity with the combination of symptoms. Astringents, aromatics, and moderate opiates are indicated when diarrhoea is present. If acidity is troublesome, attended with loss of appetite, one of the best remedies is a combination of lime water with porter or strong beer. If with costiveness there is distress from food, the aromatic tincture of Guaiacum is little less than a specific, when given in doses sufficiently large to prove laxative. In recent cases of dysentery and diarrhoea, emetics of Ipecac and sulphate of zinc often prove useful, followed by opiates, nitrate of silver, Capsicum and other aromatics. In chronic cases, in addition to these remedies the tincture of Zanthorrhiza is found very useful given in brandy and water or milk. Severe dyspepsia complicated with insanity often results in fatal marasmus, of which diarrhoea is usually one of the most troublesome symptoms. This disease is probably the most frequent fatal termination of insanity.

PULMONARY CONSUMPTION

This is the second on the list of fatal diseases with the insane, showing that the character of disease of the brain is often scrofulous in its origin. In some cases disease of the lungs and of the brain alternate. When the excitement is great, the cough and expectoration abate or cease; when the excitement subsides the cough returns and the expectoration is abundant. The occurrence of insanity occasionally suspends the symptoms of pulmonary disease, but they recur and prove fatal when the insanity is cured.

A rapid consumption is frequently the fatal event of insanity. The form of dyspeptic Phthisis is also frequent with the insane. This disease requires no peculiarity of treatment.

Erysipelas is a troublesome disease with the insane, and often assumes a dangerous and fatal form. Erysipelas of the extremities is much more to be dreaded than that of the face. When it is suppurative it is rapid and requires very prompt treatment.

The application of strong tincture of Iodine to the inflamed surface and beyond the margin, on the very commencement of the disease, is an exceedingly successful remedy. Should the disease pass the line made by the application of the Iodine, it may be extended farther, till it shall arrest the progress of the inflammation and convert a disease which might have been dangerous and fatal, into a comparatively mild and harmless affection. A circle made beyond the boundary of disease, by the nitrate of silver or of the Lytta, often answers the same valuable purpose. Another useful practice is, to puncture the inflamed limb repeatedly with numerous incisions, thus allowing the infiltrated pus to escape, and removing the distention which greatly aggravates the suffering of the patient. The constitutional remedies in this form of disease are, first, alteratives and laxatives, followed by tonics, stimulants, narcotics, and good liquid nourishment.

Disease of the heart, of the uterus, and neuralgia, often attend insanity but require no peculiar treatment.

Amenorrhoea is frequently considered a cause of insanity, and its removal is looked to as a sure indication of cure. In this there is often disappointment. Whatever indicates returning health is favorable in insanity. When the health improves, in recent cases, before there is any particular change in the state of the mind, the indication is favorable. So far the return of the menses gives encouragement. They are restored in many cases, however, without any very obvious change in the symptoms. The menstrual period is often attended by increased excitement, and this is quite as likely to follow, as to precede or accompany discharge. In such cases the suspension of the menses is attended by favorable results till the general health is improved and the irritable state of the uterus, and general nervous system is allayed or removed. In cases where the periods of excitement are connected with the menstrual visitation the occurrence of pregnancy and the final cessation of the menses has been attended by favorable results, even by a radical cure.

Mercurial and aloetic purges, tincture of Guaiacum, the various preparations of Iron with or without Conium, are to be relied upon in amenorrhoea, but they effect a cure by improving the general health rather than by any specific effect upon the uterus itself.

It has been remarked that the insane are peculiarly liable to neuralgia, especially when the disease is paroxysmal.

It is most successfully treated by narcotics and tonics. Morphia, Conium, Nux Vomica, Belladonna, arsenical solution, Quinine, Iron, Zinc, and Nitrate of Silver, are all valuable remedies, and should be if necessary, administered freely. Belladonna, Veratrine, and cold water, applied externally, often relieve the pain remarkably.

There are cases of insanity in which there is at first high excitement, but in a few days there is an alarming collapse with symptoms of great exhaustion and debility. The head and chest are usually hot, while the extremities are cold, purple, and covered with perspiration. The action of the heart is feeble, often irregular. The pulse is exceedingly weak, and, in fatal cases, ceases at the wrist long before the brain dies. These cases indicate danger from the first, and must be treated promptly or fatal symptoms will occur unexpectedly. The bowels should be gently moved by calomel, and small doses of this remedy may be continued for a few days. Cold should be applied to the head, and blisters, sinapisms and rubefacients to the extremities and the chest. Great care should be taken not to exhaust the strength, and the vital powers should be sustained by a free use of volatile and diffusible stimulants, and good liquid nourishment. If opium is given, it should be in small doses combined with calomel, and at short intervals. Large doses fail to quiet the excitement, and in some cases seem to coincide with other influences to increase the delirium and irritation of the brain.

The views of experienced men at the present day, as to the treatment of insanity, differ greatly from those that were usually promulgated at the commencement of the present century. If there is a difference in opinion as to the necessity of medical treatment in various cases of insanity, there is great unanimity of sentiment in this country and in Great Britain, as to the indications of cure and the kind of remedies most to be relied upon when they are to be used.

The abandonment of depletion, external irritants, drastic purges and starvation, and the substitution of baths, narcotics, tonics, and generous diet, is not less to be appreciated in the improved condition of the insane, than the change from manacles, chains, by-locks and confining chairs, to the present system of kindness, confidence, social intercourse, labor, religious teaching, and freedom from restraint. In this age of improvement, no class of mankind have felt its influence more favorably than the insane. But we should not be satisfied with present attainments. Much undoubtedly remains to be done for them. Good influences are everywhere operating, and we may confidently hope that what is overlooked by the passing generation, which might have been beneficial to them, will be supplied by their successors.

THE HISTORY OF THE MALARIA TREATMENT
OF GENERAL PARALYSIS

By Julius Wagner-Jauregg, M.D.
Late Professor of Psychiatry and Neurology of the University of Vienna

COMMENT AND TRANSLATION FROM THE GERMAN
Walter L. Bruetsch, M.D.

I n an editorial of the *Journal of the American Medical Association* of April 8, 1944, it is stated that priority for the use of malaria and relapsing fever in the treatment of general paralysis (dementia paralytica) should belong to Rosenblum. This editorial statement is based on the publication by Zakon and Neymann, entitled "Alexander Samoilovich Rosenblum, His Contribution to Fever Therapy" (*Arch. Dermat. & Syph.*, 48:52, 1943).

Enthusiasm over the beneficial effect of fever in psychoses was common among psychiatrists of the middle of the last century. Several papers on this subject, some of which were quoted by Neymann and Zakon, had appeared a decade before the communication of A. S. Rosenblum was published in 1877. It is true that Rosenblum inoculated a group of mental patients with relapsing fever, but he did not continue this mode of treatment and there was no fever therapy, as we know it today, until Wagner-Jauregg on August 31, 1918, published the results of the studies on the first patients with dementia paralytica, who had been treated a year previously with inoculation malaria.

The merit of Wagner-Jauregg was that he soon realized that the beneficial effect of fever was restricted to cases of dementia paralytica. For over 20 years he then focused all his efforts on this type of mental illness, using tuberculin, typhoid vaccines and even streptococci of erysipelas to produce fever.

Wagner-Jauregg was well aware of the work of Rosenblum. I have in my possession a manuscript by Wagner-Jauregg, entitled, "The History of the Malaria Treatment of General Paralysis," which was written by him for a monograph dealing with the malaria therapy of neurosyphilis. The publication of the monograph has been postponed several times because of other important work. Later the war intervened. It is now doubtful whether the monograph will appear at all.

Dr. Bruetsch is Clinical Professor of Psychiatry and Neurology, Indiana University School of Medicine; Clinical Director and Head of the Research Department, Central State Hospital, Indianapolis, Ind.

Wagner-Jauregg died October 1, 1940. In 1927 he was awarded the Nobel Prize for his work in the use of malaria fever in the treatment of dementia paralytica. He was the first and so far the only psychiatrist to have been the winner of this prize.

"The History of the Malaria Treatment of General Paralysis," written by him in August 1935, is a valuable document. For the benefit of future medical historians, Wagner-Jauregg's version in this matter is published.

THE HISTORY OF THE MALARIA TREATMENT
OF GENERAL PARALYSIS

Julius Wagner-Jauregg, M.D.

It is a great pleasure to contribute to this monograph the chapter on the History of Malaria Therapy. I can add a few interesting details and also will take this opportunity to correct erroneous statements which have been made on this subject.

The origin of the malaria treatment of general paralysis of the insane goes back to the centuries-old observation that mental patients following an incidental febrile disease occasionally show great improvement, which may go on to complete recovery. After having made similar observations, I proposed in 1887 in a publication (1) to produce intentionally febrile diseases as a treatment method for psychiatric patients. I had in mind malaria and erysipelas. Either one of these conditions could be transmitted to other individuals without great danger. Already at that time I did not share the prevalent idea that elevated temperature is the main factor which is responsible for the favorable results of this mode of therapy. I said: "Some authors are inclined to attribute to the fever, *i.e.*, to the increase in body temperature a particular effect upon the mental condition. This theory may possibly be correct in those cases in which an improvement of the mental symptoms takes place during the fever. But this view is certainly not justified in those instances in which the improvement of the mental symptoms sets in after the febrile disease is terminated, for instance, in typhoid fever during the period of reconvalescence or in erysipelas in the stage of desquamation. And it is in this group that the greatest number of permanent recoveries occur. Furthermore, in not a few instances the mental symptoms become worse during the period of fever."

Being anxious to have my proposals put into practice, I infected several mental patients—among these were no general paralytics—with a culture of the streptococcus of erysipelas, which had proven to be very virulent in a patient with an inoperable carcinoma of the breast. But in my patients neither erysipelas nor fever developed. There was only slight redness at the site of inoculation, which disappeared after a few days.

The experiments were discontinued because, in the meantime, I had been appointed professor of psychiatry at the University of Graz (Austria). Furthermore, medical science of that period looked with disfavor at experimentation on human beings. This spirit showed itself openly in the hostile attitude of the public and of the authorities when Hirschl (2) inoculated 9 general paralytic patients with syphilis. Today this would be a matter of course, but at that time the teaching of Fournier of the syphilitic etiology of general paralysis had not been generally accepted. Hirschl almost went to prison for his zealous scientific endeavors.

With the development of tuberculin in 1890 by Robert Koch, a substance was at hand with which one could produce fever without resorting to an infectious disease. I began treating patients of the Psychiatric Clinic at Graz (Austria) with injections of tuberculin. These experiments also had to be stopped prematurely because tuberculin was soon considered a dangerous preparation. For several years tuberculin was banned from good medical practice. It had almost become a crime to use it. At this time I was called to Vienna as the head of the University Hospital for Nervous and Mental Diseases. The vehement dispute over the use of tuberculin was calming down and its value was slowly recognized. In 1894 I resumed the experimental work with tuberculin fever, and a year later reported my experiences (3). I reiterated in this paper my previous statement that elevated temperature is not the fundamental factor of the treatment.

The experiments with tuberculin, using all types of mental patients, were continued. Many therapeutic successes were observed in patients who fell in diagnostic groups which have a high percentage of spontaneous recoveries. It was therefore difficult to evaluate the exact effect of this treatment method. Among the apparently cured patients, however, were a few cases of general paralysis. This was something unusual and attracted my attention. From this time on the main interest was focused on general paralytic patients. First, a comparative study was carried out to determine whether tuberculin really influenced the course of general paralysis in a favorable way. Sixty-nine general paralytics were given bouts of fever by injecting increasing doses of tuberculin until a dose of 0.1 was reached. They were compared with 69 patients who remained untreated.

The same experiment was repeated with a group of 60 general paralytics, receiving tuberculin injections until the amount of 0.3 was given (4). Four years later the tuberculin-treated patients were compared with those who were left untreated. The result was that the general paralytics who were given tuberculin fever had more and better remissions and also a longer duration of life (5). In the meantime I had begun treating with tuberculin general paralytic patients of my private practice, using doses up to 0.3 and later up to 1.00. These cases were, as a rule, not as far advanced as the hospital patients. At the same time I combined the tuberculin injections with mercurial inunctions, because I never could convince myself that specific anti-syphilitic treatment of general paralysis was without any value whatsoever, a view held by most psychiatrists of that period. With this combined tuberculin-mercury treatment, a complete remission was obtained in quite a few instances with the return of the patients to their former occupation. A report of this work was made in 1909 at the International Medical Congress in Budapest (6).

The tuberculin-mercury therapy of general paralysis, however, was never widely used. The medical scientists of that period were hypnotized by the discovery of the syphilitic etiology of general paralysis and could see the solution of this special problem only in a specific treatment. And yet in 1909 and later the tuberculin-mercury treatment gave better results than any other form of therapy. Today several cases of general paralysis are still alive which were successfully treated with tuberculin and mercury in the second decade of 1900. The number of full remissions in early cases was by no means small. But the relapses were frequent, and only a small number of the complete remissions remained permanent. To make the treatment more effective, I searched for other means. I tried various vaccines, and finally used typhoid vaccines which, when injected intravenously, produced marked febrile reactions. In addition, I replaced mercury by the recently introduced salvarsan. In 1913 I still hoped to work out a satisfactory treatment method without having to resort to the use of inoculation with malaria. In the same year I received a letter from Dr. E. van Dieren of Amsterdam asking me what I thought of the idea of inoculating with malaria general paralytic patients. As a family doctor he had recommended this procedure on several occasions, but the specialists had advised against it. I wrote him to make such experiments which, in my opinion, should be very promising. I added that I might try it myself, if my hopes of treating general paralysis more successfully with typhoid vaccines and salvarsan should not materialize. Dr. van Dieren to my knowledge never inoculated patients with malaria.

The psychologic moment which induced me to try malaria inoculation was prompted by the following incident. A prominent oil-well engineer was admitted to the Psychiatric Hospital with symptoms of incipient general paralysis. He was given treatment consisting of a combined course of typhoid vaccines and arsphenamines. He recovered to such a degree that he was able to return to the province of Galicia, where he was supervising the drilling of oil-wells. However, several months later he was back in Vienna with all the manifestations of general paralysis. I realized that with the methods of treatment at hand little could be accomplished and that the disease would now rapidly progress to the inevitable fatal outcome. (This was the same engineer whom de Kruif (7) had mentioned in his book.) It was the tragic outlook for this man which again forced on my mind the thought of producing intentionally an infectious disease in general paralytic patients. In addition, other evidence had accumulated that the original idea might well be justified, to produce artificially an infectious disease in these patients. During my work with tuberculin fever I had noted that those patients who by incident developed an abscess, a phlegmonous cellulitis, lobar pneumonia, or a tuberculous infection had frequently the best and most prolonged remissions.

At about the same time, in June 1917, when the hospital was full of wounded military personnel, my assistant Dr. Alfred Fuchs reported to me one morning that a slightly injured soldier had been admitted with chills and fever, apparently having contracted malaria fever on the Balkan front line. "Should he be given quinine?" he asked. I immediately said: "No." This I regarded as a sign of destiny. Because soldiers with malaria were usually not admitted to my wards, which accepted only cases suffering from a psychosis or patients with injuries to the central nervous system. I gave the order to make a blood smear and to examine for malarial parasites. At the same time I asked a shell-shocked soldier, who was very useful for doing odd jobs, to catch all the mosquitoes he could find on the hospital grounds. He returned with a great number of them, and I convinced myself that all the mosquitoes belonged to the species of culex. There were no anopheles in this random sample.

The examination of the blood smear of the soldier with chills and fever had revealed the presence of malarial parasites of the tertian type. It was June 14, 1917. On that day I obtained during a paroxysm a small sample of the soldier's blood, and I inoculated 3 general paralytic patients by rubbing a few drops into several superficial scarifications of the skin. Then the malaria of the soldier was stopped with quinine.

Of the 3 inoculated patients only 2 developed malaria. Additional cases were inoculated subcutaneously with blood obtained from the veins of the originally inoculated general paralytic patients, who by this time were ill with malaria fever. Altogether 9 general paralytics were inoculated in the summer of 1917. Then the inoculations were discontinued because I wanted to see whether this experiment would prove to be a real therapeutic success.

A year later malaria therapy was resumed. This time malaria blood for inoculation was obtained through the courtesy of the physician-in-chief of the ward for malaria patients, who were mostly soldiers from the Balkan armies. Of 4 inoculated patients 3 succumbed to malaria. Soon after inoculation it became apparent that estivo-autumnal parasites (malaria tropica) had been hidden in the strain of tertian malaria and had been used for the inoculations. After this misfortune no new cases were inoculated until September 1919, when Dr. Doerr (now professor of public health and hygiene at the University of Basel, Switzerland) furnished the clinic with an unquestionable strain of tertian malaria. From that time on malaria therapy has been prac-

ticed uninterruptedly at the Psychiatric Clinic of Vienna. The malaria strain of September 1919 has been maintained up to the present day—more than 16 years—in continuous human passage. I do not know of any other strain in the world which has been used for so many years. Not even the strain of the New York Psychiatric Institute, which has been maintained for 9 years, from 1923 to 1932, at the time of the report by Kopeloff, Blackman and McGinn (8), can compete with the record of the Vienna strain.

I have been asked how my inner feelings were during the first days and weeks which followed the first inoculations with malaria. My emotional life at that time and already during the era of the tuberculin experiments has been described by de Kruif somewhat more turbulent than it actually was. The unusual experiment of human malaria inoculations moved me very little. From the previous work I was accustomed to seeing remissions following fever treatment, and the measure of success which might be obtained by the malaria experiment could not be anticipated. Furthermore, we were already in the third year of the war, and its emotional implications became more manifest from day to day. Against such a background a therapeutic experiment could stir me little, in particular since its success could not be foreseen. What meant a few paralytics, who could possibly be saved, in comparison to the thousands of able-bodied and capable men who often died on a single day as the result of the prolongation of the war.

How sceptical I was toward the early successes with the malaria treatment is shown by the fact that I waited a year until the publication of the first report. Very likely I would have hesitated even longer, if the editor of the *Psychiatrisch-Neurologische Wochenschrift*, in which my preliminary communication appeared (9), had not urged me to make a contribution for the *Festschrift* in honor of my friend Dr. Anton, professor of psychiatry at the University of Halle (Germany).

I must add here that already in 1917 malaria therapy was followed up with arsphenamine injections in the same way as salvarsan had previously been given as an adjunct to the tuberculin treatment. It was difficult to convince even the co-workers of my own clinic of the soundness of the combined treatment, and I had to defend vehemently this principle in scientific discussions, until it was generally recognized. Today barely anyone doubts the correctness of this procedure.

Now one may ask the question: Were the inoculations of the summer of 1917 the first attempts of this sort ever made? Sometime after the malaria treatment had spread from Vienna to every corner of the world, I became aware that French physician, Dr. Émil Legrain, several years previously had advocated in a publication the use of therapeutic malaria inoculations. On my desk lies a book by this author, consisting of 612 pages. It was published in 1913 by Maloine in Paris and is entitled: "Traité clinique des fièvres des pay chauds." In the last 12 pages of the book, which deals mainly with the intermittent fevers, the author states that malaria frequently has a good effect upon other diseases. He asserts that it is but a step from this knowledge to the actual use of malaria as a therapeutic means, and he claims to have taken that step. He reported on 13 cases which he had inoculated with malaria followed by beneficial results. Among these were no cases of general paralysis. The group consisted of 2 patients with malignant syphilis, 1 case with luetic ulcers, 4 patients with pulmonary tuberculosis, 1 with an abscess of the testicles, a case with a slow healing wound, an obstinate general eczema, an arthropathy of the knee, and 2 cases with syphilis of the liver. He also recommended inoculation with quartan malaria in the following instances: inoperable carcinoma, tuberculosis of the larynx, tuberculous meningitis, sleeping sickness, epilepsy, certain forms of melancholia, incipient general paralysis and tabes.

It is astounding that such proposals, although no one had taken them up, were forgotten so completely that they entirely should have been lost sight of by contemporaries, when the malaria therapy of general paralysis became known. Even in France, where Pagniez in 1920 without much response directed attention to the malaria treatment and whose article in *La Presse Médicale* of May 30, 1925, finally was responsible for its introduction in Paris, the name of Legrain was not mentioned in spite of a rapidly increasing literature on malaria therapy. (Malaria treatment found its way to Paris via Brussels.) In 1931, I became acquainted, for the first time, with my predecessor Legrain from the introduction to the book by Leroy and Médakovitch (10).

Now I acquired Legrain's book and after having read it, I realized why he had been so completely forgotten. Legrain was evidently an individual given to vagaries, who in 1913 still held concepts on malaria which were utterly antiquated. He ridiculed Laveran with his plasmodia and Donald Ross with his mosquitoes and scorned the use of quinine. Legrain was not taken seriously, there was no one who believed in his successes, and soon he faded from the memory of his colleagues.

It is not in accordance with facts, when Riser (11) makes the statement that since 1910 Legrain had systematically inoculated general paralytic patients with malaria. Legrain has never infected general paralytics with malaria, nor has he treated in a systematic way with inoculation malaria other diseases.

In the literature Rosenblum is usually credited with being the first who inoculated general paralytics for therapeutic purposes, using recurrent fever and not malaria. The facts,

however, are that Rosenblum has never inoculated his patients with the idea of treating their mental illness. What he did was to make available his mental patients—among whom were no general paralytics—to the bacteriologist Motschutkoffsky, who in Odessa in the year of 1876 studied the transmissibility of recurrent fever to human beings. Subsequently, a few of these patients recovered from their psychoses and Rosenblum reported this later under an assumed name (12). Rosenblum never continued these experiments.

The suggestion to treat mental cases with malaria was really made by Raggi (13) in 1876, but he never put this idea into practice. Indirect malaria therapy was carried out by Galloni, director of an Italian mental institution, who withheld quinine in psychotic patients who incidentally had contracted malaria because he had observed that such mental patients frequently recovered from their psychoses.

BIBLIOGRAPHY

1. Wagner, J. Ueber die Einwirkung fieberhafter Erkrankungen auf Psychosen. Jahrb. f. Psychiat. u. Neurol., 7:94, 1887.
2. Quoted by Krafft-Ebing, von, R. Arbeiten aus dem Gesamtgebiet der Psychiatrie und Neuropathologie, II. Heft, Leipzig, J. A. Barth, 1897, pp. 12-14. Hirschl is the anonymous person in this paper by Krafft-Ebing.
3. Wagner v. Jauregg. Psychiatrische Heilbestrebungen. Wien. klin. Wchnschr., 8:155, 1895.
4. Pilcz A. Ueber Heilversuche an Paralytikern. Jahrb. f. Psychiat. u. Neurol., 25:141, 1905.
5. Pilcz, A. Zur Tuberkulinbehandlung der Paralytiker. Psychiat.-neurol. Wchnschr., 11:431, 1910.
6. Wagner v. Jauregg. Ueber die Behandlung der progressiven Paralyse. Wien. med. Wchnschr., 59:2124, 1909.
7. de Kruif, P. Men against death. 9. Wagner-Jauregg, The friendly fever. New York: Harcourt, Brace and Company, 1932, p. 249.
8. Kopeloff, N., Blackman, N., and McGinn, B. "Asexualization" of the plasmodium in induced malaria. Am. J. M. Sc., 184:262, 1932.
9. Wagner v. Jauregg. Ueber die Einwirkung der Malaria auf die progressive Paralyse. Psychiat.-neurol. Wchnschr., 20:132 and 251, 1918/19.
10. Leroy, R., and Médakovitch, G. Paralysie générale et malariathérapie. Paris: G. Doin & Cie., 1931.
11. Riser. La prophylaxie de la syphilis nerveuse et l'organisation d'un centre régional de malaria-thérapie. Prophylax antiven., 3:507, 1931.
12. Oks, B. Ueber die Wirkung fieberhafter Krankheiten auf Heilung von Psychosen. Arch. f. Psychiat., 10:249, 1880.
13. Raggi, A. Il processo febbrile nei pazzi. Riv. clin. di Bologna, 6:163, 1876.

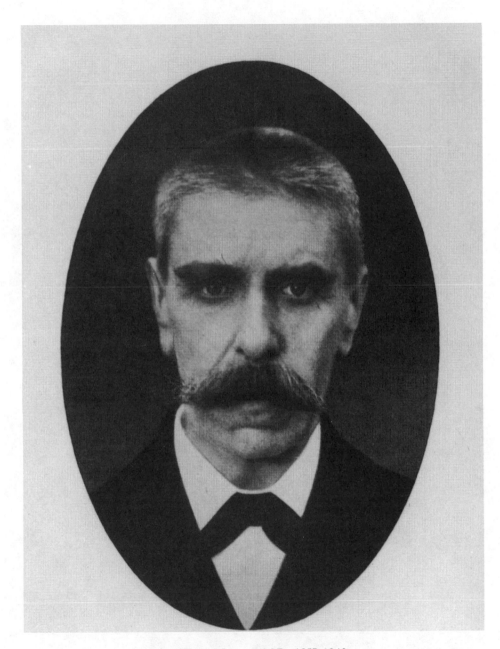

Julius Wagner-Jauregg, M.D., 1857–1940

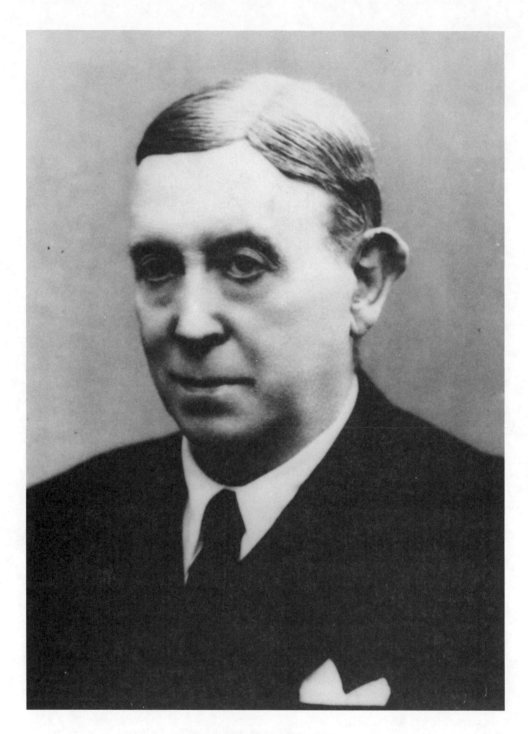

Dr. Egas Moniz, 1874–1955

Prefrontal Leucotomy in the Treatment of Mental Disorders

By Egas Moniz

Professor of Neurology, University of Lisbon, Portugal.

A year has elapsed since I inaugurated a surgical procedure in the treatment of certain psychoses. Guided by certain physiologic and clinical data, I suggested that by interrupting some of the connections between the prefrontal lobes and other parts of the brain, some modifications might be brought about in the mental processes of psychotic individuals. The first results were encouraging and I published them in a monograph.[1] Subsequent observations, moreover, showed that we were following a procedure that was of benefit to mental patients.

The idea was to operate upon the brains of the patients, not directly upon the cell groups of the cortex or of other regions, but rather by interrupting the connecting fibers between cells of the prefrontal area and other regions, that is to say by sectioning the subcortical white matter. As a result of the interruption of the cylinder axes the cells of the prefrontal area and of other regions of the brain connected with these would be affected secondarily.

The hypotheses underlying the procedure might be called in question; the surgical intervention might be considered very audacious; but such arguments occupy a secondary position because it can be affirmed now that these operations are not prejudicial to either physical or psychic life of the patient, and also that recovery or improvement may be obtained frequently in this way.

Certain symptoms have been observed following the intervention in the prefrontal area, both on the neurological and on the mental side, and these have been discussed both in my book and before the Neurological Society of Paris. However, these disturbances are transitory and none of these symptoms has persisted beyond a few days or weeks. Two or three of the patients in my first series have remained somewhat apathetic but even in these cases there is some doubt as to the effect of the operation, because the personality of the patient was not very well known before the operation.

The procedure as first developed consisted in the injection of alcohol into the subcortical white matter of the prefrontal area but subsequently sections were made in the subcortical white matter by a leucotome with a steel loop, tending to crush the white matter a little in this area. At the present time we are using a leucotome with a steel band that cuts rather than compresses, and this has given great satisfaction.[2]

The present technique is also slightly different from that of the early operations. The trephine openings are made a little farther posteriorly, that is about 1 to 1.5 cm. in front of a vertical line passing through the base of the tragus, and 3 cm. to either side of the midsagittal line. The leucotome is introduced to a depth of 4.5 cm. in an anterolateral direction, the loop is opened and the instrument turned so as to cut a core about 1 cm. in diameter in the white matter. The blade is retracted into the instrument which is withdrawn one centimeter and a second core is cut at 3.5 cm., and finally a third at 2.5 cm. from the surface of the brain. No tissue is removed. The leucotome is then withdrawn entirely and re-introduced in an anteromesial direction to a depth of 4 cm. where the first section is made, withdrawn 1 cm. in order to cut a second core at 3 cm., and a final section is made at a distance of 2 cm. from the surface of the brain.

The cores are cut at two different depths in the anterolateral and anteromesial direction for two reasons. In the first place the angle in the lateral direction is wider and the white matter lies farther below the surface; and in the second place, in separating the distances between the cores there is less probability that a single cavity will be formed at least as far as the two superficial sections are concerned. There would be no likelihood of this occurring in the deep sections, but if these two cores came together in the superficial region, the fasciculus from the paracentral lobule to the medial and posterior portions of the prefrontal lobe might be injured. The destruction of this fasciculus brings about certain vesical disturbances that may sometimes be quite severe even though they are only transitory.

In this article I do not wish to emphasize the technical details described in the monograph, but I do wish to pay tribute to the splendid cooperation of the neurosurgeon, Dr. Almeida Lima. Furthermore I wish to draw attention to the modifications that have brought us better results. In this new technique I have seen only minor and temporary disturbances referable to injury of the frontal lobes, the sphincter disorders have been avoided, and except for certain ocular signs (sluggish pupils, anisocoria) that last only a few days, all the other symptoms that I previously de-

---

1 Tentatives Operatoires dans le Traitement de Certaines Psychoses, Paris, 1936, Masson et Cie.
2 The leucotome is made by Gentile et Cie. of Paris.

scribed are rarely observed. The explanation probably lies in the use of the cutting leucotome.

I am now attacking the prefrontal lobes more extensively, making six cores on each side. Not only have the complications been fewer, but the clinical results have been better.

Eighteen patients were subjected to operation in the second series of cases (I previously reported 20 cases). The patients have been drawn from the mental hospital directed by Prof. Sobral Cid and from the clinic of Dr. Diego Furtado at Telhal. We can already draw one conclusion both from the first attempt and from the later operations. Deteriorated patients obtain slight or no benefit from the treatment. Nevertheless one of the cases described below had lasted for five and a half years. In more recent cases, even in those diagnosed schizophrenia, clinical recoveries have been observed. Some of the patients have left the hospital and have resumed their usual occupations. This article presents a summary of the clinical observations on three patients from the Bombarda Hospital directed by Prof. Sobral Cid whose cooperation I wish to acknowledge with thanks. By means of these summaries the diagnoses may be arrived at and the treatment evaluated.

REPORT OF CASES

CASE I.—B. V. J., female, aged 36. Family history: The mother was hysterical and attempted suicide when she found that her husband was seriously ill. Personal history: The patient was well until the time of marriage at 27 years. She had a miscarriage, and two daughters born at term. In the Belgian Congo where she went with her husband, she became sad, interested in nothing, and incapable of running her household. Her husband said he would have to send her back to Lisbon and this made her very angry. She attempted suicide twice, by hanging and by swallowing sulphuric acid. During the voyage she threw her clothes overboard and a knife was found hidden beneath her pillow.

She arrived in Lisbon in January, 1931, very anxious, expecting horrible events. Everything that happened around her was directed toward her person and her situation. She was sure of the truth of her ideas. At first she was confined to a nursing home and returned after some time to her own home without improvement in her mental status. Her daughters were in school and the patient believed that the school had been destroyed in a conflagration and her daughters burned up; the letters that they wrote her did not come from them. The patient was agitated and was admitted again to the Bombarda Hospital. There she was perpetually anxious, with great lamentation, resistive, sometimes hysterical, and her mood was depressed. She was oriented as to place and surroundings but disoriented in time. She always watched closely what was going on around her in order to defend herself from imaginary dangers. She thought the nurse belonged to a sect that would persecute her. The blood that she thought she saw was the blood of her daughters who had been killed. She was always waiting for somebody to come and kill her. She made attempts at flight. She blamed herself for the misfortunes of her sister. She said that the sister had been assassinated in the hospital when she came to visit the patient, that she herself was surrounded by bad women, etc. When her condition improved in the hospital she was allowed to go home on a trial visit, but during this short period at home she was agitated and fearful that somebody was coming to kill her. She re-entered the hospital in the same condition four days after her

departure. Her situation remained substantially the same during four years.

In summary: The patient showed a systematized paraphrenia with chronic delusions of persecution. At the onset there was depression, change of character, suicidal attempts; later on anxiety, excitement, delusional state, with fear of imminent danger, despondency, and then physical persecutions radiating from herself to the persons of her family. There was a tendency toward isolation, and toward flight, motivated by her delusional ideas.

She was referred to the Hospital Santa Marta May 9, 1936, very agitated. She was immediately operated on under avertin anesthesia by Dr. Almeida Lima according to the technique described. The next day she was more tranquil. On the 12th she felt well; "It's all over. I've been locked up now for five and a half years but I wasn't crazy. I want to go back to live with my daughters."

May 16 she was observed by Prof. Sobral Cid who found her in good condition although possibly a little reticent. She would not admit, at least frankly, that she had been insane. The family found her in excellent condition, just as she had been before the psychosis. She left the hospital and now after six months she remains in entirely normal condition.

CASE II.—J. R. G., aged 36, police officer. In the family history it is noted that an uncle had epileptic attacks. In his personal history there were frequent nosebleeds but no alcoholism nor syphilis. In 1928 after working in the sun all day the patient had insomnia and in the following days psychomotor agitation developed; he wished to escape, to jump out of the window, to attack people who restrained him; but he became calm after some luminal and warm baths. He walked about constantly although slowly, and stopped eating. After a few days trembling, anxiety, and following this, psychomotor agitation developed and he was admitted to the Bombarda Hospital. Status on June 28, 1928: disorientation as to time and space, retardation in replies always preceded by movements of the lips, sometimes mutism, stereotyped movements, inexpressive face and refusal of food; uncertain, swaying walk, the trunk bent forward, the head flexed; waxy flexibility. Later on there were periods of excitement alternating with shorter periods of apathy and mutism. He never responded except in monosyllables and in a low voice. He remained in this state until October 28, 1928, when he left the hospital in custody of his brother. The patient improved outside the hospital and during seven years he remained in good health. He performed his military service and finally joined the police force where he had a good record.

In 1935 he developed gonorrhoea and accused the doctors of having poisoned him, and of having conspired together to do him harm.

He again entered the hospital July 26, 1935, in a very agitated condition, tearing his clothes with his teeth, beating his head against the pillows, swinging his arms and legs violently about, in spite of restraint. He wept aloud, crying: "You're robbers. You want to kill me and my whole family. The doctors want to assassinate me without letting anybody know about it." He was well oriented in place and time. He replied slowly or not at all to questions. The temperature was a little elevated on account of generalized furunculosis but subsided when this was cured. The patient remained, however, in a very disturbed state.

In February and March, 1936, he still showed the same agitation. He continued to tear clothes with his teeth. He threw himself out of bed without any precaution. He ran about, he jumped, he cried, he wept, he repeated his complaints in stereotyped fashion but he was not violent toward others. There was no fever and there seemed to be considerable organic deterioration.

His condition seemed to warrant the diagnosis of schizophrenia. He was transferred to the Hospital Santa Marta March 21, 1936, and operated upon the same day under avertin anesthesia, prefrontal leucotomy being performed according to the technique described.

The agitation of the patient diminished immediately after the operation and disappeared completely in three days. On April 9 the patient was in good condition, talked relevantly and coherently, and was correctly oriented. He desired to go home in order to resume his work. He was sent to the mental hospital where he was observed by Prof. Sobral Cid who considered him well and permitted him to leave April 12. Information obtained recently indicates that he is maintaining his recovery now seven months after operation.

CASE III.—J. J. S., aged 36, newsboy. The family history was negative. The patient had sold newspapers since his childhood. In 1922 he suffered from alcoholism and auditory hallucinations and hunted about for people whose voices he heard. "But I was never able to find them." Ideas of jealousy were present but not severe enough to be termed delusions. The patient improved after a month but shortly after that he returned to excessive drinking and in April, 1935, had an attack of delirium tremens of short duration. Following the development of auditory hallucinations there was marked anxiety and psychomotor agitation. He cried out that he believed in God, that his thoughts were being influenced, that he wished to be let alone. He heard voices that menaced him and made him afraid. These voices incited him to injure others but he did not wish to give his soul to the devil and on that account did not harm anyone. He beat on the walls to make the voices go away. He poured water on the floor because the voices told him that there was no water present, etc., and he showed insomnia and marked anxiety. He struck his wife and children because, as he said, they wished to poison him. He continued to sell the papers but did this badly. He often abandoned his work to go to various churches. He locked himself in a room isolating himself from the family. He ate in various places away from home, always saying grace over his food before taking it.

One day he drew his money from the sale of papers during the preceding month and took it to an unknown place. He was committed to the Bombarda Hospital July 8, 1935.

General and neurologic examinations were negative. He was calm on entering the hospital but when he found out that he was committed he demanded his discharge, saying he was well and wished to work. There was good rapport, and he replied readily. He was oriented in place and time. His attitude was that of a person listening for someone. He confessed that he heard voices and he was convinced that spirits entered into his body. He said, "They talk, talk, but I don't understand at all what they are saying. I want to sleep but they won't let me. They come to me by radio." When asked if these voices spoke of his wife he replied, "Yes. Some say that she is not my wife, others say that she is acting badly, that my children are not my children; but, nevertheless (he added) things that I don't see I can't swear to." The patient made crosses on his chest, on his head, etc., saying they were stars; he went through stereotyped movements with his arms, and sometimes when he was sitting he would rise and take a turn or two around the room before sitting down. He employed incomprehensible neologisms. On one occasion he took off his coat and jumped into the fish pond. He always gave peurile explanations or made irrelevant remarks concerning his gestures and movements. The Wassermann reaction in both blood and cerebrospinal fluid was negative. In spite of this he received antisyphilitic treatment and gained weight, but the hallucinations and the disturbed conduct persisted. On November 4, 1935, he was reticent in regard to his auditory hallucinations. He was unsociable, walking slowly from one side of the room to the other. He picked up and placed in his pocket pieces of wood, nails, twigs that he tore off from the shrubs in the garden. On one day he attacked an attendant saying that the attendant was persecuting him, and he had to be restrained. He continued to assault this attendant and to say that the attendant was going to kill him.

During his stay in the hospital he received his wife and children with indifference but he ate what was brought to him.

The diagnosis was hebephrenic dementia praecox which appeared to be pursuing a chronic course. He was transferred to the Hospital Santa Marta where a leucotomy was done July 10, 1936, according to the technique described above: three sections anterointernally and three anteroexternally in the white matter of each prefrontal lobe. The next day the patient was a little less agitated than formerly. On the 15th he was more tranquil but his statements in regard to his home and his affairs were still inaccurate. He did not give sufficient indication to permit the examiner to know whether he was still having auditory hallucinations. The condition of the patient improved during the following days. He had never confessed, in spite of the solicitation of his wife and of the resident physician of the hospital, where he had placed the money that he had withdrawn a few days before his commitment, but six days after the operation when he was asked about this in the presence of his wife he replied that he had entrusted it to the woman who supplied him with the newspapers. Since his wife was not sure of this information, the patient said, "That's true. She is a lady of high character with whom I trust much more than that." At my request the wife hunted up this lady and she came immediately to the hospital bringing with her the money that she had deposited in the bank for the patient.

On the first of August it was noted that the patient was getting along well and we were convinced that the hallucinations of hearing had disappeared. We wished to send him to the hospital to be examined by Prof. Sobral Cid but the patient considered himself cured and he was sent home. We saw him most recently November 11 altogether well and he had already undertaken his usual occupation.

SUMMARY

Following this exposition I do not wish to make any comment since the facts speak for themselves. These were hospital patients who were well studied and well followed. The recoveries have been maintained. I cannot believe that the recoveries can be explained upon simple coincidence. Prefrontal leucotomy is a simple operation, always safe, which may prove to be an effective surgical treatment in certain cases of mental disorder.

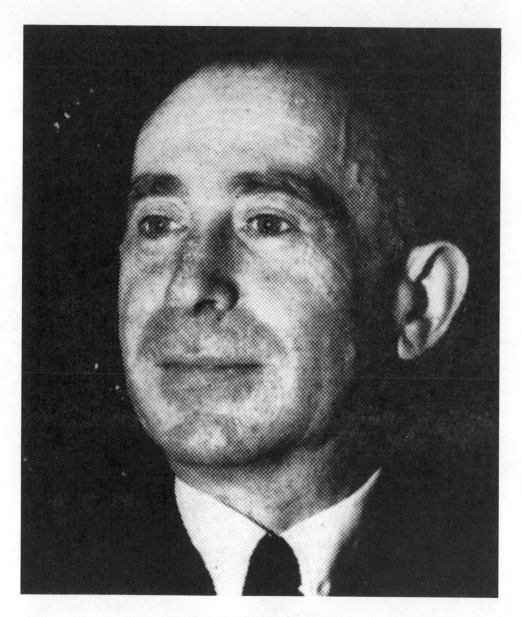

Manfred Sakel, M.D., 1900–1957

THE METHODICAL USE OF HYPOGLYCEMIA
IN THE TREATMENT OF PSYCHOSES

By Manfred Sakel, M.D.
Vienna, Austria

The American literature has lately contained reports of the therapeutic results and possibilities of the methodical use of hypoglycemia in the treatment of psychoses; it is nevertheless understandable that serious and critical scientists still wait to be convinced, and continue to retain a cautious attitude toward this new therapy. It is not only because an inadequate number of confirmatory reports of the value or soundness of the treatment have so far appeared. I think there are other reasons that could be given and before I proceed to the real subject of this talk, namely the origin and theoretical basis of this therapy, I think it would be well to discuss briefly these other reasons for the prevalence of an attitude of cautious scepticism.

The instinctively cautious attitude adopted by the profession toward this special kind of therapeutic procedure is due to the fact that the basic idea behind it is fundamentally at variance with the biological principles which are ordinarily involved in other therapeutic procedures. The great advances in treatment made by modern medicine in recent years have taught us to expect that every successful treatment has to be based on sound biological principles: a treatment has to fit somehow into the physiological processes with which we are already acquainted. A treatment ought either to eliminate some recognized functional disturbance in the physiological mechanism, or else destroy the actual causative agent of a disease—an infectious agent, for example, can be made innocuous by certain medicines, or a recognized poison, which disturbs the normal physiological processes can be eliminated or neutralized in some way. Modern therapy in recent years has developed consistently along such lines, and even the fever therapy, for example, was neither an unexpected nor an illogical development. When Wagner-Jauregg so brilliantly called the attention of the medical profession to the therapeutic effect of fever, physicians could recall instances in their own clinical experience when one or another psychotic subject was helped or cured by an attack of fever. It was not difficult to come to realize that fever was not a meaningless accompaniment of the organism's struggle against some toxin, but was instead an essential and perhaps indispensable part of the organism's defenses. The discipline of modern science nowadays demands that the first step in the development of a treatment is either to find the toxin that causes the disease, or else to discover what constitutional or functional disturbance is responsible for the symptoms of the disease. It is clear that when a science such as medicine has reached its present high degree of scientific objectivity, there is no room for therapeutic mysticism, or for anything which even suggests it.

Now, how does the hypoglycemic treatment of the psychoses fit into this picture? Does it stand in any kind of analogous relation to the kind of biological or physiological principles we have just mentioned? No, it certainly does not. And this is precisely the difference, which I have just attempted to describe, which all strictly scientifically minded physicians must feel, consciously or unconsciously, in regard to this treatment. But it is nevertheless justifiable to allow an exception in the case of the hypoglycemic treatment, for it has a special and unique position and should not be measured by ordinary standards. This must be so because the fundamental fact is that we do not know the nature of underlying processes of the disease called schizophrenia. In fact, it is still a debatable question whether we are dealing with a disease entity in the ordinary sense at all or simply with a symptomatic clinical picture. And we not only know nothing of the schizophrenic process and schizophrenic diseases, but we know nothing either about the conditions or processes involved in normal thinking, to say nothing of the complicated process that must be involved in an hallucination or delusion.

When we consider our experiences with the hypoglycemic treatment, and more particularly with the hypoglycemic state itself I think we can now say without much fear of contradiction that psychological factors are not likely to be the only ones involved in a mental dislocation as serious as that found in schizophrenia. There must be some injury to the deeper vital processes as well, perhaps a pathophysiological disturbance, or something perhaps even more complicated. We cannot however dispense with the psychological analysis and understanding of the delusions. There is no substitute for a thorough analysis of the delusions, for that is the only way we can begin to understand the complexes and difficulties of our patient. These problems and preoccupations are merely distorted and transformed by the disease process before appearing in the delusions, but by un-

From the Harlem Valley State Hospital, Wingdale, N.Y.
Translated from the German by Joseph Wortis, M.D.

derstanding them, we are enabled to diminish their force and thus relieve the patient.

I have a high regard for strict scientific procedure, and would be glad if we could follow the accustomed path in solving this special problem: it would have been preferable to have been able to trace the cause of the disease first, and then to follow the path by looking for a suitable treatment. But since it has so happened that we by chance hit upon the wrong end of the right path, shall we undertake to leave it before better alternatives present themselves? For even if the hypoglycemic treatment of psychoses accomplishes only a part of what it promises, it nevertheless has a value beyond its therapeutic claims, for it should perhaps now enable us to work backwards from it to the nature and cause of schizophrenia itself.

I am aware that this may prove to be a larger and more difficult undertaking, but I believe it can be said that it is well worth the effort, even though my own theoretical premises, on which the treatment has been based, should finally prove to be wrong. The mistakes in theory should not be counted against the treatment itself, which seems to be accomplishing more than the theory behind it.

The working hypothesis is schematic. The scheme involves a picture of the biological processes and activity of the nerve cell itself, about which we actually know nothing, in contrast to our extensive knowledge of the anatomy, histology and functional localization of modern neurology. The working hypothesis is based on the assumption that the nerve cell is functionally comparable to a fuel engine, so that each of its various functions may be placed in analogy to the functions of such an engine. The nerve cell in other words, like an engine, must have a certain potential energy comparable to that of a running engine that is disengaged. Furthermore the nerve cell, if it is to retain this potential energy, must depend on a continuous supply of endogenous excitant material comparable to the engine's fuel. Every individual has his own normal nerve cell functional capacity or state of tension, which is sustained by a corresponding amount of excitant hormones. The intensity of potential energy of the nerve cell depends on the proportional mixture of excitant and inhibiting hormones. The level which is normal for each individual is sustained by an automatic regulation. Should the automatic regulation be disturbed by some disease process, then an excess of excitant hormone in the mixture—like too much gas in a motor—can cause an overactivity and therefore a pathological activity of the cell. If the inhibitory factors dominate, then the reaction is weaker, like that of a motor with too little gas. The continuation of the normal tonus of the nerve cell is, in other words, conditioned like the activity of a fuel engine, by both the amount of gas or fuel, and by the kind of regulation. I at first applied this schema to the abstinence symptoms of morphinists. The symptoms that an abstinent morphinist displayed seemed to me to be not primarily but rather secondarily psychological, with the real origin in the vegetative sphere. Since most of the physical symptoms resembled the symptoms of a severe Grave's disease, I concluded that there must be an overstimulation of the sympathetic part of the vegetative nervous system. The sudden onset of the symptoms and their inevitable spontaneous

disappearance without treatment in a few days led me to believe that the stimulation of the vegetative nervous system was due to some pathological change in the nerve cell rather than an excess of the excitant hormone, such as we know exists in Grave's disease. I thought that the nerve cell, because of some pathological change, was able to attract more of the circulatory excitant hormone than it usually does. In order to visualize this sudden and transitory affinity of the nerve cell for the excitant hormone, I assumed that the nerve cell was changed by the morphine and that it acquired, to use another figure, additional valences in this way. Let us assume that the normal nerve cell has two valences which have to be saturated with the excitant hormone in order to preserve a normal tonus. If moderate amounts of morphine are administered then one of the valences, having an equal affinity for morphine, becomes saturated with morphine instead of with the excitant hormone and the result is an abnormal relaxation of the cell. If still more morphine is administered the cell must be stimulated to produce new valences in order to preserve its tone. If, for example, another valence is produced, then there are again two valences which can be saturated with the excitant hormone, so that in spite of the morphine there is no abnormal relaxation of the cell. That is why the morphinist has to keep increasing the dose. This process can repeat itself indefinitely.

The function of the insulin in this abstinence treatment is on the one hand to neutralize the excitant material, and on the other, to cover the unsaturated valences. The success of the treatment with morphinists readily suggested the possibility of using a non-alkaloid to pacify the nerve cell in other excited states. The working hypothesis was up to now proving serviceable.

While using these moderate doses of insulin, it was observed clinically that certain mental or even characterological changes accidentally appeared in certain patients. The assumption of a simply quantitative diminution of cellular function could no longer explain these changes. As such clinical observations were repeated, they could no longer be regarded as accidents but had to be related intimately to the hypoglycemia. Observations like the following could not be overlooked: Patients of an extreme egoism, with an egocentric attitude verging on autism, would become extroverted after an accidental hypoglycemic shock and would become extremely accessible and friendly. This even occurred quite frequently during the first days of abstinence when we were accustomed to see the patients, who were usually quite psychopathic to begin with, become even more asocial than ever.

The fact that stubbornly fixated psychotic character anomalies could be relieved during hypoglycemia and the observation that the rigidity of the personality could be relaxed, sometimes for a sustained period, all led me to think of the possibility of using hypoglycemia as such in the treatment of the psychoses.

I shall later have occasion to talk of the development of the method which made it possible to reach this goal. But for the present I wish to sketch briefly the working hypothesis which guided me in varying the method in different psychotic states.

The assumption that insulin diminished the activity of the nerve cell was sufficient explanation of the sedative effect on excited states but did not serve to explain the mental changes during and after hypoglycemia. The schematic picture which helped me to explain these phenomena was the following:

Activity in the sphere of the nervous system always consists of reactions to stimuli which flow in certain pathways. The changes occurring during hypoglycemia could be explained by the assumption that the hypoglycemia blockades the pathways which happen to be most active at a given time, so that the reactions to the same stimuli now come through pathways which had previously been inactive.

In order to make this picture clear I will take the example of a unicellular organism: Every reaction in this organism too must be regarded as a response to stimulus, and each cellular function is induced by a signal or stimulus. Each different reaction is dependent on the nature of the stimulus, and both reaction and stimulus are appropriate to each other. In order that this may be possible it is necessary that the whole course of the reaction, from the point of entry of the stimulus to the final end effect, should run through the appropriate intracellular pathway. The more primitive the cell, the fewer the possible varieties of reaction, and the fewer appropriate pathways there must be. At a higher level of development, as new varieties of reaction appear, it becomes necessary for new pathways to develop. When this happens, those pathways which are older in the evolutionary scale are overshadowed by the new pathways that develop and the former fall into the background. In multicellular organisms it becomes necessary to transmit stimuli from one cell to another along fixed pathways in order to allow a given functional activity. At any one stage of development these intracellular pathways are specialized and fixated, and insure a precise performance of the most complicated functions in response to appropriate stimuli, and of course the thinking process is such a function. A stimulus can provoke a reaction only when the stimulus is applied at the appropriate pathway, but not when it is applied to another. If an inappropriate stimulus reaches a certain pathway, it provokes no reaction; a sound wave, for example, produces no reaction on the optic nerve. In the course of long periods of evolution, the course of reactions and the responses to stimuli become more complicated. The stimuli themselves change in time too—so that it becomes necessary for new pathways to develop. The more ancient pathways sink into the background, but the appropriate relation between stimulus and nerve pathway continues. The most recent pathways to develop are therefore the youngest in the evolutionary scale, and are at the same time the most complicated pathways and those most frequently used.

We know from experience that the youngest and most active organs are most sensitive to injury, and this applies to the nerve pathways. Whenever the nerve cell is injured by some disease process in the organism, either qualitative or quantitative changes may occur. Qualitative injury to the nerve call causes injury to the youngest pathways first of all, just as the most recently developed organs in the body are the first to respond to injury. The more severe the injury, the older the pathways are which become involved.

The result is that the older pathways must again be activated, and the reactions to stimuli again run across these older pathways. If the injury is very violent there is a distortion and confusion of the intracellular pathways. The former change becomes apparent in the patient's primitive attitude toward the outside world, the latter change manifests itself in the patients disorientation and disorganization. By the process of short circuiting, inappropriate pathways and reactions are involved in the response to given stimuli. A stimulus for example instead of producing a reaction along its appropriate pathway, by means of a short circuit induces reactions over another or several other afferent or efferent pathways. Thus a response may take place over a false pathway by means of a short circuit in spite of the absence of the appropriate stimulus, so that a false sensation is experienced. An olfactory stimulus for example may at the same time, because of a short circuit, induce reactions along both acoustic and visual pathways. This represents the schematic picture of the nature of hallucinations in psychotics, developed from observations on the effect of hypoglycemia on hallucinations.

A clinical example:

A patient who had been having auditory hallucinations for decades, and who had developed a whole delusional system, was subjected to treatment. In four weeks the shock dose was reached. During hypoglycemia, just before the development of coma, the hallucinations disappeared completely for about an hour. After further treatment the hallucinations not only disappeared for an hour before the onset of coma, but also for another three hours after the termination of hypoglycemia. The patient meanwhile had no physical complaints whatever. This transitory disappearance of the hallucination was not due to any change in environment or to any physical disturbance, as the following experience shows: For the first few days the patient explained the disappearance of the hallucinations by saying that his enemy was being kept away from him. Later, as he began to observe that the hallucinations disappeared regularly during and immediately after the hypoglycemia, he concluded himself, without any suggestion from others, that "It must be due to some change in me, when those voices disappear during the treatments. It can't be due to something that is being done to my enemy."

I would not call that insight, for the patient's paranoia has lasted too many years for that, but it was interesting to observe the conflict between the paranoid attitude which he could not abandon, and his attempt at a logical solution of the facts.

The following case shows that there are no elements of suggestion or physical change involved in the disappearance of the hallucinations during and after hypoglycemia even in the transitory reactions.

A female patient who presented a picture of paranoid schizophrenia for about a year, associated with purely auditory hallucinations, lost her auditory hallucinations completely after four weeks of hypoglycemic treatment in spite of the fact that she had not yet recovered. She showed no insight, spoke of her hallucinations as of a simple fact, but talked of them in the past tense. She said for example: "I am healthy again, I can go back to my job in Washington. You know that it's been said on the radio that my job is being held for me. You can hear it too." When the examiner paused as if to listen a moment and then said: "No, I don't hear anything. What do you hear?" the patient listened intently for a minute and then said: "Yes, I don't hear anything now either. I haven't heard it for the past few days but it's true anyway."

I shall now only give a short example involving visual hallucinations.

A young girl who had been in the hospital for a few months with a whole system of bizarre delusions which we cannot discuss at present, kept seeing designs, letters and figures on her arm which she imagined that her supposed husband had tattooed there by remote control. She experienced her first shock about 16 days after treatment started and her visual hallucinations thereupon disappeared. When asked again that day, "What about those drawings on your arm?" She thought a while and said" "I think my sight is getting bad, I can't see them now. I've got to give my eyes a rest and then I'll see them again." After her hypoglycemic state was terminated the hallucinations again reappeared but would disappear thereafter during each hypoglycemic treatment for longer and longer periods, and finally disappeared completely. But it still took some time before the patient could look back and appreciate the fact that these delusions were not real.

In all of the examples which I have just given it seems that the hypoglycemia had disconnected the most recent pathways and isolated the short circuits, and thus prevented the false discharge of reactions from appropriate pathways to inappropriate ones. After further manipulation of the hypoglycemic treatment it was possible to blockade and isolate the short circuited pathways so that finally the reactions to stimuli traveled exclusively over appropriate pathways. This picture of the mechanism involved in hallucinations is again merely meant to be schematic.

It is much more difficult to apply this scheme to the abstract and intangible problems involved in the processes of thought or of consciousness. At the risk of getting involved in mythology, the absence of any other helpful picture obliges us to resort again to an hypothesis which will enable us to explain the effect of hypoglycemia on the purely mental processes of thought. We should picture these processes as involving separate cellular units analogous to those of our previous working hypothesis, and these units are again related to different stages of development. To justify, but not to prove, this assumption I shall start with the more concrete and easily observable neurological analogies: I refer to the disappearance of the various reflexes during hypoglycemia and coma in the order of their evolutionary development, as well as the reappearance of these reflexes in reverse order. It cannot be overlooked that the first organic functions to be eliminated are those which are phylogenetically and ontogenetically most recent, with these followed in turn by the older and older ones in regular order. The cremasteric reflex for example disappears first, a Babinski appears at the first sign of coma, while the corneal reflex—which is more ancient—remains active longest, remains in other words most resistant to the hypoglycemia. Similarly, all the other functions are put out of action, layer by layer, as coma deepens and grows more prolonged, with the respiratory center last to be involved. The temperature center, which I may call a more recent development, is involved earlier. When hypoglycemia is terminated and normal relations are again revived, the first centers to re-

spond are again the older and more resistant ones, for example, respiration, temperature, then the older corneal reflex as the first reflex, the Babinski much later, etc. The special sensitivity of everything that is of more recent development, more complicated and more dominant, is also revealed by the fact that the dominant left hemisphere is more quickly and more completely eliminated.

If we apply all this to mental processes, we may undertake to explain the various reactions to the selfsame hypoglycemic state by saying that here too those components of the mind which happen to be most dominant and active are most quickly and effectively eliminated. In accordance with this assumption we often see that a depression often changes during hypoglycemia to its opposite, so that the patient becomes manic; a manic patient becomes depressed, a confused patient becomes clear or lucid, an excited patient grows calm, or a stuporous patient becomes active again during hypoglycemia. I have therefore been led to assume that the hypoglycemic state first eliminates and inhibits that portion of consciousness in a psychotic subject which happens to be most active at the time, with the result that the other portions—which I may perhaps call the antagonistic part of the patient's mentality—again rise to the surface to again achieve dominance, even if only for a short time. In cases which progress favorably, repeated and correctly managed hypoglycemic states finally serve to produce a permanent dominance of those psychic components which hitherto have been repressed. In this way those portions which had been active before begin to retreat and fall into the background themselves. The remarkable observation of the so-called "activated psychosis" or "reversal of reaction" which I shall later describe, also fits into this picture. All these complicated attempted explanations, however incorrect they may prove to be, were necessary as a working hypothesis in order to develop the extremely complicated hypoglycemic method and technique. This method involves a modification in the time of termination of the hypoglycemic state in various psychotic states, for the most favorable results. This working hypothesis is only a schematic representation of apparently inconsistent clinical observations gathered over a period of years, before they could be used to clarify the modifications of technique.

I will only briefly discuss the nature of this technique, since I feel that even the best description cannot serve to convey more than a vague picture to an audience. Even the most complete description without practical training and experience is not sufficient for a successful trial. Before hypoglycemia could be recommended as a therapeutic principle a technique had to be developed which allowed its systematic use with a minimum of danger. I must however emphasize that the mere technique of the hypoglycemic treatment of the psychoses is only comparable to a knowledge of ligature and asepsis in an operation. That is, it is an absolutely essential condition if dangers are to be avoided. But the success of an operation also depends on sufficient knowledge and experience on the part of the surgeon. In order to handle a hypoglycemic treatment successfully one has to be able to act quickly in accordance with each new situation while the avoidance of dangers ought to take place automatically almost without intruding on consciousness. The technical side of the hypoglycemic treatment in itself tells us nothing about the most important factors in the treatment, namely how each individual case has to be managed. However, the rules for the technique and method have to be strictly followed throughout the treatment, for they are the products of years of experience and careful observation. The fact that we do not yet know the factors which are operative in this treatment does not justify our arbitrarily erecting new principles. Too great an optimism in regard to this method is more dangerous than an overcautious pessimism, since it leads to an amateurish and unsuccessful use of the technique, with the failure finally falsely attributed to the therapy itself. The dangers of the treatment have to be avoided of course, but they ought not preoccupy the physician so much that he forgets the treatment itself, for in many cases favorable results can only be attained when the danger zone is reached.

THE TECHNIQUE

The technique requires that the patient be given increasing doses of insulin until the so-called shock dose is reached, the size of the shock dose varies considerably in different individuals and may be anything from 15 to 450 units. The initial dose varies from 15 to 50 a day depending on the physical condition of the patient and the duration of his illness, and the doses are increased by 5 to 20 units daily until the shock dose is reached. This constitutes phase 1. By shock dose we understand that amount of insulin which in any individual produces deep coma and areflexia within 4 or 5 hours after one injection. (This is not always necessary.) A shock dose is given 3 to 6 times a week until the desired result is attained but if the patient does not respond no more than 50 injections need be given. This constitutes phase 2. After severe physical manifestations of shock, one or more rest days may intervene, but at least one to three days of rest are allowed every week. These constitute phase 3. Phase 4, which can often be omitted in chronic cases, consists of the administration of a fraction of the shock dose for about eight days, during which marked hypoglycemic reactions are avoided. The insulin injection is always given fasting and is followed in four or five hours by a sufficient amount of carbohydrates. It is often well to give the patient as many grams of sugar as he has had units of insulin. I should like to mention in passing that the blood sugar level, regardless of the amount of insulin given, does not drop beyond a certain level. The neurological symptoms of hypoglycemia or coma are not dependent on any one blood sugar level. I shall not undertake here to give an exact description or definition of the concept of coma or of the somewhat misleading term "shock," as these are things which can be learned in the course of practical experience. I shall only say, to prevent any misunderstanding, that coma should be associated with the absence of the corneal reflex, or at least with the presence of a Bakinski. Individual variations have to be made continuously, as therapeutic results cannot be achieved by a stereotyped repetition of hypoglycemic states measured by so many hours, but depends instead on the correct management of each individual hypoglycemic state, and especially on its termination at the right moment. These are matters which can be learned only through long experience.

It would not be proper to neglect psychiatric factors in discussing the treatment of psychoses. Even in an essentially physical treatment of psychoses such as this is, a consideration of psychological and other psychiatric factors is especially necessary. For however strong the impression may be that we are somehow influencing the psychic processes by means of biochemical processes, it must always be remembered that the opposite is possible as well. The activity of the brain and the very material it deals with in the course of normal physiological processes, are after all purely psychological. It is therefore not a matter of indifference to the mentally sick patient what his psychic problems and conflicts are, for this material must be elaborated under peculiarly difficult conditions, and the preoccupations and problems which he is forced to solve now under such difficult circumstances demand our special attention.

When for example we treat a patient with a peptic ulcer which is not due to a dietary error, it is nevertheless important to consider the patient's diet in the course of treatment, for this can facilitate, disturb or neutralize the cure which we achieve by other means. It is not otherwise in the treatment of psychoses. An incorrect psychological management of the patient's complexes in any psychosis, however organically or pathophysiologically determined, can cause great harm.

What has been said up to now is intended merely to chronologically summarize the development of the hypoglycemic treatment. The same holds true for the hypothetical considerations which served as a working basis for the further development of the treatment. However, mere theoretical considerations which may prove to be incorrect, or a statement of the difficulties of the technique are no proof that the treatment is useful or practicable. I am well aware that serious workers can be convinced only by definite clinical evidence of the value of the treatment. Since I shall not have time here to fully present the clinical evidence of results, I shall only attempt to review a few typical facts which demonstrate both the value and perhaps too the logical soundness of this therapeutic approach.

Even the small doses given at the beginning of treatment often produce marked changes in the psychotic subject. They become calmer and less tense. But these changes do not differ essentially, except perhaps in the quality of the sedative effect from the pacification achieved by other therapeutic measures. But these changes become dramatic and striking when more intense degrees of hypoglycemia are reached. These changes are so specific and dramatic that it is difficult to do justice to them in words. From one minute to the next, the mental picture changes, so to speak, at a single stroke. One cannot escape the impression that the mental changes move consistently in a single direction. It almost looks as if the patient suddenly acquired, so to speak, a different style of thinking. Completely confused patients suddenly become lucid, even if only for a short time at first. Patients absorbed in their hallucinations suddenly lose them, excited patients grow calm, and in the same hypoglycemic state stuporous patients may be aroused. A paranoid patient for example will suddenly lose his delusions and ideas of reference when the hypoglycemia has reached a certain depth. In fact he gains insight into the abnormal nature of his previous hallucinations. In the early stages of treatment the patients become psychotic again as soon as the hypoglycemic state is ended. This change is so complete and abrupt that it almost seems as if one kind of consciousness had been replaced by another. As the treatment progresses these lucid periods last longer and longer, and the normal personality, so to speak, stays with the patient longer. When one sees over and over again how a patient of this sort achieves lucidity during hypoglycemia, and then becomes psychotic again after he has been given some sugar, how can one doubt that this change is intimately related to the hypoglycemia? The periods of lucidity during hypoglycemia become longer and longer and then begin to extend beyond the period of termination of the hypoglycemia. The periods after hypoglycemia during which the former personality dominates become longer and longer, and qualitatively better, until finally the periods last until the next following hypoglycemic state. One cannot escape the impression that each hypoglycemic period serves to remove another portion of the psychosis, so that the former normal personality can be more and more readily revived. When this has happened, a curious phenomenon develops. A patient that showed his normal personality for a short period during hypoglycemia when treatment began, now at the end of treatment, after he has improved, begins to show psychotic symptoms during hypoglycemia. I have called that the reversal of reaction. One practically witnesses the struggle for dominance between two kinds of consciousness. The consciousness which happens to be most active at a given time is paralyzed during hypoglycemia, so that the repressed consciousness again achieves dominance. The activated symptoms which appear in the course of this reversal of reaction represent an abbreviated version of the patient's own past psychotic development. Those patients for example who do not respond to hypoglycemia with a complete and sudden even if temporary loss of their schizophrenic shell, may at least respond sufficiently to return for a while to some previous stage in their psychotic development. One can force the psychosis, so to speak, back step by step to its previous stages, and in favorable cases back again to the original prepsychotic personality. It would therefore be incorrect to conclude that the hypoglycemia has a specific anti-psychotic action; it is more correct, as the phenomena of the reversal of reaction and of activated symptoms show, to say that it is that part of the mind which happens to be most active and dominant at a given time which is subdued, to the advantage of the repressed portion. As treatment advances, however, the psychotic residue which is reactivated during hypoglycemia, diminishes and disappears in time. A clinical example:

N.N. A 21-year-old female university student of philology. Her family history seemed to show some taint, but the patient's family was hesitant about giving information. The patient herself was an excellent and unusually talented student up to two years before treatment started. In addition to her studies the patient was also socially active, was brilliant and likable and was always the center of her group. Gradually the patient began to neglect her studies, grew irritable and withdrawn, kept more and more to herself under the pretext that she did not get on with people, but gradually definite ideas of reference developed. It became clear in time that the patient was hallucinating. She finally had to be brought to a hospital where she remained for a year and a half. During this time her condition grew gradually but clearly worse. She was apathetic and unemotional, completely absorbed in the hallucinations and could scarcely be distracted from them for more than a few minutes at a time, to establish contact. She would always sink back into her autism, refused to answer concrete questions to the point, but referred instead to her hallucinations. She said Christ was communicating with her from the cross and was giving her commands, that He accompanied her on an aeroplane but had now multiplied Himself, because there was somebody at each window talking to her in a strange language. The patient herself knew several languages. The patient had no wish to work at all, kept muttering to herself, and conversed with her visions. She took no interest in the outside world, or in her relatives, was untidy and had to be fed. The outlook seemed very poor, and I did not at first expect a response to insulin treatment.

During Phase I the patient showed little response to small doses of insulin, both during and after hypoglycemia. It took a long time—about four weeks—before shock doses were reached at all. The type of shock reaction looked prognostically poor too. The patient responded to shock doses with extreme excitement, and this appeared to be rather favorable evidence of an emotional response, even though of a pathological nature. Still more time was required until the hallucinations began to disappear for a short time at least during hypoglycemia. In the seventh week of treatment the patient responded to 170 units of insulin by losing her hallucinations about three hours after the injection. At this time she was able to establish contact, but was still emotionally flat and uninterested. She admitted that she no longer saw Christ nor heard his voice, but He had only gone away and would come back again. Half an hour later during hypoglycemia the patient suddenly became very emotional and excited for about half an hour. She then went into coma, which could not however be continued for long, because the patient would always develop sudden respiratory distress. The poor prognosis in the first place, and the unfavorable hypoglycemic reactions made me wonder whether it would be worthwhile to continue treatment at all. But since the mother of the patient insisted, treatment was continued. The patient's hypoglycemic reactions remained the same, but she slowly but surely began to show improvement. For several hours after the termination of hypoglycemia, the patient was sufficiently free of her hallucinations to begin to read papers again, which she had not done for two years. It was also possible to converse with her again. However, she showed hardly any insight into her illness, and was not interested to know why she was brought to a sanatorium in a foreign country. In the course of further treatment the patient developed epileptic seizures on three separate occasions, followed always with retrograde amnesia of short duration. After 12 weeks of treatment the patient began to be symptom-free both during hypoglycemia and thereafter. She no longer had hallucinations or delusions, began to act in a way appropriate to her training and surroundings, played tennis and visited the museums and cinema; she did not do these things spontaneously on her own initiative, but she was interested, and could converse sensibly. Except for a certain loss of spontaneity she was by now almost completely recovered. Since this already exceeded our expectations and since the patient was already under treatment more than three months, the treatment was concluded, to allow the patient to show the further improvement which we often see after treatment is concluded, with the possibility in mind that she could be given a second course of treatment if this did not occur. But after a few weeks she showed so much further improvement that she not only appeared normal to her family and friends but also to the physician after close examination. She no longer had the least trace of abnormality. Two years have since passed and the patient is still perfectly well.

The cases I have discussed were not chosen from the large clinical material because they were particularly favorable. I have had many cases that proved to be failures and in still other cases the treatment did not proceed without setbacks and difficulties. I chose these cases not because they were successful but because they were good clinical examples of the relation between hypoglycemia and the changes in the mental or psychotic state. I hope that I have been at least somewhat successful in conveying to you the absolutely inescapable impression that one gets in following a case through treatment: that there is undoubtedly an intimate relation between improvement and hypoglycemic treatment. Psychiatrists need no longer have that paralyzing feeling of insufficiency toward their psychotic patients that they used to have. They can now have instead a feeling that they now possess an instrument with which they can break through the barrier and attack the psychosis, so to speak, at its vital point. This fact alone would mean a great deal even if the statistical results were not as good as they are. When I think again of my own clinical material, which comprises about 300 cases which I have treated myself, to say nothing of at least as many cases which I have seen treated elsewhere, and consider how often I have seen improvement follow the treatment, improvement in many cases amounting to recovery, to an extent which has up to now been unprecedented in schizophrenics, and when I consider the numerous transitory reactions in which schizophrenics suddenly become accessible again, or when I consider the other various changes in the psychotic picture which occur during treatment, the conclusion becomes inescapable that these changes and these improvements were actually caused by the treatment. Regular and repeated changes of this sort cannot be due to mere coincidence. I shall only briefly summarize the results:

In spite of the difficulties there are in preparing statistics in the case of a disease like schizophrenia where there are no objective symptoms with which we can establish the diagnosis or evaluate the results, nevertheless I think that with material as large as mine, it is possible to avoid the errors involved in a smaller group of cases.

I have divided the case material into three groups: recent cases of less than six months' duration, cases of less than one and one-half years' duration and chronic cases of over one and one-half years' duration.

In the successfully treated cases the concept of a full re-

mission is very strictly defined. We have only included those patients in this group who were not only symptom-free, with full insight into their illness, and with full capacity for return to their former work, but also where one had no intuitive feeling that there might have been some change in personality.

We called those patients good remissions who were completely symptom-free and who had insight and were able to go back to their work, but where one had the intuitive feeling that there was some personality change.

Under social remissions we understand the third group of patients with more or less marked improvement, but who are not however included in the group of successfully treated cases.

In recent cases the treatment has given us over 80 per cent of good remissions with capacity for work of which about 70 per cent are full remissions.

In chronic cases the results are all poorer in direct relation to the duration of the illness. In our group of cases we have had 40 per cent of remissions with capacity for work. The statistics for spontaneous remissions vary with different authors from approximately 5 to 25 per cent. When we consider that the results in our treated cases are several times better than the most optimistic statistics for spontaneous remissions, and when we consider further that the quality of remission in our treated cases is far superior than that of spontaneous remissions, then we are entitled to conclude that the treatment is effective. The impressive reintegration of personality that we saw in the course of treatment of recent cases, led us at first to treat only recent cases and we at first neglected the chronic cases where the chances of recovery seemed so much poorer. But after more intensive experience with chronic schizophrenics in hospitals, my therapeutic experiences led me to change my views.

In the course of the introduction of the treatment to this country I had the opportunity, through the invitation of State Commissioner Dr. F.W. Parsons to conduct a course for the State Hospital System of New York. The case material which was available at the time of the demonstration of the technique to the physicians was not particularly favorable. However, in spite of the unfavorable material it was possible to allow about half of the twenty patients to return to their homes again, in some cases with capacity for work, and a few others with good remissions, while the rest of the patients were at least sufficiently improved to allow them to lead a tolerably human existence in the institution, so that even these results can now be said to be by no means a matter of indifference, and from a humane medical point of view, definitely positive.

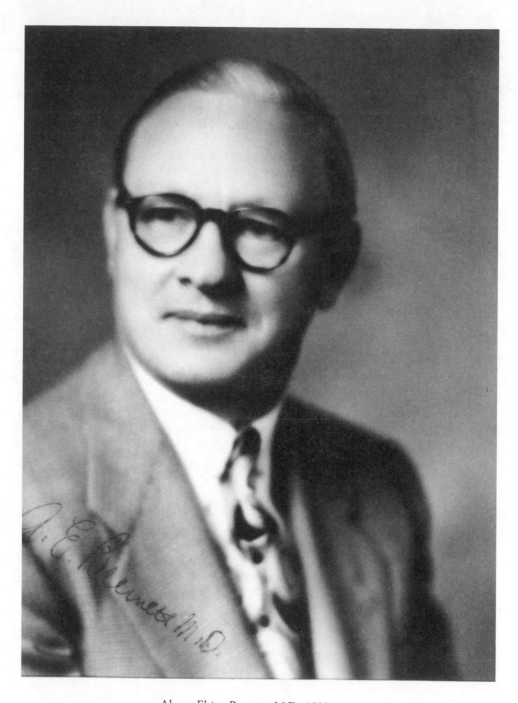

Abram Elting Bennett, M.D., 1898–

CURARE: A PREVENTIVE OF TRAUMATIC COMPLICATIONS IN CONVULSIVE SHOCK THERAPY

(Including a Preliminary Report on a Synthetic Curare-Like Drug)

By A.E. Bennett, M.D.

Omaha, Nebraska

Since L. Meduna, (1) in 1935, introduced convulsive (metrazol) shock therapy for schizophrenia, over 1000 articles attempting to evaluate its usefulness have appeared in the world's literature. The immediate results in early schizophrenic states appeared to be at least equal to those reported from Sakel's hypoglycemic shock therapy. The follow-up reports, however, indicated that sustained results are inferior to those of insulin shock therapy and possibly no greater than those of previous psychiatric treatment methods.

Since my preliminary report (2) on 21 cases of chronic resistant affective disorders in February of 1938, many others have confirmed its usefulness. A recent follow-up study (3) of 70 cases, after six months to two years, indicates that 90 per cent of severe depressive reactions can be terminated within two to three weeks of treatment with about 10 to 15 per cent of relapses, The results obtained in the midlife, involutional and presenile depressive states over a long period of time suggest that in these forms of mental illness convulsive shock therapy offers the greatest field of usefulness.

In spite of these results, because of certain hazards in the treatment—particularly the traumatic complications, this revolutionary psychiatric treatment has been seriously condemned by many workers and totally abandoned by some. Recently at prominent national meetings such remarks as these have been made by neuropsychiatrists whose opinions bear great weight: "I give the treatment just one more year to survive," "I think we should wake up now to the fact that this is not real therapy. Anything that actually injures the patient whom we are supposed to be looking after should be stopped. The use of metrazol is the use of a perfectly dreadful drug."

I can only conclude that such remarks are made by individuals who have not had extensive experience with this therapy. In my opinion, it is one of the real revolutionary therapies of modern psychiatry. Its use is still empiric, as was

malarial therapy 20 years ago, with its hazards and complications, until replaced by safer, less hazardous, more efficient artificial fever combined with chemotherapy. (4) Convulsive shock therapy will remain until replaced by some more specific measure, since there is something fundamentally sound in this therapy, never approached heretofore in effectiveness, in depressive stupor, mixed catatonic or chronic manic excitement states.

The problem of traumatic complications, because of the severity of the convulsion induced by metrazol, has greatly restricted its usefulness and has raised the question whether the treatment could survive in its raw state. The incidence of serious extremity fractures of humerus or femur has been 1.5 to 2 per cent and dislocations 17.2 per cent. (5) Compressive fractures of the spine have been carefully evaluated as 43 to 51 per cent. (6)

For the past two years the seriousness of this problem has prevented my giving any metrazol treatment without instituting prophylactic measures. We first tried hyperextensive procedures of the spine, under orthopedic guidance, restraining the pelvis, hips and shoulders to prevent flexor spasms of the spine and adducting the arms, without complete success. In addition, we tried administering metrazol after first inducing insulin coma, on the theory that insulin shock produced hypotonia sufficient to prevent fracture complications. Later, we added spinal anesthesia (7) to paralyze back and lower extremities, thus adequately preventing spinal and lower extremity fractures. But this method had obvious objections; it left the arms unprotected and a shoulder fracture occurred in one case. None of these measures—orthopedic restraint, preliminary upbuilding (calcium, viosterol, etc.), or even spinal anesthesia would prevent all complications. The fundamental problem was still the severity of the convulsive seizures.

We then attempted to find less severe convulsant drugs and experimented with tutin, picrotoxin and coriamyrtin. We found none of these drugs would produce seizures sufficiently mild to prevent fractures. We also tried total nitrogen inhalation, as recommended by Alexander and Himwich, (8) but found it therapeutically ineffective.

The problem resolved itself into finding some method of softening or lessening the convulsive seizure and still preserving the therapeutic effectiveness.

Read at the ninety-sixth annual meeting of The American Psychiatric Association, Cincinnati, Ohio, May 20-24, 1940. From the psychiatric departments of the Bishop Clarkson Memorial Hospital, University of Nebraska College of Medicine, Omaha, and the Lincoln State Hospital, Lincoln, Nebraska.

The principle of curarization or blocking the neuromuscular junction to prevent excessive nerve impulses from reaching the muscles seemed theoretically feasible. Through the courtesy of Mr. Richard C. Gill, who had recently returned from South America with the largest amount of curare ever available for experimental research, and E. R. Squibb and Sons, together with the assistance of Dr. A. R. McIntyre, professor of pharmacology at the University of Nebraska, we have been able to carry out extensive studies with the drug.

HISTORICAL RÉSUMÉ OF AVAILABLE INFORMATION ON CURARE

Since time immemorial, South American Indians of the upper Amazon region have used gum curare on the tips of arrows, darts and spears to paralyze their game in hunting. Generalized muscular paralysis, respiratory failure and death occur within a few minutes after injection. The edibility of animals killed by so called Indian arrow poison is not affected. The secrets of curare preparation have been carefully guarded by the Indian witch doctors (curare makers) of the tribes and much mystery or "black magic" clouds its manufacture.

Crude gum curare is prepared by the natives by brewing the stems, bark, root and leaves of certain plants in water. The resultant infusion is strained and concentrated by boiling to a consistency adaptable to adhering to spear and blow gum dart points.

The first record of the primitive use of curare is in Hakluyt's description of Sir Walter Raleigh's contact with the Indians of the Orinoco plain in 1595. Alexander Humboldt (1859) first witnessed the manufacture of Indian made curare.

Sir Robert Schomburgh (1844) first named the plant group which enters into the making of the poison. He believed that animals hit by it died in convulsions similar to those produced by strychnine and named the plant strychnos toxifera. Consequently we find it listed in botany in the strychnine family despite the fact that pure curare is diametrically opposed to strychnine in action and is even an antidote for strychnine poisoning. Watterton and Brodie in 1815 demonstrated asphyxia to be the cause of death from curare poisoning.

Boussingault and Roulin, in 1824, first extracted the alkaloid curarin. Later, in 1864, Preyer isolated it in crystalline form. Claude Bernard, in 1844, first described the physiological action of the drug upon the neuromuscular junction and confirmed asphyxia as the cause of death. In 1849 he proved the drug harmless when administered by mouth. With M. Pelouze he reported a series of observations on experiments with animals: 1) The drug must enter the body by a wound to produce paralysis. 2) The action is upon the myoneural junction. 3) Sensory nerves and cardiovascular systems are relatively unaffected. 4) The drug does not injure muscle or nerve.

Thus, the drug became a useful tool for physiologic study. Lapique later found that curare lowered the excitability of muscle while leaving the excitability of nerve unimpaired. He showed that curarized muscle was still able to contract with vigorous stimulation, but the charges induced by the natural nerve impulse were too feeble to produce contraction.

Jousset, Demine and Busch in 1867 first attempted to apply the drug in clinical medical therapy. They treated convulsive states, epilepsy, rabies, chorea, strychnine poisoning and various tics. Hoffman, 1879, Hoche, 1894, and Cash, 1901, also experimented with curare. Tsocanakis, in 1923, tried curare in spastic paralysis. Bremer, in 1927, proved that the drug exhibited a selective action in reduction of local tetanus and decerebrate rigidity. West (1931-1935) and Cole (1934) reported partial results in relief of tetanus convulsions, relief of rigidity of Parkinsonism, causalgia, and spastic paraplegia. Burman (1938-1939) reported extensively upon its relaxing effect in spastic, athetoid, and dystonic states of muscular rigidity and tremor.

A great drawback to experimental and clinical investigation of the drug has been inaccurate information from native curare makers, because no gourd or tube of crude curare made by one witch doctor would duplicate the ingredients of another. Also, different curare plants from various areas give varying toxic action. Other lethal substances such as venom were added from time to time. These contaminants have snarled chemical and physiologic research. On the whole, the impression gained from pharmacologic literature is that the drug is highly toxic and dangerous, not applicable to clinical medicine. Furthermore, until recently, no large quantities of authenticated curare have been available at any one time for experimental research.

In 1934, Mr. Richard C. Gill, after exhaustive studies and prolonged contact with South American Indians, was able to learn the actual botanical ingredients and the secrets of manufacture. In 1938 he brought back to this country the largest amount of authentic and field tested curare ever gathered and brought back to the civilized world. In addition, he brought back a large amount of unauthenticated curare, that is, curare from regions he had not personally visited. This supply was turned over to the E. R. Squibb and Sons' research department.

STANDARDIZATION OF THE DRUG

After considerable experimentation by Dr. A. R. McIntyre, professor of pharmacology at the University of Nebraska, and Mr. H. A. Holaday, head of the biological development and control division of Squibb's biological laboratories, working independently, the technic of standardization, at first difficult, has been simplified. Biologic methods of assay are necessary with each new batch of the drug. An aqueous infusion or hot alcoholic extract of the drug is prepared. The curare itself is extraordinarily stable, not destroyed by autoclaving. Assay by a variety of methods gives a result so precise that recheck reveals an error within the limit of one per cent.

Methods and Assay.—Curare-acetylcholine antagonism upon a frog gastrocnemius preparation has been applied. A frog gastrocnemius preparation is made which, with addition of acetylcholine produces an isometric type of contraction which furnishes a reference height for comparisons

FIGURE 1. Bio-Assay of Curare

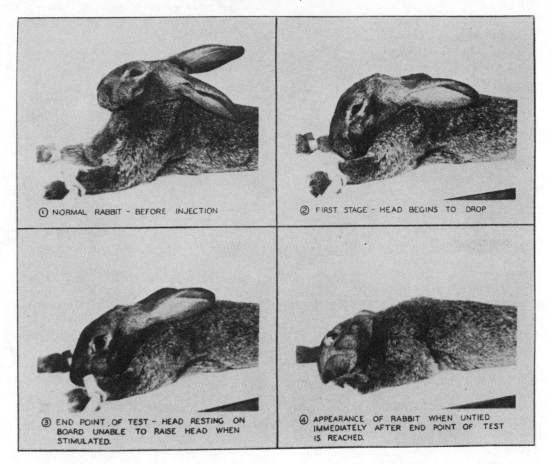

① NORMAL RABBIT - BEFORE INJECTION

② FIRST STAGE - HEAD BEGINS TO DROP

③ END POINT OF TEST - HEAD RESTING ON BOARD UNABLE TO RAISE HEAD WHEN STIMULATED.

④ APPEARANCE OF RABBIT WHEN UNTIED IMMEDIATELY AFTER END POINT OF TEST IS REACHED.

with a decreased height contraction obtained through the inhibiting effect of the curare solution.

Another method of assay is the head-drop method in the rabbit, developed by Holaday. The curare solution is injected slowly into the ear vein of the rabbit and the dose adjusted so that the neck muscles after two and one-half to three minutes reach a degree of flaccidity which just prevents the animal from raising the head and keeps the chin down. This end point is very clear-cut and a typical curare effect occurs exactly as seen in the human after injection of a curarizing dose. The amount per kilogram necessary to produce this effect in rabbits is estimated and the dosage is figured according to body weight of the patient. (See Fig. 1.)

Still another method, now abandoned, was to determine the lethal dose required for one-half of a certain number of mice. The estimated human dose was calculated by starting with one-sixth of the lethal dose for mice and finding the effective physiologic dose. The rabbit method is by far the best method in our experience.

PHYSIOLOGIC ACTION OF CURARE

Action of pure curare is upon the neuromuscular mechanism. In certain impure preparations, another action is seen, ascribed by Burman (9) to curin. This side-effect is a histamine-like action producing sudden fall in blood pressure, bronchial spasm, facial pallor, erythema and urticaria; which are relieved by epinephrine. These preparations we have not employed clinically but are investigating them further. We believe them unsafe for clinical use.

The action of curare is upon the net-like structure of fine nerve fibers at the terminus called the motor end plate. It is here that acetylcholine, the chemical mediator or regulator of chronaxie of nerve impulses to voluntary muscle, acts. Curare prevents acetylcholine from acting on the nerve muscle junction and inhibits its action, thus producing a paresis of muscle. Curare poisoning (curarization) thus prevents the transmission of natural nerve impulses from motor nerves to the muscles. This peripheral motor flaccid paralysis affects nerve endings generally of all striated or voluntary musculature, but selectively affects first fine, fast-moving muscles of high chronaxie, such as short muscles of the eyes, and throat, later, the larger, slower-moving muscles of head, neck, extremities, intercostals and diaphragm.

The circulation is relatively unaffected and sensory nerves are not affected. While reflexes may be somewhat diminished they are not abolished. Death occurs from asphyxia due to respiratory paralysis. The so-called lethal point of the drug is questionable because large doses are tolerated if respiration can be continued. The drug is quick acting and very rapidly eliminated. The rapidity of absorption has much to do with lethality. Small amounts of the

FIGURE 2. A Straight Unrestrained Metrazol Convulsion

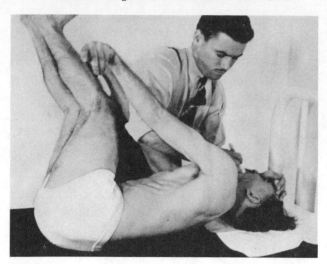

FIGURE 3. The Same Patient as Shown in Figure 2 After Curarization Followed by Metrazol, Illustrating the Remarkable Diminution of Muscular Contraction

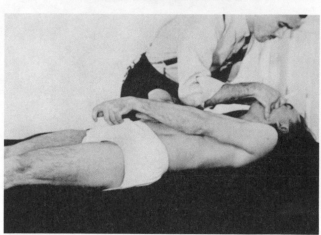

drug injected rapidly are toxic and produce cardiac failure in animals while large amounts may be given slowly without toxic symptoms. Fifty times the lethal dose has been given to dogs by Dr. A. R. McIntyre without fatality by keeping up artificial respiration.

The physiologic effects are noted immediately at the end of an intravenous injection given over a period of one to two minutes. In about two more minutes the peak of curarization is reached, whereupon the effect slowly recedes and seems to vanish in fifteen to twenty minutes. The same effect occurs in fifteen to twenty minutes after intramuscular injection. Physiologic symptoms are seen in the following sequences: The patient first complains of haziness or fuzziness of vision. Next, bilateral ptosis appears with slight nystagmoid movements, relaxation of the face and heaviness, with relaxation of the jaws. The patient at this point complains of tightness of the throat and huskiness of the voice. Generalized heaviness and weakness of the neck muscles with inability to raise the head are followed by weakness to complete paresis of the spinal muscles, legs and arms. Last, appears shallowness of respiration from weakness of the intercostal and the diaphragm.

These symptoms follow the same order as the progressive symptoms of a patient with myasthenia gravis; double ptosis and nasal smile also simulate the myasthenic. Excess saliva may accumulate in the throat and the patient complain of difficulty in breathing, but this occurrence is counteracted considerably if the relaxed jaws and tongue are held forward. Injections of epinephrine, prostigmin or metrazol all seem to counteract quickly the action of curare. Burman (9) believes that a sustained, clinically relaxing effect upon hyperkinetic or spastic muscles remains for a long period of time after the toxic deacetylcholinizing effect of curare has disappeared. We have not been convinced of any such prolonged action from curare. In fact this temporary effect is a drawback to its usefulness in spastic states. It is essentially a very transiently acting drug because of its rapid elimination.

There are a number of drugs known to have a curare-like action: quinine methochloride, erythroidine hydrochloride, ammonium bases, amides and amines, choline, muscarin, snake venoms, methyl strychnine, aromatic series, pyridin, quinolin, thallin, nicotine series, piperdin, putrefactive ptomains and products of muscular metabolism.

Curare, as yet, has not gained a definitely useful application in clinical medicine. Attempts have been made from time to time to apply the curarization principle in treatment of spasmodic disorders. West (11) and others have reported partial results in tetanus. The most encouraging recent report is that of Burman in infantile cerebral palsies, spastic pyramidal states, and extrapyramidal rigidity states which are associated with involuntary movements, athetosis and tremor.

After an extensive use upon spastic paralytic children, of carefully assayed products of aqueous and alcoholic extracts of crude curare prepared by Dr. A. R. McIntyre, I became convinced of the safety of the drug. Experiments begun at the Lincoln State Mental Hospital were soon extended to my private patients; for the past nine months, (10) I have not administered convulsive shock therapy without preliminary curarization.

Up to April 15, 1940, 74 patients were given 466 treatments in my private practice; 27 patients were given 163 treatments under my supervision at the State Hospital without experiencing accidents or complications with one exception (see Table III). At the present time we are using a concentrated aqueous extract of curare known as intocostrin, biologically assayed and prepared by E. R. Squibb and Sons.

TECHNIC OF CURARIZATION PRELIMINARY TO CONVULSIVE SHOCK THERAPY

An intravenous injection of an aqueous solution of intocostrin containing 10 mg. of active curare principle per cc. is given over a period of one to two minutes. It has been found that 1 cc. curarizes 15 to 20 pounds of body weight. Females take less than males; older patients more than

FIGURE 4. EEG Patterns of Curarized Patient Subjected to Metrazol Shock Therapy[a]

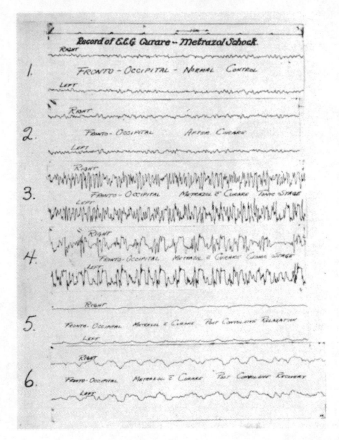

[a]First tracing shows normal control record. Second tracing shows normal pattern persists after curare. Third and fourth tracings show waves of increased frequency and high amplitude following metrazol. Fifth tracing shows complete absence of rhythmic activity. Sixth tracing shows slow waves of 2–3 per second that persist during confusional state.

younger patients. After a few injections, this individual variation in dosage can be easily calculated. On an average, 5 to 8 cc. is needed for a 100 to 150 pound woman and 8 to 12 cc. for a 150 to 200 pound male. The speed of injection influences the dose necessary. With a rapid injection, curarization is accomplished with a smaller dose. At first we gave injections within three to five minutes; lately injections of smaller dosage have been given within one to two minutes, with perfect safety.

One to two minutes after the injection, physiologic curarization effect is seen as described above. When the patient is barely able to lift the head or legs, the peak reaction has occurred. About two minutes after the curare injection, the estimated convulsant dose of metrazol is given.

Since my preliminary report, (10) we have gained more confidence in the treatment and find that we no longer need take any precautions such as hyperextension or the use of tongue gag, recommended at first to prevent complications. By the time the patient regains consciousness, the effect of curare has disappeared. Metrazol seems to be at least partially antidotal in its action.

Although patients are not able to thrash about after ad-

TABLE I. From September 1937 to September 1939 (99 Cases—89 Depressive and 10 Manic)

Diagnosis	Number of Cases	Results*	Relapse
All types of depressions	89	46 A	
		39 B	11 (1 suicide)
		4 C	
Manic excitement	10	5 A	
		4 B	2
		1 C	

*Results:

A—complete remission with full insight; return to former social level.

B—Social remission, able to adjust at home but with some residual symptoms, usually anxiety. Incomplete insight.

C—Unimproved.

Comment.—Of 89 depressed patients, 46, or 51 per cent, obtained a full remission lasting up to two years; 39, or 44 per cent, obtained a social recovery, but 11, or 12 per cent, relapsed requiring repeated treatment. Five of these were again improved to a good social level. Four patients, or 4 per cent, were unimproved by treatment. Five, or 50 per cent, of 10 manic states obtained a full clinical remission lasting up to two years. Four, or 40 per cent, obtained a social remission, but two relapsed, requiring state hospital commitment; one was unimproved.

We are unable to give accurately the percentage of traumatic spinal lesions in this series because routine radiographic studies were not made. We believe the incidence of traumatic spinal lesions was at least 25 per cent, judging by the frequency of subjective symptoms—mainly back pain. The incidence of extremity fractures was four, two femur and two humeri; and two dislocations.

ministration of metrazol, they should be carefully watched for evidence of respiratory embarrassment until consciousness is fully regained. Ampoules of epinephrin and prostigmin should be available for injection as an antidote. If respiratory failure should occur, artificial respiration should be effective, since the excretion of the drug is rapid and the patient will spontaneously regain breathing power within a short time. It is doubtful whether respiratory failure need be feared unless too large a dose or too rapid an injection of curare is employed. The criterion to be followed is sufficient curare to paralyze the muscles of the neck and back—when the patient is unable to raise the head, sufficient motor paresis has been produced for metrazol to be given. Care must be used not to allow the patient's head to fall backwards as his neck muscles are powerless. Advice has been given to hold the relaxed jaw forward if the patient's tongue interferes with respiration. As experience is gained with the method, less curare is used. It is not necessary to produce complete paresis of the neck or legs in order to soften the convulsive shock sufficiently to prevent fractures.

There is no increased tolerance to repeated doses of curare, nor are larger doses of metrazol required to induce a convulsion. However, to avoid failure, we usually give one-half to one cc. more metrazol than estimated, since the effect of curare may begin to wear off before a second metrazol injection can be given. If a sub-convulsive dose of metrazol is given, a one cc. larger dose than the original should be given as soon as possible before the curare effect disappears.

The patient's dread of treatment and postconvulsive discomfort is much less from combined curare-metrazol than from metrazol alone. The nursing problem is likewise simplified. Patients upon regaining consciousness have less

TABLE II. Results Obtained in 74 Cases by Combined Curare-Metrazol Shock Therapy (October 1939–April 15, 1940)

Diagnosis	Number of Cases/ Sex	Age	Duration of Psychosis	Average Shocks	Average Hospital Days	Total Curare-Metrazol Shocks	*Results	Remarks
(A) AFFECTIVE DISORDERS—(52 Depressive and 6 Manic States)								
Reactive depression	10 4—F 6—M	19–76	2 wks.–5 yrs.	4.8	46.4	48	7—A 3—B	1—Relapse (recovered second course). 2—Had serious organic disease.
Manic depressive	29 18—F 11—M	21–77	2 mo.–5 yrs.	6.5	41.5	188	18—A 10—B 1—C	2—Had serious organic disease. 2—did not finish treatment. 3—Treated as out-patients.
Involutional melancholia	13 7—F 6—M	41–68	2wks.–2yrs. 5 over 1 yr.	6.3	48.6	82	6—A 7—B	2—Had serious organic disease
Manic states	6 3—F 3—M	22–59	1 wk.–4 mo.	5.4	31.4	32	3—A 3—B	
Total	58	19–77	1 wk.–5 yrs.	5.7	41.9	350	34—A 23—B 1—C	29, 40%, were over 45 yrs. 17, 30%, were over 55 yrs. 8, 14%, were over 60 yrs. 4, 7%, were over 65 yrs.
(B) SCHIZOPHRENIA AND PSYCHONEUROSES—(11 Schizophrenics, 5 Psychoneuroses)								
Schizophrenia	11 6—F 5—M	16–52	5 da.–8 yrs.	8.5	60.6	93	1—A 6—B 4—C	2—Treated as out-patients.
	4—F		6 mo.–20 yrs.	5.5	49.5	23	1—A	
	1—M						2—B	2—Treated as out-patients
Psychoneuroses	5	35–42					2—C	1—Discontinued treatment.

*Results:

A—Complete remission with full insight,, return to former social level.

B—Social remission,, able to adjust at home,, but with some residual symptoms,, usually anxiety.

C—Unimproved.

Comment on Entire Series—74 patients received 466 curare-metrazol shocks. No complications occurred. Dosage of metrazol was from 4 to 10 cc. Three patients did not finish course of treatment; 7 patients were treated as out-patients.

nausea and headache and no muscular aching, thus eliminating much post-convulsive treatment, such as external heat or drugs for pain. Furthermore, other patients on the ward are less disturbed, because there are no remarks about severity or dreadfulness of shock treatment. Patients having had both methods much prefer the combined curare-metrazol procedure.

Figs. 2 and 3 show the contrast between a straight metrazol convulsion and a combined curare-metrazol seizure in the same patient, illustrating the remarkable diminution of muscular contraction.

Since the preliminary report (10) on the actual technic of this method, the demand for curare has been difficult to supply. Through the gratuity of E. R. Squibb and Sons, concentrated aqueous extract of curare (intocostrin) has been supplied to several leading psychiatric institutions: New York Psychiatric Institute and Hospital, under the direction of Drs. Nolan Lewis, E. Barrera and M. Harris; George Washington University, Dr. Walter Freeman; Philadelphia General Hospital, Dr. J. F. Stouffer; Sheppard & Enoch Pratt Hospital, Dr. L. F. Woolley, Colorado Psychopathic Hospital, Dr. F. G. Ebaugh; University of Wisconsin, Dr. Hans Reese; Menninger Clinic, Dr. William Menninger; Milwaukee Sanitarium, Dr. L. H. Ziegler; Neurological Institute, Dr. Paul Hoefer; Hartford Hospital, Dr. Ralph

Tovell; The Tucker Sanatorium, Dr. Geo. S. Fultz, Jr.; Worcester State Hospital, Dr. Erel L. Guidone; Longview Hospital, Dr. D. Goldman.

While we have had no subjective symptoms even suggestive of traumatic skeletal lesions, with one exception, since instituting combined curare-metrazol shock therapy, we have carried out a series of roentgenographic studies to ascertain if spinal lesions have occurred. In 26 consecutive patients we have x-rayed the vertebral columns before and after a series of curare-metrazol shocks and in only one of these patients have we been able to demonstrate any evidence of compressive fracture. In this case a compressive fracture of the 7th dorsal vertebra occurred. This accident occurred in the state hospital series (see Table III). Difficulty in injecting metrazol, because of the patient's poor veins, allowed the protective effect of the curare to wear off. Therefore the patient had a very hard seizure. In a few other patients compression fractures were found, the result of previous metrazol therapy.

We have been satisfied from clinical experience that the same therapeutic effectiveness occurs with the combined treatment as reported previously in affective disorders with straight metrazol shock therapy. This opinion was confirmed by brain wave studies made by W. E. Rahm, research assistant in neurophysiology, New York Psychiatric Insti-

TABLE III. Lincoln State Hospital, Lincoln, Nebraska*—Combined Curare-Metrazol Shock Therapy

Diagnosis	Number of Cases/Sex	Age	Average Number of Shocks	Total Curare-Metrazol Shocks	Results	Complications
Schizophrenia	21 8—F 13—M	17–53	6	139	3—A 7—B 11—C	One compression fracture of 7th dorsal. Metrazol given after curarization had worn off.
Depressions	5 3—F 2—M	53–62	5.4	27	4—B 1—C	
Manic	1—M	32	4	4	1—C	
Total	27	17–62	5.1	163	3—A 11—B 13—C	

Comment.—This series of chronic state hospital patients was treated with smaller amounts of curare given by a more rapid injection, obtaining a maximum effect within 1½ minutes after injection. X-rays were taken before and after treatment. One spinal fracture occurred after the curare effect had disappeared. Poor veins caused inability to give metrazol promptly. The dosage of metrazol varied from 5 cc. to 12 cc. Previously in this hospital, spinal fractures were frequent and a few extremity fractures occurred.

*Treatments in this series were carried out by Drs. R. W. Gray and G. W. Russell under the direction of Dr. A. H. Fechner, superintendent.

tute, at a demonstration of the treatment at the Institute. The E. E. G. patterns made upon curarized patients subjected to metrazol shock therapy showed essentially the same pattern (see Fig. 4) as from metrazol alone. These findings simply corroborate the clinical observations that curare in no way influences the convulsive shock treatment except to lessen the severity of the spasmodic treatment and thus to eliminate the traumatic hazard.

In Table I the results obtained in affective disorders by metrazol treatment alone prior to curare therapy are listed.

In Table II we have evaluated the number of patients who have received in private practice at the Bishop Clarkson Memorial Hospital, combined curare and metrazol shock therapy; in Table III, those in the Lincoln State Hospital. These tables do not include experience with many spastic, athetoid, dystonic and hyperkinetic children and adult patients who have received curare treatments. In no institution, although the treatments have been administered by a number of physicians, have any toxic accidents occurred from administration of curare.

An attempt was made to procure data from collaborating institutions carrying on studies with combined curare-metrazol therapy. In most instances the series of completed cases is still too small to draw useful conclusions.

Up to April 15, 1940, reports upon 21 patients who received 109 curare-metrazol shocks have been sent from the following institutions: Philadelphia General Hospital, Dr. J. F. Stouffer; Sheppard & Enoch Pratt, Dr. L. F. Woolley; Milwaukee Sanitarium, Dr. L. H. Ziegler; and George Washington University, Dr. Walter Freeman. In general, these groups report the same good results in affective disorders with indifferent to poor results in schizophrenia. None observed any toxic symptoms from curare and no complications occurred.

The introduction of this improved method of therapy has enabled us to widen the scope of usefulness of convulsive shock therapy. We have had experience with a number of cases of depressive psychoses complicated by age factors or severe organic disease. These cases are worthy of report to illustrate the safety of treatment and the recovery of pa-

tients who would never have been able to withstand metrazol shock therapy alone. In my opinion hardly any of these patients could have made spontaneous recoveries without this therapy. They are all socially well adjusted individuals at the present time.

CASE HISTORIES OF UNUSUAL CASES HAVING RECEIVED CURARE-METRAZOL SHOCK TREATMENT

CASE I.—Male, age 61, developed a severe reactive agitated depression following a diagnosis of rectal carcinoma and the first stage colostomy. This mental state made the second stage operation impossible. Radium was then applied to the tumor, a progressive weight loss of 25 pounds occurred, and during convalescence the patient fell in a bathroom and sustained compression fracture of the spine. He was referred for psychiatric treatment.

Physical examination revealed undernutrition, anemia and good functioning colostomy with a bleeding mass high up in the rectum. The mental reaction was a characteristic agitated depression with fearful hypochondriacal delusions: "Everyone talks about me; all the bones in my body are broken; I'm going to be drowned, dissected, or put away," he begged to "get it over with" and wished to end it all. There were no sensorium changes.

Progress.—Three weeks of symptomatic treatment—nutritional, sedative and anti-anemic vitamin therapy made no change in the physical or mental state. Then over a period of one month, nine combined curare-metrazol shocks were given. Steady sustained mental improvement progressed to complete recovery with a rapid gain of weight. Three weeks after the last shock treatment, the rectal carcinoma was removed by abdomino-perineal resection. Post-operative convalescence was uneventful and the patient resumed full occupation as a business executive six weeks after the operation.

CASE II.—Female, age 54, had been handicapped by posterolateral sclerosis from pernicious anemia for 15 years. Excellent management had kept the blood count at high level, but the patient's ataxia required the use of a cane. Fifteen years before, upon learning she had pernicious anemia, the patient had a reactive depression lasting two months. Following a strenuous year of teaching and a physical examination in July, 1939, when it was suggested she might have hypertension and Bright's disease from

TABLE IV. Unusual Cases of Depression Complicated by Organic Disease

Case	Sex	Age	Organic Disease	Mental Status	Treatment	Result
1	M	61	Carcinoma (rectum). Colostomy—radiation sickness—compression fracture of the spine.	Reactive depression, making removal of carcinoma impossible.	Full mental recovery after 9 combined curare-metrazol shocks.	Carcinoma removed—able to return to full occupation as an executive.
2	F	54	Pernicious anemia, combined sclerosis of 14 yrs. duration. Patient ambulatory with cane.	Reactive depression.	Full recovery after five curare-metrazol shocks.	Resumed full occupation as college teacher.
3	M	64	Diabetes mellitus.	Severe agitated depression.	Full recovery after failure to improve on insulin. Recovery after 6 curare-metrazol shocks.	Returned to former social status.
4	F	77	Arteriosclerosis.	Reactive depression.	Full recovery after 7 curare-metrazol shocks.	Returned to former social status.
5	M	76	Right hemiplegia aphasia—coronary artery disease.	Severe agitated depression.	Three curare-metrazol shocks. Improved depressive reaction.	Able to be transferred to nursing home for custodial care.

Comment.—Five cases illustrate the increased safety of modified convulsive therapy by curare. All represent cases that would have been serious risks from straight metrazol; showing that this safer method enlarges the scope of usefulness of the therapy.

which her mother had died, the patient reacted at once with anxiety and depression. The patient was unable to resume college teaching the fall term of 1939.

Progress.—For three months, psychotherapeutic office treatment was given, but the depressive features became more marked; hypochondriacal fears of "constitutional diseases, insanity and incurability" with a persistent suicide drive continued. The economic problem was important, since the patient's source of livelihood would be gone unless teaching could be resumed by 1940. Convulsive shock therapy was advised. After five combined curare-metrazol shocks, the patient made a full and complete recovery and within five weeks after beginning treatment, she returned to full occupation as a college teacher.

CASE III.—Male, age 64, for six months had progressive weakness, weight loss and mental depression. He gave up work and self-accusatory delusions developed: He was a thief, people were coming to punish him. He shut himself from all contacts and threatened suicide. Observation in another institution revealed a 30 pound weight loss, arteriosclerosis and diabetes mellitus. He was referred for psychiatric treatment.

Progress.—The mental reaction was characterized by marked depression, inactivity, attempts to seclude himself in dark places, at times mutism and other times restlessness with extreme apprehension. Three weeks of diabetic high caloric diet therapy with adequate insulin failed to produce a weight gain or influence the mental state. After six combined curare-metrazol shocks the patient gained 20 pounds and made a complete recovery. The diabetic condition was then readily controlled by protamine zinc insulin. This recovery was effected within a two months hospitalization period.

CASE IV.—Female, age 77, had had a previous reactive depression at 63 years of age, lasting a few weeks. Following the sudden death of her husband in August, 1939, the patient again became depressed, apprehensive, agitated and uninterested. After four months she was hospitalized for treatment.

Progress.—Within five weeks, after seven combined curare-metrazol shocks, the patient made a full and complete recovery.

CASE V.—Male, aged 76, had suffered at age 72 a cerebral thrombosis with right sided involvement and aphasia. After several months he was able to be up in a wheel chair. For the past two years he had given up completely, was depressed, tearful, blamed his family for mistreatment and remained constantly in bed. He was admitted for psychiatric observation.

Examination showed a marked spastic right hemiplegia, motor aphasia, coronary artery disease and hypertension of 190/110. The mental reaction was that of extreme emotionalism, irritability, paranoidal ideas and a wish to die.

Progress.—Three combined curare-metrazol shocks were given for the purpose of removing the depressive features. The patient withstood these treatments without ill effect. Improvement in the mental attitude was so marked that the patient became ambulatory in a wheel chair and could be transferred to a nursing home for permanent custodial care.

COMMENT ON THE FIVE CASES

The results obtained illustrate the increased safety of combined curare-metrazol therapy as shown by its successful use with Cases IV and V, ages 77 and 76. These aged patients would have been serious risks if treated by metrazol alone. The effect of the treatment upon patients II and III, with diabetes and pernicious anemia was extremely interesting, illustrating the fact that serious organic diseases do not influence the therapeutic effectiveness. I would not have had the courage to treat either patient with straight metrazol. Case I looked particularly hopeless because of the complication of rectal carcinoma, radiation sickness, and fractured vertebral column. The outcome here speaks for the extreme value of the therapy. I doubt if recovery, physical or mental, could have been accomplished by any other method.

SYNTHETIC CURARE

The problem of collecting and preparing curare entails considerable difficulty, as already discussed. A synthetic preparation would be an important advance in therapy, especially if a sustained curare-like effect followed oral administration.

Quinine has been known for some time to have a curariform action as shown by its relaxing effect upon myotonia congenita and dystonia musculorum deformans. It also aggravates myasthenia gravis symptoms. The commercially available quinine salts, however, have too weak a curarelike action to be useful in convulsive shock therapy. Prior to using curare I tried quinine sulphate, but could not demonstrate any reduction in severity of convulsions by its use.

King has shown that in curare there are certain tertiary ammonium bases. It has also been known that quaternary ammonium compounds formed by the addition of alkyl radicles to the nitrogen atom of the quinoline ring have a curare-like action. Dr. H. King (13) has prepared a synthetic compound called quinine methochloride, formed by the addition of a methyl group to the quinuclidine nucleus of the quinine molecule. Harvey (14) has shown that this drug has a strong curare-like action when administered either orally or parenterally.

Through the courtesy of E. R. Squibb and Sons' research department, I was furnished quinine methochloride for experimentation. An aqueous solution was prepared containing 18 mg. per cc. In spastic paralysis immediate complete curariform action was seen after intravenous injection with 10-15 mg. per kilo of weight. Prior to convulsive shock therapy a complete relaxation of body musculature was obtained in all patients with 7-10 mg. per kilo of weight similar to that seen under curare. This curare-like effect, dependent upon the amount of drug used, markedly reduced the severity of the convulsive seizure.

From our experience so far, with this drug, we believe it will adequately prevent traumatic complications of convulsive shock therapy. However, we are not as yet certain about its margin of safety. In some instances after the convulsion the period of apnea was prolonged, suggesting more respiratory embarrassment than seen from curare; artificial respiration and prostigmin were necessary to restore normal breathing. Following intravenous injection there was also a decided drop in blood pressure that we have not seen from curare unless it is injected too rapidly. By the end of the metrazol shock, however, the blood pressure was back to original or higher levels. Whether the action of the drug is a pure curare effect is still not settled. The quinine may have other side effects. The curare-like action from quinine methochloride is transient and wears off as rapidly as from straight curare. Because of the relative insolubility of the drug, larger volumes of solution have to be given.

Further experimentation will be necessary before the drug can be safely recommended; also, to ascertain whether the drug can be successfully used orally to diminish metrazol convulsive seizures.

CONCLUSIONS

1. Convulsive shock therapy has proved most useful as a means of terminating chronic resistant affective psychoses.

2. The usefulness of this therapy has been restricted and has been in danger of abandonment because of the severity of the convulsive shock with the hazards of traumatic complications.

3. There is something fundamentally sound in the application of this therapy. The problem has been to eliminate the traumatic hazards.

4. Previous attempts to eliminate traumatic complications have not been successful.

5. The principle of preliminary curarization before induction of metrazol shock has proved successful in eliminating all traumatic hazards.

6. A uniform standardized curare preparation has now been perfected that is non-toxic in physiologic doses and has proved to be a safe treatment.

7. The physiologic and pharmacologic effects of the drug have been discussed. The technic of this combined therapy is described.

8. Roentgenographic evidence and electro-encephalographic evidence are presented to show that the curare protects from traumatic complications, yet leaves the therapeutic effectiveness of metrazol undisturbed.

9. The results of previous metrazol therapy in affective psychoses are compared with curare-metrazol results to show the same therapeutic results are obtained without complication. Other investigators have confirmed our results with this new treatment.

10. A series of cases of depressive psychoses complicated with severe organic diseases are shown that widen the scope of usefulness of this modified therapy. A number of cases can now be salvaged that formerly could not have taken the treatment.

11. Curare is "tailor made" as a "shock absorber" for convulsive shock therapy.

12. A synthetic curare-like drug, quinine methochloride, has been prepared that has been shown to have a strong curare-like action. After intravenous injection it produces effective motor paresis sufficient to prevent traumatic complications of convulsive shock therapy. Further experimentation will be necessary, however, to determine the safety factor, before its use can be recommended.

13. If a continued, sustained supply of pure curare or a safe synthetic curare-like drug can be obtained, it will soon be illegitimate to administer convulsive shock therapy without this safeguard against the all too frequent and serious traumatic accidents.

BIBLIOGRAPHY

1. Meduna, Ladislaus: Versuche über die biologische Beeinflüssung des Ablaufes der Schizophrenie; Campher und Cardiazalkrampfe. Ztschr. f.d. ges. Neurol. u. Psychiat., 152:253–262 (Feb. 19), 1935.

2. Bennett, A.E.: Convulsive shock therapy in chronic depressive psychoses, Bull. Menninger Clinic, 2:97, 1938; Am. J. Med. Sci., 1936:420 (Sept.), 1938.

3. Bennett, A.E.: Metrazol convulsive shock therapy in affective psychoses, Am. J. Med. Sci., 198:695–701 (Nov.), 1939.

4. Bennett, A.E., Nielsen, J.C., Fechner, A.H., and Cash, P.T.: Combined artificial fever and chemotherapy in dementia paralytica. Arch. Phys. Therapy, 20:620–627 (Oct.), 1939.

5. Carp, Louis: Fracture and dislocations by muscular violence, complication convulsions induced by metrazol for schizophrenia. Ann. of Surg., 110:107–118 (July), 1939.

6. Polatin, Philip, Friedman, M.M., and Harris, M.M.: Vertebral fractures produced by metrazol induced convulsions, J. A. M. A., 112: 1684–1687 (April 29), 1939.

7. Hamsa, W.R., and Bennett, A.E.: Traumatic complications of convulsive shock therapy. J. A. M. A., 112:2244–2246 (June 3), 1939.
8. Alexander, F.A.D., and Himwich, H.E.: Nitrogen inhalation therapy for schizophrenia. Am. J. Psychiat., 96:3 (Nov.), 1939.
9. Burman, M.S.: Therapeutic use of curare and erythroidine hydrochloride for spastic and dystonic states. Arch. Neurol. and Psych., 41:307–327 (Feb.), 1939.
10. West, Ranyard: The pharmacology and therapeutic action of curare and its constituents. Proc. Royal Med. Soc., London, 28:565–578 (Jan. 8), 1935.

11. Bennett, A.E.: Preventing traumatic complications in convulsive shock therapy by curare, J. A. M. A., 114:322–324 (Jan. 27), 1940.
12. Strauss, Hans, and Rahm, W.E. Jr.: The effect of metrazol injections on the electroencephalogram. Psychiat. Quart., 14:43–48 (Jan.), 1940.
13. King, Dr. H.: Nature, 135:469 (1935), quoted by Harvey, A.M.: The action of quinine methochloride on neuromuscular transmission. Bull. Johns Hopkins Hospital, LXVI:52–59 (Jan.), 1940.
14. Harvey, A.M.: The action of quinine methochloride on neuromuscular transmission. Bull. Johns Hopkins Hospital, LXVI: 52–59 (Jan.), 1940.

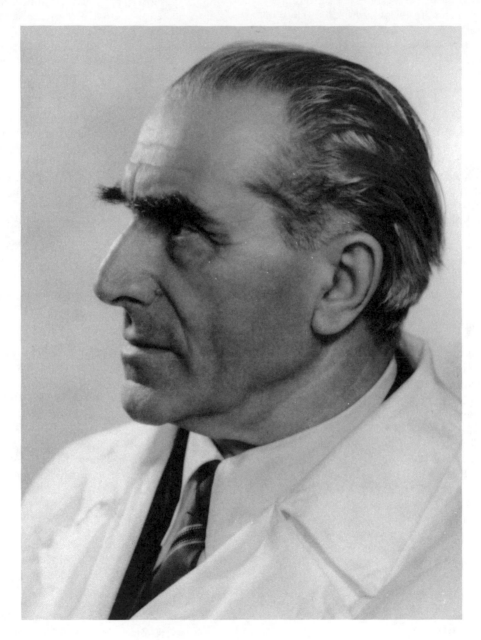

Ugo Cerletti, M.D., 1877–1963

Ugo Cerletti, working with L. Bini, was the first to demonstrate the superiority of electroconvulsive treatment to Metrazol. The first ECT was administered in 1938 to a patient with schizophrenia.

THE SOCIETY OF ALCOHOLICS ANONYMOUS

By William W.

Co-founder

Alcoholics Anonymous is grateful for this invitation to appear before The American Psychiatric Association. It is a most happy circumstance. Being laymen we have naught but a story to tell, hence the quite personal and unscientific character of this narrative. Whatever their deeper implications the attitudes and events leading to the formation of Alcoholics Anonymous are easy to portray.

Two alcoholics talk across a kitchen table. One is drinking, the other not. Severe chronics, the threat of commitment hangs over both. The time is November 1934. The active drinker became, years later, the writer of this paper. My sober visitor was an old friend and schoolmate, long catalogued by physicians and family as hopeless. I enjoyed the same rating and well knew it.

My friend had arrived to tell how he had been released from alcohol. In truth, the quality of his sobriety seemed "different." Having made contact with the Oxford Group, a nondenominational, evangelical movement, my friend had been specially impressed by an alcoholic he had met, a former patient of C. G. Jung. Unsuccessfully treating this individual for a year, Dr. Jung had finally advised him to try religious conversion as his last chance. While disagreeing with many tenets of the Oxford Group, my former schoolmate did, however, ascribe his new sobriety to certain ideas that this alcoholic and other Oxford people had given him. The particular practices my friend had selected for himself were simple:

1. He admitted he was powerless to solve his own problem.

2. He got honest with himself as never before; made an examination of conscience.

3. He made a rigorous confession of his personal defects.

4. He surveyed his distorted relations with people, visiting them to make restitution.

5. He resolved to devote himself to helping others in need, without the usual demand for personal prestige or material gain.

6. By meditation he sought God's direction for his life and help to practice these principles at all times.

This sounded pretty naive to me. Nevertheless my friend stuck to the plain tale of what had happened—no evangelizing. He related how, practicing these precepts, his drinking had unaccountably stopped. Fear and isolation left and he had received considerable peace of mind. With no hard disciplines nor any great resolves, these attributes began to appear the moment he conformed. His release was a by-product. Though sober but months, he felt he had a basic answer. Wisely avoiding any argument, he then took leave. The spark that was to become Alcoholics Anonymous had been struck.

What then did happen at the kitchen table? Perhaps this speculation were better left to medicine and religion. I confess I do not know. Possibly conversion will never be fully understood. Looking outward from such an experience, I can only say with fidelity what seemed to happen. Yet something did happen that instantly changed the current of my life. I haven't had a drink for over 14 years. All else will be mere personal opinion—or just fancy.

My friend's story had generated mixed emotions; I was drawn and revolted by turns. My solitary drinking went on, but I could not forget his visit. Several themes coursed in my mind: First, that his evident state of release was strangely and immensely convincing. Second, that he had been pronounced hopeless by competent medicos. Third, that those age-old precepts, *when transmitted by him*, had struck me with great power. Fourth, that I could not, and would not, go along with any God concept. No conversion nonsense for me. Thus did I ponder. Trying to divert my thoughts, I found it no use. By cords of understanding, suffering, and simple verity, another alcoholic had bound me to him. I could not break away.

One morning after my gin a realization welled up. "Who are you," I asked, "to choose how you are going to get well? Beggars are not choosers. Suppose medicine said carcinoma was your trouble. You would not turn to Pond's extract. In abject haste you would beg a doctor to kill those hellish cancer cells. If he didn't stop them, and you thought conversion could, your pride would fly away. You would soon stand in public squares crying 'Amen' along with the other victims. What difference then," I reflected, "between you and the cancer victim? His sick body crumbles. Likewise your personality crumbles, your obsession consigns you to madness or the undertaker. Are you going to try your friend's formula—or not?"

Of course I did try. In December, 1934, I appeared at Towns Hospital, New York. My old friend, Dr. W. D. Silkworth, shook his head. Soon free of sedation and alcohol, I felt horribly depressed. My alcoholic friend turned up.

Read at the 105th annual meeting of The American Psychiatric Association, Montreal, Quebec, May 23-27, 1949.

Though glad to see him, I shrank a little. I feared evangelism. Nothing of this sort happened. After small talk, I again asked him about the Oxford Groups. Quietly, sanely enough, he told me, and then departed.

Lying there in conflict, I dropped into black depression. Momentarily my prideful obstinacy was crushed. I cried out, "Now I'm ready to do anything—anything to receive what my good friend has." Expecting naught, I made this frantic appeal: "If there be a God, will he show himself!" The result was instant, electric, beyond description. The place lit up, blinding white. I knew only ecstasy and seemed on a mountain. A great wind blew, enveloping and permeating me. It was not of air, but of Spirit. Blazing, came the tremendous thought, "You are a free man!" Then ecstasy subsided. Still on the bed, I was now in another world of consciousness which was suffused by a Presence. One with the Universe, a great peace stole over me and I thought, "So this is the God of the preachers; this is the Great Reality." But reason returned, my modern education took over. Obviously I had gone crazy. I became terribly frightened.

Dr. Silkworth came in to hear my trembling account of the phenomenon. He assured me I was not mad; that I had perhaps undergone an experience which might solve my problem. Skeptical man of science he then was; this was most kind and astute. If he had said "hallucination" I might now be dead. To him I shall be eternally grateful.

Good fortune pursued me. Somebody brought a book entitled "Varieties of Religious Experience" and I devoured it. Written by James, the psychologist, it suggests that conversion can have objective reality. Conversion does alter motivation, and does semi-automatically enable a person to be and do the formerly impossible. Significant it was, that marked conversion experiences come mostly to individuals who know complete defeat in a controlling area. The book certainly showed variety. But bright or dim, cataclysmic or gradual, theological or intellectual in bearing, such conversions did have common denominators, they did change utterly defeated people. And so declared William James. The shoe fitted. I have tried to wear it ever since. For drunks, the obvious answer was deflation *at depth* and more of it. That seemed plain as a pikestaff. I had been trained as an engineer, so the views of this authoritative psychologist meant everything to me.

Armored now by utter conviction, and fortified by my characteristic power drive, I took off to cure alcoholics wholesale. It was twin jet propulsion; difficulties meant nothing. The vast conceit of my project never occurred to me. I pressed my assault for 6 months; my home was filled with alcoholics. Harangues with scores produced not the slightest result. None of them got it. Disappointingly, my friend of the kitchen table, who was sicker than I realized, took little interest in these other alcoholics. This fact may have caused his endless backslides later on. For I had found that working with alcoholics had a huge bearing on my own sobriety. But why wouldn't any of my new prospects sober up?

Slowly the bugs came to light. Like a religious crank, I was obsessed with the idea that everybody must have a "spiritual experience" just like mine. I'd forgotten that there were many varieties. So my brother alcoholics just stared incredulously or kidded me about my "hot flash." This had spoiled the potent identification so easy to get with them. I had turned evangelist. Clearly the deal had to be streamlined. What came to me in 6 minutes might require 6 months in others. It was to be learned that words are things, that one must be prudent. It was also certain that something ailed the deflationary technique. It definitely lacked wallop. Reasoning that the alcoholic's "hex," or compulsion, must issue from some deep level, it followed that ego deflation must also go deep or else there couldn't be any fundamental release. Apparently religious practice would not touch the alcoholic until his underlying situation was made ready. Fortunately all the tools were right at hand. You doctors supplied them.

The emphasis was straightway shifted from "sin" to "sickness"—the *"fatal malady,"* alcoholism. We quoted doctors that alcoholism was more lethal than cancer; that it consisted of an obsession of the mind coupled to increasing body sensitivity. These were our Twin Ogres of Madness and Death. We leaned heavily on Dr. Jung's statement how hopeless the condition could be and then poured that devastating dose into every drunk within range. To modern man, science is omnipotent; it is a god. Hence if science would pass a death sentence on the drunk, and we placed that verdict on our alcoholic transmission belt, it might shatter him completely. Perhaps he would then turn to the God of the theologian, there being no place else to go. Whatever truth in this device, it certainly had practical merit. Immediately our whole atmosphere changed. Things began to look up.

Bankrupt at the time, I stumbled into a business venture. It took me to Akron, Ohio, where the deal quickly collapsed leaving me dispirited. Alone, I panicked in fear of getting drunk. *This was something new for I realized that I hadn't thought of drinking since the December 1934 experience.* I could now see my peril clearly and thus brush off the usual rationalizations. With relief, I perceived that my new spiritual conditioning really meant something now that the heat was on. But that didn't stop the compulsive uprush of drinking desire. I needed to talk to another alcoholic, and quickly.

Shortly I was introduced to Dr. Robert S., a surgeon. He was an alcoholic in a bad way. This time there was no preachment from me. I told him my experience, and what I thought I knew about alcoholism. Needing him as much as he did me, there was genuine mutuality for the first time and, as we now say in AA, he soon "clicked" never to drink again. That was June 1935. We began to spend long hours on drunks at a local hospital. One of them is sober yet, no relapse. Though nameless, the first AA Group had actually started. Dr. S. has since hospitalized some 4,000 cases at Akron. The bulk have recovered. All this too without a cent of monetary return to him. Thus he became co-founder of Alcoholics Anonymous. As I left Akron in September 1935 three alcoholics were staying sober. Arrived at New York, I set to work and another AA group took shape. But nothing was very sure; we still flew blind.

It was soon necessary to retire from the Oxford Group. The good people there had disapproved us. For our purpose, the Oxford Group atmosphere wasn't entirely right. Their demands for absolute moral rectitude encouraged guilt and rebellion. Either will get alcoholics drunk, and did. As non-alcoholic evangelists, they couldn't understand that. Good friends, these, we owed them much. From them we had learned what, and what not, to do.

Then commenced a 3-year season of trial and error eventuating in our textbook, "Alcoholics Anonymous," published in 1939.

That book, now backbone of our AA society, opens with a typical story of drinking and recovery. Next comes a chapter of hope, entitled "There Is A Solution." In AA vernacular 2 chapters describe alcoholism and the alcoholic, their object being of course to first identify and then deflate. A chapter is devoted to softening up the agnostic. This leads to the "Twelve Steps" of present-day Alcoholics Anonymous. The heart of our therapy, and a practical way of life, these "Steps" are little but an amplified and streamlined version of the principles enumerated by my friend of the kitchen table. These being quite well known, I shall leave them to a footnote.[1]

The balance of the text is mostly devoted to practical application of these "Twelve Steps," and to reducing inner resistances of the reader. Working with other alcoholics is very heavily emphasized. Chapters are devoted to wives, family relations, and employers. The final chapter pictures the new society and begs the recovered alcoholic to form a group himself. This ideology is then shored up by 30 case histories, or rather stories, written by AA members. These complete the identification and stir hope. The 400 pages of "Alcoholics Anonymous" contain no theory; they narrate experience only.

When the book appeared in April 1939, we had about 100 members. One-third of these had impressive sobriety records. The movement had spread to Cleveland and drifted toward Chicago and Detroit. In the East it inclined to Philadelphia and Washington. There was an extraordinary event at Cleveland. The *Plain Dealer* published strong pieces about us backed by editorials. A barrage of telephone calls descended on 20 AA members, mostly new people. AA book in hand, they took on all comers. New members worked with the still newer. Two years later, Cleveland had garnered by this chain reaction hundreds of new members. The batting average was excellent. It was our first evidence that we might digest huge members rapidly.

Then came great national publicity. The *Saturday Evening Post* piece (March 1941) shot thousands of frantic inquiries into our tiny New York office. This gave us lists of alcoholics in hundreds of cities. Business men traveling

out of established AA centers used these names to start new groups. By sending literature and writing often, AA groups sprung up by mail. With no personal contact whatever, this was astounding. Clergy and medical men began to give their approval. I wish to say that Dr. Harry Tiebout, chairman of our discussion today, was the first psychiatrist ever to observe and befriend us. Alcoholics Anonymous mushroomed. The pioneering had ended. We were on the U. S. map.

As of 1949 our quantity results are these: The 14-year-old society of Alcoholics Anonymous has 80,000 members in about 3,000 groups. We have entry into 30 foreign countries and U. S. possessions; translations are going forward. By occupation we are an accurate cross section of America. By religious affiliation we are about 40% Catholic; nominal and active Protestants, also many former agnostics, and a sprinkling of Jews comprise the remainder. Ten to 15% are women. Some Negroes are recovering without undue difficulty. Top medical and religious endorsements are almost universal. AA membership is pyramiding, chain style, at the rate of about 30% a year. During 1949, we expect 20,000 permanent recoveries, at least. Half of these will be medium or mild cases (average age about 36)—a fairly recent development.

Of alcoholics who stay with us and really try, 50% get sober at once and stay that way, 25% do so after some relapses and the remainder usually show improvement. But many problem drinkers do quit AA after a brief contact, maybe three or four out of five. Some are too psychopathic or damaged. But the majority have powerful rationalizations yet to be broken down. Exactly this does happen providing they get what AA calls a "good exposure," on first contact. Alcohol then builds such a hot fire that they are finally driven back to us, often years later. These tell us that they *had* to return; it was AA or else. They had learned about alcoholism from alcoholics; they were hit harder than they had known. Such cases leave us the agreeable impression that half our original exposures will eventually return, most of them to recover. So we just indoctrinate the newcomer. We never evangelize; Barleycorn will look after that. The clergy declare we have capitalized the Devil. These claims are considerable but we think them conservative. The ultimate recovery rate will certainly be larger than once supposed.

Such is a glimpse of our origin, central therapeutic idea, and quantity result. The qualitative result is assuredly too large a subject for this paper.

Alcoholics Anonymous is not a religious organization;

---

1 Here are the steps we took which are *suggested* as a Program of Recovery:

    1. We admitted we were powerless over alcohol—that our lives had become unmanageable.

    2. Came to believe that a Power greater than ourselves could restore us to sanity.

    3. Made a decision to turn our will and our lives over to the care of God *As We Understood Him*.

    4. Made a searching and fearless moral inventory of ourselves.

    5. Admitted to God, to ourselves, and to another human being the exact nature of our wrongs.

    6. Were entirely ready to have God remove all these defects of character.

    7. Humbly asked Him to remove our shortcomings.

    8. Made a list of all persons we had harmed, and became willing to make amends to them all.

    9. Made direct amends to such people wherever possible, except when to do so would injure them or others.

    10. Continued to take personal inventory and when we were wrong promptly admitted it.

    11. Sought through prayer and meditation to improve or conscious contact with God as we understood Him, praying only for knowledge of His will for us and the power to carry that out.

    12. Having had a spiritual experience as the result of these steps, we tried to carry this message to alcoholics, and to practice these principles in all our affairs.

there is no dogma. The one theological proposition is a "Power greater than one's self." Even this concept is forced on no one. The newcomer merely immerses himself in our society and tries the program as best he can. Left alone, he will surely report the gradual onset of a transforming experience, call it what he may. Observers once thought AA could appeal only to the religiously susceptible. Yet our membership includes a former member of the American Atheist Society and about 20,000 others almost as tough. The dying can become remarkably open minded. Of course we speak little of conversion nowadays because so many people really dread being God-bitten. But conversion, as broadly described by James, does seem to be our basic process; all other devices are but the foundation. When one alcoholic works with another he but consolidates and sustains that essential experience.

The forces of anarchy, democracy, and dictatorship play impressive roles in the structure and containment of our society; Barleycorn the Tyrant Dictator is quite impersonal. But Hitler never did have a Gestapo half so effective. When the anarchy of the alcoholic faces his tyrant, that alcoholic must become a social animal or perish. Perforce, our society has settled for the purest kind of democracy. Naturally, the explosive potential of our rather neurotic fellowship is enormous. As elsewhere, it gathers closely around those external provocators: power, money, and sex. Throughout AA these subterranean volcanos erupt at least a thousand times daily; explosions we now view with some humor, considerable magnanimity, and little fear at all. We think them valuable object lessons for development. Our deep kinship, the urgency of our mission, the need to abate our neurosis for contented survival; all these, together with love for God and man, have contained us in surprising unity. There seems safety in numbers. Enough sand bags muffle any amount of dynamite. We think we are a pretty secure, happy family. Drop by any AA meeting for a look.

Many AA members see that psychiatry may some day greatly enlarge our present resources.

For example: As you observe, I am a person of depressive and paranoid tendency. Surely you must ask, "What is going to happen to that man when his power drive wears off or hits something too hard? Minus alcohol, won't he explode?" A very good question, that. Some years ago, my power drive did wear off and I hit frustration hard. But I neither exploded nor turned to alcohol. That comfortable fact may be due to long AA conditioning which had probably cut off my neurosis somewhere below the compulsive drinking level; but 18 months' psychiatry did remove certain festering neurotic roots, and hence my heavy depression. Numbers of AA's, thus bedeviled, are trying psychiatry. Most of us, though, are getting off far easier.

There isn't the slightest evidence that violent neurosis, drunkenness, or lunacy is to be the destiny of Alcoholics Anonymous. Such dark forecasts have not materialized.

Many an alcoholic is now sent to AA by his own psychiatrist. Relieved of his drinking, he returns to the doctor a far easier subject. Practically every alcoholic's wife has become, to a degree, his possessive mother. Most alcoholic women, if they still have a husband, live with a baffled father. This sometimes spells trouble aplenty. We AA's certainly ought to know! So, gentlemen, here is a big problem right up your alley.

Now to conclude: We of AA try to be aware that we may never touch but a segment of the total alcohol problem. We try to remember that our growing success may prove a heady wine; that our own resources will always be limited. So then, will you men and women of medicine be our partners; physicians wielding well your invisible scalpels; workers all, in our common cause? We like to think Alcoholics Anonymous a middle ground between medicine and religion, the missing catalyst of a new synthesis. This to the end that the millions who will suffer may presently issue from their darkness into the light of day!

I am sure that none, attending this great Hall of Medicine will feel it untoward if I leave the last word to our silent partner, Religion:

God grant us the serenity to accept the things we cannot change, courage to change the things we can, and wisdom to know the difference.

NOTE.—Following the reading of this paper time did not permit me a word of appreciation for the generous comment by Dr. G. Kirby Collier, one of our earliest friends and a most steadfast supporter of our cause. Nor, on behalf of Alcoholics Anonymous as a whole, could I express the deep gratitude we feel for having had the opportunity of presenting our point of view before the American Psychiatric Association at Montreal.

The Use of Antabuse (Tetraethylthiuramdisulphide) in Chronic Alcoholics

By S. Eugene Barrera, M.D., Walter A. Osinski, M.D., and Eugene Davidoff, M.D.

Albany, New York

Renewed widespread interest in the drug therapy of chronic alcoholism has been awakened recently by studies of Jacobsen and his collaborators (1–6) concerning Antabuse (tetraethylthiuramdisulfide). The reports of these Scandinavian investigators suggested that Antabuse was potentially more effective than previous pharmacotherapeutic procedures in the treatment of chronic alcoholism. Papers concerning the physiology and pharmacology of Antabuse have also been published by these observers (7–10).

According to Martensen-Larsen (3), Antabuse taken in doses 2–3 grams gives no symptoms, except fatigue. After consumption of even small amounts of alcohol, however, a series of unpleasant symptoms develops. With a blood alcohol concentration of 10–20 mg%, a deep flushing of the face results with consequent rise in skin temperature. The pulse is accelerated and increase in the cardiac impulse is observed. At somewhat higher doses, 30–60 mg%, nausea and vomiting may occur. As a rule blood pressure is unchanged or slightly reduced. The cardiac output increases about 50%, and the ventilation increases 100% or more. The carbon dioxide percentage in the alveolar air falls from about 5% to 4%. The symptom complex is accompanied with unpleasant subjective symptoms of uneasiness, fatigue, a pounding sensation of the heart, and shortness of breath.

The symptoms are considered to be due to a formation of acetaldehyde because intravenous infusions of acetaldehyde, resulting in concentrations corresponding to those observed after ingestion of Antabuse and alcohol, give the same symptoms. In the blood, an increase of acetaldehyde is seen (5–10 times that obtained after the same dose of alcohol is taken by individuals not treated with Antabuse).

The condition described above persists for ½–4 hours after consumption of alcohol and is followed by a state of fatigue and sleepiness. The "hypersensitivity" to alcohol, after the ingestion of Antabuse, begins as a rule within a few hours and can be traced for 10–14 days after discontinuing the drug.

Some patients may suffer fatigue for several months, but otherwise the treatment results in no undesirable aftereffects. No severe pathological changes have been noted in urine analysis, liver function tests, electrocardiograms, and blood counts.

If treated with adequate doses of Antabuse, all patients develop the described symptoms after consumption of alcohol. No habituation to the drug occurs. On the contrary, the sensitivity of alcohol increases with continued or repeated treatment, and the dose of Antabuse can be decreased accordingly.

METHOD OF PROCEDURE

This phase of the preliminary report conducted at the Albany Hospital and the Mental Hygiene Clinic, Veterans Administration Center, Watervliet, New York, is purely clinical and psychiatric in nature. Thus far, 21 patients have been studied for a minimum of 2 months and a maximum of 4 months. They were all habitual drinkers. Fourteen patients had initial periods of hospitalization and were later followed in the outpatient clinic. Seven of the patients were followed in the outpatient clinic throughout their treatment and observation. All patients received careful and complete physical, neurologic, neuropsychiatric, and routine laboratory examinations before drug therapy was started.

The first group of 5 patients treated with Antabuse was started on the medication shortly after admission to the hospital. At that time, the acute symptoms resulting from a recent alcoholic debauch had not yet completely subsided. As a test procedure a minimum of psychotherapy was used. The patients were merely told the drug might help them overcome the alcoholism, that there might be some unpleasant effects, and that, if they chose to, it was up to them to take the drug for an indefinite period of time.

These first 5 patients treated were given 1.5 grams of Antabuse on the first day, 0.75 gram each morning for the next 2 days, and then were placed on a maintenance dose of 0.5 gram of Antabuse for one week. These patients were carefully observed for toxic effects in view of the fact that they were still under the influence of liquor when the Antabuse was given. All subjective and objective changes were noted.

Read at the 105th annual meeting of The American Psychiatric Association, Montreal, Quebec, May 23–27, 1949.

From the Department of Neurology and Psychiatry, Albany Medical College and Hospital, and The Veterans Administration Mental Hygiene Clinic, Watervliet, N.Y.

The second group of 16 patients consisted of 9 who had an initial period of hospitalization and 7 who were under treatment and observation in the clinics. In this group psychotherapeutic procedures were employed after treatment was thoroughly explained. Treatment with Antabuse was deferred until the patients had fully recovered from the effects of acute alcoholism. The cooperation of relatives, social service agencies, and Alcoholics Anonymous was enlisted. Several talks were held with leading members of the A.A. group and their cooperation in the follow-up care of patients was obtained.

These 16 patients were given 2 grams of Antabuse on the first day, 1.5 grams on the second day, and 1 gram on the third day. On the morning of the fourth day, 0.75 gram of Antabuse were given. In the afternoon or the evening of the fourth day a trial dose of alcohol was administered under controlled conditions. Preference was given to the patient's choice of beverage. If whiskey was preferred 40–80 cc. were given; if beer was preferred, 350 cc. were given. The amount of Antabuse administered after the fourth day varied with each patient. Range of dosage was from 0.5 gram to 0.75 gram daily. Patients were then given a second trial of alcohol on the eight or tenth day of treatment. The dose of Antabuse was then decreased slowly at weekly intervals until the optimum maintenance dose was determined. This was considered to be the amount of Antabuse necessary to produce slight flushing of the head, mild dyspnea, and slight increase in pulse rate.

The treatment procedure was adjusted to the individual patient. However, the average maintenance dose varied from 0.125 gram to 0.5 gram daily.

The results obtained in these 21 cases treated with Antabuse were compared with 21 cases of chronic alcoholism admitted to the Albany Hospital during the last months of 1948.

RESULTS

1. Effect on Alcoholic Habits

Of the 21 patients treated for a period of 2–4 months 14 discontinued the use of alcohol entirely. Seven resumed their alcoholic habits; six of these were abstinent for a period of one month before discontinuing the use of Antabuse.

Of the first 5 patients treated who had not recovered from their alcoholic state and who were given Antabuse soon after admission to the hospital, 2 have abstained from the use of alcohol for a period of 4 months. Two resumed their alcoholic habits after one month had elapsed. One was lost sight of. In the 2 cases who discontinued drinking, psychotherapeutic procedures were employed subsequently.

Of the 16 patients in the second group who received Antabuse after recovery from their alcoholic state and for whom a careful, more adequate dosage schedule and psychotherapeutic regime were worked out to suit their individual needs, 12 have discontinued the use of alcohol for periods of 2 to 4 months.

Of the 4 who resumed their alcoholic habits, one had been making fair progress for a while, but resumed drinking and was committed to a state mental hospital. Another failed to respond and has not returned. The 2 other patients discontinued drinking for one month but resumed their alcoholic habits and took the Antabuse sporadically.

In the control group of 21 cases treated by routine psychotherapeutic procedures only 5 remained sober during a 3-month period of observation. The others resumed their alcoholic habits within a month after discharge from the Albany Hospital.

2. Physiologic Effects

Under the controlled conditions of observation outlined, none of the patients experienced severe toxic effects of the combination of Antabuse and alcohol. The first 5 patients treated before they had recovered from their alcoholic debauch complained of a warm feeling about the head and neck and a heaviness in the chest during the first 2 days of treatment. Subsequently these symptoms subsided but a feeling of fatigue persisted during the first month.

Three patients in this group displayed no subjective or objective symptoms after the first test dose of alcohol (40 cc. of whiskey). However, when the dose of Antabuse was increased from 0.5 gram to 0.75 gram daily for another week, the desired reaction to 40–80 cc. of alcohol followed. The dose of Antabuse was then decreased to 0.5 gram daily. One week later, a test dose of 40–50 cc. still produced a substantial reaction.

One of these 3 drinkers, who was 60 years of age and had had 58 admissions to the Albany Hospital for acute and chronic alcoholism, discontinued the use of Antabuse because of its unpleasant effects and because of his desire to continue drinking, which was interfered with by Antabuse.

Another patient who had had 5 admissions for early delirium tremens waited for the unpleasant effects of Antabuse and the test dose to wear off and then resumed drinking after discontinuing Antabuse.

The other 2 of the first 5 patients became so apprehensive after experiencing the flushing sensation of the head and the dyspnea during the initial administration of Antabuse prior to their recovery from the effects of acute alcoholism that they refused to take a test dose of alcohol. A brief summary of their case records is presented below:

CASE 1.—M.W. Age 27. The patient was admitted after alcoholic debauch and was taking paraldehyde upon admission. He was given 1.5 grams of Antabuse. He immediately experienced shortness of breath, flushing of the face, and tired feeling. The next day, he was given 0.75 gram and the symptoms were repeated. He was placed on a maintenance dose of 0.5 gram daily and since then has refused to take a drink, and even delined to take the test dose, because he said he had made up his mind to stop drinking and was afraid he might be started again by the test alcohol. However, he was obviously apprehensive. He is still taking 0.5 gram of Antabuse and has not had a drink in 4 months. He said he had lost his desire for alcohol.

CASE 2.—A.K. Age 49. The patient was admitted after alcoholic debauch and he also had been taking paraldehyde. Following

TABLE 1. Results in Case With Coronary Artery Disease

	B.P.	Pulse	R	EKG
Before trial dose of alcohol administered	140/90	90	14	Essentially as on admission
40 cc of alcohol administered at 7:45 PM				
8:00 PM	90/60	100	16	
8:05 PM	88/55	110	16	No change from
8:10 PM	88/55	100	16	previous EKG
8:15 PM	85/60	100	16	
8:20 PM	95/65	90	16	
8:25 PM	100/65	92	16	
8:30 PM	110/70	92	16	
8:45 PM	120/70	90	16	
9:00 PM	135/78	90	16	No change from
9:15 PM	140/88	90	16	previous EKG

the first dose of 1.5 grams of Antabuse, he felt very tired and sleepy, experienced dyspnea, pressure in the chest, flushing of the face, and a "feeling of heat" in his head. As in Case 1, he was placed on a maintenance dose of 0.5 gram after the third day. He refused to take a drink of alcohol for one month and would not even take a test dose. His blood pressure upon admission was 140/85 and there was no change following Antabuse. However, his respirations increased from 16 to 20 and his pulse rate from 80 to 100. Although he had stated that he refused the test dose of alcohol because he might start drinking, he discontinued taking Antabuse after a month had elapsed. Recent social service investigation revealed that he was imbibing heavily again.

The other patient in this group of 5 who discontinued drinking after taking the test doses said he was afraid to take alcohol because of the effect it might have on him again while he was taking Antabuse. He has abstained for 4 months now.

In the second group of 16 cases, after the test dose, greater flushing of face, increased loss of appetite, gastrointestinal reactions associated with nausea and vomiting, and more fatigue were noted. However, there was less shortness of breath than in the first 5 cases. Other subjective features noted included a gripping feeling in the chest, uncomfortable sensations in the stomach, pounding of the heart, and a feeling of weakness.

In summary, the most prevalent symptoms were flushing of the face, conjunctival injection, dizziness, headache, palpitation of the heart, a feeling of pressure in the chest, some dyspnea and nausea. Four of the patients developed transient vomiting of mild degree 8–10 hours after the test dose of alcohol was administered. Most of the unpleasant symptoms subsided after 45 to 75 minutes.

Of particular interest were the pulse and blood pressure changes. In all cases, the pulse rate ranged from 100 to 120 with an increase in rate of 20 to 40. Falls in blood pressure were noted in 12 of the cases. In 11 patients the fall averaged from 25 to 35 mms. In one case suffering from coronary artery disease a fall in blood pressure of 50 mms. was noted. This case is described in detail below:

This 58-year-old white male was admitted to the Albany Hospital after an alcoholic debauch of 2 weeks' duration. He was extremely restless, apprehensive, dehydrated, and complained of insomnia.

Past history revealed that he had had 6 other admissions for acute and chronic alcoholism. Three years before this admission he had a posterior myocardial infarction from which he recovered uneventfully but 2 years later developed auricular fibrillation with mild congestive failure. He was digitalized but auricular fibrillation continued. Numerous domestic and occupational conflicts remained unresolved and he continued his drinking habits.

Physical examination on admission for his recent alcoholic state revealed the following positive findings: B.P. 148/94, P-98, R 24, T 100.8. Conjunctivae were injected and his face was slightly flushed. He was very dehydrated. Heart was enlarged. Auricular fibrillation with pulse deficit of 10 was present. Lungs were clear. Liver was 1 finger below costal margin but was not tender.

Laboratory studies on admission revealed normal blood count, Hb 15 grams, Rbc 5.1 million, WBC 9,500, 65% polys, 33% lymphs, 2 eosinophiles. Urine was negative except for specific gravity 1.025. Blood nonprotein nitrogen 35 mg%. Sedimentation rate 5 mm/hr. Cephalin flocculation test and icteric index were normal. EKG showed evidence of posterior wall infarction and auricular fibrillation.

He was placed on a high carbohydrate, high protein diet, and parenteral B complex. After one week of treatment he recovered from his alcoholic episode.

Antabuse was started on the eight hospital day. After 5.25 grams of Antabuse a trial dose of 40 cc. of alcohol was administered under controlled conditions and results were obtained as listed in Table 1.

The complete reaction subsided in 75 minutes. The desired test reaction was obtained. He was then started on daily doses of Antabuse 0.5 gram daily.

There were no significant changes in blood count, urine, N.P.N. of the blood, sedimentation rate, and cephalin flocculation or icteric index. He has been responding well to treatment and psychotherapy.

DISCUSSION

The rationale of this therapy appears to be as follows:

1. It is a variation of the conditioned reflex emetine aversion method. The favorable response to the conditioned reflex treatment alone has been summarized and reported favorably by Voegtlin (11).

2. The unpleasant effects produced when both alcohol and Antabuse are given together are most likely due to the increased concentration of acetaldehyde.

3. In contrast to other forms of drug therapy or continued

reflex methods, the unpleasant effects are present not only each time the individual takes a small but adequate dose of Antabuse and imbibes alcohol but actually increases with continued treatment with Antabuse.

4. The medical treatment with Antabuse for short periods not only induces the patient to cease consumption of alcohol temporarily but if continued helps overcome the craving. The prolonged effect of Antabuse is a factor to be considered here.

The Antabuse effects lasts 10–14 days after discontinuance of the drug and sometimes longer. In addition, the patient feels the effect each time he tries to fool himself by taking a drink surreptitiously. In this manner, people who are being treated by psychotherapeutic methods or in Alcoholics Anonymous are prevented from initial "backsliding."

5. The most important aspect is that it prepares the patient for psychotherapeutic procedures and paves the way for these procedures during the period of temporary abstinence and recovery from his alcoholic state. He is made amenable to the psychotherapeutic procedures, which are accompanied by efforts to secure the necessary changes in his habits, to readjust him socially, to give him confidence in his ability, to help him solve his conflicts, and to overcome the escape and other mechanisms involved in his alcoholism. Without psychotherapeutic procedures, the treatment is of little value, as was indicated in our first 5 cases. The 2 patients among the 5 who ceased drinking did so only because they were amenable to subsequent psychotherapy. The use of social service department educational conferences with the family and the aid of Alcoholics Anonymous are of considerable value.

As Dr. Norman Brill has so aptly stated, the value of the drug seems to depend upon two other things: 1) a desire on the part of the patient to be helped, and 2) a willingness to take the drug with consistency. As long as the patient's basic difficulties are not resolved, the desire for alcohol will persist and together with it a lack of desire to take the medication. In some instances, it would seem that the conflict over whether "Should I or should I not drink" will be displaced to "Should I or should I not take the drug." When the need for drink is strong enough the drug will not be taken unless psychotherapeutic procedures are used.

Therefore, it is important to emphasize that the chief value of Antabuse lies in the fact that it paves the way for psychotherapeutic procedures. Because of its rather prolonged aftereffect and relatively mild reaction, as compared to emetine, particularly when given under controlled conditions, Antabuse in conjunction with psychotherapy may prove superior to other methods of treatment of chronic alcoholism. Its primary value used alone is to prevent backsliding of the patient and it overcomes the initial craving for alcohol.

CONTRAINDICATIONS

Except for cases of myocardial failure or coronary disease, there are no definite contraindications to the drug as yet. Moreover, under controlled conditions of hospitalization

and careful medical checkup including electrocardiographic study, it is possible to administer the drug to individuals who have early myocardial failure. We have done so in one case without any harmful results. However, the drug should be given with caution in the following conditions: 1) enlarged thyroid, 2) cirrhosis of the liver, 3) nephritis, 4) diabetes mellitus, 5) pregnancy, 6) epilepsy.

The following studies are needed in order to determine delayed toxic effects: 1) periodic acetaldehyde blood levels before, during, and after reaction to the alcohol Antabuse test; 2) complete blood count and urinalysis; 3) routine blood pressure readings and pulse rate recordings; 4) electrocardiogram; 5) liver and kidney function tests; 6) serum bicarbonate levels; 7) wherever possible special respiratory studies in addition to objective routine check on respiratory rate and depth; 8) basal metabolic rate; 9) electroencephalographic studies; 10) studies on goitregenic effect.

CONCLUSIONS

At present the drug should be used under controlled conditions of observation and should be given under the aegis of the psychiatrist at this time until further knowledge is obtained. If and when the value of the drug is further established, it may be released to use by physicians but periodic psychiatric consultations and psychotherapeutic procedures should be instituted.

Coordinated research studies by pharmacologist, physiologist, internist, and psychiatrist are now in progress. The value of the controlled, carefully planned study, and preliminary complete check-up preferably in a hospital including psychotherapeutic procedures, is indicated in our study particularly by the difference in reaction between the first 5 patients treated as compared with the subsequent group of 16 patients.

Under controlled conditions, severe untoward effects are minimal. We observed no toxic effects of alarming proportions in any of our cases. However, indiscriminate use of the drug without careful planning is to be condemned.

A battery of psychologic tests before and after Antabuse are valuable. The importance of follow-up and aid in the therapy by the social service department, when the patient is returned to the community, has been mentioned. A complete team evaluation of the patient's personality, including psychiatric examination, psychologic inventory and projective tests, and social service estimate of the patient's adaptation in the family and community, is essential. The value of this psychiatric team in follow-up treatment cannot be overestimated. The determination of which type of personality and under which conditions Antabuse may be most effective can then be established.

SUMMARY

1. Fourteen of 21 cases treated with Antabuse abstained from alcohol for periods of 2 to 4 months. Twenty-one cases represent too small a group from which to draw many general conclusions. However, the drug appears to have value

in the treatment of chronic alcoholism but it has to be given under controlled conditions and in conjunction with psychotherapy. It appears to be more effective than other drug or conditioned reflex therapies used previously.

2. Further coordinate research including internal medical, pharmacologic, psychologic, and social service studies in conjunction with the psychiatric observations are indicated on a greater number of cases to establish the value of the drug. Furthermore, the patients should be studied over a longer period of time, *i.e.*, about a year, to determine the permanency of their abstinence.

3. Under controlled conditions no severe untoward effects were noted.

BIBLIOGRAPHY

1. Hald, Jens, et al. The sensitizing effect of tetraethylthiuramdisulphide (Antabuse) to Ethyl-alcohol. Acta Pharmacol, 4:285, 1948.
2. Hald, Jens, and Jacobsen, Erik. A drug sensitizing the organism to ethyl alcohol. Lancet, 255:1001, Dec. 25, 1948.
3. Martensen-Larsen, O. A new method in the treatment of alcoholics. Nye Linier i Alkholistbehandlingen, Ugeskrift for Laeger, 110:1207, 1948.
4. Glud, Erik. Personal communication.
5. Jacobsen, Erik, and Martensen-Larsen, O. Treatment of alcoholism with Antabuse. J.A.M.A., 139:918, April 2, 1949.
6. Scott, J. Murray. Antabuse for alcoholism. Correspondence reprinted from J.A.M.A., 139:954, April 2, 1949.
7. Asmussen, Erling, et al. Studies on the effect of tetraethylthiuramdisulphide (Antabuse) and alcohol on respiration and circulation in normal human subjects. Acta Pharmacol. 4:297, 1948.
8. Hald, Jens, and Jacobsen, Erik. The formation of acetaldehyde in the organism after ingestion of Antabuse (tetraethylthiuramdisulphide) and alcohol. Acta Pharmacol, 4:305, 1948.
9. Asmussen, Erling, et al. The pharmacological action of acetaldehyde on the human organism. Acta Pharmacol., 4:311, 1948.
10. Larsen, Valdemar. The effect on experimental animals of Antabuse (tetraethylthiuramdisulphide) in combination with alcohol. Acta Pharmacol., 4:321, 1948.
11. Voegtlin, Walter L., and Broz, William R. The conditioned reflex treatment of chronic alcoholism. X. An analysis of 3125 admissions over a period of ten and a half years. Ann. Int. Med., 30:580, March 1949.

Chlorpromazine Treatment of Mental Disorders

By Vernon Kinross-Wright, M.D.

Associate Professor of Psychiatry, Baylor College of Medicine, Houston, Texas

Chlorpromazine,[1] a derivative of phenothiazine, was developed in France by the Rhone-Poulenc Research Laboratories. Under its trade names of Largactil and Megaphon it has been the object of much interest and experimentation in Europe, during the past 2 years. In this country where it is known as Thorazine it has been accepted for its superior antiemetic properties. More recently it has been used in the treatment of psychiatric disorders.

Pharmacology

Courvoisier, *et al.* (1) have conducted extensive animal and chemical investigations and find that chlorpromazine exhibits the following properties: 1) Anticholinergic action; 2) antiadrenergic action; though there is no inhibition of the hyperglycemic response of adrenalin; 3) central effect which is sedative, anticonvulsive, hypothermic, and antiemetic. The drug is also said to lower the metabolic rate. 4) There is a mild antihistaminic and local anesthetic activity. 5) The compound potentiates certain drugs, especially morphine and barbiturate derivatives.

The fate of chlorpromazine in the organism is unknown but probably it is degraded in the liver (2). Little is excreted through the kidneys.

The work of Moyer, *et al.* (3) in this country indicated that chlorpromazine in dogs is a hypotensive agent which decreases peripheral resistance with a variable effect upon cardiac output. These authors found no evidence of acute renal toxicity, though parenteral administration increased sodium and water excretion.

Clinical Studies

There appears to be considerable variability in the human response to chlorpromazine. The central depressant effects have been universally noted. There is usually a striking drop in blood pressure, particularly during the first few days of administration of the drug, with a compensatory tachy-cardia. Changes in body temperature, basal metabolism, urinary excretion have been variable. Other effects of sympathetic and parasympathetic inhibition have been noted. Increase of appetite may occur. No significant changes in the body biochemistry have been reported.

Clinical Uses

Chlorpromazine has been used in Europe for a wide range of conditions in the fields of surgery, anesthesia, gynecology and medicine. It was introduced into psychiatry in combination with barbiturates in prolonged sleep treatment (4). Hamon, *et al.* first used chlorpromazine alone in the treatment of manic illness (5). Their good results were reproduced by Delay and his associates, who have treated a variety of psychotic patients with success (6). Of the increasing number of publications, mention should be made of that of Staehelin and Kielholz in Switzerland and more recently of Lehmann and Hanrahan in Canada (7, 8). Improvement, and often cure, has been described in practically every type of mental illness. As might be expected with a new therapy dosages and uses have differed considerably, but more authors have agreed that initial parenteral administration speeds up improvement. Treatment has been continued for months in some cases.

The present study concerns an unselected group of admissions to the psychiatric service of a general hospital together with a lesser number of outpatients, 95 in all. A majority of the patients received initially a minimum of 50 mgms. of chlorpromazine intramuscularly 4 times daily. The effects of the drug are cumulative and it is usually possible to switch to oral dosage after a few days. Intramuscular administration is often painful and produces marked induration at the site of injection, particularly if the solution escapes into fatty tissue.

The total daily amount of chlorpromazine may be increased by as much as 100 mgms *per diem* until optimum effect is achieved, Increasing familiarity with the effects of the drug has led to the use of higher dosages. In one case improvement was delayed until 1,600 mgms. a day had been given for 10 days. However the average therapeutic dose for psychotic patients is about 800 mgms. each 24 hours. In neurotic patients and in children treatment is started by the oral route and in doses as low as 30 mgms. daily. Once im-

---

Read at the 110th annual meeting of The American Psychiatric Association, St. Louis, Mo., May 3–7, 1954.

From the Department of Psychiatry, Baylor University College of Medicine.

---

1 Supplied through the courtesy of Smith, Kline and French Laboratories as Thorazine.

provement was manifested medication was given solely by mouth and progressively reduced over a period of weeks. In a few patients who showed a tendency to relapse higher dosage was again instituted.

Although most of the expected clinical phenomena were observed during treatment there was a surprising inconstancy in degree in different patients. All the patients who responded to chlorpromazine showed an initial somnolence from which, however, they could be easily aroused. After the first few days of treatment the lethargy decreased. Some patients presented a rather striking similarity to patients a few days after prefrontal lobotomy—a fact remarked on by some of the European writers.

In spite of the lack of spontaneous activity, patients are fully oriented and even severely withdrawn patients showed a rapid increase in their contact with reality. Some said that they had never felt so relaxed and very few of the psychotic patients made any complaints about the treatment. Neurotic patients on the other hand were aware of the hypotension and described themselves as "lightheaded, dizzy, and faint." None of the patients experienced frank syncopal attacks but these have been reported elsewhere (9). Some patients complained of a dry nose and mouth. Nausea and epigastric distress occurred occasionally in patients on oral therapy though this was somewhat unexpected in view of the well-established antiemetic properties. Three patients mentioned aching eyes and experienced some difficulty in focusing on close objects. Occasionally injection is painful and in these cases procaine is added. While on intramuscular dosage many of the patients exhibited a marked grayish pallor which is quite characteristic.

The hypotensive response was always apparent, the systolic pressure often dropped by 40 to 60 points and diastolic reading by as much as 40 points. In no case was it found necessary to withdraw chlorpromazine on this account even in ambulatory patients. Two of the patients were hypertensive before treatment and in both of these blood pressure dropped to normal levels without bad effects. After the withdrawal of chlorpromazine the blood pressure returned to pretreatment levels within 48 hours.

The compensatory tachycardia is often conspicuous but does not worry the patients. One woman suffering from an anxiety state commented on it but said that it was not nearly as unpleasant as the palpitations she had experienced for years.

No consistent temperature changes were noted. A consistent reduction of body temperature did not occur. In 5 cases there was a marked elevation of temperature for a few days during chlorpromazine administration, without leucytosis or other clinical findings. These patients had few complaints and the pyrexia promptly subsided when chlorpromazine was discontinued. In 2 cases replacement of the drug was accompanied by return of the fever for a short time. Measurement of metabolic rate was not attempted but there was no clinical evidence of significant decrease. Increase of appetite was the rule and some patients became ravenously hungry and gained weight. This was true even where other signs of clinical improvements were meager.

Sleep was greatly improved in almost all the patients in

spite of the fact that those on large intramuscular dosage were lethargic throughout the day. Improved sleep is often associated with heightened dream activity. It is worth noting that the total sedative requirements for the service have been greatly reduced since this new treatment was instituted. Also worth mentioning is the strange, striking quiet which has come over the ward with its population of acutely disturbed patients. On one occasion when supplies of the drug were exhausted this was brought home to us with particular emphasis.

When patients are on chlorpromazine the vital signs and blood pressure are recorded at 6 hourly intervals. All barbiturate sedation is avoided. When necessary, paraldehyde, whose action does not seem to be potentiated by chlorpromazine, is used for sedation. As part of an investigation into possible hepatic toxicity many patients are given a battery of liver function tests before and every 4 days during treatment. Electrocardiogram and a thorough physical examination are prerequisites of treatment.

RESULTS

Table 1 briefly summarizes the results obtained to date with 95 patients. Many of these patients are still receiving chlorpromazine on an outpatient basis and are continuing to make progress. Some have been under treatment for over 3 months. Others have required but a few doses to relieve their major symptoms. In agreement with general experience states of psychomotor excitement and agitation have been quickly controlled with 200–400 mgms. daily. This seems to be true regardless of the type of psychomotor excitement. In one case of schizophrenic excitement, and one case of acute mania, however, chlorpromazine did not ameliorate the symptoms. The addition of 3 electric shock treatments on successive days produced a prompt remission in both these patients. This experience was duplicated with another case of involutional melancholia. It seems as though the combination of EST and chlorpromazine does well in certain instances since all 3 of these patients had previous attacks of lesser severity, which has required a greater number of EST's for improvement. Delirious states are notably responsive, often clearing up in a matter of hours. The series includes cases of toxic deliria due to alcohol, bromides, ACTH, and brain lesions.

The results in the schizophrenic patients have been gratifying, particularly in those paranoid symptomatology. Of 14 paranoid schizophrenics, only 3 were not improved. Six of these have already returned home and are making good adjustments. In 3 patients with delusional ideas the hallucinations seem to have entirely disappeared. The following case history is illustrative:

A 32-year-old colored, married female was admitted because of combativeness, refusal to wear clothes, ideas of being poisoned, hearing persecutory voices, and generally disorganized behavior of 4 months duration.

Patient had an unhappy childhood and had always been introverted with compulsive habits, episodes of nervousness and severe dysmenorrhea. She was highly ambitious and never made friends, always hypersensitive and suspicious. Four months prior to admis-

TABLE 1. Results of Chlorpromazine Treatment

	Total	In Remission	Much Improved	Slightly Improved	Unchanged
Schizophrenia	29				
Paranoid		4	5	2	3
Hebephrenic		1	2	1	
Catatonic		1	3	1	
Simple					1
Unclassified		2	3		
Depression	18				
Manic depressive		4	2	1	
Reactive		1	4	2	1
With cerebral vascular disease		1			
Involutional melancholia		1	1		
Mania	2	2			
Anxiety State	9	2	4	3	
Hysteria	8				
Conversion		1	2	1	2
Dissociation		2			
Delirium	10				
Bromide		1			
ACTH		1			
Alcohol		5			
With organic brain disease		2	1		
Psychosis	2				
Unclassified			1	1	
Posttraumatic Neurosis	5		2	3	
Alcoholism	2		1	1	
Psychopathic Personality	2				
Aggressive			1		
Inadequate				1	
Emotional Immaturity	1				1
Neurodermatitis	1		1		
Childhood Behavior Disturbance	3	1	1	1	
Narcolepsy (Idiopathic)	1		1		
Convulsive Disorder	2		1		1
Total	95	32	36	18	9

sion the patient accused her husband and sister of trying to poison her, made violent assaults on her husband. She believed her mind was being controlled by others, heard voices plotting to kill her, was unable to sleep and refused to care for herself.

On admission she was acutely disturbed and presented a picture of paranoid schizophrenia. Physical examination was unremarkable and laboratory findings within normal limits. Her condition grew worse during first 4 days; totally disorganized in behavior with many paranoid ideas, she was extremely belligerent. She was given chlorpromazine 50 mgm., I.M., q.i.d. After 6 days there was slight lessening of activity and paranoid delusions but she was still very disorganized, slept little, but ate better. Chlorpromazine was increased to 100 mgm, q.i.d. Within 24 hours there was marked improvement, she seemed euphoric, slept well, and ate with enormous appetite. There was moderate hypotension. Within 48 hours the patient was rational and cooperative, sleep rhythm was restored. Oral chlorpromazine was substituted after 4 days with continued improvement, and tapered off over the next 10 days. Patient continued to improve. She was discharged 23 days after admission in good health. She was friendly toward her husband, had no ideas of persecution or reference, showed good affect and had some insight into her illness. She has continued to do well at home.

All the cases of depression have shown some improvement and several have returned home and are doing well. Depressed patients, particularly those who showed much psychomotor retardation, did not demonstrate the striking results seen in the schizophrenic and manic group. However, improvement in depressed patients is often masked by the effects of chlorpromazine itself, and only when it is withdrawn or reduced in amount is the improvement apparent. The following case history is illustrative:

A 42-year-old married, colored man was well until 3 years ago, when he broke his ankle at work. Following this he was confused for 3 weeks and was thought by his doctor to have had a cerebral vascular accident. Since then he has been seclusive, nervous, and progressively more depressed, profoundly depressed in the past few months. He would not eat, slept little, cried, and read the Bible. He talked frequently of suicide, complained of backache. He had not been able to work.

On admission the patient presented a picture of retarded depression. Physical examination showed B.P. of 240/118 with hypertensive heart disease and grade ii retinal arteriosclerosis. Routine investigation and liver function tests were within normal limits. EKG showed left axis deviation; x-ray of spine was negative. Diagnosis was depression secondary to hypertension and possible cerebral vascular accident.

The patient remained depressed and almost mute for the first 10 days. During this period his B.P. dropped to an average of 210/110. Chlorpromazine was instituted, increased gradually by 50 mgm. steps each day up to 200 mgm. daily, by mouth (to avoid sudden hypotension). The patient improved at once; appetite increased and he slept well. He had no diurnal lethargy and was more sociable. Blood pressure dropped in 24 hours to 130/90 and in one week to 120/70. He was discharged 17 days later on 75 mgm. daily with B.P. 110/80. He was cheerful and considering a return to work. He had no complaints referable to reduction in B.P. He continued to have backaches but did not spontaneously mention this.

Among the neurotic group response has been more variable. Most of the patients report some improvement but as mentioned above the side effects of chlorpromazine sometimes cause patients to refuse larger doses. The improved sleep habits and increased appetite in this group suggest that chlorpromazine would be of value as an adjuvant to psychotherapy. This case of conversion hysteria, though, appears specially noteworthy.

A 31-year-old married, white mechanic was referred because of painful paralysis of the left leg, nervousness and headaches of 3 months duration. His symptoms developed 30 minutes after a heavy truck transmission had fallen on his abdomen and left leg. His previous adjustment had been good though there were marital difficulties and he had been living for some months previously in a setting of tension on this account.

Following his accident he had been conservatively treated. Aside from the paralysis and extensive bruising there were no injuries. Neurological examination was negative except for stocking anesthesia of the lower extremity. He received osteopathic treatments and when these did not help was given a bad prognosis. After seeing several other medical men he was finally referred for psychiatric help by his lawyer. A diagnosis of conversion hysteria with tension state was made and psychotherapy instituted some 3 months after injury. Probably because of the compensation and legal issues the patient did not progress. Sodium amytal interviews were unrewarding. For over 5 months after his accident his leg was still paralyzed and very painful. He developed numbness in his right leg, was depressed, and losing weight. He entertained paranoid ideas against his physicians.

He was hospitalized and treated with chlorpromazine, 200 mgm. daily by injection. He became extremely drowsy for 24 hours. The next day he said that his leg no longer was numb and that he felt good. By the third day he was ambulatory with a slight limp. He was happy and elated over his improvement. He continued to improve while chlorpromazine was tapered off over a 2-week period. Three weeks after the termination of treatment he was back at work, eating and sleeping well. He stated that he had never felt so well in his life. He had fair insight into his illness and was unconcerned about the possible loss of a large financial settlement.

Two patients with convulsive disorder associated with behavioral disturbance are included in the series. One of these has fewer seizures with chlorpromazine than on any other anticonvulsant regime. This finding has been noted by others (10, 11).

Few undesirable reactions other than those attributable to the physiological effects of chlorpromazine have been encountered so far. Moyer, et al. in a study of renal and hepatic functions have found no evidence of toxicity in their patients who were, however, on smaller dosage. They also did not find abnormalities of the electrocardiogram or blood elements attributable to the drug. Lehmann and Hanrahan noted slight changes in liver function tests in some of their patients with clinical evidence of hepatic dysfunction in 3. In this series no conclusive evidence of hepatic toxicity has been found, even in patients with pre-existent liver damage of moderate degree. This aspect of chlorpromazine is being more extensively investigated.

Three patients developed more or less generalized skin eruption of an urticarial nature associated with malaise. More powerful antihistamines did not bring relief, but in each case cessation of chlorpromazine for a few days only allowed the skin to clear. One schizophrenic patient became very euphoric with outspoken erotic tendencies which subsided with discontinuance of treatment for 10 days. Two patients on high doses developed coarse tremor, muscular rigidity, and immobile expression. This Parkinson-like syndrome disappeared quickly after reduction of dosage.

There do not appear to be any absolute contraindications to chlorpromazine treatment. It should be used with caution in patients with hepatic, cardiac or renal disease and in those who have recently taken barbiturates or opiates.

COMMENT

Chlorpromazine has a diverse pharmacological action on the human organism. A considerable body of evidence has been accumulated pointing to its therapeutic efficacy in many kinds of mental disorders. It is a drug of low toxicity even in large doses and one which may be administered over long periods of time without an undesirable increase of tolerance.

It appears to be a highly effective agent for controlling psychomotor excitement of all kinds without the undesirable effects of the standard methods and maintaining the patient in a fairly accessible state at all times. Its action on other types of mental illness is not so remarkable but is certainly worthy of further investigation, particularly in the chronic schizophrenic patients in whom most treatments are unrewarding. Facilitation of communication together with a remarkable objectivity towards significant ideas and feelings has occurred in many of this group.

Speculation about the mode and site of action of the drug seems premature but such evidence as there is suggests that it is a subcortical one. While in the initial states of treatment there is a definite resemblance in the behavior of these patients to those who have been lobotomized there are none of the deficits found in the latter. Neither the dosage nor the mode of administration of the drug is in any way standardized. The initial results obtained in Europe and this country have been satisfactory enough to justify a thorough clinical investigation of chlorpromazine and a search for even more powerful related compounds.

BIBLIOGRAPHY

1. Courvoisier, S., Foumel, J., Ducrot, R., Kolsky, M., and Koetschet, P. Propriétés Pharmacodynamiques du Chlorhydrate de Chloro-2 (diméthylemino-3" propyl)—10 phénothiazine Arch. Internationales de Pharmacodynamie et de Thérapie. Vol. XCII, Jan. 1953.
2. Largactil. Rhone-Poulenc Research Laboratories publication.
3. Moyer, J. H., Kent, B., Knight, R., Morris, G., Huggins, R., and Handley, C. A. Am. J. Med. Sci., (in press), 1954.
4. Deschamps, A. Hibernation Artificielle en Psychiatrie—Presse Medicale 43-21st June, 1952.

5. Hamon, J., Paraire, J., and Velluz, J. Remarques sur l'Action du 4560 R P sur l'Agitation maniaque Ann. Med. Psychol., 100 (1:3) 331, 1952.
6. Delay, J., Deniker, P., Harl, J.M.—Utilisation en Thérapeutique Psychiatrique d'une Phénothiazine d'Action Centrale Elective. Ann. Med. Psychol., 110 (2:1) 12–7, 1952.
7. Staehelin, J.E., and Kielholz, P. Schweiz. Med. Wchrschr 83:581, 1953.

8. Lehmann, H.E., and Hanrahan, C.E. Arch. Neur. and Psych., 71:227, 1954.
9. Moyer, J.H. Personal Communication, 1954.
10. Davis, M., Benda, P., and Klein, F. Bull mém Soc. Med. Hopitaux, Paris, 69:691, June 1953.
11. Finney, R.M. Personal Communication, 1954.

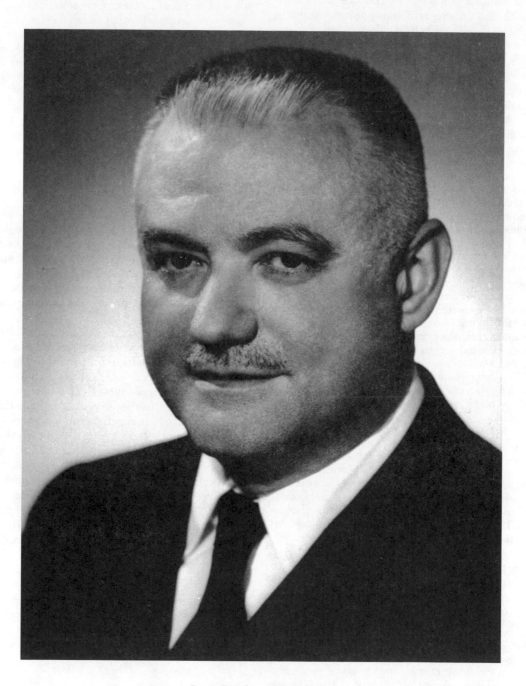

Pierre Deniker, M.D., 1917–

In 1952 Pierre Deniker, working with the French psychiatrist Jean Delay, reported the beneficial results of chlorpromazine for treating psychotic patients.

CLINICAL FINDINGS IN THE USE OF TOFRANIL IN DEPRESSIVE AND OTHER PSYCHIATRIC STATES

Benjamin Pollack, M.D.

Assistant Director of Clinical Psychiatry, Rochester State Hospital, Rochester, New York

Roland Kuhn (1) of Zurich, Switzerland, reporting a large series of cases with promising results in the use of Tofränil in the treatment of depressive states, has indicated that this drug is more or less a specific anti-depressive drug although not primarily a stimulant and not a monamine oxidase inhibitor. To date there has been no satisfactory replacement for electroshock therapy in the typical depressive state. The discovery of a drug which would be helpful in such conditions would be of paramount importance, and would permit more extensive treatment in the psychiatrist's office and avoid the necessity for hospitalization. The interest produced by iproniazid and other monamine oxidase inhibitors has furthered the research in this field in an attempt to elaborate a compound which would be free of dangerous complications.

Tofränil (2), known also as imipramine and G 22355, is a recently synthesized psychotherapeutic agent which has now had fairly extensive trials in Europe and more recently in this country. The mode of action of this drug is not quite clear, except for its central nervous system action. It is, however, not essentially a stimulant but in exceedingly high doses in animals can cause tremors, rigidity and respiratory arrest. To do so it is necessary to use doses 20 to 30 times the therapeutic dose used in clinical treatment. This drug produces only a slight potentiation of barbiturates and little or no hypothermic effect. In animals there is evidence of some anti-convulsive effect which protects against metrazol and electroshock in animals when used in very high doses, but here again in humans electroshock can be given readily with little or no change in the dose. It does not increase norepinephrine or serotonin in the brain and is not a monamine oxidase inhibitor. There are some slight peripheral anesthetic qualities and it may therefore produce some peripheral paresthesias or some slight anesthesia of the cornea. Forty percent is excreted as 2 metabolites in the urine and less than 2% is excreted unchanged. It is rapidly absorbed and it likewise disappears from the body in 24 hours. The Forrest reagent test of the urine is negative. It has no influence on conditioned responses.

Long-term observations with injections in animals of huge doses have not produced hematological or hepatic changes. The lethal dose in animals is estimated as somewhere between 400 and 1200 mgs. per kilo which, of course, would far exceed the clinical dosage, so that there is a very wide margin of safety. It would appear that it is absorbed almost as rapidly orally as parenterally. It can be used both intramuscularly and intravenously, but in the former it is quite irritating.

Its formula resembles that of promazine in which the sulphur atom has been replaced by a dimethyl chain. (Graph 1)

The use of Tofränil was first begun at the Rochester State Hospital in September 1958, 6 months ago. Since this was a new drug which had had few clinical trials in this country, an attempt was made to ascertain its usefulness by giving it not only to patients suffering from various depressions but to those who had a variety of other mental illnesses. Approximately 273 patients are involved in the results. These patients consist of acute and chronic disorders. The drug was administered in practically every newly admitted patient who was suffering from depressive symptoms without regard to the diagnosis. It was also used for various schizophrenic conditions and organic conditions, particularly where there were elements of anxiety or depression. The diagnoses of the treated cases are shown in Table 1.

Treatment was given in various parts of the hospital, and this report is a compilation of the observations of many of the personnel from the various services. For the most part, the patients were treated with relatively low doses of 25 mgs. of Tofränil t.i.d., particularly in the acute cases and with 50 mgs. t.i.d. in the more chronic cases. It was readily determined that there was a direct relationship between the dosage and the intensity and frequency of side effects. Side effects increased proportionately with age, and many were noted, particularly in patients 60 years of age and over. In the younger group relatively few side effects were noted. Except for dizziness, side effects were almost infrequent in dosages of 75 mgs. and under, and more frequent in dosages between 75 to 200 mgs. Most of the side effects were more annoying than dangerous and consisted of dryness of the mouth, perspiration, tremors, especially of the upper extremities, dizziness and occasional blurred vision, and in some patients some tendency to gastrointestinal disturbances. Some patients complained of marked constipation, but in the author's experiences this was not as prominent a symptom as reported by other investigators. Increased agitation occurred in a small number of patients. Because of this, certain of the treatment schedules included the use of both tranquilizers, such as Thorazine, and

GRAPH 1

TABLE 1

DIAGNOSIS	
Involutional Depression without agitation	25
Involutional Depression with agitation	21
Manic-Depression	44
Reactive Depression	7
Organic Depression	52
Psychoneurotic Depression	19
Senile Depression	5
Schizoaffective Depression	41
Unspecified Depression	21
Schizophrenia	19
Alchoholism	10
Other not Depressed	9
	273

Two-thirds of the treated patients were over 45 years of age (Table 2).

TABLE 2

Age	Male	Female	Total
15–24	1	7	8
25–34	12	25	37
35–44	15	28	43
45–54	19	34	53
55–64	25	32	57
65+	8	67	75
	80	193	273

stimulants such as Ritalin. With the combination of such drugs it is, of course, much more difficult to evaluate the role of Tofrānil. There did not appear to be any particular tendency toward hypotensive attacks with this drug, in spite of the complaints of dizziness which apparently are due to other causes as is vertigo. One serious side effect which has not been reported in the literature is the factor of sudden falls which occur apparently only in treated patients who are 60 or over. These are of a peculiar type in that the patient falls without any prior warning or previous episode of dizziness or vertigo. Because of this he may fall suddenly as a dead weight with possible consequent injuries. Such falls occurred only in patients who were receiving Tofrānil in doses in excess of 75 mgs. per day, and were entirely abolished in dosages below this level. A further peculiarity is that the patients are amazed to find them-

selves suddenly falling. There is no loss of consciousness nor do the falls appear to be due to hypotensive episodes as no particular alteration in blood pressure can be seen in such individuals. Experimentally, it has been reported that Tofrānil may upset the carotid sinus mechanism in animals, and this may perhaps offer an explanation for such falls. It can be seen from Table 3 that dizziness and tremors constituted the largest number of side effects. These, however, are seldom of sufficient severity to require discontinuing the medication since lowering the dosage, as a rule, will abolish these symptoms. The literature contains two reports of the occurrence of jaundice with the use of Tofrānil. So far no cases of agranulocytosis has been reported. Unlike Marsilid, Tofrānil does not cause states of euphoria which may reverse the depressive states into manic excitements. There is a greater tendency to a more normal type of feeling so that the patient does not feel stimulated or overactive. This is an important differential since it permits a patient to act with good judgment and to partake of social activities in an acceptable manner.

CLINICAL RESULTS

All research workers who used this drug initially were unanimous in the conclusion that, unlike many other psychopharmacological agents, it specifically affects depressive conditions and has a very little effect on paranoid states or disturbed behavior, particularly in schizophrenics. This initial impression is rather intriguing and a unique finding, and should be investigated more widely for a longer period of time. Since depressive states frequently have a natural tendency towards recovery, it is much more difficult to evaluate the results produced by Tofrānil as compared to the results noted in the use of phenothiazines in schizophrenics and allied conditions. It would, however, appear that proportionately a larger number of patients are improved clinically than could be anticipated without the drug and that such improvement occurs more rapidly. The specificity of the effect can also be demonstrated in that in early cases the patient will quickly relapse if the drug is removed since there is very little storage of this drug in the body beyond 24 hours. Its effect is much less spectacular than the results produced by ECT, but is much more acceptable to most patients. It would appear evident that the greatest value of the drug is in conditions of pure retarded depression which are unassociated with somatic complaints, agitation or paranoid tendencies. The greater frequency or intensity of such symptoms accompanying the depression will, as a rule, lessen the therapeutic benefits of Tofrānil. However, it seems to be almost impossible to point with any degree of consistency to certain target symptoms which are affected most promptly and effectively by this medication. Endogenous depressions appear to do well and a number of agitated depressions respond quite well. However, in some it often is necessary to use certain other drugs such as Thorazine or Ritalin. Tofrānil appears to remove the depressive elements and to free anxiety which requires control by tranquilizers. These are best given at night in a single dose, to promote sleep and to avoid leth-

TABLE 3

Side Effects	Total	Required Discontinuation
Agitation	7	
Hypomanic	0	
Seizures in Epileptics	0	
Parkinsonism	0	
Dystonia	1	
Syncope	5	
Hypotension	1	
Palpitation	2	
Cardiovascular	0	
Tremor	28	1
Diplopia	7	
Perspiration	16	
Dry Mucous Membranes	19	
Jaundice	0	
Photosensitization	0	
Dermatologic	2	
Constipation	0	
Excessive Weight Gain	0	
Urinary Frequency	0	
Nausea	5	
Dizziness	22	1
Falls	17	3
Insomnia	2	
Total patients with side effects—67		

TABLE 4. Depressions, Female Reception Service (All Treated Patients)

Recovered	0
Much Improved	30%
Improved	56%
Unimproved	14%
Worse	0

TABLE 5. Schizophrenias

Recovered	0
Much Improved	14%
Improved	24%
Unimproved	38%
Worse	24%

TABLE 6. Depression in 57 Cases of CAS-Senile or Organic

Recovered	0
Much Improved	28%
Improved	40%
Unimproved	20%
Worse	12%

argy or drowsiness during the daytime. When the drug is effective, results may be seen as early as the first or second day and usually within a week. Occasionally little effect will be noted for 2 or 3 weeks. One articulate, intelligent patient who had had much experience with the effects of other drugs stated in speaking of Tofrānil that its effect is "sneaky; without realizing it you suddenly find yourself doing and enjoying things which you were too tired to do the day before." There is no dramatic change but many of the patients state that they feel normal or that they feel good. There appears to be a general release of the depressive attitudes even though at the same time some patients may continue to talk of various feelings of guilt or sinfulness. In this connection the drug may relax the patient sufficiently so that they are more responsive and available for concomitant psychotherapy. They gradually become more remote or detached from their thought content with subsequent improvement in affect. The drug was used in association with ECT without any particular increase in side effects or complications. It appeared to be also effective in recurrent depression which previously had been treated by electroshock. It was found that the use of Tofrānil in such cases diminished the frequency of relapses.

The drug was also used on 60 schizophrenics, many of whom had depressions associated with paranoid ideas. Others were catatonics or withdrawn or mute. It was quickly evident that Tofrānil was not of great value in schizophrenics and in fact in many cases was contraindicated because at least half of them became worse. It would appear that a compensated paranoid schizophrenic who is given this drug may be relieved of depression or anxiety, but the paranoid elements become exaggerated. Such patients became much more disturbed, suspicious, hostile and aggressive.

An example of this reaction was a male patient who prior to treatment had been somewhat surly and inappropriate, hostile, suspicious, occasionally defiant, but on the whole able to control his symptoms and in general quite cooperative. He received 100 mgm. of Tofrānil and within a week became restless, agitated, sullen, argumentative, combative and unable to control the symptoms or the emotional state which previously was held under some degree of control.

A number of depressions in arteriosclerotics and seniles were treated with rather impressive results. In about 50% to 65% of the patients the depression cleared or become ameliorated. The organic symptoms of confusion and disorientation, of course were not affected. It must be realized, however, that there are many patients in the older age group who develop depression without precipitating organic etiology. This type appears to respond quite well to the use of this drug.

It must again be emphasized that in the older person the drug should not be used in large doses, an effective dose usually varying between 25 and 75 mgm.

The results of treatment are briefly summarized in Tables 4-7. On the reception service most of the patients treated were either readmissions or acute admissions and most of them were suffering from an involutional psychosis, a manic-depressive depression or an acute psychoneurosis. There were also a few depressions associated with psychosis with cerebral arteriosclerosis.

A group of seniles or arteriosclerotic patients were selected from a chronic area for treatment for a single symptom which they commonly displayed, namely depression. For the 57 in this group, the results are shown in Table 6.

It is, of course realized that the results quoted in this group are based upon the improvement in only one symptom, namely depression.

TABLE 7. Results of Tofrānil Therapy in 273 Acute and Chronic Patients

Diagnosis	Much Improved	Improved	Unimproved or Worse
All treated patients	56%	16%	28%
Involutional Depression	58%	16%	26%
(a) Without Agitation	58%	17%	25%
(b) With Agitation	60%	13%	27%
(c) Combined with Chlorpromazine	63%	18%	19%
(d) Combined with Chlorpromazine and Ritalin	69%	8%	23%
Manic-Depressive	70%	13%	17%
Reactive Depression	72%	7%	21%
Organic and Senile Depression	56%	14%	30%
Psychoneurotic Depression	59%	14%	27%
Schizophrenia	14%	24%	62%

These tables vividly display the specificity of this drug in treatment and indicate why it has been labelled by many research workers as an anti-depressive drug which produces promptly or gradually a change in the depressive state. Some patients fail to respond to treatment and show no improvement in their depression and it seems impossible to determine the difference among patients since they apparently display the same type of symptom. No study was made of the environmental situations or previous personality patterns. Table 7 includes a number of private patients seen in office practice by some of the psychiatrists participating in this study.

There are sufficient indications, however, that Tofrānil is a useful drug and that somewhere between 50% and 70% of patients displaying depressive symptoms will improve. Where no improvement occurred, a tranquilizer, usually chlorpromazine, and a stimulant, usually Ritalin, were added to the treatment schedule. This combined form of treatment resulted in 10% higher improvement rate than when Tofrānil was used alone. When the depression failed to clear adequately or to sufficient degree, an occasional electric shock was given in conjunction with the use of Tofrānil. Indications are that the addition of Tofrānil to such therapy will reduce the relapse rate and permit a more stable course. The use of this drug has reduced the need for ECT to almost the vanishing point, except for an occasional concurrent shock treatment.

Of the patients treated who are now out of the hospital, (approximately 50) the vast majority of pure depressive states were released from the hospital within one or two months. It is interesting to note that some of these include patients who failed to respond to electric shock previously or whose improvement lasted for only a short period of time.

SUMMARY

1. Preliminary observation would indicate that Tofrānil is a useful drug in the treatment of depressive states. It is not a tranquilizer and, therefore, is of little value in other conditions. It is a promising drug which can be used as an antidepressant. However, its indication and scope must be studied for a longer period to determine what symptoms respond best to it.

2. The effect of Tofrānil in many patients can be increased by the concomitant use of a tranquilizer or a stimulant. In a number of patients Tofrānil, by removing the depressive elements, frees and exaggerates anxiety.

3. It can be used in combination with electric shock or after electric shock as a maintenance dose.

4. It is of little value in the treatment of schizophrenics and in paranoid types may often aggravate the condition and break down an unstable equilibrium to which the patient has become adjusted.

5. The combined use of Tofrānil and a tranquilizer is helpful in certain psychoneurotic states, associated with anxiety or with reactive depressions.

6. It is of value in the treatment of depressions occurring in the older age group.

7. High doses are unnecessary and the effective range is somewhere between 75 and 150 mgm. per day.

8. For the most part, side effects are minimal, particularly in the younger age group. As one approaches the older age group, the frequency of such side effects increases, but usually they are more uncomfortable than serious. In patients over 60 there may be a tendency to sudden falls which occur without warning. It is recommended that in older patients the dosage be limited to 75 mgm. or less.

9. Side effects can usually be reduced in frequency or intensity by a reduction in the dosage.

10. Long-term use of the drug is apparently necessary as patients may relapse, at least in the early stages when the drug is prematurely removed. Since the drug is rapidly excreted, it is necessary to give the medication 3 times a day.

BIBLIOGRAPHY

1. Kuhn, Roland: Schweiz. Med. Wchnschr., 87:1135, Aug. 1, 1957.
2. Unpublished sources.

THE USE OF LITHIUM IN THE AFFECTIVE PSYCHOSES

By Ralph N. Wharton, M.D., and Ronald R. Fieve, M.D.

New York State Psychiatric Institute, New York, New York

Lithium carbonate has been used with caution and control at the New York State Psychiatric Institute for the past six years. Nineteen patients, 15 of whom had at least two well-documented prior manic attacks, were given 25 trials of lithium after therapeutic refractoriness on phenothiazines. Eleven of the 25 manic episodes had good responses to lithium treatment; the individual manic attack was definitely shortened as compared with the patient's past attacks. The authors suggest that lithium may be the treatment of choice for phenothiazine-refractory or phenothiazine-allergic manic patients treated in a research setting.

Since the initial work of Cade (5) in 1949, there have been a number of articles in the world literature from Australia (17), Denmark (2), England (13, 15), France (10), and Russia (3, 16) concerning the use of lithium for the treatment of manic behavior. In the United States, Gershon (11), Colbert (6), Kingstone (14), and Schlagenhauf (19) have written about the use of lithium for the treatment of manic states.

A number of authorities (including Wikler [24]) have decried the use of lithium as a therapeutic agent in the field of general medicine, reporting it as inhumane. Only one current pharmacologic text mentions its therapeutic use. Since reports of death following its use as a salt substitute in the 1940s in the treatment of hypertension (8, 23), it has been generally shunned as a therapeutic agent in the United States.

Despite the clinical enthusiasm of some observers regarding the effectiveness of this salt in the treatment of mania, there is yet to be reported a carefully documented study clearly demonstrating the efficacy of lithium as compared with other treatment modalities, including the phenothiazines.

Our interest in lithium stems not only from an attempt to test the validity of the clinical impression that this drug is useful in the treatment of manic-depressive psychoses but also from the theoretical implications of the actions of this salt as a new agent of an *entirely different chemical nature* than phenothiazines. The ease of determination with the

flame photometer makes comparisons between blood level and behavior possible. The mechanism of the action of the salt is unknown, in terms of its capacity to act as a depressant of nervous activity.

METHODOLOGY

In this study, a total of 19 patients with manic-depressive psychosis, manic phase, were treated with lithium between the years 1959 and 1965.

The patients selected for treatment manifested hyperactivity, pressure of speech, and elation state. They were accepted only when the diagnosis of a manic state was agreed upon by two clinical psychiatrists.

The only patients excluded were those with serious physical illnesses or with known renal or cardiac disease in which the natural history of those illnesses might interfere with our evaluation of lithium. Patients tending to remit spontaneously during the initial observational period of

TABLE 1. Psychiatric History of 19 Patients

History	Males (N=9)	Females (N=10)
Number of prior manic attacks		
One	2	2
Two to five	6	7
Six to nine	0	0
Ten or more	1	1
Prior treatment in other manic phases		
Electroconvulsive therapy		
Improved	2	1
Not improved	0	2
Phenothiazines		
Improved	1	4
Not improved	7	5
Allergic	1	1

Read at the 122nd annual meeting of the American Psychiatric Association, Atlantic City, N.J., May 9-13, 1966.

The authors are with the New York State Psychiatric Institute, 722 West 168th Street, New York, N. Y., where Dr. Wharton is Senior Research Psychiatrist, and Dr. Fieve is Chief of Psychiatric Research, Department of Internal Medicine.

The authors wish to thank Lawrence C. Kolb, M.D., for his advice and encouragement in the preparation of this paper, and Bernice Blumenthal and Barbara Little for the lithium determinations.

TABLE 2. Chlorpromazine-Refractory Patients Responsive to Lithium

Patient	Age	Sex	Prior Manic Attacks		Lithium-Treated Attacks	
			Duration	Treatment	Duration	Evaluation
H.G.S.	57	M	1 month 1½ months	Chlorpromazine, 600 mg. Fluphenazine, 30 mg. Prolixin, 30 mg.	2 weeks	32-month follow-up without relapse.
E.P.	52	F	5 months 4 months	Chlorpromazine, 1200 mg. Chlorpromazine, 1400 mg.	2 weeks	36-month follow-up without relapse on lithium maintenance.
W.L.	26	M	1½ months	Chlorpromazine, 1500 mg.	2 weeks	Lithium treatment stopped. Patient relapsed and second lithium treatment induced remission. 24-month follow-up without relapse. Lithium treatment stopped.
D.S.	20	F	3 months 3 months 1½ months	Spontaneous improvement 5 ECT Chlorpromazine, 800 mg.	2 weeks	Placebo relapse. Maintenance treatment for 6 months without relapse. Follow-up physician treated next relapse with ECT.
P.A.	26	F	3 months 3 months 2 months	Chlorpromazine, 2200 mg. Chlorpromazine, 1000 mg. Chlorpromazine, 1000 mg. Perphenazine, 16 mg.	2 weeks	Relapse in 17 months. Second lithium treatment induced remission in 4 days. 15-month follow-up.
F.L.	58	F	3-month average, 10 attacks	10 prior attacks treated with ECT and chlorpromazine	2 weeks	Relapse in 3 months. Second course of lithium with good response. Seizure while on lithium. No relapse in 24 months on maintenance thioridazine.
E.F.	35	M	1½ months 2 months	Spontaneous remission Chlorpromazine, 800 mg., allergic to drug	2 weeks	21-month follow-up without relapse.
C.G.	45	M	4-6 month average, 10 attacks	1st: no drug treatment 2nd: 7 ECT 3rd: 14 ECT 4th: chlorpromazine, 300 mg. 5th: chlorpromazine, 600 mg. 6th: chlorpromazine, 600 mg.. 7th: chlorpromazine, 600 mg. 8th: chlorpromazine, 2000 mg. 9th: chlorpromazine, 1600 mg. 10th: chlorpromazine, 1600 mg.	2 weeks	11th attack treated with lithium. 18-month follow-up without relapse.
E.H.	52	F	3 months 3 months	Chlorpromazine, 300 mg. Fluphenazine, 20 mg.	2 weeks	Relapse in 9 months. Second response to lithium in 2 weeks.

TABLE 3. Manic Attacks in 19 Patients Treated With Lithium Carbonate

Quality of Response	Number of Trials
Good	11
Equivocal	6
Inadequate	3
Poor	5
Total trials	25

ten days were excluded from the study; therefore, no patient was started on active medication within ten days of admission to the acute service. In this way, baseline behavioral observations were made, and the influence of the ward milieu became a constant. During the first ten days, a placebo was given. Patients were given a full medical and neurological examination and evaluation. Initial physical examination, blood count, urinalysis, electrolytes, chest X-ray, EKG, and weight were recorded within 48 hours of admission.

Three patients initially admitted for study and treatment were excluded: one had Stoke-Adams attacks and myocardial disease; another was too assaultive and destructive to take oral medication; and the third patient spontaneously remitted after transfer from another hospital.

The clinical state of each patient was carefully evaluated by two clinical members of the psychiatric staff and the charge nurse weekly. A global evaluation of behavior and response to medication was made throughout the trial period. Patients were rated on a five-point weekly scale as: much improved, minimally improved, no change, minimally worse, and much worse. At the end of the study, an over-all rating of change was made in four categories including: good, equivocal, inadequate, and poor; both minimally worse and much worse were rated as poor response.

In all, there were 25 trials with lithium carbonate in 19 patients, consisting of nine men and ten women. The age of the women averaged 36.3 years with a range of 19-52 and that of the men averaged 44.5 years with a range of 25-66. Fifteen of the 19 had individually experienced two to ten manic attacks prior to their admission to the study; thus their pattern of frequency and duration was established and known. All patients (with one exception) had been treated with phenothiazines previously for at least two weeks at doses of over 800 mg. daily with no appreciable effect on their manic state (see Tables 1 and 2).

Baseline electrolytes were done before the start of treatment and repeated twice weekly after treatment was under way. Lithium determinations were done twice weekly on all patients from fasting blood specimens. The method of

FIGURE 1. History of Manic Attacks in One Patient With Annual Psychotic Episodes of Known Periodicity

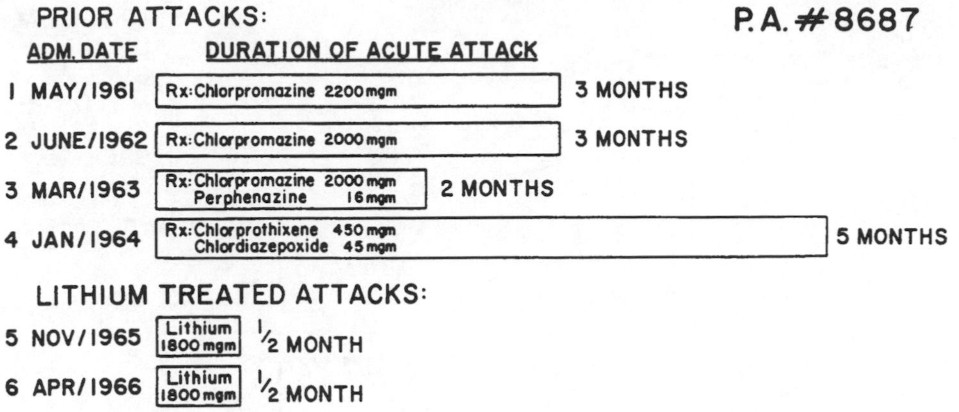

PRIOR ATTACKS:　　　　　　　　　　　　　P.A. #8687

ADM. DATE　　DURATION OF ACUTE ATTACK

1 MAY/1961　Rx: Chlorpromazine 2200 mgm　　　　3 MONTHS

2 JUNE/1962　Rx: Chlorpromazine 2000 mgm　　　3 MONTHS

3 MAR/1963　Rx: Chlorpromazine 2000 mgm
　　　　　　　Perphenazine　　16 mgm　2 MONTHS

4 JAN/1964　Rx: Chlorprothixene　450 mgm
　　　　　　　Chlordiazepoxide　45 mgm　　　　5 MONTHS

LITHIUM TREATED ATTACKS:

5 NOV/1965　Lithium 1800 mgm　1/2 MONTH

6 APR/1966　Lithium 1800 mgm　1/2 MONTH

---

determination, using the EEL flame photometer and Titan yellow, was that described by Barrow (4). All patients were allowed to be fully ambulatory on a closed ten-bed acute psychiatric service and were encouraged to take at least two quarts of fluid daily. An additional one-gram salt supplement was given daily.

After the observation period of ten days, patients were treated with lithium carbonate for a two-week period at a dosage that maintained the blood level between 1-2 meq/liter. If severe nausea supervened the level was reduced, but this problem only arose with one patient. In that instance intravenous fluids were given for 48 hours on two occasions.

After two weeks, a maintenance level of .5-1.0 meq/liter was utilized. The dose, which averaged between 1200 and 1800 mg. per day during the first days of treatment, was divided into three doses given after meals; subsequently it was tapered off to an average of 900 mg. once the blood level of 1-2 meq/liter was achieved. The nurses were trained in the use of a checklist of the more common toxic effects. This checklist was used with each patient prior to each dose. The clinical toxic effects (20) of the drug are well known. It is clear that in the early deaths associated with its use, blood levels were not followed.

The known human toxic effects, which have been fully elaborated by Schou (21), Gershon, and Maggs, include gastrointestinal upset, tremor, ataxia, dizziness, decreased blood pressure, and rarely, epileptiform seizures. At high levels in vitro, lithium may block carbohydrate and amino acid metabolism by affecting specific enzyme systems; at high levels in tissue culture, lithium may affect astrocyte metabolism (9). However, no information is available as to lithium's action at these usual doses in man.

RESULTS

In the 25 trials on 19 patients only three were excluded. Responses were separated into four categories: good re-

TABLE 4. Comparative Results of Lithium Treatment

Study	Results
Wharton and Fieve	11 out of 25 trials=44 percent good response 17 out of 25 trials=68 percent over-all improved
Schou	18 out of 39 trials=46 percent "+ positive effective group" 39 out of 48 trials=80 percent "positive and possible effect"

sponse, equivocal response, inadequate trial, and poor response[1] (see Table 3).

An attack was considered aborted when a significant change was noted in all three parameters under observation, i.e., decreased motor hyperactivity, altered mood, and decreased pressure of speech.

Good responses were rated as such in those patients who had recurrent manic attacks that were *definitely aborted* (i.e., shortened duration of present attack compared to prior attack by at least two weeks).

Other patients, despite apparent striking responses, were rated only as equivocal when the prior history was not fully detailed enough to clarify the precise duration of prior attacks. Two outpatient department patients were also rated as equivocal because of inadequate documentation of the duration of previous attacks (despite the clinician's impression of striking change).

For example, a good response was so recorded in patient WL #9369 after lithium following his spending 16 days on a closed ward for disturbed behavior when 1400 mg. of chlorpromazine (Thorazine) had previously failed. Furthermore, he relapsed when treatment was stopped for ten days, and he responded a second time to the lithium prior to an operative procedure.

Typical is another patient, PA #8687 (followed for over five years), with four previous annual successive attacks, each with a fixed periodicity of 8-15 weeks' duration (see Figure 1). The fifth and sixth attacks, treated with lithium, each lasted only two weeks. E.P. (also known for over five years), suffered three serial Christmas attacks, each beginning at the holiday season and lasting three to four months.

---

[1] Our "good response" group approximates Schou's "(+) positive effect" group. Our "equivocal response" group approximates Schou's "possible effect" group.

FIGURE 2. Results of Behavioral Rating Scale Correlated With Lithium Treatment

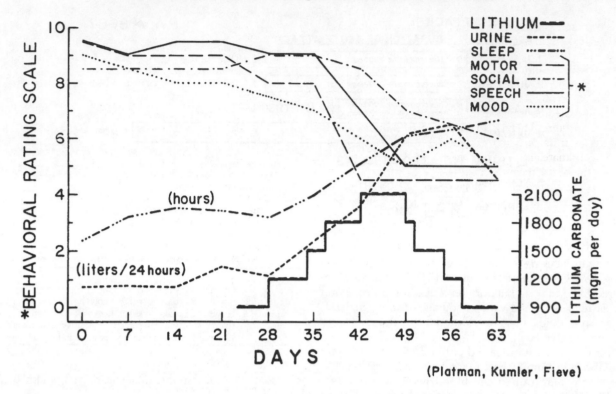

(Platman, Kumler, Fieve)

On lithium carbonate treatment she had her briefest attack and on maintenance she had had no attacks for the past two Christmas seasons.

Only in one case was it necessary to terminate lithium treatment because of toxicity. The patient with an alcoholic history had one grand mal and two focal Jacksonian seizures on the day when her serum lithium was 2.6 meq/liter, following an erroneous double dose of medication. With cessation of treatment, seizures did not recur. Another patient required intravenous fluids for 48 hours on two occasions during two separate trials. Mild tremor was noted in 40 percent of the group. Over 80 percent had transient anorexia and nausea, and 33 percent vomited on one or more occasions but not persistently.

Equivocally treated attacks were so rated when there was an improvement in the patient's clinical state but the total duration of the attacks was not significantly shortened. Inadequate trials were those where the lithium was not given for a long enough period to fully rate its efficacy. Poor responses were those in which the attacks were not clearly controlled in two weeks and further treatment measures were subsequently utilized. Of note is the failure of lithium to modify one clearly demonstrated drug-induced mania on 300 mg. of imipramine.

DISCUSSION

The prognosis and natural history of the individual manic attack are uncertain. Strecker comments that "between ages 15 to 25, the average duration is three-six months with future attacks in general of greater length" (22). Noyes and Kolb

state the "average duration of the attack is six months" (18). Arieti comments generally that "the prognosis is almost always good, but uncertain as to recurrence" (1).

Our patients who had good responses all did so within two weeks of lithium carbonate treatment. However, none of the untreated attacks lasted six months. They varied in duration from the spontaneous remission within ten days to five months. Untreated "control" attacks were not available for comparison in this phenothiazine era. Three patients were given placebos after the 14-day treatment period and all relapsed.

Certainly it is clear that current treatment, whether lithium, phenothiazines, or ECT, shortens duration of manic attacks as the natural history is reported in the earlier literature and in texts.

Maggs used *intensity* of the symptoms of the attack as measured by the Wittenborn scale to evaluate the effects of lithium treatment; he reported his results as statistically significant compared with placebo in 18 of 28 patients treated. Schou in his data demonstrated decreased *frequency* of attacks as well as the capacity to abort attacks in 39 of 48 patients treated, or approximately an 80 percent improvement, including both his "(+) positive effect" and "possible effect" groups. We have used shortening of the duration of the attack as the measure of efficacy, and found an unequivocal and conservative 44 percent improvement after two weeks on lithium. If we include our equivocal response group, 17 out of 25 (68 percent) improved (see Table 4)

Following these clinical results, we have started a more intensive study of manic patients on our metabolic and behavioral ward with other controls, employing the Burdock clinical profile and specific scales for measuring activity, mood, social interaction, and sleep, as well as physiological and biochemical parameters.

It is premature at this time to report the biochemical and physiological findings of this more detailed study. However, Figure 2 illustrates this more detailed technique correlating behavior with lithium salt treatment.

It is our impression that this kind of closer correlation between observable body activity, social behavior, mood, speech, and metabolism is needed to further evaluate the effects of lithium. There is no question that lithium is a potent drug in its capacity to alter mood in some unusual way. The ultimate aim is to gain more understanding of the mechanisms of the recently reported ionic shifts in sodium as well as the altered electrophysiology that occurs during affective states. Whether these early reports of increased exchangeable sodium in depression, as reported by Coppen and associates (7) and Gibbons (12), represent a primary affective biochemical lesion or are epiphenomena remains a question. It is hoped that these unsettled issues can be further elucidated by using lithium as an important research tool.

SUMMARY

Nineteen patients refractory or allergic to phenothiazine treatment were given 25 trials of lithium treatment for a manic state with hyperactivity, elation, and pressure of speech. Effective dose ranges for most patients were between 1200 and 1800 mg. per day on initial treatment, with maintenance at 900 mg. per day. A ten-day control period of observation preceded treatment. Each patient's own past history of duration of attack was used to evaluate the effective shortening of the lithium-treated attack.

Eleven of 25 (44 percent) of the manic episodes had good responses, characterized by definite shortening of the duration of the individual manic attack as compared with past manic attacks. Seventeen of 25 (68 percent) of the manic attacks (including both good and equivocal response) in our series responded to lithium, which may be the drug of choice for phenothiazine-refractory or phenothiazine-allergic manic patients treated in a research setting.

REFERENCES

1. Arieti, S., ed.: American Handbook of Psychiatry, New York: Basic Books, 1959.
2. Baastrup, P.C.: Use of Lithium in Manic-Depressive Psychosis, Compr. Psychiat. 5:396–408, 1964.
3. Baichikov, A.G., et al.: Use of Rare Metals in Various Disease States, Med. Promyshl. SSSR 8:18–25, 1962.
4. Barrow, G.R.: Estimation of Lithium in Blood, J. Med. Lab. Techn. 17:236–238, 1960.
5. Cade, J.F.J.: Lithium Salts in the Treatment of Psychotic Excitement, Med. J. Aust. 2:349–352, 1949.
6. Colbert, E.G.: Lithium Salts (Letter to the Editor), J.A.M.A. 176: 744, 1961.
7. Coppen, A., Shaw, D.M., and Mangoni, A.: Total Exchangeable Sodium in Depressive Illness, Brit. Med. J. 2:295–298, 1962.
8. Corcoran, A.C., et al.: Lithium Poisoning from the Use of Salt Substitutes, J.A.M.A. 139:685–688, 1949.
9. Friede, R.L.: The Enzymatic Response of Astrocytes to Various Ions in Vitro, J. Cell. Biol. 20:5–15, 1964.
10. Gerest, F.: Le Traitement de l'Access Maniaque, Lyon Med. 86:3–15, 1954.
11. Gershon, S., and Yuwiler, A.: The Lithium Ion: A Specific Pharmacological Approach to the Treatment of Mania, J. Neuropsychiat. 1:229–2411, 1960.
12. Gibbons, J.L.: Total Body Sodium and Potassium in Depressive Illness, Clin. Sci. 19:133–138, 1960.
13. Hartigan, G.P.: Use of Lithium Salts in Affective Disorders, Brit. J. Psychiat. 109:810–814, 1963.
14. Kingstone, E.: The Lithium Treatment of Hypomanic and Manic States, Compr. Psychiat. 1:317–320, 1960.
15. Maggs, R.: Treatment of Manic Illness with Lithium Carbonate, Brit. J. Psychiat. 109:56–65, 1963.
16. Mosketikv, K., and Belskaya, G.M.: Results of Lithium Iodide in Treatment of Some Psychotic States, Neuropath. I. Psikhiat. 63:92–95, 1963.
17. Noack, C.H., and Trautner, E.M.: Lithium Treatment of Manic Psychosis, Med. J. Aust. 2:219–222, 1951.
18. Noyes, A.P., and Kolb, L.C.: Modern Clinical Psychiatry, 6th ed. Philadelphia: W. B. Saunders Co., 1963.
19. Schlagenhauf, G., Tupin, J., and White, R.B.: The Use of Lithium Carbonate in the Treatment of Manic Psychoses, Amer. J. Psychiat. 123:201–206, 1966.
20. Schou, M.: Biology and Pharmacology of the Lithium Ion, Pharmacol. Rev. 9:17–58, 1957.
21. Schou, M.: Lithium in Psychiatric Therapy, Psychopharmacologia 1: 65–78, 1959.
22. Strecker, E.A., Ebaugh, F.G., and Ewalt, J.R.: Practical Clinical Psychiatry, 6th ed. Philadelphia: Blakiston, 1947.
23. Talbott, J.H.: Use of Lithium Salts as a Substitute for Sodium Chloride, Arch. Intern. Med. 85:1–10, 1950.
24. Wikler, A.: The Relation of Psychiatry to Pharmacology. Baltimore: Williams & Wilkins, 1957.

THE AMERICAN JOURNAL OF PSYCHIATRY
GRATEFULLY ACKNOWLEDGES THE SUPPORT OF THE SPONSORS
OF THE SESQUICENTENNIAL ANNIVERSARY SUPPLEMENT.

Abbott Laboratories

Astra/Merck Group of Merck & Co., Inc.

Bristol-Myers Squibb Company

Burroughs Wellcome Co.

Cerenex Pharmaceuticals, Division of Glaxo Inc.

Ciba Pharma Division

Dista Products Company, a Division of Eli Lilly and Company

Gate Pharmaceuticals

Hoechst-Roussel Pharmaceuticals Inc.

Janssen Pharmaceutica Inc.

McNeil Pharmaceutical

Parke-Davis, Division of Warner Lambert Company

Roche Laboratories

Roerig Division/Pfizer Inc.

Sandoz Pharmaceuticals Corporation

Scios-NOVA Pharmaceuticals

Searle Pharmaceuticals

SmithKline Beecham Pharmaceuticals

Solvay Pharmaceuticals

The Upjohn Company

Wyeth-Ayerst Laboratories

Zeneca Pharmaceuticals Group

The following is a list of sources for the illustrations
in the Sesquicentennial Anniversary Supplement.

ISBN 0-89042-275